# Emergency Medicine: Applications of Artificial Intelligence

# Emergency Medicine: Applications of Artificial Intelligence

Editor: Sonja Andersen

AMERICAN
MEDICAL PUBLISHERS
www.americanmedicalpublishers.com

AMERICAN
MEDICAL PUBLISHERS
www.americanmedicalpublishers.com

**Cataloging-in-Publication Data**

Emergency medicine : applications of artificial intelligence / edited by Sonja Andersen.
p. cm.
Includes bibliographical references and index.
ISBN 979-8-88740-087-7
1. Emergency medicine. 2. Artificial intelligence--Medical applications.
3. Medical emergencies. 4. Critical care medicine. I. Andersen, Sonja.
RC86.7 .E44 2023
616.025--dc23



American Medical Publishers,
41 Flatbush Avenue,
1st Floor, New York,
NY 11217, USA

ISBN 979-8-88740-087-7 (Hardback)

# Contents

# Preface

The rapid advancements in artificial intelligence technology have paved the way for the use of machine learning applications in health care. These applications address existing challenges in the emergency department such as triage and disposition, early detection of conditions and outcomes, emergency department operations, and therapeutic interventions. Artificial intelligence can be used in three ways in the context of emergency and critical care. The first one is to build risk stratification prediction models in critical care. The second use of AI involves utilizing unsupervised machine learning techniques to divide the varied population into homogeneous subgroups. The third use of AI is for reinforcement learning algorithms to prescribe treatment regimens in a sequential way. The dynamic treatment regime (DTR) model uses reinforcement learning to estimate a set of decision rules, one for each step of intervention. It specifies how to tailor treatments to patients considering their treatment and covariate histories. DTR lowers model complexity and is considered more appropriate for medical epidemiology. This book is a vital tool for all researching or studying the role of AI in emergency and critical care medicine. It aims to equip students and experts with the advanced topics and upcoming concepts in this subject.

Various studies have approached the subject by analyzing it with a single perspective, but the present book provides diverse methodologies and techniques to address this field. This book contains theories and applications needed for understanding the subject from different perspectives. The aim is to keep the readers informed about the progresses in the field; therefore, the contributions were carefully examined to compile novel researches by specialists from across the globe.

Indeed, the job of the editor is the most crucial and challenging in compiling all chapters into a single book. In the end, I would extend my sincere thanks to the chapter authors for their profound work. I am also thankful for the support provided by my family and colleagues during the compilation of this book.

**Editor**

1

# Identification and Prediction of Novel Clinical Phenotypes for Intensive Care Patients with SARS-CoV-2 Pneumonia

*Hui Chen[1*†], Zhu Zhu[2†], Nan Su[3], Jun Wang[1], Jun Gu[4], Shu Lu[5], Li Zhang[6], Xuesong Chen[7], Lei Xu[8], Xiangrong Shao[9], Jiangtao Yin[10], Jinghui Yang[11], Baodi Sun[12] and Yongsheng Li[13*]*

*[1] Department of Critical Care Medicine, The First Affiliated Hospital of Soochow University, Soochow University, Suzhou, China, [2] Department of General Surgery, The Affiliated Suzhou Science & Technology Town Hospital of Nanjing Medical University, Suzhou, China, [3] Department of Respiratory and Critical Care Medicine, The First Affiliated Hospital of Soochow University, Soochow University, Suzhou, China, [4] Department of Respiratory Medicine, Affiliated Hospital of Nantong University, Nantong, China, [5] Department of Intensive Care Unit, Affiliated Hospital of Nantong University, Nantong, China, [6] Department of Respiratory Medicine, Zhongda Hospital Southeast University, Nanjing, China, [7] Department of Respiratory and Critical Care Medicine, The First Affiliated Hospital of Nanjing Medical University, Nanjing, China, [8] Department of Emergency Medicine, The Affiliated Hospital of Xuzhou Medical University, Xuzhou, China, [9] Department of Respiratory Medicine, The Affiliation Hospital of Yangzhou University, Yangzhou, China, [10] Department of Intensive Care Unit, The Affiliated Hospital of Jiangsu University, Zhenjiang, China, [11] Department of Critical Care Medicine, Sir Run Run Hospital, Nanjing Medical University, Nanjing, China, [12] Department of Emergency, Sir Run Run Hospital, Nanjing Medical University, Nanjing, China, [13] Department of Intensive Care Medicine, Tongji Medical College, Tongji Hospital, Huazhong University of Science and Technology, Wuhan, China*

***Correspondence:**
*Yongsheng Li*
*dr_ysli@126.com*
*Hui Chen*
*15905162429@163.com*

*† These authors have contributed equally to this work*

**Background:** Phenotypes have been identified within heterogeneous disease, such as acute respiratory distress syndrome and sepsis, which are associated with important prognostic and therapeutic implications. The present study sought to assess whether phenotypes can be derived from intensive care patients with coronavirus disease 2019 (COVID-19), to assess the correlation with prognosis, and to develop a parsimonious model for phenotype identification.

**Methods:** Adult patients with COVID-19 from Tongji hospital between January 2020 and March 2020 were included. The consensus k means clustering and latent class analysis (LCA) were applied to identify phenotypes using 26 clinical variables. We then employed machine learning algorithms to select a maximum of five important classifier variables, which were further used to establish a nested logistic regression model for phenotype identification.

**Results:** Both consensus k means clustering and LCA showed that a two-phenotype model was the best fit for the present cohort ($N = 504$). A total of 182 patients (36.1%) were classified as hyperactive phenotype, who exhibited a higher 28-day mortality and higher rates of organ dysfunction than did those in hypoactive phenotype. The top five variables used to assign phenotypes were neutrophil-to-lymphocyte ratio (NLR), ratio of pulse oxygen saturation to the fractional concentration of oxygen in inspired air ($Spo_2/Fio_2$) ratio, lactate dehydrogenase (LDH), tumor necrosis factor $\alpha$ (TNF-$\alpha$), and urea nitrogen. From the nested logistic models, three-variable (NLR, $Spo_2/Fio_2$ ratio, and LDH) and four-variable (three-variable plus TNF-α) models were adjudicated to be the best performing, with the area under the curve of 0.95 [95% confidence interval (CI) = 0.94–0.97] and 0.97 (95% CI = 0.96–0.98), respectively.

**Conclusion:** We identified two phenotypes within COVID-19, with different host responses and outcomes. The phenotypes can be accurately identified with parsimonious classifier models using three or four variables.

**Keywords: COVID-19, phenotypes, machine learning, intensive care unit, 28-day mortality**

## INTRODUCTION

Severe acute respiratory syndrome coronavirus 2 (SARS-CoV-2) pneumonia is a newly recognized infectious disease first reported in Wuhan, China, and expeditiously spread to hundreds of countries with massive mortality rate (1–4). The clinical spectrum of coronavirus disease 2019 (COVID-19) ranges from asymptomatic infection to critical illness and results in high rates of hospitalization and intensive care unit (ICU) admission (5). However, COVID-19 ICU mortality was various (6–8), and the treatment responses were disparate (9–11), indicating that COVID-19 is clinically and biologically heterogeneous.

Various studies have proposed different phenotypes of COVID-19. According to 85 consecutive ICU COVID-19 patients, Azoulay et al. identified three clinical and biological phenotypes at ICU admission using hierarchical clustering. ICU mortality rates were 8, 18, and 39% in clusters 1, 2, and 3, respectively (12). Gattinoni et al. identified two primary phenotypes based on respiratory mechanics and response to ventilatory support (13). Rello et al. classified COVID-19 patients into five specific individual phenotypes, according to the disease severity and hypoxemia management strategy (14). Whereas these phenotypes were isolated and limited by sample size, host responses to SARS-CoV-2 infection were vast and multidimensional and include immune dysfunction, abnormal coagulation, and varying degrees of organ failure (15). Different combinations of these features may cluster into novel clinical phenotypes, and patients in each phenotype may respond differently to treatments. However, whether such COVID-19 phenotypes can be derived from clinical data have never been explored.

Unsupervised machine learning approaches, such as consensus k means clustering (16) and latent class analysis (LCA) (17), have been used to identify distinct phenotypes in sepsis (18), acute respiratory distress syndrome (ARDS) (19) and other critical illnesses (20). Consensus clustering is a partitioning approach in which the clustering framework incorporates results from multiple runs of an inner-loop clustering algorithm. LCA is a well-validated statistical technique, which is a form of distribution mixture modeling used to estimate the best-fitting model for a dataset, based on the hypothesis that the data contain several unobserved groups or classes that are concealed within the observed multivariate distribution. Here, we used consensus k means clustering to derive phenotypes and assessed the reproducibility of the phenotypes using LCA.

The first goal of the study was to identify novel clinical phenotypes in ICU COVID-19 patients, using consensus k means clustering and LCA. The second goal was to develop parsimonious models that could ultimately be used prospectively to identify COVID-19 phenotypes.

## MATERIALS AND METHODS

### Study Design and Participants

This single-center, retrospective, observational study was performed at Tongji Hospital, which was designated to admit patients with SARS-CoV-2 infection in Wuhan. Adult patients (≥18 years) with laboratory-confirmed SARS-CoV-2 infection and admitted to ICUs between January 2020 and March 2020 were included in the present study. According to the World Health Organization guidance (21), laboratory confirmation for SARS-Cov-2 was defined as a positive result of real-time reverse transcriptase–polymerase chain reaction assay of nasal and pharyngeal swabs.

This study was approved by the Research Ethics Commission of Tongji Hospital. Written informed consent was waived by the Ethics Commission because of the emergency circumstance. Patient-level informed consent was not required. Part of present patients have been described previously by Chen et al. (22) and Wang et al. (23).

### Data Collection

All data were drawn from electronic health record data at Tongji hospital (Tongji cohort). Demographic data, chronic comorbidities, vital signs, and laboratory results within the first 24 h after ICU admission were collected, as well as treatments and outcomes. Because of incomplete measurement and recording of arterial oxygen partial pressure ($Pao_2$), we adopted pulse oxygen saturation ($Spo_2$) instead of $Pao_2$, as well as the fraction of inspired oxygen ($Fio_2$). Sequential Organ Failure Assessment (SOFA) scores were calculated to determine the severity of illness using data from the first 24 h of ICU admission. All patients were closely followed until 28 days after ICU admission. Data were collected using a case record form modified from the standardized International Severe Acute Respiratory and Emerging Infection Consort.

## Outcomes

The primary outcome in the present study was 28-day mortality. Secondary outcomes were the duration of hospital stay and complications during hospitalization, which included ARDS, septic shock, acute kidney injury, acute cardiac injury, and coagulopathy. The diagnosis of complications is presented in the **Supplementary Material**.

## Clinical Variables for Phenotyping

We selected 26 candidate clinical variables based on their association with severity or outcome of COVID-19, including age, vital signs (heart rate, respiratory rate, temperature, mean blood pressure), markers of inflammation [white blood cell count (WBC count), neutrophil-to-lymphocyte ratio (NLR), high-sensitivity C-reactive protein (hs-CRP), interleukin 2R (IL-2R), IL-6, IL-8, and tumor necrosis factor α (TNF-α)], markers of organ dysfunction [hypersensitive troponin I (hs-TnI), international normalized ratio (INR), platelet (PLT) count, total bilirubin, creatinine, urea nitrogen, lactate dehydrogenase (LDH), and $SpO_2/FIO_2$ ratio], hemoglobin, red blood cell distribution width (RDW), D-dimer, fibrinogen, albumin, and glucose. All variables were collected within 24 h of ICU admission, and we recorded the most abnormal value if a variable was recorded more than once.

## Consensus k Means Clustering

Consensus k means clustering was conducted to 26 variables using a partitioning approach. We first assessed the candidate variable distributions, missingness, and correlation. Multiple imputations with chained equations (Additional Methods in **Supplementary Material**) were used to account for missing data; standardized transformation was used for the dataset, and non-normally distributed variables were log-transformed prior to standardized transformation. We then determine the optimal number of phenotypes with consensus k means clustering, according to the gap statistics, consensus matrix heatmaps, and adequate pairwise-consensus values between cluster members (>0.8). Once the optimal number was determined, we selected rank plots of variables by mean standardized difference between phenotypes to visualize the patterns of clinical variables. We also conducted a sensitivity analysis after excluding highly correlated variables using rank-order statistics ($r > 0.5$). Additional details of consensus k means clustering are presented in **Supplementary Material**.

## Latent Class Analysis

We further employed LCA to assess the reproducibility of the phenotypes. Similarly, all variables underwent standardized transformation and were log-transformed as appropriate. In the LCA, we estimated models ranging from to five classes. Akaike information criterion (AIC), Bayesian information criteria, entropy, class size (classes containing relatively small numbers were not considered clinically meaningful), and the Vuong–Lo–Mendell–Rubin (VLMR) likelihood ratio test (which compares fit of model k classes to k-1 classes) were used to determine the optimal number of classes. Once determined, each individual was assigned a class according to model-generated probabilities. More details of LCA are presented in the **Supplementary Material**.

## Parsimonious Algorithms to Classify COVID-19

Based on previous research, we attempted to construct a parsimonious model (three-variable or four-variable model) to predict phenotypes. First, machine learning algorithms, including classification tree with bootstrapped aggregating (bagging), extreme gradient boosting (XGBoost), and gradient boosted model (GBM), were used to identify the most important classifier variables. To select the most important variables, variable importance was used for the bagging model and XGBoost. Relative influence factor of variable was used for GBM. More details of machine learning algorithms are presented in the **Supplementary Material**. Second, the five most important classifier variables common to all three machine learning algorithms were then used to generate five logistic regression models (generated by sequential addition of the variables), and the receiver operating characteristic curve and area under the curve (AUC) were calculated for each model. AIC and DeLong's test were used to compare model performance. The best model was determined by a combination of accuracy, parsimony, and simplicity in clinical. Additionally, to assess the clinical usefulness of the best model, decision curve analysis (DCA) was conducted by quantifying the net benefits at different threshold probabilities. Finally, after the best model selected, a 10-fold cross-validation was applied to internally validate the stability of the model. This was performed by randomly splitting the patients into 10 equal samples. Nine-tenths of these samples were used to construct logistic regression models, and the model coefficients were applied to the remaining sample (1/10). This process was repeated 10 times, and the AUC to each fold was generated.

## Statistical Analysis

Values are presented as the mean (standard deviation) or median (interquartile range) for continuous variables as appropriate and as the total number (percentage) for categorical variables. Comparisons between groups were made using the $\chi^2$ test or Fisher exact test for categorical variables and Student *t*-test or Mann–Whitney *U*-test for continuous variables as appropriate. A $p < 0.05$ was used to determine statistical significance for all tests. LCA was conducted using Mplus software (version 8.3). All other analyses were done using R (version 3.6.0).

# RESULTS

## Patients

During the study period, a total of 504 patients with COVID-19 were included in the Tongji cohort. The schematic of study is shown in **Figure 1**. Among the Tongji cohort, 259 patients (51.4%) were male, the age was 64 (52–72) years, and the SOFA score was 3 (2–6). Within the first 24 h after ICU admission, 16 patients (3.2%) received vasopressor therapy, and 23 patients (4.6%) received invasive

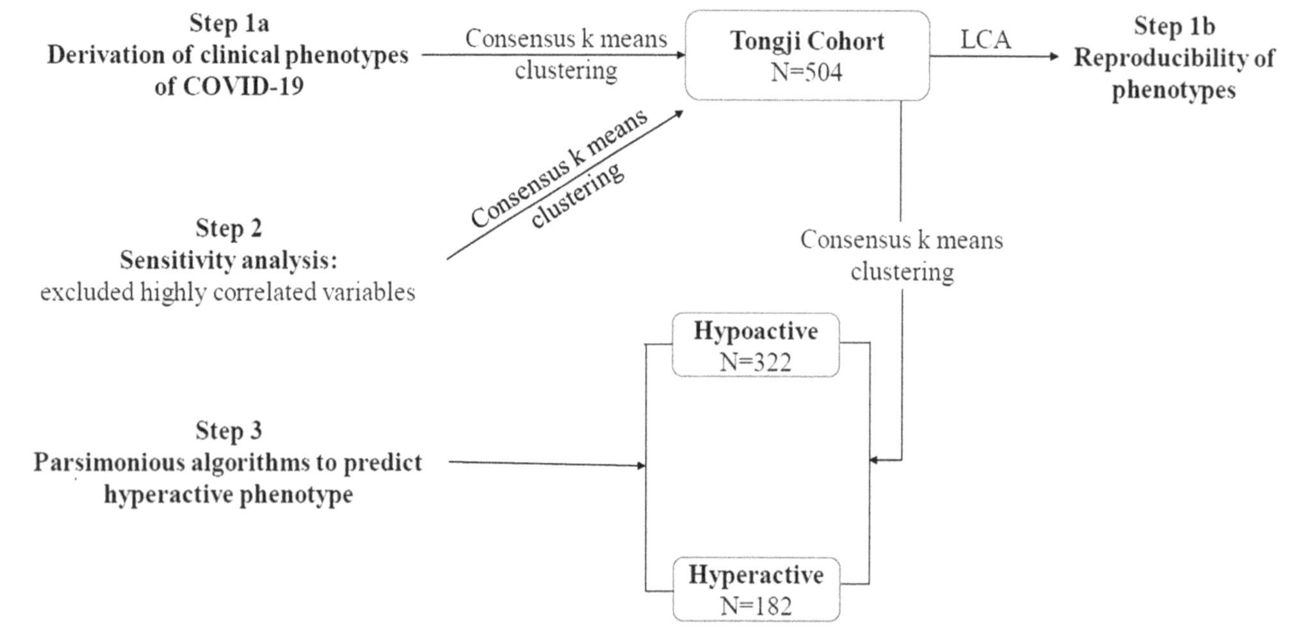


**FIGURE 1** | Schematic of study. LCA, latent class analysis.

mechanical ventilation. The overall 28-day mortality rate was 33.7%.

## Derivation of Clinical Phenotypes for COVID-19

In Tongji cohort, based on gap statistics, consensus matrix plots, and consensus values (**Supplementary Figure 1**), the consensus k means clustering found that a two-class model was the optimal fit with the two distinct phenotypes of COVID-19. Ultimately, 322 patients (63.9%) were classified as hypoactive phenotype, and 182 (36.1%) were classified as hyperactive phenotype. Sensitivity analysis indicated that no substantial changes were evident after excluding variables with high correlation (**Supplementary Table 3** and **Supplementary Figure 2**).

The characteristics of phenotypes in the two-class model are shown in **Table 1** and **Supplementary Figure 3**. Rank plots of variables by the standardized mean difference between phenotypes are presented in **Figure 2**. Most variables were significantly different between the two phenotypes. Compared to patients with the hypoactive phenotype, those with the hyperactive phenotype were older, prone to have elevated measures of inflammation (e.g., WBC count, NLR, hs-CRP, IL-2R, IL-6, IL-8, TNF-α), higher D-dimer, higher heart rate, higher respiratory rate, and extreme laboratory values regarding the organ dysfunction (e.g., hs-TnI, INR, PLT count, total bilirubin, creatinine, urea nitrogen, LDH, and $SpO_2/FIO_2$). Additionally, in comparison with the hypoactive phenotype, the hyperactive phenotype had significantly higher SOFA score on ICU admission and higher comorbidity rates (**Supplementary Table 4**).

## Treatments and Outcomes in COVID-19 Phenotypes

A large proportion of patients with the hyperactive phenotype received corticosteroid therapy (78.6 vs. 44.1%; $p < 0.001$), high-flow nasal cannula oxygen therapy (17.0 vs. 4.7%; $p < 0.001$), non-invasive mechanical ventilation (45.6 vs. 7.1%; $p < 0.001$), invasive mechanical ventilation (59.3 vs. 3.4%; $p < 0.001$), and renal replacement therapy (11.5 vs. 1.6%; $p < 0.001$) during their ICU stay, compared to those with hypoactive phenotype (**Supplementary Table 4**). Patients assigned to hyperactive phenotype had significantly higher 28-day mortality (74.3 vs. 10.8%; $p < 0.001$) and higher rates of organ dysfunction during their ICU stay compared to those assigned to hypoactive phenotype (**Table 2**).

## Reproducibility Using LCA

LCA confirmed statistical fit of the two-class model. In LCA, using the VLMR test, a two-class model showed significantly improved fit compared with one-class mode ($p = 0.0066$), and no further improvement in model fit was observed when the three-class ($p = 0.058$), four-class ($p = 0.41$), or five-class model ($p = 0.40$) was involved. Good class separation was observed in the two-class model (entropy > 0.80), indicating strong separation between the classes (**Supplementary Table 5**). The two-class model classified 341 patients (67.7%) in class 1 (referred as hypoactive phenotype) and 163 patients (32.3%) in class 2 (referred as hyperactive phenotype). Average latent class probabilities were 0.98 for class 1 and 0.96 for class 2. The clinical characteristics of the phenotypes were similar when derived using this method, as well as by rank plots (**Figure 2** and **Supplementary Table 6**).

**TABLE 1** | Class-defining variables of phenotypes using consensus k means clustering.

| Variables | Hypoactive phenotype (*n* = 322) | Hyperactive phenotype (*n* = 182) | *p*-value |
|---|---|---|---|
| Age (years) | 58 (48–69) | 69 (62–77) | <0.001 |
| Heart rate (bpm) | 89 (78–101) | 95 (82–108) | <0.001 |
| Respiratory rate (bpm) | 20 (20–22) | 24 (20–32) | <0.001 |
| Temperature (°C) | 37.0 (36.5–37.8) | 37.2 (36.5–38.0) | 0.063 |
| MAP | 96.0 (89.7–104.7) | 99.7 (89.0–106.0) | 0.209 |
| $Spo_2/Fio_2$ ratio | 297 (259–433) | 131 (90–229) | <0.001 |
| WBC count ($\times 10^9$/L) | 5.2 (4.0–6.6) | 9.4 (7.0–13.1) | <0.001 |
| NLR | 3.4 (2.0–5.4) | 13.5 (8.6–25.3) | <0.001 |
| Platelet count ($\times 10^9$/L) | 213 (159–278) | 164 (121–225) | <0.001 |
| Hemoglobin (g/L) | 126 (115–137) | 129 (115–143) | 0.043 |
| RDW (%) | 12.4 (11.9–13.2) | 13.0 (12.2–13.9) | <0.001 |
| High-sensitivity C-reactive protein (mg/L) | 26.2 (5.6–65.2) | 104.6 (65.0–163.4) | <0.001 |
| Interleukin 2R (U/mL) | 658 (426–906) | 1,262 (904–1648) | <0.001 |
| Interleukin 6 (pg/mL) | 10.2 (2.3–31.1) | 64.8 (31.0–157.0) | <0.001 |
| Interleukin 8 (pg/mL) | 11.4 (6.5–19.5) | 32.3 (20.0–66.4) | <0.001 |
| Tumor necrosis factor α (pg/mL) | 7.8 (5.8–10.0) | 12.8 (8.9–18.8) | <0.001 |
| d-Dimer (μg/mL) | 0.7 (0.4–1.4) | 5.3 (1.8–21.0) | <0.001 |
| Fibrinogen (g/L) | 4.8 (4.0–5.9) | 5.4 (3.3–6.5) | 0.152 |
| INR | 1.0 (1.0–1.1) | 1.2 (1.1–1.4) | <0.001 |
| Hypersensitive troponin I (pg/mL) | 3.8 (1.9–8.4) | 40.1 (13.3–296.2) | <0.001 |
| Albumin (g/L) | 36.0 (33.3–38.6) | 29.9 (27.1–32.7) | <0.001 |
| Total bilirubin (μmol/L) | 8.7 (6.5–11.7) | 13.2 (9.9–19.2) | <0.001 |
| Creatinine (μmol/L) | 66.0 (55.8–82.0) | 89.0 (71.5–119.0) | <0.001 |
| Urea nitrogen (mmol/L) | 4.2 (3.2–5.5) | 9.3 (6.4–15.2) | <0.001 |
| Lactate dehydrogenase (U/L) | 260 (203–334) | 511 (415–678) | <0.001 |
| Glucose (mmol/L) | 6.1 (5.2–7.2) | 8.1 (6.3–11.8) | <0.001 |

*MAP, mean arterial pressure; $Spo_2/Fio_2$ ratio, ratio of pulse oxygen saturation to the fractional concentration of oxygen in inspired air; WBC, white blood cell count; NLR, neutrophil-to-lymphocyte ratio; RDW, red blood cell distribution width; INR, international normalized ratio.*

## Parsimonious Algorithms to Predict Phenotypes of COVID-19

The most important classifier variables from the bagging, XGBoost, and GBM are presented (**Supplementary Table 7**, **Supplementary Figures 4, 5**). The top five variables were consistent across all three machine learning models, which included NLR, $Spo_2/Fio_2$ ratio, LDH, TNF-α, and urea nitrogen, and were therefore selected as the best predictors for the parsimonious models. After five logistic models constructed by sequential addition of the best predictors, an improved model performance, increased AUC, and decreased AIC were observed when model 1 went to model 4 (**Supplementary Table 8**). Considering that TNF-α was not routinely tested in other hospitals, therefore, the three-variable (NLR, $Spo_2/Fio_2$ ratio, and LDH) and four-variable models (NLR, $Spo_2/Fio_2$ ratio, LDH, TNF-α) were both the best in terms of balancing classifying accuracy and model simplicity.

Multivariable analyses showed that three variables or four variables in the model were all predictors of the phenotypes (**Supplementary Table 9**). The AUC was 0.95 [95% confidence interval (95% CI) = 0.94–0.97] for the three-variable model and 0.97 (95% CI = 0.96–0.98) for the four-variable model. The DCA curves indicated that the threshold probabilities were 0–0.95 for the three-variable model and 0–0.94 for the four-variable model (**Figure 3**). The mean AUCs of cross-validation for the three- and four-variable models were 0.95 (0.03) and 0.97 (0.02), respectively.

## DISCUSSION

The novel findings of our analyses can be summarized as follows. We identified two distinct COVID-19 phenotypes with different clinical and biological characteristics, mortality, and other clinical outcomes. We also developed a parsimonious model to predict phenotypes of COVID-19 using machine learning algorithms. These findings have important implications for early detection of patients who are likely to develop critical illness, as well as future researches in COVID-19.

Clinical and biological heterogeneity of critical illness (e.g., ARDS, sepsis) is thought to be dead ends for pharmacotherapy trials. Not a single clinical or biological variable was sufficient to identify phenotype (24). To put it simple, none of the clinical variables could be used to subdivide COVID-19. By contrast, based on 26 candidate clinical variables, we found two

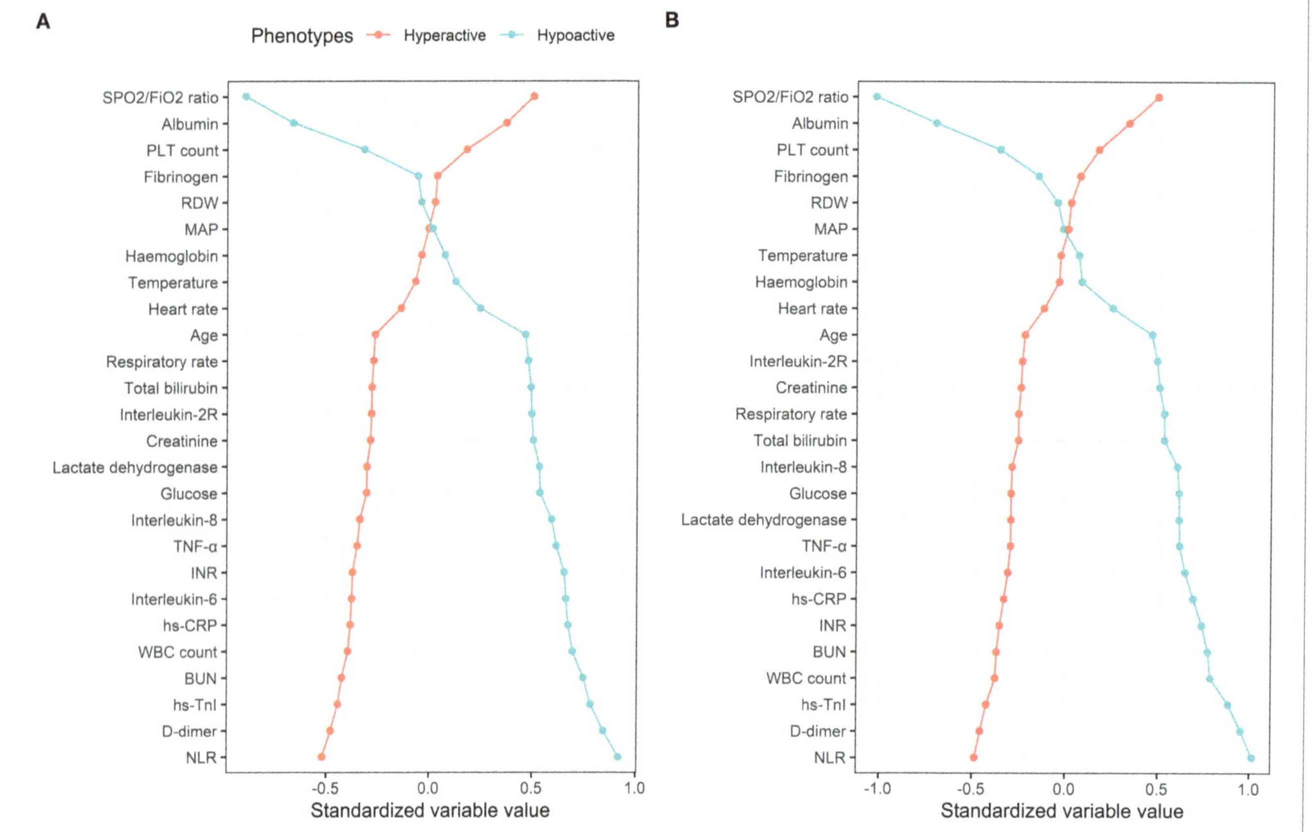


**FIGURE 2 |** Comparison of variables that contribute to clinical phenotypes in the Tongji cohort. Clinical phenotypes were derived from consensus k means clustering **(A)** and LCA **(B)**. In all panels, the variables are standardized such that all means are scaled to 0 and SDs to 1. A value of 1 for the standardized variable value (*x*-axis) signifies that the mean value for the phenotype was 1 SD higher than the mean value for both phenotypes shown in the graph as a whole. RDW, red blood cell distribution width; MAP, mean arterial pressure; TNF-α, tumor necrosis factor α; INR, international normalized ratio; hs-CRP, high-sensitivity C-reactive protein; BUN, urea nitrogen; hs-TnI, hypersensitive troponin I; NLR, neutrophil-to-lymphocyte ratio.

**TABLE 2 |** Comparison of clinical outcomes according to phenotypes using consensus k means clustering.

| | Hypoactive phenotype ($n = 322$) | Hyperactive phenotype ($n = 182$) | *p*-value |
|---|---|---|---|
| ARDS | 46 (14.3%) | 149 (81.9%) | <0.001 |
| Septic shock | 25 (7.8%) | 128 (70.3%) | <0.001 |
| Coagulopathy | 14 (4.3%) | 84 (46.2%) | <0.001 |
| Acute kidney injury | 16 (5.0%) | 96 (52.7%) | <0.001 |
| Acute cardiac injury | 32 (10.0%) | 120 (65.9%) | <0.001 |
| 28-d mortality | 35 (10.8%) | 135 (74.3%) | <0.001 |

*ARDS, acute respiratory distress syndrome.*

distinct phenotypes of COVID-19 most sufficiently describing the present cohort using consensus k means clustering, which strongly correlated with degrees of the host response to SARS-CoV-2 infection. Specifically, compared to patients with hypoactive phenotype, the host response of patients with hyperactive phenotype seems to be more dysregulated, characterized by high plasma concentrations of inflammatory biomarkers, extreme coagulation, and high proportion of organ failure or injury on ICU admission. Furthermore, replication of these findings using LCA substantiates the robustness of the two phenotypes in the present cohort.

Several phenotypes of COVID-19 have been documented, with the aim to receive "precision therapy." Patients with COVID-19 pneumonia presents with low elastance, low ventilation-to-perfusion ratio, low lung weight, and low lung recruitability were classified as type L, whereas type H patients were characterized by high elastance, high ventilation-to-perfusion ratio, high lung weight, and high lung recruitability. Response to treatments, including higher $FIO_2$ and higher positive end-expiratory pressure (PEEP), and prone positioning may differ in type L and type H (13). Compared to phenotypes in the present study, similarly, hyperactive phenotype and type H seemed to represent a subset of COVID-19 patients who were severely ill. Unlike previous COVID-19 phenotypes, the COVID-19 phenotypes in the present study only used routinely available data associated with the degrees of host response, regardless of the characteristics of chest imaging or the respiratory mechanics, which can be identified at the time of patient admitted to the

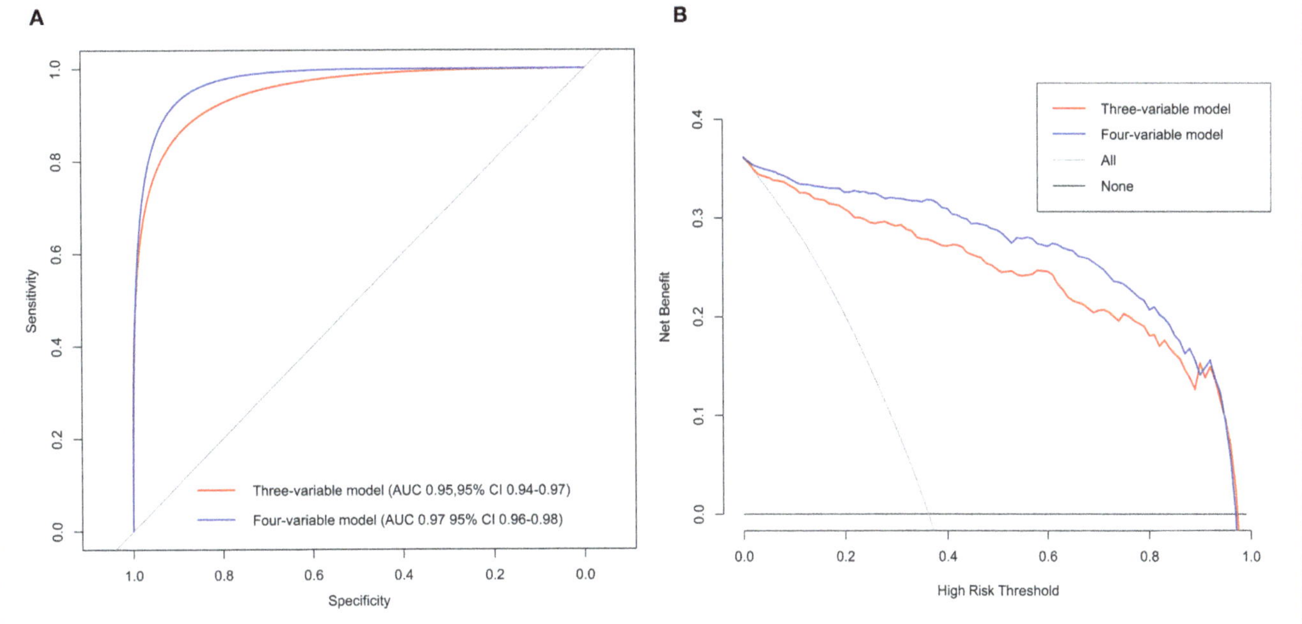


**FIGURE 3** | Receiver operating characteristic curves **(A)** and DCA **(B)** of the two best-performing regression models in Tongji cohort.

ICU. Besides, these phenotypes were multidimensional, differed in their laboratory abnormalities, patterns of organ dysfunction, and were not homologous with traditional patient groupings such as by severity score or a single variable.

We proposed a three-variable (NLR, $SpO_2/FIO_2$ ratio, and LDH) and four-variable model (NLR, $SpO_2/FIO_2$ ratio, LDH, and TNF-α) for identifying the hyperactive phenotype of COVID-19. Unlike traditional forward stepwise modeling, we used three machine algorithms to identify the most important classifier variables. The ability to identify phenotypes using a small set of variables is a crucial step toward their clinical application. On the one hand, to predict the occurrence of critical illness in COVID-19: according to 1,590 COVID-19 patients, Wenhua Liang et al. (25) constructed a predictive risk score including 10 variables to predict a patient's risk of developing critical illness; likewise, NLR [odds ratio (OR) = 1.06; 95% CI = 1.02–1.10] and LDH (OR = 1.002; 95% CI = 1.001–1.004) were included in the risk model. However, the definition of "critical illness" was obscure, which was described as a composite of admission to the ICU, invasive ventilation, or death. Besides, the overall mortality was only 3.2%, implying that such risk score may not be validated in real intensive care patients with COVID-19. In the present study, the ICU mortality of Tongji cohort was in line with prior reports, and critically ill patients (hyperactive phenotype) were identified based on the clustering analysis and LCA, which maximized the differences between patients, without taking the clinical outcome into account (26). On the other hand, to select more homogeneity patients for clinical trials: hypothetically, like the series research of ARDS, the interactions between phenotypes and treatments (PEEP, fluid management, and simvastatin) were significant.

Interestingly, different from the ARDS phenotypes (24, 27), we observed that none of inflammatory cytokines could predict COVID-19 phenotypes, except for TNF-α. Proinflammatory cytokines levels (IL-6, IL-8) in hyperinflammatory ARDS were at least 20-fold higher than hyperactive COVID-19 in our study, suggesting that COVID-19 is associated with only mild inflammatory cytokine elevation. An alternative mechanism of disease therefore seems likely (28) and warrants further researches. Additionally, pulmonary-specific variables, such as $PaO_2/FIO_2$ ratio, seem to contribute less to phenotype identification in ARDS; nevertheless, $SpO_2/FIO_2$ ratio is a primary variable to classify COVID-19 phenotype in the present study. A potential explanation for this finding is that patients were enrolled into ARDS clinical trials based on specific pulmonary criteria (e.g., $PaO_2/FIO_2$ ratio), but COVID-19 patients in Tongji cohort are more heterogeneous with respect to pulmonary variables (e.g., $SpO_2/FIO_2$ ratio).

The first strength of our study is the identification of two class phenotypes for intensive care patients with COVID-19 and development of the first parsimonious model for predicting hyperactive phenotype. The observational nature of the present study is another strength as it included all consecutive patients with COVID-19 during 3 months, and the results are therefore more likely to represent the population as encountered in the ICU in clinical practice.

This study also has several limitations. First, our study is a single-center, retrospective, observational study, and we lack the external validation of the phenotypes and the parsimonious model. Testing for COVID-19 phenotypes in more heterogeneous samples is an important direction in future researches. Second, the 26 candidate clinical variables did not fully reflect the host response to SARS-CoV-2 infection; we cannot exclude that adding other markers would provide different phenotypes. Third, whether these phenotypes are dynamic and change over time, resulting in distinct COVID-19 trajectories, is unknown. Finally, although a three- or four-variable model has a good accuracy in predicting the phenotypes, when phenotypes are defined by the parsimonious model rather than the clustering analysis or LCA, we may no longer detect the statistically significant differences in outcomes and treatment responses.

## CONCLUSION

In summary, this analysis confirmed the existence of two distinct phenotypes for intensive care patients with COVID-19. We also provide evidence for accurate parsimonious classifier models of COVID-19 phenotypes. Promisingly, these simple models may aid clinicians in predicting which COVID-19 patients are likely to develop critical illness, delivering timely treatments, and improving patient selection in clinical trials, which in turn could significantly impact patient outcomes.

## ETHICS STATEMENT

The studies involving human participants were reviewed and approved by Tongji Hospital Ethics Committee. Written informed consent for participation was not required for this study in accordance with the national legislation and the institutional requirements.

## AUTHOR CONTRIBUTIONS

YL and HC conceptualized the research aims, design the study, take responsibility for the integrity of the data and the accuracy of the data analysis. HC did the statistical analysis. HC and ZZ wrote the first draft of the manuscript. All authors contributed to acquisition of data, provided comments and approved the final manuscript.

## ACKNOWLEDGMENTS

We thank all doctors who worked in the hospital during the period of patient recruitment as well as the patients who were involved in this study.

## REFERENCES

1. Huang C, Wang Y, Li X, Ren L, Zhao J, Hu Y, et al. Clinical features of patients infected with 2019 novel coronavirus in Wuhan, China. *Lancet.* (2020) 395:497–506. doi: 10.1016/S0140-6736(20)30183-5
2. Guan WJ, Ni ZY, Hu Y, Liang WH, Ou CQ, He JX, et al. Clinical characteristics of coronavirus disease 2019 in China. *New Engl J Med.* (2020) 382:1708–20. doi: 10.1056/NEJMoa2002032
3. Richardson S, Hirsch JS, Narasimhan M, Crawford JM, McGinn T, Davidson KW, et al. Presenting characteristics, comorbidities, and outcomes among 5700 patients hospitalized with COVID-19 in the New York City area. *JAMA.* (2020) 323:2052–9. doi: 10.1001/jama.2020.6775
4. Chen N, Zhou M, Dong X, Qu J, Gong F, Han Y, et al. Epidemiological and clinical characteristics of 99 cases of 2019 novel coronavirus pneumonia in Wuhan, China: a descriptive study. *Lancet.* (2020) 395:507–13. doi: 10.1016/S0140-6736(20)30211-7
5. Grasselli G, Pesenti A, Cecconi M. Critical care utilization for the COVID-19 outbreak in Lombardy, Italy: early experience and forecast during an emergency response. *JAMA.* (2020) 323:1545–6. doi: 10.1001/jama.2020.4031
6. Yang X, Yu Y, Xu J, Shu H, Liu H, Wu Y, et al. Clinical course and outcomes of critically ill patients with SARS-CoV-2 pneumonia in Wuhan, China: a single-centered, retrospective, observational study. *Lancet Respir Med.* (2020) 8:475–81. doi: 10.1016/S2213-2600(20)30079-5
7. Grasselli G, Zangrillo A, Zanella A, Antonelli M, Cabrini L, Castelli A, et al. Baseline characteristics and outcomes of 1591 patients infected with SARS-CoV-2 admitted to ICUs of the Lombardy Region, Italy. *JAMA.* (2020) 323:1574–81. doi: 10.1001/jama.2020.5394
8. Wang D, Hu B, Hu C, Zhu F, Liu X, Zhang J, et al. Clinical characteristics of 138 hospitalized patients with 2019 novel coronavirus-infected pneumonia in Wuhan, China. *JAMA.* (2020) 323:1061–9. doi: 10.1001/jama.2020.1585
9. Shang L, Zhao J, Hu Y, Du R, Cao B. On the use of corticosteroids for 2019-nCoV pneumonia. *Lancet.* (2020) 395:683–4. doi: 10.1016/S0140-6736(20)30361-5
10. Russell CD, Millar JE, Baillie JK. Clinical evidence does not support corticosteroid treatment for 2019-nCoV lung injury. *Lancet.* (2020) 395:473–5. doi: 10.1016/S0140-6736(20)30317-2
11. Gattinoni L, Chiumello D, Rossi S. COVID-19 pneumonia: ARDS or not? *Crit Care.* (2020) 24:154. doi: 10.1186/s13054-020-02880-z
12. Azoulay E, Zafrani L, Mirouse A, Lengliné E, Darmon M, Chevret S. Clinical phenotypes of critically ill COVID-19 patients. *Intens Care Med.* (2020) 46:1651–2. doi: 10.1007/s00134-020-06120-4
13. Gattinoni L, Chiumello D, Caironi P, Busana M, Romitti F, Brazzi L, et al. COVID-19 pneumonia: different respiratory treatments for different phenotypes? *Intens Care Med.* (2020) 46:1099–102. doi: 10.1007/s00134-020-06033-2
14. Rello J, Storti E, Belliato M, Serrano R. Clinical phenotypes of SARS-CoV-2: implications for clinicians and researchers. *Eur Respir J.* (2020) 55:2001028. doi: 10.1183/13993003.01028-2020
15. Li H, Liu L, Zhang D, Xu J, Dai H, Tang N, et al. SARS-CoV-2 and viral sepsis: observations and hypotheses. *Lancet.* (2020) 395:1517–20. doi: 10.1016/S0140-6736(20)30920-X
16. Wilkerson MD, Hayes DN. ConsensusClusterPlus: a class discovery tool with confidence assessments and item tracking. *Bioinformatics.* (2010) 26:1572–3. doi: 10.1093/bioinformatics/btq170
17. Rindskopf D, Rindskopf W. The value of latent class analysis in medical diagnosis. *Stat Med.* (1986) 5:21–7. doi: 10.1002/sim.4780050105
18. Seymour CW, Kennedy JN, Wang S, Chang CC, Elliott CF, Xu Z, et al. Derivation, validation, and potential treatment implications of novel clinical phenotypes for sepsis. *JAMA.* (2019) 321:2003–17. doi: 10.1001/jama.2019.5791
19. Sinha P, Delucchi KL, McAuley DF, O'Kane CM, Matthay MA, Calfee CS. Development and validation of parsimonious algorithms to classify acute respiratory distress syndrome phenotypes: a secondary analysis of randomised controlled trials. *Lancet Respir Med.* (2020) 8:247–57. doi: 10.1016/S2213-2600(19)30369-8
20. Vranas KC, Jopling JK, Sweeney TE, Ramsey MC, Milstein AS, Slatore CG, et al. Identifying distinct subgroups of ICU patients: a machine learning approach. *Crit Care Med.* (2017) 45:1607–15. doi: 10.1097/CCM.0000000000002548
21. Arabi YM, Mandourah Y, Al-Hameed F, Sindi AA, Almekhlafi GA, Hussein MA, et al. Corticosteroid therapy for critically ill patients with middle east respiratory syndrome. *Am J Respir Crit Care Med.* (2018) 197:757–67. doi: 10.1164/rccm.201706-1172OC

22. Chen H, Wang J, Su N, Bao X, Li Y, Jin J. Simplified immune-dysregulation index: a novel marker predicts 28-day mortality of intensive care patients with COVID-19. *Intens Care Med.* (2020) 6:1645–7. doi: 10.1007/s00134-020-06 114-2
23. Wang Y, Lu X, Li Y, Chen H, Chen T, Su N, et al. Clinical course and outcomes of 344 intensive care patients with COVID-19. *Am J Respir Crit Care Med.* (2020) 201:1430–4. doi: 10.1164/rccm.202003-0736LE
24. Sinha P, Delucchi KL, Thompson BT, McAuley DF, Matthay MA, Calfee CS. Latent class analysis of ARDS subphenotypes: a secondary analysis of the statins for acutely injured lungs from sepsis (SAILS) study. *Intens Care Med.* (2018) 44:1859–69. doi: 10.1007/s00134-018-5378-3
25. Liang W, Liang H, Ou L, Chen B, Chen A, Li C, et al. Development and validation of a clinical risk score to predict the occurrence of critical illness in hospitalized patients with COVID-19. *JAMA Intern Med.* (2020) 180:1–9. doi: 10.1001/jamainternmed.2020.2033
26. Bos LD, Schouten LR, Van Vught LA, Wiewel MA, Ong DS, Cremer O, et al. Identification and validation of distinct biological phenotypes in patients with acute respiratory distress syndrome by cluster analysis. *Thorax.* (2017) 72:876–83. doi: 10.1136/thoraxjnl-2016-209719
27. Calfee CS, Delucchi K, Parsons PE, Thompson BT, Ware LB, Matthay MA. Subphenotypes in acute respiratory distress syndrome: latent class analysis of data from two randomised controlled trials. *Lancet Respir Med.* (2014) 2:611–20. doi: 10.1016/S2213-2600(14)70097-9
28. Leisman DE, Deutschman CS, Legrand M. Facing COVID-19 in the ICU: vascular dysfunction, thrombosis, and dysregulated inflammation. *Intens Care Med.* (2020) 6:1105–8. doi: 10.1007/s00134-020-06059-6

# 2

# Machine Learning Approach to Predict Positive Screening of Methicillin-Resistant *Staphylococcus aureus* During Mechanical Ventilation Using Synthetic Dataset From MIMIC-IV Database

*Yohei Hirano [1]*, Keito Shinmoto [2], Yohei Okada [3], Kazuhiro Suga [4], Jeffrey Bombard [5], Shogo Murahata [5], Manoj Shrestha [6], Patrick Ocheja [7] and Aiko Tanaka [8]*

*[1] Department of Emergency and Critical Care Medicine, Juntendo University Urayasu Hospital, Chiba, Japan, [2] Department of Internal Medicine, Tokyo bay Ichikawa Urayasu Medical Center, Chiba, Japan, [3] Department of Primary Care and Emergency Medicine, Graduate School of Medicine, Kyoto University, Kyoto, Japan, [4] Department of Mechanical Engineering, Faculty of Engineering, Kogakuin University, Tokyo, Japan, [5] Dowell Co., Ltd., Hokkaido, Japan, [6] DeerWalk Japan, Tokyo, Japan, [7] Graduate School of Informatics, Kyoto University, Kyoto, Japan, [8] Department of Anesthesiology and Intensive Care Medicine, Osaka University Graduate School of Medicine, Osaka, Japan*

***Correspondence:**
*Yohei Hirano*
*yhirano@juntendo-urayasu.jp*

**Background:** Mechanically ventilated patients are susceptible to nosocomial infections such as ventilator-associated pneumonia. To treat ventilated patients with suspected infection, clinicians select appropriate antibiotics. However, decision-making regarding the use of antibiotics for methicillin-resistant *Staphylococcus aureus* (MRSA) is challenging, because of the lack of evidence-supported criteria. This study aims to derive a machine learning model to predict MRSA as a possible pathogen responsible for infection in mechanically ventilated patients.

**Methods:** Data were collected from the Medical Information Mart for Intensive Care (MIMIC)-IV database (an openly available database of patients treated at the Beth Israel Deaconess Medical Center in the period 2008–2019). Of 26,409 mechanically ventilated patients, 809 were screened for MRSA during the mechanical ventilation period and included in the study. The outcome was positivity to MRSA on screening, which was highly imbalanced in the dataset, with 93.9% positive outcomes. Therefore, after dividing the dataset into a training set ($n = 566$) and a test set ($n = 243$) for validation by stratified random sampling with a 7:3 allocation ratio, synthetic datasets with 50% positive outcomes were created by synthetic minority over-sampling for both sets individually (synthetic training set: $n = 1,064$; synthetic test set: $n = 456$). Using these synthetic datasets, we trained and validated an XGBoost machine learning model using 28 predictor variables for outcome prediction. Model performance was evaluated by area under the receiver operating characteristic (AUROC), sensitivity, specificity, and other statistical measurements. Feature importance was computed by the Gini method.

**Results:** In validation, the XGBoost model demonstrated reliable outcome prediction with an AUROC value of 0.89 [95% confidence interval (CI): 0.83–0.95]. The model showed a high sensitivity of 0.98 [CI: 0.95–0.99], but a low specificity of 0.47 [CI: 0.41–0.54] and a positive predictive value of 0.65 [CI: 0.62–0.68]. Important predictor variables included admission from the emergency department, insertion of arterial lines, prior quinolone use, hemodialysis, and admission to a surgical intensive care unit.

**Conclusions:** We were able to develop an effective machine learning model to predict positive MRSA screening during mechanical ventilation using synthetic datasets, thus encouraging further research to develop a clinically relevant machine learning model for antibiotics stewardship.

**Keywords: prediction, machine learning, mechanical ventilation, Methicillin-Resistant *Staphylococcus aureus*—MRSA, outcome**

## INTRODUCTION

Selection of antibiotics for critically-ill patients undergoing mechanical ventilation in the intensive care unit (ICU) is challenging (1, 2), as these patients are susceptible to nosocomial infections such as ventilator-associated pneumonia (VAP), catheter-related blood site infection, and catheter-associated urinary tract infection (3–5). Thus, multiple anti-bacterial agents with broad spectrum are often empirically selected for the treatment of this population. However, the inappropriate use of broad-spectrum antibiotics could lead to the emergence of resistant bacteria (6, 7). The incorrect usage of antibiotics might also cause adverse effects outweighing their benefits (8). Therefore, optimized antibiotics selection would be beneficial for patient outcomes.

In particular, the decision-making regarding the use of antibiotics for methicillin-resistant *staphylococcus aureus* (MRSA) is a source of distress for clinicians, due to their harmful complications such as hypersensitivity reactions, neutropenia, thrombocytopenia, and acute kidney injury (9–11). Although a variety of risk factors for MRSA colonization have been identified and reported (12, 13), there are currently no specific criteria for the use of antibiotics for MRSA.

To identify patients carrying MRSA, a specific screening test is often used. MRSA detection could be helpful for clinicians not only to determine the choice of antibiotics, but also to identify the patients who could potentially spread MRSA to other patients. However, the commonly used culture screening method for MRSA requires several days to obtain the result, and thus cannot be used to obtain information in real time (14). Hence, the accurate and timely prediction of the presence of MRSA in mechanically ventilated patients would have great significance and impact in the clinical setting.

Recently, machine learning methods have demonstrated their usefulness for clinical decision support in infectious diseases (15). This study aimed to develop and validate a machine learning-based model to predict the presence of MRSA in mechanically ventilated patients by using only available patient data obtained before MRSA screening.

**Abbreviations:** VAP, Ventilator-Associated Pneumonia; ICU, Intensive Care Unit; MRSA, Methicillin-Resistant *Staphylococcus aureus*; MIMIC, Medical Information Mart for Intensive Care; COPD, Chronic Obstructive Pulmonary Disease; SOFA, Sequential Organ Failure Assessment; APACHE, Acute Physiology and Chronic Health Evaluation; ED, Emergency Department; SICU, Surgical Intensive Care Unit; TSICU, Trauma Surgical Intensive Care Unit; CCU, Coronary Care Unit; AUROC, Area Under the Receiver Operating Characteristic; CI, Confidence Interval.

## MATERIALS AND METHODS

### Data Sources and Ethical Approval

The data for the current retrospective study were obtained from the Medical Information Mart for Intensive Care (MIMIC)-IV database, version 1.4. This publicly available relational database is provided by the Laboratory for Computational Physiology at the Massachusetts Institute of Technology (MIT, Cambridge, MA, USA), and includes information on critical care patients who were admitted to the ICU at the Beth Israel Deaconess Medical Center (BIDMC, Boston, MA, USA) during the period 2008–2019. Patient identifiers were removed according to the Health Insurance Portability and Accountability Act (HIPAA) Safe Harbor provision. Details of the MIMIC-IV database have been described elsewhere (16, 17). The MIMIC-IV project was approved by the Institutional Review Boards of BIDMC and MIT. Requirement for individual patient consent was waived because the project did not impact clinical care and all protected health information was deidentified. Data were extracted by Yohei Hirano, MD, who completed the requested online training course of the Collaborative Institutional Training Initiative (CITI) program (record ID: 38943363) and was approved as credentialed user to access the MIMIC-IV database. The current study was conducted in accordance with the Declaration of Helsinki.

### Study Population and Outcomes

The study population were adult patients screened for MRSA during mechanical ventilation. The outcome was a MRSA-positive result on the screening test. A flow diagram of patient inclusion is shown in **Figure 1A**. Overall, 26,409 patients with invasive ventilation were identified from the MIMIC-IV database. Of these, 25,600 patients who were not screened for MRSA during the ventilated period were excluded. We meant to exclude also non-adult patients, aged 17 years and under, but no patients met this criterion. Thus, 809 adult patients MRSA-screened during mechanical ventilation were our included cohort. Finally, the subjects were divided into two groups by

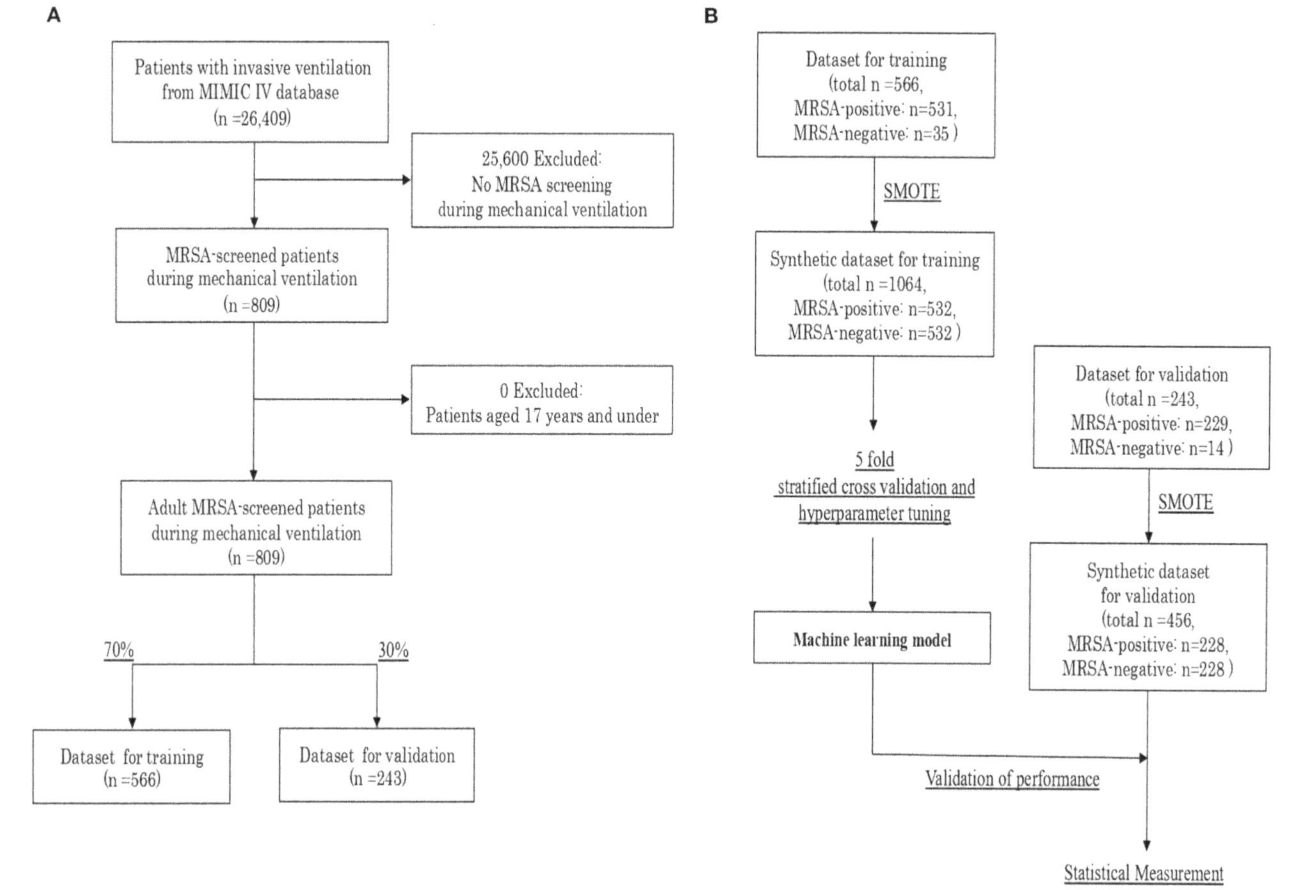


**FIGURE 1 | (A)** Flow diagram of patient inclusion. **(B)** Procedure for creating the synthetic datasets and validating the machine learning model. MIMIC, Medical Information Mart for Intensive Care; MRSA, Methicillin-Resistant *Staphylococcus aureus*; SMOTE, Synthetic Minority Over-sampling Technique.

stratified random sampling with a 7:3 allocation ratio: a dataset for training ($n = 566$) and a dataset for validation ($n = 243$).

## Generation of Synthetic Datasets

The characteristics of the included cohort are shown in **Supplemental Table 1**. The outcome was highly imbalanced, with 93.9% of the patient classified as MRSA-positive by the screening test. As the imbalanced classification task is hard for predictive modeling due to the severely skewed class distribution and unequal misclassification costs, we created synthetic datasets with 50% of positive outcomes by synthetic minority over-sampling technique (SMOTE), independently for the training and validation datasets. SMOTE offers more related minority class samples to learn from, which leads to more coverage of the minority class (18). As the prevalence of MRSA screening test generally varies in individual countries and facilities, we set the outcome balance setting for the synthetic dataset at 50%, which is most balanced. We could generate a synthetic training dataset with a total of 1,064 samples, and a synthetic validation dataset with 456 samples (**Figure 1B**).

## Predictor Variables

In this study, 28 variables concerning pre-hospitalization information were selected as outcome predictors according to the availability of data from the MIMIC-IV and previous literature reviews on risk factors for MRSA (9, 12, 13, 19). These variables included age, sex, ICU locations, past medical history (diabetes mellitus, chronic obstructive pulmonary disease (COPD), chronic heart disease, cerebrovascular disease, peripheral vascular disease), Charlson comorbidity index, cellulitis, pressure ulcer, sequential organ failure assessment (SOFA) score at MRSA screening, acute physiology and chronic health evaluation (APACHE) III score on admission, admission from emergency department (ED), days spent at the hospital at the time of MRSA screening, days of ventilator use at MRSA screening, prior use of corticosteroids or antibiotics such as quinolone, macrolide, carbapenem, and interventional procedures (peripheral line, peripherally inserted central catheter (PICC) line, central venous catheter (CVC) line, pulmonary artery catheter (PAC) line, arterial line, urinary catheter, hemodialysis, and tracheostomy) before MRSA screening. ICU locations were handled as dummy variables, including medical intensive care unit (MICU), surgical intensive care unit (SICU),

MICU/SICU, trauma surgical intensive care unit (TSICU), coronary care unit (CCU), cardiac vascular intensive care unit (CVICU), and other ICUs [neuro surgical intensive care unit (NSICU) or post anesthesia care unit (PACU)].

## Development and Validation of Machine-Learning Models

Using the synthetic training datasets, we trained and developed an XGBoost machine learning model as a classifier for outcome prediction. To avoid overfitting the model, we used five-fold stratified cross-validation. In addition, optimization of hyperparameters was performed to obtain the best performance in outcome prediction.

After the algorithm training process, the performance of the developed model was validated using the synthetic validation dataset. As statistical measures of performance, we calculated the area under the receiver operating characteristic (AUROC) curve, sensitivity, specificity, positive likelihood ratio, negative likelihood ratio, positive predictive value, negative predictive value, and accuracy. The process of machine learning and validation is described in **Figure 1B**. In addition, feature importance was computed as the normalized total reduction of the criterion brought by the feature, which is known as Gini importance.

## Statistical Analysis and Software Library for Machine Learning

Data were extracted from MIMIC-IV using structured query language (SQL) through Google Cloud's BigQuery platform. Statistical analyses of the characteristics of the cohorts were performed using SciPy (version 1.4.1) with Python (version 3.7.4, in Anaconda 2019.10). Age, as a continuous variable, was reported as mean and standard deviation. All categorical variables were reported as counts and percentages. The *t*-test was used to compare means between two samples. The chi-square test was used to compare frequencies. All tests were two-sided, and the significance level was set at 5% ($p < 0.05$). For model development, scikit-learn (version 0.21.3) with Python was employed.

# RESULTS

## Characteristics of the Synthetic Datasets Used for Machine Learning

The characteristics of the synthetic datasets used for machine learning are shown in **Table 1**. The mean age in the synthetic training data was 66.6 ± 14.0 years, significantly older than that of the synthetic validation data (62.9 ± 15.6 years). A smaller fraction of patients admitted from ED or hospitalized in the CCU was present in the synthetic training data compared with the synthetic validation data (41.3% vs. 54.4% and 5.6% vs. 13.8%, respectively). Among procedures, peripheral line placement was performed significantly less frequently in the synthetic training data than in the synthetic validation data. The Charlson comorbidity index and the number of days of ventilator use at MRSA screening were also significantly different between the two datasets.

## Performance of the Machine Learning Model

**Figure 2** presents the ROC curve, AUROC value, confusion matrix, and statistical measures used to evaluate the performance of the machine learning model in the validation dataset. The ROC curve and its AUROC value showed good predictive ability of the model for MRSA-positivity in the screening test (AUROC: 0.89 [95% confidence interval (CI): 0.83–0.95]). Although the accuracy, specificity, and positive predictive value were relatively low (0.73 [CI: 0.68–0.77], 0.47 [CI: 0.41–0.54], and 0.65 [CI: 0.62–0.68], respectively), the model demonstrated a high sensitivity of 0.98 [CI: 0.95–0.99] and a high negative predictive value (0.96 [CI: 0.90–0.98]).

## Feature Importance

The importance of the XGBoost model features is shown in **Figure 3**. Admission from ED was the most important variable in predicting MRSA-positivity in the screening test during mechanical ventilation. The five most important variables also included insertion of previous arterial lines, prior quinolone use, hemodialysis, and admission in the SICU, although they were far less important than admission from ED. Co-existing diseases such as peripheral vascular disease, diabetes mellitus, and chronic heart disease were also relatively important predictors. However, prior use of macrolide or carbapenem, tracheostomy, COPD, and cellulitis were of no importance in the predictive model.

# DISCUSSION

In the current study, we undertook the development of a machine learning model to predict MRSA colonization during mechanical ventilation using the MIMIC-IV, a large open relational database containing data derived from the ICUs of a single center. As the extracted data were found to be highly imbalanced in terms of outcome, we created independent synthetic balanced datasets for training and validation by an oversampling technique. The machine learning-based model thus developed showed good performance in predicting MRSA screening positivity, with the reasonably high AUROC of 0.89.

Although previous large-scale studies have clarified the risk factors for MRSA colonization or infection, decision-making for the antimicrobial coverage of MRSA by critical care physician is still challenging. These risk factors are not specific, but rather common in critically ill patients, so that clinical practitioners cannot discriminate between MRSA-positive and negative patients without specimen testing. In this context, our current study supports the potential use of a machine learning model, which could be superior to human learning in predicting outcomes depending on complexly intertwined factors. Previously, Hartvigsen et al. reported the results of their challenge toward the prediction of MRSA-positive patients by machine learning models (20). They succeeded in developing a machine learning-based model which showed high predictive performance in the ICU patients. However, our study is novel

**TABLE 1** | Characteristics of the synthetic dataset used for machine learning.

| Variable | Synthetic training data ($n$ = 1,064) | Synthetic validation data ($n$ = 456) | *P*-value |
|---|---|---|---|
| Age (years) | 66.6 [14.0] | 62.9 [15.6] | <0.001 |
| Gender (male) | 528 (49.6%) | 234 (51.3%) | 0.73 |
| **ICU location** | | | |
| MICU | 213 (20.0%) | 73 (16.0%) | 0.13 |
| MICU/SICU | 92 (8.6%) | 33 (7.2%) | 0.40 |
| SICU | 105 (9.9%) | 47 (10.3%) | 0.81 |
| TSICU | 76 (7.1%) | 33 (7.2%) | 0.95 |
| CCU | 60 (5.6%) | 63 (13.8%) | <0.001 |
| CVICU | 137 (12.9%) | 45 (9.9%) | 0.14 |
| Other (NSICU or PACU) | 4 (0.4%) | 3 (0.7%) | 0.46 |
| **Past medical history** | | | |
| Diabetes Mellitus | 162 (15.2%) | 72 (15.8%) | 0.81 |
| COPD | 15 (1.4%) | 6 (1.3%) | 0.89 |
| Chronic heart disease | 210 (19.7%) | 77 (16.9%) | 0.28 |
| Cerebrovascular disease | 88 (8.3%) | 25 (5.5%) | 0.08 |
| Peripheral vascular disease | 33 (3.1%) | 14 (3.1%) | 0.97 |
| Charlson comorbidity index | 5 (3–7) | 6 (4–7) | 0.01 |
| Cellulitis | 22 (2.1%) | 9 (2.0%) | 0.91 |
| Pressure ulcer | 381 (35.8%) | 142 (31.1%) | 0.22 |
| SOFA score (at MRSA screening) | 4 (2–6) | 4 (2–7) | 0.11 |
| APACHE III score (on admission) | 58 (41–78) | 55(40–75) | 0.26 |
| Admision from ED | 439 (41.3%) | 248 (54.4%) | 0.004 |
| Length of hospital days (at MRSA screening) | 3.0 [4.5] | 2.9 [4.0] | 0.39 |
| Length of ventilator days (at MRSA screening) | 1.9 [2.9] | 1.9 [2.6] | 0.03 |
| **Prior antibitics use (before MRSA screening)** | | | |
| Quinolone | 75 (7.0%) | 30 (6.6%) | 0.76 |
| Macrolide | 25 (2.3%) | 9 (2.0%) | 0.66 |
| Carbapenem | 24 (2.3%) | 12 (2.6%) | 0.67 |
| Prior corticosteroids use (before MRSA screening) | 11 (1.0%) | 5 (1.1%) | 0.91 |
| **Procedures (before MRSA screening)** | | | |
| Peripheral line | 675 (63.4%) | 348 (76.3%) | 0.03 |
| PICC line | 62 (5.8%) | 36 (7.9%) | 0.16 |
| CVC line | 284 (26.7%) | 96 (21.1%) | 0.07 |
| PAC line | 51 (4.8%) | 32 (7.0%) | 0.10 |
| Arterial line | 293 (27.5%) | 146 (32.0%) | 0.19 |
| Urinary catheter | 144 (13.5%) | 66 (14.5%) | 0.67 |
| Hemodialysis | 109 (10.2%) | 44 (9.6%) | 0.75 |
| Tracheostomy | 8 (0.8%) | 1 (0.2%) | 0.22 |
| **Outcome** | | | |
| MRSA-positive on screening test | 532 (50.0%) | 228 (50.0%) | 1.0 |

*All categorical variables are shown as n (%). A continuous variable (Age) is shown as mean [standard deviation]. ICU, Intensive Care Unit, MICU, Medical Intensive Care Unit, SICU, Surgical Intensive Care Unit, TSICU, Trauma Surgical Intensive Care Unit, CCU, Coronary Care Unit, CVICU, Cardiac Vascular Intensive Care Unit, NSICU, Neuro Surgical Intensive Care Unit, PACU, Post Anesthesia Care Unit, COPD:Chronic Obstructive Pulmonary Disease, SOFA, Sequential Organ Failure Assessment, MRSA, Methicillin-Resistant Staphylococcus aureus, APACHE, Acute Physiology And Chronic Health Evaluation, ED, Emergency Department, PICC, Peripherally Inserted Central Catheter, CVC, Central Venous Catheter, PAC, Pulmonary Artery Catheter.*

in that we targeted the specific population of mechanically ventilated patients, who exhibit more severe conditions and are more susceptible to nosocomial infections, such as VAP, than those analyzed in the previous study. Broad-spectrum antibiotics including coverage for MRSA are frequently the initial choice by practitioners to treat these patients at high risk of death, thus the reliable prediction of MRSA colonization would more likely lead to a reduction of unnecessary antibiotics use.

Our prediction model showed low specificity and positive predictive value to predict MRSA colonization, indicating that

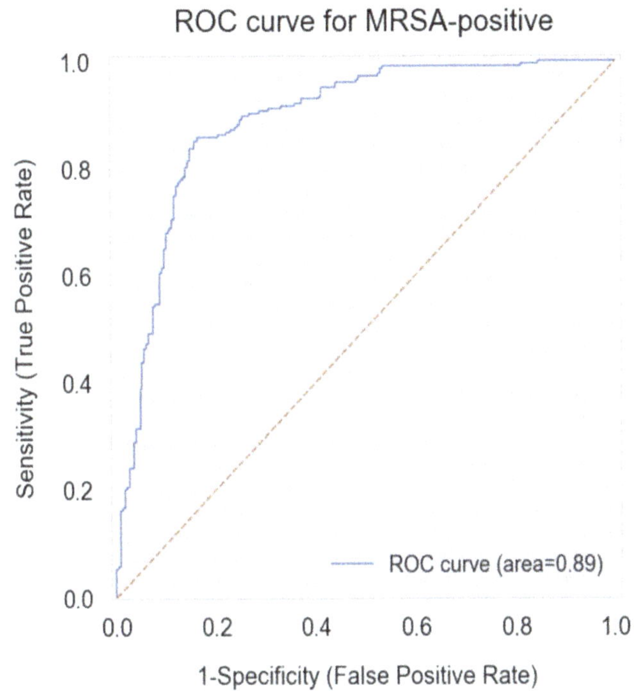


**Confusion Matrix**

| | Predict MRSA-negative | Predict MRSA-positive |
|---|---|---|
| True MRSA-negative | 108 | 120 |
| True MRSA-positive | 5 | 223 |

**Statistical Measures**

| Statistical measures | Value | 95% CI |
|---|---|---|
| Sensitivity | 0.98 | 0.95 - 0.99 |
| Specificity | 0.47 | 0.41 - 0.54 |
| Positive Likelihood Ratio | 1.86 | 1.64 - 2.11 |
| Negative Likelihood Ratio | 0.05 | 0.02 - 0.11 |
| Positive Predictive Value | 0.65 | 0.62 - 0.68 |
| Negative Predictive Value | 0.96 | 0.90 - 0.98 |
| Accuracy | 0.73 | 0.68 - 0.77 |
| AUROC | 0.89 | 0.83 - 0.95 |

**FIGURE 2 |** ROC curve, confusion matrix, and statistical measures of performance of the machine learning model. MRSA, Methicillin-Resistant *Staphylococcus aureus*; CI, Confidence interval; AUROC, Area Under the Receiver Operating Characteristic.

the prediction of MRSA-positivity by the model does not guarantee positivity of the MRSA screening test. On the other hand, our model demonstrated high sensitivity and negative predictive value, implying that predicted MRSA negativity strongly supports the actual absence of MRSA colonization. The result of MRSA screening test does not promise the necessity of antibiotics coverage for MRSA. However, MRSA colonization is a high risk factor to develop MRSA infections in ICU patients (19). Therefore, acknowledgment of the presence of MRSA colonization as early as possible before the result of MRSA-screening test comes out might be helpful as one of the risk evaluations for MRSA infection, although other clinical conditions or examinations such as gram staining of the patients should be definitely considered to decide the use of antibiotics with coverage of MRSA. Real-time identification of the mechanically-ventilated patients who could potentially spread MRSA is also beneficial because this patient population requires medical practitioners to provide many contact opportunities for cares.

In this study, the model was created using 28 features that have been reported to be risk factors for MRSA colonization or infection in the previous literature, and that could be accurately extracted from the MIMIC-IV database. Among these features, admission from ED contributed the most to the prediction model. As the population of the study consisted of mechanically-ventilated patients, we presumed that patients admitted from ED might constitute an epidemiologically unique patient subgroup, distinct from those who were admitted in the ICU for the purpose of surgical operations. Patient admitted from ED could have more complex combinations of risk factors for MRSA colonization, including not only medical conditions or existing diseases, but also social backgrounds, such as transfer from residential care homes or homelessness (21, 22). In contrast, patient severity scores such as SOFA or APACHE III were less important predictors. It is reassuring that well known risk factors for MRSA, such as hemodialysis and arterial lines, were detected as important features for the prediction. The ICU location of admission (SICU or MICU/SICU) was also highly relevant to the prediction, although we cannot determine whether this was related to the transmission of MRSA itself or to differences in patient diagnosis in each ICU. As previously described elsewhere (23), the model identified prior use of quinolones as an important risk factors for MRSA, compared to carbapenem or macrolide. However, caution is required in the interpretation of the feature importance of each variable, because the percentage of positives for some of the assessed features was very low.

Our study has several limitations. First, we trained the model and validated it using synthetic datasets due to the severe class imbalance of the extracted datasets. The evaluation of the model on unrealistic data is the strongest limitation of the study, and could have led to an overly optimistic assessment of its performance, thus absolutely requiring external validation using real-world datasets with more balanced outcomes in the future. Second, we could not take into account how and why MRSA screening tests were performed in the included patients. In our dataset, the MRSA screening positivity rate was extremely high. Moreover, only 809 out of 26,409 patients were screened for MRSA during mechanical ventilation. These facts implied that

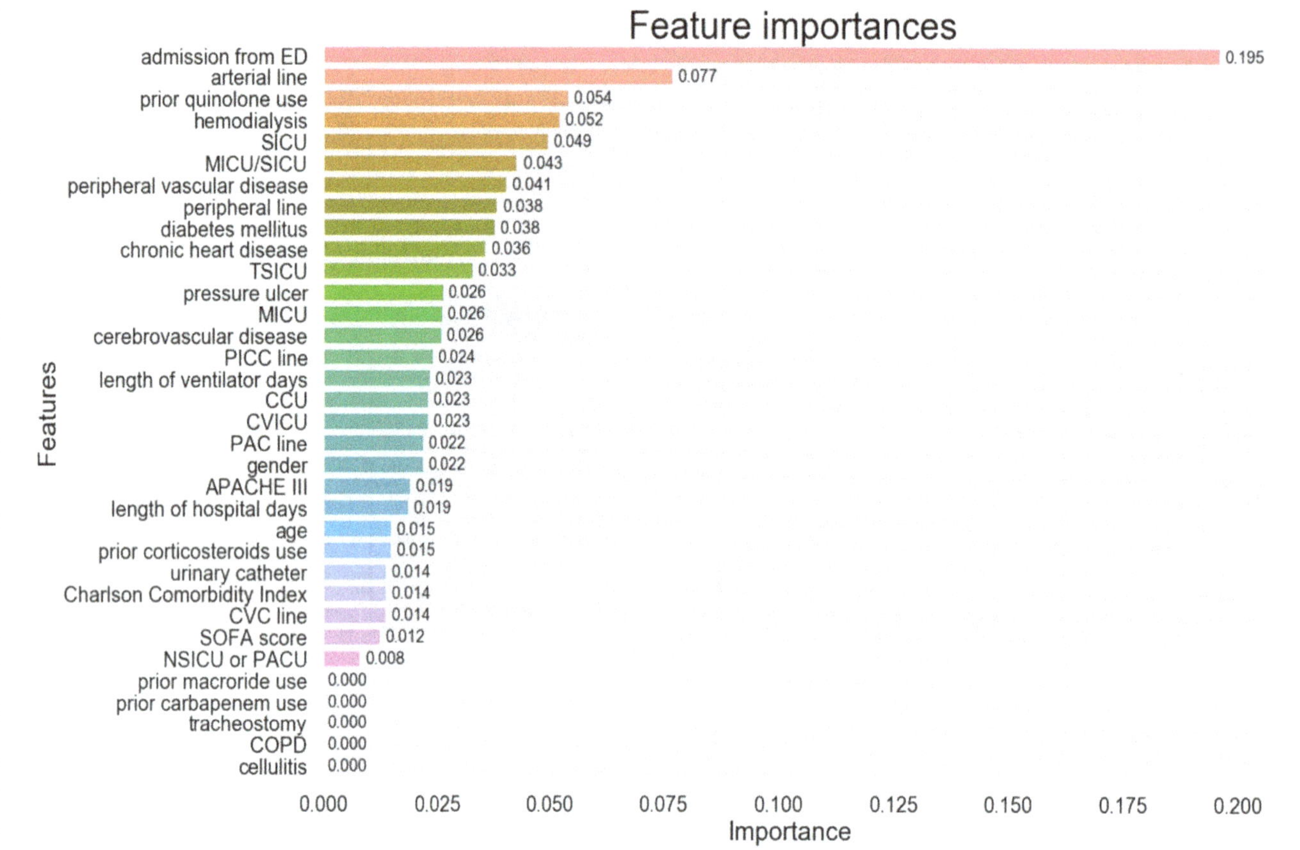


**FIGURE 3 |** Feature importance of the model variables. ED, Emergency Department, SICU, Surgical Intensive Care Unit; MICU, Medical Intensive Care Unit; TSICU, Trauma Surgical Intensive Care Unit; PICC, Peripherally Inserted Central Catheter; CCU, Coronary Care Unit; CVICU, Cardiac Vascular Intensive Care Unit; PAC, Pulmonary Artery Catheter; APACHE, Acute Physiology and Chronic Health Evaluation; CVC, Central Venous Catheter; SOFA, Sequential Organ Failure Assessment; NSICU, Neuro Surgical Intensive Care Unit; PACU, Post Anesthesia Care Unit; COPD, Chronic Obstructive Pulmonary Disease.

clinicians might have decided to screen a patient for MRSA based on specific reasons such as clinically strong suspicion of MRSA positivity or MRSA screening protocol for the facility. The reasons physicians in the facility consider selecting patients for screening can also overlap with the predictors used to develop the model. These might have caused bias. Third, we could not include well-known risk factors for MRSA colonization such as pre-existing cancer, HIV infection, and intravenous drug use as predictive features, due to the insufficient information available from the dataset. Hence, the model is amenable to further improvements in performance. Finally, the model might not have worldwide generalizability because it was trained on a dataset derived from a single center, while the epidemiology of antimicrobial resistance differs among countries, hospitals and ethnicities (24, 25). It might be preferable to develop and use microbiome prediction models specific for each region or hospital.

## CONCLUSIONS

In conclusion, we were able to develop a machine learning model to predict positive screening for MRSA during mechanical ventilation using a synthetically augmented dataset from single center/MIMIC-IV database. Although external validation using more balanced, real-world datasets is required, the result of the current study demonstrated the possibility of early detection of MRSA in mechanically-ventilated patients by a machine learning approach, which might lead to optimized antibiotic selection by clinicians.

## ETHICS STATEMENT

The studies involving human participants were reviewed and approved by the Institutional Review Boards of the Beth Israel Deaconess Medical Center (BIDMC) and the Massachusetts Institute of Technology (MIT). Written informed consent for participation was not required for this study in accordance with the national legislation and the institutional requirements.

## AUTHOR CONTRIBUTIONS

YH, JB, SM, MS, and PO: extracted data and conducted data cleaning. YH, KS, MS, and PO: analyzed the data. YH, KS, YO, and AT: interpreted the data. YH drafted the manuscript. All authors reviewed and discussed the manuscript. All authors read and approved the final manuscript. All authors jointly conceived of and designated this study.

## ACKNOWLEDGMENTS

We would like to thank Ohno Kunihisa, Ryo Uchimido, and Satoru Hashimoto for their guidance and support on this work. We also thank Editage (www.editage.jp) for English language editing.

## REFERENCES

1. Wunderink RG, Srinivasan A, Barie PS, Chastre J, Dela Cruz CS, Douglas IS, et al. Antibiotic stewardship in the intensive care unit. An Official American Thoracic Society Workshop Report in Collaboration with the AACN, CHEST, CDC, and SCCM. *Ann Am Thorac Soc.* (2020) 17:531–40. doi: 10.1513/AnnalsATS.202003-188ST
2. Fernando SM, Tran A, Cheng W, Klompas M, Kyeremanteng K, Mehta S, et al. Diagnosis of ventilator-associated pneumonia in critically ill adult patients-a systematic review and meta-analysis. *Intensive Care Med.* (2020) 46:1170–9. doi: 10.1007/s00134-020-06036-z
3. Papazian L, Klompas M, Luyt C-E. Ventilator-associated pneumonia in adults: a narrative review. *Intensive Care Med.* (2020) 46:888–906. doi: 10.1007/s00134-020-05980-0
4. Rupp ME, Karnatak R. Intravascular catheter-related bloodstream infections. *Infect Dis Clin North Am.* (2018) 32:765–87. doi: 10.1016/j.idc.2018.06.002
5. Luzum M, Sebolt J, Chopra V. Catheter-associated urinary tract infection, clostridioides difficile colitis, central line-associated bloodstream infection, and methicillin-resistant *Staphylococcus aureus*. *Med Clin North Am.* (2020) 104:663–79. doi: 10.1016/j.mcna.2020.02.004
6. Magalhães C, Lima M, Trieu-Cuot P, Ferreira P. To give or not to give antibiotics is not the only question. *Lancet Infect Dis.* (2020) 21:e191–201. doi: 10.1016/S1473-3099(20)30602-2
7. Laxminarayan R, Van Boeckel T, Frost I, Kariuki S, Khan EA, Limmathurotsakul D, et al. The Lancet Infectious Diseases Commission on antimicrobial resistance: 6 years later. *Lancet Infect Dis.* (2020) 20:e51–60. doi: 10.1016/S1473-3099(20)30003-7
8. Arulkumaran N, Routledge M, Schlebusch S, Lipman J, Conway Morris A. Antimicrobial-associated harm in critical care: a narrative review. *Intensive Care Med.* (2020) 46:225–35. doi: 10.1007/s00134-020-05929-3
9. Hassoun A, Linden PK, Friedman B. Incidence, prevalence, and management of MRSA bacteremia across patient populations—a review of recent developments in MRSA management and treatment. *Critical Care.* (2017) 21:211. doi: 10.1186/s13054-017-1801-3
10. Falagas ME, Vardakas KZ. Benefit-risk assessment of linezolid for serious gram-positive bacterial infections. *Drug Saf.* (2008) 31:753–68. doi: 10.2165/00002018-200831090-00004
11. Bruniera FR, Ferreira FM, Saviolli LRM, Bacci MR, Feder D, da Luz Gonçalves Pedreira M, et al. The use of vancomycin with its therapeutic and adverse effects: a review. *Eur Rev Med Pharmacol Sci.* (2015) 19:694–700.
12. Graffunder EM, Venezia RA. Risk factors associated with nosocomial methicillin-resistant *Staphylococcus aureus* (MRSA) infection including previous use of antimicrobials. *J Antimicrob Chemother.* (2002) 49:999–1005. doi: 10.1093/jac/dkf009
13. Hidron AI, Kourbatova EV, Halvosa JS, Terrell BJ, McDougal LK, Tenover FC, et al. Risk factors for colonization with Methicillin-Resistant *Staphylococcus aureus* (MRSA) in patients admitted to an urban hospital: emergence of community-associated MRSA nasal carriage. *Clin Infect Dis.* (2005) 41:159–66. doi: 10.1086/430910
14. French GL. Methods for screening for methicillin-resistant *Staphylococcus aureus* carriage. *Clin Microbiol Infect.* (2009) 15:10–6. doi: 10.1111/j.1469-0691.2009.03092.x
15. Peiffer-Smadja N, Rawson TM, Ahmad R, Buchard A, Georgiou P, Lescure F-X, et al. Machine learning for clinical decision support in infectious diseases: a narrative review of current applications. *Clin Microbiol Infect.* (2020) 26:584–95. doi: 10.1016/j.cmi.2019.09.009
16. Johnson A, Bulgarelli L, Pollard T, Horng S, Celi LA, Mark R. MIMIC-IV (version 0.4). *PhysioNet.* (2020). Available at:https://doi.org/10.13026/a3wn-hq05
17. Goldberger A, Amaral L, Glass L, Hausdorff J, Ivanov P, Mark R, et al. Components of a new research resource for complex physiologic signals. *Circulation.* 101:e215220. doi: 10.1161/01.CIR.101.23.e215
18. Chawla NV, Bowyer KW, Hall LO, Kegelmeyer WP, SMOTE. Synthetic minority over-sampling technique. *JAIR.* (2002) 16:321–57. doi: 10.1613/jair.953
19. Fukuta Y, Cunningham CA, Harris PL, Wagener MM, Muder RR. Identifying the risk factors for hospital-acquired Methicillin-Resistant *Staphylococcus aureus* (MRSA) infection among patients colonized with MRSA on admission. *Inf Control Hosp Epidemiol.* (2012) 33:1219–25. doi: 10.1086/668420
20. Hartvigsen T, Sen C, Brownell S, Teeple E, Kong X, Rundensteiner E. Early prediction of MRSA infections using electronic health records. In *Proceedings of the 11th International Joint Conference on Biomedical Engineering Systems and Technologies.* Funchal, Madeira, Portugal: SCITEPRESS—Science and Technology Publications. p. 156–67.
21. Crnich CJ. Impact and management of MRSA in the long-term care setting. *Curr Transl Geriatr and Exp Gerontol Rep.* (2013) 2:125–35. doi: 10.1007/s13670-013-0047-4
22. Leibler JH, León C, Cardoso LJP, Morris JC, Miller NS, Nguyen DD, et al. Prevalence and risk factors for MRSA nasal colonization among persons experiencing homelessness in Boston, MA. *J Med Microbiol.* (2017) 66:1183–8. doi: 10.1099/jmm.0.000552
23. Couderc C, Jolivet S, Thiébaut ACM, Ligier C, Remy L, Alvarez A-S, et al. Fluoroquinolone use is a risk factor for methicillin-resistant *Staphylococcus aureus* acquisition in long-term care facilities: a nested case-case-control study. *Clin Infect Dis.* (2014) 59:206–15. doi: 10.1093/cid/ciu236
24. Livermore DM, Pearson A. Antibiotic resistance: location, location, location. *Clin Microbiol Inf.* (2007) 13:7–16. doi: 10.1111/j.1469-0691.2007.01724.x
25. Nadimpalli ML, Chan CW, Doron S. Antibiotic resistance: a call to action to prevent the next epidemic of inequality. *Nat Med.* (2021) 27:187–8. doi: 10.1038/s41591-020-01201-9

# 3

# Prediction of Mortality in Surgical Intensive Care Unit Patients Using Machine Learning Algorithms

*Kyongsik Yun [1†], Jihoon Oh [2†], Tae Ho Hong [3] and Eun Young Kim [4*]*

*[1] Computation and Neural Systems, California Institute of Technology, Pasadena, CA, United States, [2] Department of Psychiatry, College of Medicine, Seoul St. Mary's Hospital, The Catholic University of Korea, Seoul, South Korea, [3] Division of Hepato-Biliary and Pancreas Surgery, Department of Surgery, College of Medicine, Seoul St. Mary's Hospital, The Catholic University of Korea, Seoul, South Korea, [4] Division of Trauma and Surgical Critical Care, Department of Surgery, College of Medicine, Seoul St. Mary's Hospital, The Catholic University of Korea, Seoul, South Korea*

***Correspondence:***
*Eun Young Kim*
*freesshs@naver.com*

*† These authors have contributed equally to this work*

**Objective:** Predicting prognosis of in-hospital patients is critical. However, it is challenging to accurately predict the life and death of certain patients at certain period. To determine whether machine learning algorithms could predict in-hospital death of critically ill patients with considerable accuracy and identify factors contributing to the prediction power.

**Materials and Methods:** Using medical data of 1,384 patients admitted to the Surgical Intensive Care Unit (SICU) of our institution, we investigated whether machine learning algorithms could predict in-hospital death using demographic, laboratory, and other disease-related variables, and compared predictions using three different algorithmic methods. The outcome measurement was the incidence of unexpected postoperative mortality which was defined as mortality without pre-existing not-for-resuscitation order that occurred within 30 days of the surgery or within the same hospital stay as the surgery.

**Results:** Machine learning algorithms trained with 43 variables successfully classified dead and live patients with very high accuracy. Most notably, the decision tree showed the higher classification results (Area Under the Receiver Operating Curve, AUC = 0.96) than the neural network classifier (AUC = 0.80). Further analysis provided the insight that serum albumin concentration, total prenatal nutritional intake, and peak dose of dopamine drug played an important role in predicting the mortality of SICU patients.

**Conclusion:** Our results suggest that machine learning algorithms, especially the decision tree method, can provide information on structured and explainable decision flow and accurately predict hospital mortality in SICU hospitalized patients.

**Keywords: anesthesia and intensive care, informatics, intensive care, surgery, machine learning**

## INTRODUCTION

Prediction of mortality rate of patients in intensive care unit (ICU) has been a critical issue (1–3).To assess the probability of death in ICU patients, several models using routine admission variables (4) and objectively derived weights were proposed in the 1980s (5). Along with these attempts, Acute Physiology And Chronic Health Evaluation (APACHE) II was developed to assess the severity and mortality of patients admitted to ICU in 1985 (6, 7). Other scoring systems such as Simplified

Acute Physiology Score (SAPS) II that can provide a probability of hospital mortality have also been suggested (8). With new variables such as Glasgow Coma Scale and thrombolysis, APACHE was updated to APACHE IV in 2006, showing better performance in predicting mortality rate in ICU patients (9). SAPS III also added several variables that could be quickly measured at admission, showing increased prediction performance compared to SAPS II (10).

However, they have several limitations in clinical settings although APAHCE, SAPS, and other scoring systems are widely used. First, as these prediction models only use a few variables, more precise and accurate prediction is difficult. SAPS III applies only 20 variables while APACHE IV uses 26 ones. This simplicity makes it possible to quickly determine the status of patients admitted to ICU (11). Second, SAPS and APACHE IV only assess physiological states of patients on the first day of admission. Although there are other scoring systems that can repetitively measure patients' status (e.g., Sequential Organ Failure Assessment named SOFA), the prognosis and mortality could not be accurately predicted from the data measured only once at the time of admission.

For these reasons, there have been several attempts to predict the mortality rate of critically ill patients using machine learning techniques. Support vector analysis could discriminate mortality in patients with hematologic malignancies (12). Random forest model can well-predict death from in-hospital patients, showing higher accuracy rate than Modified Early Warning Scores (MEWS) (13). Latent variable models that use information from electronic healthcare records predicted in-hospital death with combined time-varying model yielding the best performance (14) and it can also accurately estimate the probability of death in 1-year for multi-condition hospitalized patients (15). These findings demonstrate that the accuracy of mortality prediction for critically ill patients can be increased when machine learning algorithms and various medical data are used. However, it is currently unknown how machine learning algorithms make decisions during the prediction process. Thus, the objective of this study was to determine whether machine learning algorithms using demographic, laboratory, and other disease-related variables could predict in-hospital death of critically ill patients who were admitted to surgical intensive care unit (SICU) with considerable accuracy and identify factors contributing to the prediction power.

## METHODS

### Participants Selection

From January 1990 to March 2017, patients admitted to SICU of our institution for postoperative management after major abdominal surgeries were included in this study. Our institution is a tertiary referral hospital and SICU has an average of 1,800 patients annually. Major abdominal surgeries were defined as operation under general anesthesia status with endotracheal tube over 4 h regardless of the type of diagnosis, the status of malignancy or benign, the type of surgery or surgical sites. Subjects who met any of the following features were excluded from study; (a) age <18 or >80 years, (b) the duration of SICU stay <24 h, (c) patient was admitted to SICU due to medical or neurological problem without operation, (d) hopeless condition of patient in medical aspects, (e) pregnant state, or (f) measurements required for our predictor were not recorded at any time during ICU stay. Finally, a total of 1,352 patients were enrolled for further analysis (**Figure 1**).

### Data Extraction

Clinical data and medical records during the study period were retrospectively reviewed. Authors used patient-level information and medical records extracted from electrical medical records (EMR) of our institution. Disease characteristics included the diagnosis of disease, origin or location of lesion, malignancy or benign status. The policy of vital sign measurement in our institution was prescribed to mandate the frequency of vital sign measurement to be two every hour unless otherwise specified. Variables of laboratory tests included results of arterial blood gas analysis and serum blood chemistry test. The usage of inotropes or vasopressors was also reviewed. The outcome measurement was the incidence of unexpected postoperative mortality defined as mortality without pre-existing not-for-resuscitation order that occurred within 30 days of the surgery or within the same hospital stay as the surgery. Finally, a total of 43 variables composed of 1,758,334 entries of enrolled patients were used for analysis. Detailed protocol of data extraction is presented in **Figure 1**. This study was approved by the Institutional Review Board of the Ethics Committee of our institution (IRB No. KC17RESI0672).

### Model Development and Validation

#### Decision Trees

Decision trees can predict classifications (life or death) from medical data and these have the advantage of being able to present decisions visually and explicitly (16). We can use the final decision tree to accurately explain why a particular prediction is performed. To predict the classification, the algorithm followed the tree's decision from the root (start) node to the leaf node (final classification). Each step of the prediction involved checking the value of one predictor variable. If predictor *x1* exceeded a certain value *n*, it would follow the right branch representing *type 1* (life). Otherwise, it would follow the left branch to indicate *type 0* (death). The purpose of training the decision tree was to create a model that could predict the value of target variable based on multiple input variables. We tried and tested multiple decision points to numerically sort all values using a greedy approach and to maximize the prediction performance of the target value. All input variables and decision points were evaluated and selected in a greedy manner based on cost function.

Tree partitioning continued until the node contained a minimum number of training examples or reached the maximum tree depth. The Gini cost function was used to indicate how

**Abbreviations:** ICU, Intensive care unit; APACHE, Acute physiology and chronic health evaluation; SAPS, Simplified acute physiology score; AUC, Area under the receiver operating characteristic curve; SICU, Surgical intensive care unit; EMR, Electrical medical records; AST, Aspartate transaminase; ALT, Alanine transaminase; MEWS, Modified early warning score; SOFA, Sequential organ failure assessment.

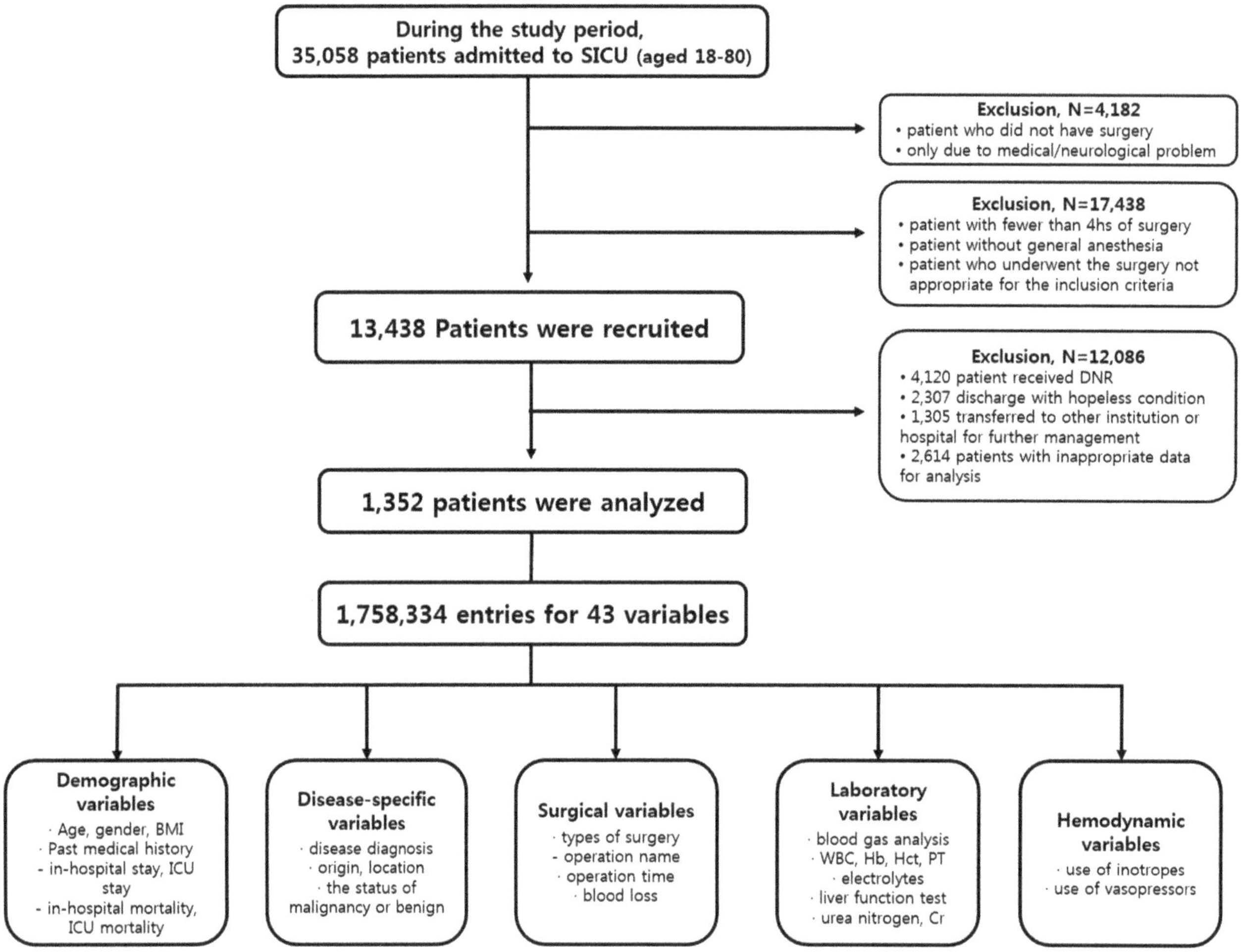


**FIGURE 1** | Flow diagram of participant selection.

good a decision split was, depending on how many classes were mixed in the two groups generated by the decision split (17). Data were divided into three sets; (1) 70% were used for training, (2) 15% were used for validating that the network was generalizing with training stopped before overfitting, and (3) 15% were used for completely independent test for network generalization. Moreover, 10-fold cross validation was used to test the stability of results by randomly shuffling training/validation/testing data sets.

## Neural Networks

Base model architecture is as follows (**Figure 2**). In this study, 43 variables were used as input variable to the neural network that consisted of one hidden layer with 100 neurons (parameters). A linear output neuron was used to obtain the final output of the regressive model. It is known that the model can fit multi-dimensional mapping problems arbitrarily well if consistent data are given with enough neurons in its hidden layer (18, 19).

We tested different number of hidden neurons (10, 20, 50, 100, 200, 300 neurons) and layers (1–5 layers), and compared the performance (**Figure 3**). We found that the area under curve (AUC) is saturated at the number of neurons of 200 or more (10-cross validations), and the AUC is maximum at the single layer with 200 neurons. Therefore, we determined 200 hidden neurons (number of parameters) and a single layer for our neural network parameters.

The network was trained with scaled conjugate gradient backpropagation algorithm (20, 21). Same training (70%), validation (15%), and testing (15%) division as decision tree was used in neural networks. Ten-fold cross validation was also used, and we compared the results with decision tree using independent *t*-test (Matlab, MathWorks Inc.).

## Naive Bayes

Naive Bayes is a classification algorithm that applies a density estimate to the data and assumes that the predicted variables are conditionally independent. Naive Bayes classifiers are known to produce a posterior distribution that is robust to biased class density estimates (22). The Naive Bayes classifier assigns observations to the most likely class (i.e., maximum post-decision rule). The algorithm first estimates the density of predicted variables within each class. It then models the posterior

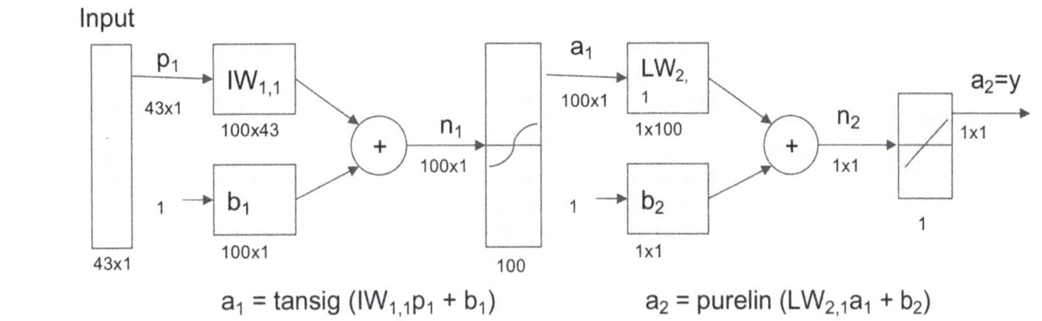


**FIGURE 2 |** Neural network model for prediction of life and death in hospital. Neural network model to transform 43 Surgical Intensive Care Unit (SICU) medical data for prediction of life and death. Tansig = hyperbolic tangent sigmoid function; Purelin = linear transfer function.

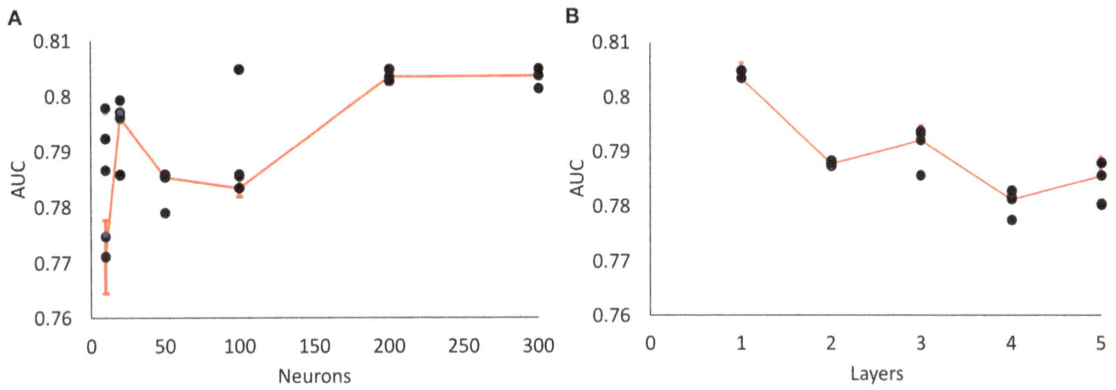


**FIGURE 3 |** Parameter optimization for neural networks. **(A)** Area Under Curve (AUC) values from different number of neurons (single layer, 10, 20, 50, 100, 200, 300 neurons) (10-fold cross validation results). Maximum AUC at 200 neurons or more. **(B)** AUC values from different number of layers with 200 neurons (10-fold cross validation results). Maximum AUC at single layer (Error bars represent standard errors).

probability according to the Bayes rule. That is, for all $k = 1, ..., K$,

$$\hat{P}\left(Y = k \middle| X_1, \ldots, X_p\right) = \frac{\pi(Y = k)\prod_{j=1}^{P} P(X_j|Y = k)}{\sum_{k=1}^{K}\pi(Y = k)\prod_{j=1}^{P} P(X_j|Y = k)} \quad (1)$$

Where $Y$ is a random variable corresponding to the class index of the observation. $X_1, ..., X_P$ are random predictors of observation. $\pi(Y = k)$ is a prior probability with class index $k$. The algorithm then classifies observations by estimating posterior probabilities for each class and assigning observations to classes that yield maximum posterior probabilities.

### Random Forests and Hellinger Distance Estimates

Furthermore, to establish the model stability of imbalanced dataset (only 10% of participants belonged to expired class), we applied the Hellinger Distance Decision Tree (23), the Hellinger Distance Random Forest (24) and the Random Forest model (25). To test the machine learning model stability, we performed a 10-fold cross-validation and tested whether the machine learning model performance was significantly different depending on the various data selections for training and testing. Since the F1 score is the harmonic mean of precision and recall, statistical tests were only performed on the AUC and F1 scores.

## RESULTS

### Participants and Variable Selection

The criteria used for patient selection and lists of variables are presented in **Figure 1**. During the inclusion period, 35,058 patients were admitted to SICU. Among them, 4,182 were excluded as they had medical or neurological problem without operation. Then 17,438 patients who underwent surgery for <4 h were excluded. Of 13,438 patients who were recruited after meeting the selection criteria, 12,086 patients with a "do not resuscitate form" or were discharged with hopeless condition were excluded. Analysis in more detail, among 12,086 patients, 4,120 patients received actual "do not resuscitate form," 2,307 patients with discharge with hopeless condition, and 1,305 patients were transferred to other institution or hospital for further management. Additionally, there were 2,614 patients who were excluded from the analysis due to insufficient medical data. Thus, data of 1,352 patients were used for training machine learning algorithms. Forty-three variables

**TABLE 1** | Comparative analysis of demographics of enrolled patients according to the survival or expire.

| Variables | Survivor* (%) | Expired** (%) | *p-value* |
|---|---|---|---|
| Number of patients | 1,232 (91.1) | 120 (8.9) | |
| Mean age (year) | 50.6 ± 9.4 | 68.8 ± 10.3 | 0.023 |
| Male/Female | 848/384 | 82/38 | 0.918 |
| Diagnosis | | | 0.015 |
| Malignancy | 1,102 (89.4) | 97 (80.8) | 0.036 |
| Upper GI tract | 141 (11.4) | 8 (6.7) | |
| Lower GI tract | 293 (23.8) | 24 (7.6) | |
| Hepatobiliary-pancreas | 663 (53.8) | 64 (8.8) | |
| Miscellaneous | 5 (0.4) | 1 (0.8) | |
| Benign | 130 (10.6) | 23 (19.2) | 0.008 |
| Hemoperitoneum | 32 (2.6) | 2 (1.7) | |
| Panperitonitis | 87 (7.1) | 8 (15) | |
| Biliary shock | 5 (0.4) | 0 | |
| Miscellaneous | 6 (0.5) | 3 (2.5) | |
| Type of surgery | | | <0.001 |
| Elective operation | 1,020 (82.8) | 78 (65) | |
| Emergency operation | 212 (17.2) | 42 (35) | |

**The patient survived more than 30 days after surgery or during the same hospital stay as the surgery.*

***The unexpected postoperative mortality which was defined as the mortality without the pre-existing not-for-resuscitation order and occurred within 30 days of the surgery or within the same hospital stay as the surgery.*

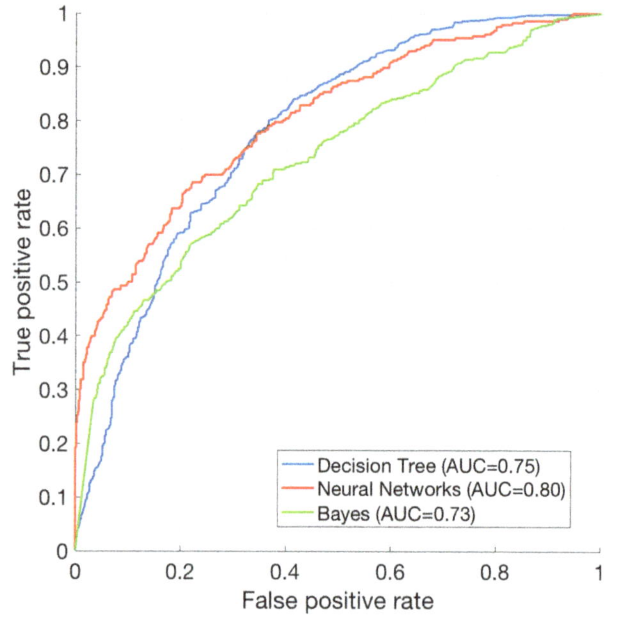


**FIGURE 4** | Receiver operating characteristics curve of machine learning algorithms. ROC curve of Decision tree (AUC = 0.75), neural net (AUC = 0.80), and Bayes (AUC = 0.73) classification algorithms. The results are based on 10-fold cross validations.

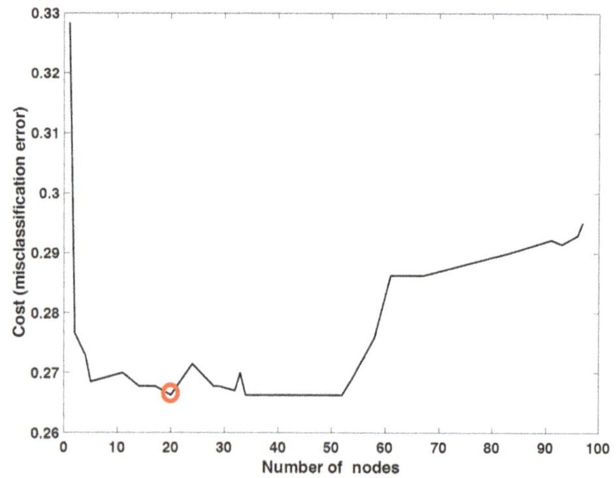


**FIGURE 5** | Optimized decision tree for the classification of life/death of patients in surgical intensive care unit.

consisting of demographic, laboratory, hemodynamic, surgical, and disease-specific variables were used to estimate mortality of SICU patients. Comparative analysis results of participants are presented in **Table 1**.

## Prediction Performance of Mortality Using Machine Learning Algorithms

The performance of mortality prediction is presented in **Figure 4**. Among decision tree, neural network, and Bayes classifier algorithms, the neural network algorithm showed the highest performance with an AUC of 0.80, followed by the decision tree with an AUC of 0.75. Bayes classifier had the least predictive accuracy, with an AUC of 0.73. As the decision tree algorithm has nodes that represent variables and conjunction that connects the nodes, the performance of this algorithm mainly depends on the number of nodes and tree size (26). Thus, we explored different ways to find the optimal performance of the decision tree algorithm by adjusting the number of nodes (**Figure 5**). We found that the optimal number of nodes that could minimize the decision tree's misclassification error rate was 77, where the classification prediction error was 0.2478 (75% classification accuracy). Using this number of nodes, decision tree structure was pruned. The results were based on the 10-fold cross validation.

We compared the 10-fold cross validation results between the neural networks and the decision tree algorithms. The AUCs among 10 validation runs were stable in that the standard deviation was 0.0012 for the decision tree, and 0.0017 for the neural networks. The independent $t$-test showed that $t_{(18)} = 68.05$ and $p < 0.00001$. Therefore, the neural network algorithm performed significantly better than decision tree.

To test whether the difference in F1 scores was significant in different machine learning models, we used the Kruskal-Wallis test, ANOVA's non-parametric counterpart. The results showed significant differences in the F1 score (Kruskal-Wallis chi square = 52.93, df = 5, $p < 0.001$). Then we tested the pairwise comparison using the Wilcoxon rank test between

**TABLE 2** | Performance metrics of each ML model (Wilcoxon rank test, *$p <$ 0.0017, adjusted $p$-value for multiple comparisons).

| | F1 score | Precision | Recall | AUC |
|---|---|---|---|---|
| Decision tree | 0.72 | 0.62 | 0.87 | 0.75 |
| Neural networks | 0.83 | 0.74 | 0.95 | **0.80** |
| Bayes | 0.82 | 0.70 | **0.98** | 0.73 |
| Random forest | **0.84** | **0.78** | 0.90 | 0.77 |
| Hellinger distance decision tree | 0.48* | 0.49 | 0.48 | 0.65* |
| Hellinger distance random forest | 0.51* | 0.51 | 0.51 | 0.74 |

*Bold value denote the highest value in each metric.*

different ML models. Although Random Forest had the highest F1 score, we found no significant difference between Random Forest, Bayes, Decision Tree, and Neural Network ML models ($p > 0.05$). Compared to the random forest, the Hellinger distance decision tree and the Hellinger distance random forest showed a significant decrease in the F1 score ($p < 0.001$). When considering multiple comparison corrections, the significance level should be adjusted to 0.0017 (0.05/30 comparison) instead of 0.05.

The Kruskal-Wallis test showed significant differences in AUC values among various machine learning models (Kruskal-Wallis chi square = 43.75, df = 5, $p < 0.001$). We also tested pairwise comparisons using the Wilcoxon rank test and found no significant differences between the Random Forest, Bayes, Decision Tree, Neural Network, and Hellinger Distance Random Forest ML models ($p > 0.05$) (**Table 2**). Compared to the neural network model, the Hellinger distance decision tree showed a significant reduction in the AUC value ($p < 0.001$).

## Optimized Decision Tree for the Classification of Life/Death

**Figure 6** shows how 43 variables are applied to predict life or death of ICU patients. Among 43 variables, serum level of albumin had a crucial role in the prediction of mortality. If albumin level was higher than 2.685 g/dL, the number of days of total parental nutrition played an important role in the next decision. If albumin level was not higher than 2.685 g/dL, the peak dose of dopamine drug was important. If patient's albumin level was higher than 2.685 g/dL and the peak dose of dopamine level was higher than 8.3 mcg/kg/min, he/she was more likely to survive.

## DISCUSSION

Herein, we showed that a certain machine learning algorithm could predict death of SICU patients using variables frequently used in clinical practice. Decision tree algorithm had a higher classification performance (AUC = 0.96) than neural network or Bayes classifier algorithm. This result might be applicable to clinical application considering results of other fields (27).

Previous studies have shown that machine learning algorithms could be used to predicting the prognosis and death of ICU patients. Both support vector machine and random forest model had an acceptable performance in predicting deaths of critically ill patients. Results of the present study showed somewhat higher performance than those of previous studies. It might be related to the number of variables used in training machine learning algorithms. In Verplancke's study, 12–17 variables were included in discriminating life and death of critically ill patients. However, our model used 43 variables (12). A small number of variables can be advantageous in helping clinician to make quick decisions as they do not require additional laboratory testing. However, since the accuracy of machine learning is related to the number of variables used, it may be more effective to use as many variables as possible to increase the prediction accuracy for mortality.

According to a recent observational cohort study comparing the performance of several machine learning algorithms using the same dataset, machine learning algorithms out-performed conventional scoring systems (e.g., MEWS) (13). In that study, random forest model had the highest performance (AUC = 0.80) whereas decision tree showed the lowest value (AUC = 0.73). Churpek et al. have also shown that basic physiological data (e.g., respiratory rate and heart rate) are the most significant predictors of deterioration of in-patients (13). These results were somewhat different from our results as laboratory test played a crucial role in our findings (**Figure 4**). This difference might be due to difference between machine learning algorithm used and outcome measurement used in different studies. While Churpek et al. focused on the deterioration of condition of in-patients, we aimed to discriminate life and deaths of SICU patients. Furthermore, we did not include basic physiological data when training machine learning algorithms to match time-resolution with other laboratory variables (laboratory tests were acquired every few days while heart rate and respiratory rates were acquired continuously in SICU). Acquisition of continuous data can inevitably lead to drawbacks of the data. Removal of electrocardiogram leads due to patient's movement can cause sustained zero heart rate which is the case of "false alarm" while under-sampling or erroneous data due to sensor fault can occur during care of ICU patients. These imprecise and missing data corruptions are primary challenges in critical care and it is still difficult to detect and correct these errors in large amounts of patient data (28). Therefore, this study included only objective variables that could be periodically measured. Thus, the present study could not confirm how physiological indicators contributed to mortality prediction. For this reason, it is difficult to directly compare results of this study with existing scoring systems (e.g., APACHE, MEWS, etc.). However, it can be compared with AUC performance reported in previous studies. APACHE II and SOFA showed AUC values of 0.81 and 0.71, respectively, in predicting prognosis in patients with ventilator-assisted pneumonia (29). MEWS and modified Mortality in Emergency Department Sepsis scores had AUC values of 0.61 and 0.77, respectively, in predicting 28-days mortality of patients in emergency department (30). Although characteristic of patients and the number of data are different, our findings suggest that mortality prediction using machine learning algorithms may have higher prediction accuracy than these classical scoring systems.

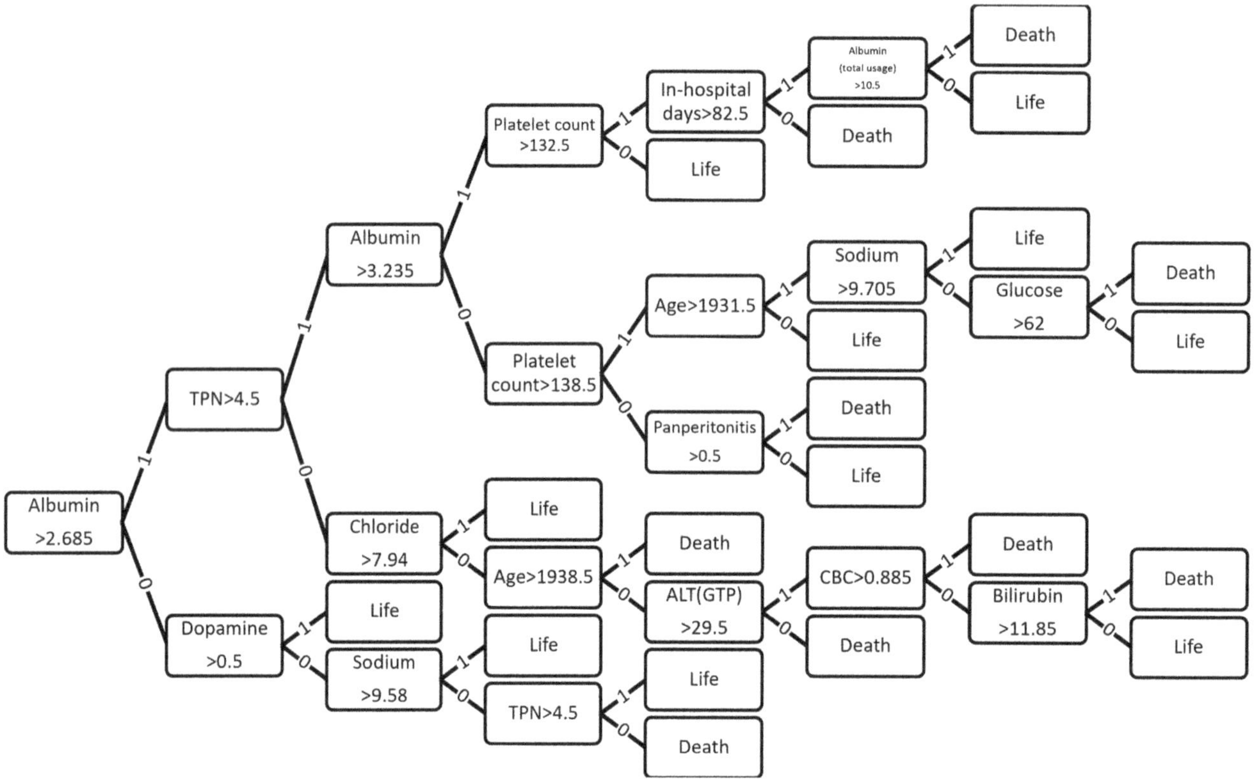


**FIGURE 6 |** Contribution of 43 variables in predicting life or death of ICU patients (32, 33).

In results of optimized decision tree method, the most important and contributing variable in predicting mortality of SICU patients was albumin (**Figure 4**). Reduced level of serum albumin is known to be an independent predictor of mortality. In a large epidemiologic study, decrement of 2.5 g/L serum albumin is associated with increased odds of deaths (31). Preoperative serum albumin concentration also well-predicted operative mortality and morbidity (32, 33). Although serum albumin concentration was an important variable for predicting the prognosis and mortality of surgical patients in previous studies, we did not give any indication of its significance while training the machine learning algorithm. Nonetheless, decision tree algorithm identified that serum albumin concentration was the most important indicator for decision-making of life and deaths. This result suggests that machine learning algorithms might be able to recognize clinically significant factors in large data sets.

This study has several limitations. First, as mentioned above, physiological indicators such as heart rate or respiratory rate were not used for prediction. This makes it difficult to compare findings of our study with classical scoring indicators. Second, as this study used dataset of a single institution, it was impossible to compare differences in various patient groups or treatment protocols. Moreover, a large number of patients enrolled were excluded from the final analysis due to the lack of essential data. But this is due to the fact that the patients who had missing these parameters were strictly excluded from the analysis to ensure a high accuracy of the model and to confirm a strong correlation with the parameters, even if the representativeness of the whole group is somewhat less. An external validation via multicenter, prospective designed study should be conducted to confirm our results in the near future. Finally, only some variables in the electronic health record were used to train the machine learning algorithm. Thus, it may be necessary to include real-time variable data to improve the accuracy for mortality prediction of critically-ill patients.

In conclusion, our results suggest that machine learning algorithms, especially the decision tree method, can provide information on structured and explainable decision flow and accurately predict hospital mortality in SICU hospitalized patients.

## ETHICS STATEMENT

The studies involving human participants were reviewed and approved by The Catholic University of Korea. Written informed consent for participation was not required for this study in accordance with the national legislation and the institutional requirements.

## AUTHOR CONTRIBUTIONS

KY and EK build research design and collected. KY, JO, and TH analyzed and interpreted the patient data. JO and KY were a major contributor in writing the manuscript. All authors read and approved the final manuscript.

## REFERENCES


1. Le Gall JR, Neumann A, Hemery F, Bleriot JP, Fulgencio JP, Garrigues B, et al. Mortality prediction using SAPS II: an update for French intensive care units. *Critical Care.* (2005) 9:R645. doi: 10.1186/cc3821
2. Pirracchio R, Petersen ML, Carone M, Rigon MR, Chevret S, van der Laan MJ. Mortality prediction in intensive care units with the Super ICU Learner Algorithm (SICULA): a population-based study. *Lancet Resp Med.* (2015) 3:42–52. doi: 10.1016/S2213-2600(14)70239-5
3. Bekelman JE, Halpern SD, Blankart CR, Bynum JP, Cohen J, Fowler R, et al. Comparison of site of death, health care utilization, and hospital expenditures for patients dying with cancer in 7 developed countries. *JAMA.* (2016) 315:272–83. doi: 10.1001/jama.2015.18603
4. Teres D, Lemeshow S, Avrunin JS, Pastides H. Validation of the mortality prediction model for ICU patients. *Critical Care Medicine.* (1987) 15:208–13.
5. Lemeshow S, Teres D, Pastides H, Avrunin JS, Steingrub JS. A method for predicting survival and mortality of ICU patients using objectively derived weights. *Critical Care Medicine.* (1985) 13:519–25.
6. Knaus WA, Draper EA, Wagner DP, Zimmerman JE. APACHE II: a severity of disease classification system. *Crit Care Med.* (1985) 13:818–29.
7. Kruse JA, Thill-Baharozian MC, Carlson RW. Comparison of clinical assessment with APACHE II for predicting mortality risk in patients admitted to a medical intensive care unit. *JAMA.* (1988) 260:1739–42. doi: 10.1001/jama.1988.03410120085032
8. Le Gall J-R, Lemeshow S, Saulnier F. A new simplified acute physiology score (SAPS II) based on a european/north american multicenter study. *JAMA.* (1993) 270:2957–63. doi: 10.1001/jama.1993.03510240069035
9. Zimmerman JE, Kramer AA, McNair DS, Malila FM. Acute Physiology and Chronic Health Evaluation (APACHE) IV: hospital mortality assessment for today's critically ill patients*. *Crit Care Med.* (2006) 34:1297–310. doi: 10.1097/01.CCM.0000215112.84523.F0
10. Sakr Y, Krauss C, Amaral ACKB, Réa-Neto A, Specht M, Reinhart K, et al. Comparison of the performance of SAPS II, SAPS 3, APACHE II, and their customized prognostic models in a surgical intensive care unit. *BJA: British Journal of Anaesthesia.* (2008) 101:798–803. doi: 10.1093/bja/aen291
11. Krizhevsky A, Sutskever I, and Hinton GE. Imagenet classification with deep convolutional neural networks. *Adv Neural Inform Process Syst.* (2012) 25:1097–5. doi: 10.1145/3065386
12. Verplancke T, Van Looy S, Benoit D, Vansteelandt S, Depuydt P, De Turck F, et al. Support vector machine versus logistic regression modeling for prediction of hospital mortality in critically ill patients with haematological malignancies. *BMC Med Inform Dec Making.* (2008) 8:56. doi: 10.1186/1472-6947-8-56
13. Churpek MM, Yuen TC, Winslow C, Meltzer DO, Kattan MW, Edelson DP. Multicenter comparison of machine learning methods and conventional regression for predicting clinical deterioration on the wards. *Crit Care Med.* (2016) 44:368–74. doi: 10.1097/CCM.0000000000001571
14. Ghassemi M, Naumann T, Doshi-Velez F, Brimmer N, Joshi R, Rumshisky A, et al. Unfolding physiological state: mortality modelling in intensive care units. In: *Proceedings of the 20th ACM SIGKDD international conference on Knowledge discovery and data mining* KDD '14. New York, NY: Association for Computing Machinery, 75–84. doi: 10.1145/2623330.2623742
15. Sahni N, Simon G, Arora R. Development and validation of machine learning models for prediction of 1-year mortality utilizing electronic medical record data available at the end of hospitalization in multicondition patients: a proof-of-concept study. *J Gen Intern Med.* (2018) 33:921–8. doi: 10.1007/s11606-018-4316-y
16. Breiman, Leo, Friedman, Jerome H, Olshen, Richard A, et al. *Classification and Regression Trees.* Monterey, CA : Wadsworth & Brooks/Cole Advanced Books & Software. (1984).
17. Drummond C, Holte RC. Exploiting the cost (In)sensitivity of decision tree splitting criteria. *ICML.* (2000) 1:8.
18. Oh J, Yun K, Hwang J-H, Chae J-H. Classification of suicide attempts through a machine learning algorithm based on multiple systemic psychiatric scales. *Front Psychiatry.* (2017) 8:192. doi: 10.3389/fpsyt.2017.00192
19. Poggio T, Girosi F. Networks for approximation and learning. *Proc IEEE.* (1990) 78:1481–97. doi: 10.1109/5.58326
20. Møller MF. A scaled conjugate gradient algorithm for fast supervised learning. *Neural Netw.* (1993) 6:525–33. doi: 10.1016/S0893-6080(05)80056-5
21. Saini LM, Soni MK. Artificial neural network-based peak load forecasting using conjugate gradient methods. *IEEE Trans Power Syst.* (2002) 17:907–12. doi: 10.1109/TPWRS.2002.800992
22. Hastie T, Tibshirani R, Friedman J. Model inference averaging. In: Hastie T, Tibshirani R, Friedman J, editors. *The Elements of Statistical Learning: Data Mining, Inference, Prediction* Springer Series in Statistics. New York, NY: Springer (2009). p. 261–94. doi: 10.1007/978-0-387-84858-7_8
23. Cieslak DA, Hoens TR, Chawla NV, Kegelmeyer WP. Hellinger distance decision trees are robust and skew-insensitive. *Data Min Knowl Disc.* (2012) 24:136–58. doi: 10.1007/s10618-011-0222-1
24. Su C, Ju S, Liu Y, Yu Z. Improving random forest and rotation forest for highly imbalanced datasets. *Intell Data Analysis.* (2015) 19:1409–32. doi: 10.3233/IDA-150789
25. Breiman L. Random Forests. *Mach Learn.* (2001) 45:5–32. doi: 10.1023/A:1010933404324
26. Bradford JP, Kunz C, Kohavi R, Brunk C, Brodley CE. Pruning decision trees with misclassification costs. In: Nédellec C, Rouveirol C, editors. *Machine Learning: ECML-98 Lecture Notes in Computer Science.* Berlin, Heidelberg: Springer (1998) 131–6. doi: 10.1007/BFb0026682
27. Gulshan V, Peng L, Coram M, Stumpe MC, Wu D, Narayanaswamy A, et al. Development and validation of a deep learning algorithm for detection of diabetic retinopathy in retinal fundus photographs. *JAMA.* (2016) 316:24 02–10. doi: 10.1001/jama.2016.17216
28. Johnson AEW, Ghassemi MM, Nemati S, Niehaus KE, Clifton DA, Clifford GD. Machine learning and decision support in critical care. *Proc IEEE.* (2016) 104:444–66. doi: 10.1109/JPROC.2015.2501978
29. Gursel G, Demirtas S. Value of APACHE II, SOFA and CPIS scores in predicting prognosis in patients with ventilator-associated pneumonia. *RES.* (2006) 73:503–8. doi: 10.1159/000088708
30. Çildir E, Bulut M, Akalin H, Kocabaş E, Ocakoglu G, Aydin SA. Evaluation of the modified MEDS, MEWS score and Charlson comorbidity index in patients with community acquired sepsis in the emergency department. *In Emerg Med.* (2013) 8:255–60. doi: 10.1007/s11739-012-0890-x
31. Goldwasser P, Feldman J. Association of serum albumin and mortality risk. *J Clin Epidem.* (1997) 50:693–703. doi: 10.1016/S0895-4356(97)00015-2
32. Garg T, Chen LY, Kim PH, Zhao PT, Herr HW, Donat SM. Preoperative serum albumin is associated with mortality and complications after radical cystectomy. *BJU Int.* (2014) 113:918–23. doi: 10.1111/bju.12405
33. Gibbs J, Cull W, Henderson W, Daley J, Hur K, Khuri SF. Preoperative serum albumin level as a predictor of operative mortality and morbidity: results from the national va surgical risk study. *Arch Surg.* (1999) 134:36–42. doi: 10.1001/archsurg.134.1.36

4

# Derivation and Validation of an Automated Search Strategy to Retrospectively Identify Acute Respiratory Distress Patients Per Berlin Definition

*Xuan Song*[1,2,3]*, Timothy J. Weister*[4]*, Yue Dong*[5]*, Kianoush B. Kashani*[6] *and Rahul Kashyap*[5*]

[1] *Division of Pulmonary and Critical Care Medicine, Department of Medicine, Mayo Clinic, Rochester, MN, United States,* [2] *Intensive Care Unit, Liaocheng Cardiac Hospital Affiliated to Shandong First Medical University, Shandong, China,* [3] *Intensive Care Unit, DongE Hospital Affiliated to Shandong First Medical University, Shandong, China,* [4] *Anesthesia Clinical Research Unit, Mayo Clinic, Rochester, MN, United States,* [5] *Department of Anesthesiology and Perioperative Medicine, Mayo Clinic, Rochester, MN, United States,* [6] *Division of Nephrology and Hypertension, Department of Medicine, Mayo Clinic, Rochester, MN, United States*

***Correspondence:***
*Rahul Kashyap*
*kashyap.rahul@mayo.edu*

**Purpose:** Acute respiratory distress syndrome (ARDS) is common in critically ill patients and linked with serious consequences. A manual chart review for ARDS diagnosis could be laborious and time-consuming. We developed an automated search strategy to retrospectively identify ARDS patients using the Berlin definition to allow for timely and accurate ARDS detection.

**Methods:** The automated search strategy was created through sequential steps, with keywords applied to an institutional electronic medical records (EMRs) database. We included all adult patients admitted to the intensive care unit (ICU) at the Mayo Clinic (Rochester, MN) from January 1, 2009 to December 31, 2017. We selected 100 patients at random to be divided into two derivation cohorts and identified 50 patients at random for the validation cohort. The sensitivity and specificity of the automated search strategy were compared with a manual medical record review (gold standard) for data extraction of ARDS patients per Berlin definition.

**Results:** On the first derivation cohort, the automated search strategy achieved a sensitivity of 91.3%, specificity of 100%, positive predictive value (PPV) of 100%, and negative predictive value (NPV) of 93.1%. On the second derivation cohort, it reached the sensitivity of 90.9%, specificity of 100%, PPV of 100%, and NPV of 93.3%. The strategy performance in the validation cohort had a sensitivity of 94.4%, specificity of 96.9%, PPV of 94.4%, and NPV of 96.9%.

**Conclusions:** This automated search strategy for ARDS with the Berlin definition is reliable and accurate, and can serve as an efficient alternative to time-consuming manual data review.

**Keywords: automation, electronic health records, acute respriatory distress syndrome, adult, ICU**

## INTRODUCTION

Acute respiratory distress syndrome (ARDS) is an acute inflammatory lung injury which occurs in the absence of cardiogenic pulmonary edema and leads to increased pulmonary vascular permeability, increased extravascular lung water, and loss of aerated lung tissue (1). Estimates of the hospital-based incidence of moderate to severe ARDS vary from 1.6 to 7.7% of all intensive care unit (ICU) admissions and 8.0–19.7% of all ventilated patients (2–5). Additionally, the reported population-based incidence of ARDS varies from 10.1 to 86.2 cases per 100,000 person-years (6–9). Overall mortality associated with ARDS is ~40%, according to the most recent observational studies (10, 11). Currently, there is no disease-specific pharmacotherapy to increase survival, and ARDS management remains supportive; therefore, the identification of ARDS with the Berlin definition in the ICU is critical, not only to identify the cases early and start primary and secondary prevention strategies but also to identify ARDS cases for potential clinical prospective studies.

Traditional paper charts have been rapidly replaced by electronic medical records (EMRs). The use of EMRs as a tool to reduce cost and improve safety has been increasing over the years in both clinical practice and health care research (12). For research, EMRs has moved medicine into the era of "big data," where an unprecedented amount of information can allow for evaluation and identification of risk factors at the population level. ARDS is often not documented in addition to respiratory failure terms. ICD-9 terms are not specific to ARDS and often code to non-specific conditions such as "respiratory distress;" therefore, it is difficult to identify ARDS cases for clinical study. A manual chart review for ARDS diagnosis could be laborious and time-consuming, so the effective and accurate use of EMRs, structured search strategies, and data capturing to identify cases are critical. In retrospective studies related to ARDS, an automated search strategy would be useful to identify cases in a timely fashion with high precision. Other similar search strategies from our team to identify sepsis, post-operative complications, acute kidney injury, and extubation failure have been developed and validated (13–16). These investigators found that by using such electronic search strategies, they were able to achieve high sensitivity and specificity in detecting patients with the syndromes and complications mentioned above.

In this study, our primary aim was to develop and validate a reliable electronic search strategy to identify cases with ARDS with the Berlin definition. Our secondary aim was to compare the sensitivity and specificity of our automated search strategy with a reference standard generated by a comprehensive, manual review of the medical record.

## MATERIALS AND METHODS

This study was approved by the Mayo Clinic Institutional Review Board (IRB) for the use of existing medical records of patients who gave prior research authorization.

### Study Population

The study population consisted of all patients admitted to the ICUs at Mayo Clinic in Rochester, MN from January 1, 2009 to December 31, 2017. Among this population, two groups of 50 patients were selected by purposeful sampling for derivation. This random purposeful sampling was done to include a random number of ARDS patients for higher yield. Both the manual reviewer and gold standard were blinded to the results of this sampling.We used separate revision cohorts to be able to test each change in the search strategy in a different group of patients, and, therefore, be able to optimize the search strategy. An additional cohort of 50 random patients was selected for the validation cohort (**Figure 1**).

We used the Berlin definition of ARDS criteria (1). The Berlin definition partitions patients by $PaO_2/FiO_2$ ratio into mild ($PaO_2/FiO_2$ 200–300), moderate ($PaO_2/FiO_2$ 100–199), and severe ARDS ($PaO_2/FiO_2$ <100) and no longer includes the term "acute lung injury." This definition also clarifies several areas, including onset, which must be within 1 week of a known clinical insult or new or worsening respiratory symptoms; chest imaging, which must include bilateral opacities that are not fully explained by effusions, lobar collapse, or nodules; and origin of edema, which cannot be fully explained by cardiac failure or fluid overload and must be objectively evaluated (e.g., by echocardiography) if no apparent predisposing factor for ARDS is present. The Berlin definition also sets a minimum positive end-expiratory pressure (PEEP) level of 5 cm $H_2O$ during $PaO_2/FiO_2$ determination because it has been recognized that changes in PEEP may reclassify patients from the current definition of ALI to ARDS (1).

### Manual Data Extraction Strategies

A manual review of patient EMRs was used for data extraction and ARDS adjudication. The manual reviewer was a practicing clinician, who reviewed the electronic medical charts with all available information. The reviewer assessed all included patients to identify patients who had ARDS per Berlin definition. The reviewer was not involved in the development or utilization of the automated electronic search strategy. Hence, the reviewer was not aware of the results of the automated search strategy.

We used the definition of Berlin ARDS criteria for manual chart review, and defined ARDS based on the presence of both of the following conditions simultaneously: (1) patients with $PaO_2/FiO_2$ ratio <300, PEEP $\geq$5 cm $H_2O$, bilateral infiltrate or edema per chest X-ray, and (2) the presence of at least one risk factor for ARDS (i.e., sepsis/septic shock, pneumonia, pancreatitis, trauma, aspiration, multiple transfusion, drug overdose, and shock). We used the final adjudicated ARDS cases based on this process as the gold standard for the study.

### Automated Electronic Search Strategy

Data were used from Mayo Clinic ICU DataMart and Unified Data Platform, which are extensive data warehouses containing a near real-time normalized replica of Mayo Clinic's EMRs. These databases contain patient information, their laboratory test results, and clinical and pathological information from sources within the institution and have been previously validated (17,

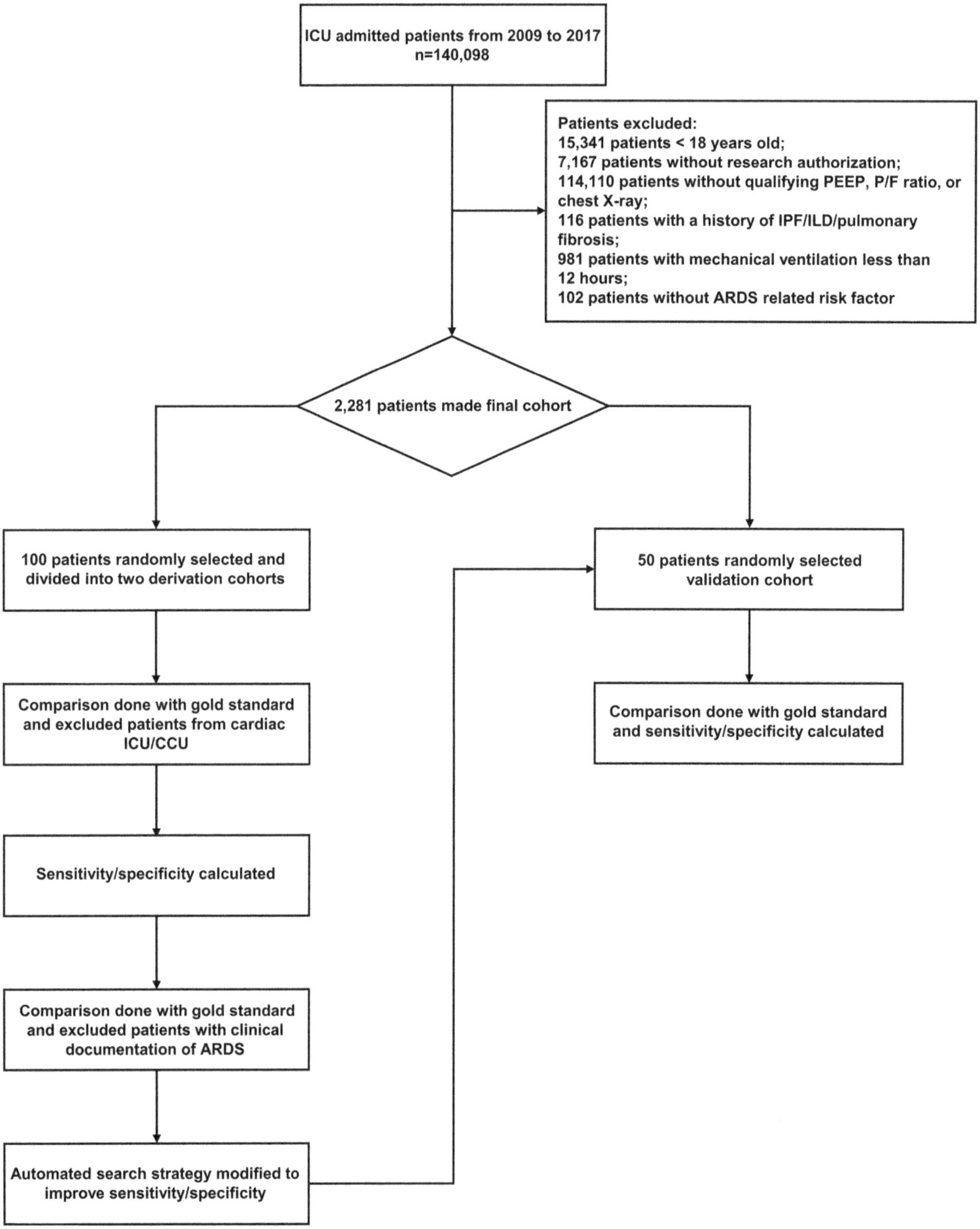


**FIGURE 1 |** Flow chart of study derivation and validation cohorts. ARDS, acute respiratory distress syndrome; IPF, idiopathic pulmonary fibrosis; ILD, interstitial lung disease; ICU, intensive care unit; CCU, cardiac care unit; PEEP, positive end expiratory pressure; P/F ratio, partial pressure of oxygen to fraction of inspired oxygen ratio.

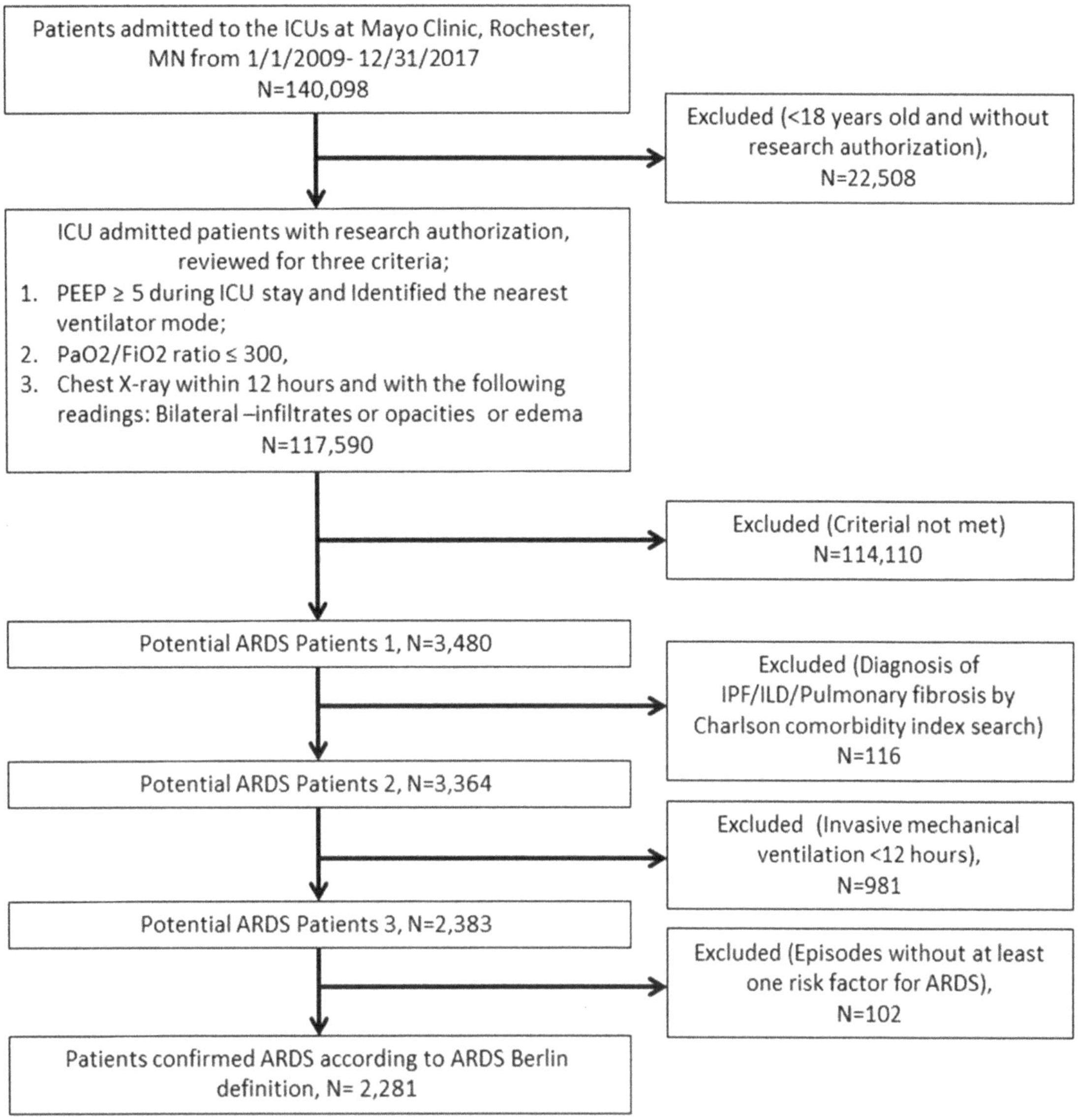


**FIGURE 2 |** The automated electronic search strategy for identifying ARDS patients per Berlin definition.

18). Ventilator parameters (such as PEEP) were captured from the ventilators.

The automated electronic search strategy for identifying ARDS patients per Berlin definition was developed in the following sequential steps (**Figure 2**). First, patients were excluded who did not provide research authorization, along with those <18 years old. Second, ARDS patients were identified according to the following criteria: (1) PEEP $\geq$5 during the ICU stay (this is "time zero") and identified the ventilator mode nearest (limited to ICU areas—procedures excluded); (2) Partial pressure of oxygen to fraction of inspired oxygen ($PaO_2/FiO_2$) ratio $\leq$300, P/F ratios were first established based on matched $PaO_2$ and $FiO_2$ from labs. If $FiO_2$ labs were missing, $FiO_2$ from vital signs within $\pm$15 min (nearest) the $PaO_2$ value were used; (3) Chest X-ray within 12 h and review radiology report for any of the following combinations: bilateral infiltrates, bilateral opacities, or bilateral edema. If one of them was present, it was considered a positive radiology report. If all 3 criteria in second step were positive, then they were classified as potential ARDS patients. Third, patients with diagnosis of Idiopathic Pulmonary Fibrosis (IPF)/Interstitial Lung Disease (ILD)/pulmonary fibrosis were excluded by Charlson comorbidity index search. Fourth, patients with invasive mechanical ventilation <12 h were excluded, and the duration of mechanical ventilation was searched according to our previously published algorithm (19). Fifth, ARDS risk factors were searched for (i.e., sepsis/septic shock, pneumonia, aspiration, pancreatitis, trauma, drug overdose, shock, and multiple transfusions), and the search strategy for each risk factor was defined. Finally, patients with cardiogenic pulmonary edema, cardiogenic shock, and positive acute decompensated

**TABLE 1** | Automated search strategy sensitivity and specificity for ARDS per Berlin definition.

| | ARDS per Berlin definition | | | |
|---|---|---|---|---|
| | Sensitivity (%) | Specificity (%) | PPV (%) | NPV (%) |
| Derivation cohort 1 | 91.3 | 100 | 100 | 93.1 |
| Derivation cohort 2 | 90.9 | 100 | 100 | 93.3 |
| Validation cohort | 94.4 | 96.9 | 94.4 | 96.9 |

*ARDS, acute respiratory distress syndrome; PPV: positive predictive value; NPV, negative predictive value.*

heart failure during ICU admission were excluded, and patients with cardiogenic pulmonary edema risk factors were also excluded by clinical note searches (20), and these risk factors include history of Coronary Heart Disease (CAD), chronic heart failure (CHF), and New ST-changes/Left bundle branch block (Electrocardiography query within ±24 h of 1st PEEP ≥5). The automated search algorithms were validated in comparison with the gold standard obtained by manual review.

## Statistical Analysis

For automation process, the only applicable analysis is sensitivity and specificity for a nominal variable (ARDS, yes/no). The sensitivity and specificity of the search algorithms were calculated by comparing the results to the gold standard obtained by manual review of the charts. We used JMP Pro 14 statistical software (SAS Institute Inc., Cary, NC, USA). *P*-values $0 < 0.05$ were considered statistically significant.

# RESULTS

Between January 1, 2009, and December 31, 2017, 140,098 adult patients with research authorization were admitted to the participating ICUs, and 2,281 patients met the ARDS Berlin definition according to the automated search strategy. A total of 100 patients were chosen after purposeful sampling to be included in the two derivation cohorts, and an additional 50 patients were selected for the validation cohort.

The automated search strategy identified ARDS patients with a sensitivity of 91.3%, specificity of 100%, positive predictive value (PPV) of 100%, and negative predictive value (NPV) of 93.1% in the first derivation cohort (**Table 1**). Disagreements between the automated search strategy and the manual review were observed in 2 patients in this data subset, both false negatives. In one of the cases, ARDS was missed by the digital algorithm as $PaO_2/FiO_2$ ratio, and chest X-ray were not found, while in the other case sepsis developed >72 h after ICU admission. In the second derivation cohort (**Table 1**), the automated search strategy reached a sensitivity of 90.9%, specificity of 100%, PPV of 100%, and NPV of 93.3%. Disagreements between the automated search strategy and the gold standard occurred in 2 patients, both false negatives. The reasons for these false-negative cases were identical to those in the first derivation cohort. The manual vs. automated cohorts had same baseline characteristics as they were exact same cohorts (data not shown).

In the validation cohort, the automatic search strategy yielded a sensitivity of 94.4%, specificity of 96.9%, PPV of 94.4%, and NPV of 96.9% (**Table 1**). Disagreements between the automated search strategy and the reference standard occurred in 2 patients, both false negatives. One case was due to missing $PaO_2/FiO_2$ ratio and chest X-ray, and the other case was because the patient used home Bilevel Positive Airways Pressure (BiPAP), and thus PEEP was not electronically recorded.

# DISCUSSION

In this study, we demonstrated an automated search strategy for ARDS that could effectively and accurately identify patients based on the accepted clinical definition (i.e., Berlin definition, among ICU patients). Several previously automated search strategies have been described in the literature (13–15, 21, 22); however, to date, the Berlin definition has not been used as a digital signature of ARDS patients.

As EMR utilization continues on an upward trajectory, the volume of available information to generate and validate digital signatures of different clinical syndromes in ICUs has grown. The accumulation of vast amounts of data provides opportunities to improve the processes of care and treatment. Manual chart review for ARDS diagnosis would likely be laborious and time-consuming; considering the significant shortage of human resources in clinical investigations, there seems to be a vital need to use EMRs for syndrome detection. Traditional ICD code searches for such conditions may not be completely sensitive or specific (18, 23), and changes in coding guidelines make them even less reliable. Thus, the development of automated search strategies can prove useful for clinical and research purposes.

Our study has several strengths. To our knowledge, this is the first study regarding the development and validation of an automated search strategy within EMRs for the identification of ARDS patients per Berlin definition. It is a valuable contribution in that it allows for a quick and reliable way to identify cases of ARDS retrospectively, which will ultimately enable pragmatic research on large cohorts of patients using existing EMRs. Using automated search strategies overcomes the barrier of time-consuming manual review and mitigates human errors that occur during manual data extraction. This electronic signature provides strong support for educational and research activities and demonstrates a simple yet effective method that can be applied to other clinical conditions.

Several limitations of our study should be acknowledged. First, the accuracy of the EMR depends on the precision of written clinical notes. As with manual chart review, we assumed clinical documentation is accurate, while errors in the documentation are possible. In our institution, periodic quality checks on clinical notes are done with frequent audits. Therefore, we believe the impact of documentation errors in this digital signature is minimal. Secondly, this is an automatic search strategy to retrospectively identify ARDS patients per the Berlin definition. It cannot identify these patients in real time, but it lays a foundation for the development of ARDS software to identify ARDS patients in real time in the future. Finally, Mayo Clinic EMR structure may be different from other institutions, thus limiting its use. The generalization of the findings is limited at this point, given that no external validation was performed. Future studies should evaluate the method in different EMR systems and in different populations.

## CONCLUSIONS

Here we reported the derivation and validation of an automated electronic search query algorithm for identifying ARDS patients according to the Berlin definition. Sensitivity and specificity approached 100% in this study and may continue to improve as processes develop around electronic notes searches, following the iterative development model previously described. The development of this type of automated search strategy is widely applicable to clinical research; it may improve the efficiency and accuracy of patient identification, thus furthering knowledge on the subjects and potentially improving outcomes. Ultimately, it may enable pragmatic research on large cohorts of patients using existing EMRs, for early and rapid identification of ARDS patients.

## ETHICS STATEMENT

This study was approved by the Mayo Clinic Institutional Review Board (IRB) for the use of existing medical records of patients who gave prior research authorization. Informed consent was obtained from all patients included in the study.

## AUTHOR CONTRIBUTIONS

RK conceptualized the study. XS and TW designed the study. XS performed data analysis and drafted the manuscript. YD and KK critically revised the article for important intellectual content. All authors read and approved the final manuscript.

## ACKNOWLEDGMENTS

We thank the Anesthesia Clinical Research Unit for their help with electronic data abstraction.

## REFERENCES


1. Force ADT, Ranieri VM, Rubenfeld GD, Thompson BT, Ferguson ND, Caldwell E, et al. Acute respiratory distress syndrome: the Berlin Definition. *JAMA.* (2012) 307:2526–33. doi: 10.1001/jama.2012.5669
2. Estenssoro E, Dubin A, Laffaire E, Canales H, Saenz G, Moseinco M, et al. Incidence, clinical course, and outcome in 217 patients with acute respiratory distress syndrome. *Crit. Care Med.* (2002) 30:2450–6. doi: 10.1097/00003246-200211000-00008
3. Roupie E, Lepage E, Wysocki M, Fagon JY, Chastre J, Dreyfuss D, et al. Prevalence, etiologies and outcome of the acute respiratory distress syndrome among hypoxemic ventilated patients. SRLF Collaborative Group on Mechanical Ventilation. Societe de Reanimation de Langue Francaise. *Intensive Care Med.* (1999) 25:920–9. doi: 10.1007/s001340050983
4. Caser EB, Zandonade E, Pereira E, Gama AM, Barbas CS. Impact of distinct definitions of acute lung injury on its incidence and outcomes in Brazilian ICUs: prospective evaluation of 7,133 patients. *Crit. Care Med.* (2014) 42:574–82. doi: 10.1097/01.ccm.0000435676.68435.56
5. Brun-Buisson C, Minelli C, Bertolini G, Brazzi L, Pimentel J, Lewandowski K, et al. Epidemiology and outcome of acute lung injury in European intensive care units. Results from the ALIVE study. *Intensive Care Med.* (2004) 30:51–61. doi: 10.1007/s00134-003-2022-6
6. Bersten AD, Edibam C, Hunt T, Moran J. Incidence and mortality of acute lung injury and the acute respiratory distress syndrome in three Australian States. *Am. J. Respir. Crit. Care Med.* (2002) 165:443–8. doi: 10.1164/ajrccm.165.4.2101124
7. Hughes M, MacKirdy FN, Ross J, Norrie J, Grant IS. Acute respiratory distress syndrome: an audit of incidence and outcome in Scottish intensive care units. *Anaesthesia.* (2003) 58:838–45. doi: 10.1046/j.1365-2044.2003.03287.x
8. Li G, Malinchoc M, Cartin-Ceba R, Venkata CV, Kor DJ, Peters SG, et al. Eight-year trend of acute respiratory distress syndrome: a population-based study in Olmsted County, Minnesota. *Am. J. Resp. Crit. Care Med.* (2011) 183:59–66. doi: 10.1164/rccm.201003-0436OC
9. Rubenfeld GD, Caldwell E, Peabody E, Weaver J, Martin DP, Neff M, et al. Incidence and outcomes of acute lung injury. *N. Engl. J. Med.* (2005) 353:1685–93. doi: 10.1056/NEJMoa050333
10. Villar J, Ambros A, Soler JA, Martinez D, Ferrando C, Solano R, et al. Age, PaO2/FIO2, and plateau pressure score: a proposal for a simple outcome score in patients with the acute respiratory distress syndrome. *Crit. Care Med.* (2016) 44:1361–9. doi: 10.1097/CCM.0000000000001653
11. Villar J, Blanco J, Anon JM, Santos-Bouza A, Blanch L, Ambros A, et al. The ALIEN study: incidence and outcome of acute respiratory distress syndrome in the era of lung protective ventilation. *Intensive Care Med.* (2011) 37:1932–41. doi: 10.1007/s00134-011-2380-4
12. Zlabek JA, Wickus JW, Mathiason MA. Early cost and safety benefits of an inpatient electronic health record. *J. Am. Med. Inform. Assoc.* (2011) 18:169–72. doi: 10.1136/jamia.2010.007229
13. Tien M, Kashyap R, Wilson GA, Hernandez-Torres V, Jacob AK, Schroeder DR, et al. Retrospective derivation and validation of an automated electronic search algorithm to identify post operative cardiovascular and thromboembolic complications. *Appl. Clin. Inform.* (2015) 6:565–76. doi: 10.4338/ACI-2015-03-RA-0026
14. Rishi MA, Kashyap R, Wilson G, Hocker S. Retrospective derivation and validation of a search algorithm to identify extubation failure in the intensive care unit. *BMC Anesthesiol.* (2014) 14:41. doi: 10.1186/1471-2253-14-41
15. Dhungana P, Serafim LP, Ruiz AL, Bruns D, Weister TJ, Smichney NJ, et al. Machine learning in data abstraction: a computable phenotype for sepsis and septic shock diagnosis in the intensive care unit. *World J. Crit. Care Med.* (2019) 8:120–6. doi: 10.5492/wjccm.v8.i7.120
16. Ahmed A, Vairavan S, Akhoundi A, Wilson G, Chiofolo C, Chbat N, et al. Development and validation of electronic surveillance tool for acute kidney injury: a retrospective analysis. *J. Crit. Care.* (2015) 30:988–93. doi: 10.1016/j.jcrc.2015.05.007
17. Herasevich V, Pickering BW, Dong Y, Peters SG, Gajic O. Informatics infrastructure for syndrome surveillance, decision support, reporting, and modeling of critical illness. *Mayo Clin. Proc.* (2010) 85:247–54. doi: 10.4065/mcp.2009.0479
18. Singh B, Singh A, Ahmed A, Wilson GA, Pickering BW, Herasevich V, et al. Derivation and validation of automated electronic search strategies to extract Charlson comorbidities from electronic medical records. *Mayo Clin. Proc.* (2012) 87:817–24. doi: 10.1016/j.mayocp.2012.04.015
19. Weister T, Singhal A, Marquez A, Smischney N, Kashyap R. Refinement of a computable phenotype for initiation of mechanical ventilation in intensive care unit. *Am. J. Respir. Crit. Care Med.* (2020) 201:A1454.
20. Kashyap R, Sarvottam K, Wilson GA, Jentzer JC, Seisa MO, Kashani KB. Derivation and validation of a computable phenotype for acute decompensated heart failure in hospitalized patients. *BMC Med. Inform. Decis. Mak.* (2020) 20:85. doi: 10.1186/s12911-020-1092-5

21. Amra S, O'Horo JC, Singh TD, Wilson GA, Kashyap R, Petersen R, et al. Derivation and validation of the automated search algorithms to identify cognitive impairment and dementia in electronic health records. *J. Crit. Care*. (2017) 37:202–5. doi: 10.1016/j.jcrc.2016.09.026
22. Guru PK, Singh TD, Passe M, Kashani KB, Schears GJ, Kashyap R. Derivation and validation of a search algorithm to retrospectively identify CRRT initiation in the ECMO patients. *Appl. Clin. Inform*. (2016) 7:596–603. doi: 10.4338/ACI-2015-12-RA-0183
23. Siew ED, Davenport A. The growth of acute kidney injury: a rising tide or just closer attention to detail? *Kidney Int*. (2015) 87:46–61. doi: 10.1038/ki.2014.293

# 5

# Ability of a Machine Learning Algorithm to Predict the Need for Perioperative Red Blood Cells Transfusion in Pelvic Fracture Patients: A Multicenter Cohort Study in China

*Xueyuan Huang[1], Yongjun Wang[2], Bingyu Chen[3], Yuanshuai Huang[4], Xinhua Wang[5], Linfeng Chen[6], Rong Gui[1]* and Xianjun Ma[7]**

*[1] Department of Blood Transfusion, The Third Xiangya Hospital, Central South University, Changsha, China, [2] Department of Blood Transfusion, The Second Xiangya Hospital, Central South University, Changsha, China, [3] Department of Transfusion, Zhejiang Provincial People's Hospital, Hangzhou, China, [4] Department of Transfusion, The Affiliated Hospital of Southwest Medical University, Luzhou, China, [5] Department of Transfusion, Beijing Aerospace Center Hospital, Beijing, China, [6] Department of Transfusion, Beijing Shijitan Hospital, Capital Medical University, Beijing, China, [7] Department of Blood Transfusion, Qilu Hospital of Shandong University, Jinan, China*

***Correspondence:**
*Rong Gui*
*guirong@csu.edu.cn*
*Xianjun Ma*
*18560087567@163.com*

**Background:** Predicting the perioperative requirement for red blood cells (RBCs) transfusion in patients with the pelvic fracture may be challenging. In this study, we constructed a perioperative RBCs transfusion predictive model (ternary classifications) based on a machine learning algorithm.

**Materials and Methods:** This study included perioperative adult patients with pelvic trauma hospitalized across six Chinese centers between September 2012 and June 2019. An extreme gradient boosting (XGBoost) algorithm was used to predict the need for perioperative RBCs transfusion, with data being split into training test (80%), which was subjected to 5-fold cross-validation, and test set (20%). The ability of the predictive transfusion model was compared with blood preparation based on surgeons' experience and other predictive models, including random forest, gradient boosting decision tree, K-nearest neighbor, logistic regression, and Gaussian naïve Bayes classifier models. Data of 33 patients from one of the hospitals were prospectively collected for model validation.

**Results:** Among 510 patients, 192 (37.65%) have not received any perioperative RBCs transfusion, 127 (24.90%) received less-transfusion (RBCs $<$ 4U), and 191 (37.45%) received more-transfusion (RBCs $\geq$ 4U). Machine learning-based transfusion predictive model produced the best performance with the accuracy of 83.34%, and Kappa coefficient of 0.7967 compared with other methods (blood preparation based on surgeons' experience with the accuracy of 65.94%, and Kappa coefficient of 0.5704; the random forest method with an accuracy of 82.35%, and Kappa coefficient of 0.7858; the gradient boosting decision tree with an accuracy of 79.41%, and Kappa coefficient of 0.7742; the K-nearest neighbor with an accuracy of 53.92%, and Kappa coefficient of 0.3341). In the prospective dataset, it also had a food performance with accuracy 81.82%.

**Conclusion:** This multicenter retrospective cohort study described the construction of an accurate model that could predict perioperative RBCs transfusion in patients with pelvic fractures.

**Keywords: pelvic fracture, perioperative, RBCs transfusion, predictive model, machine learning**

## INTRODUCTION

Pelvic fracture is a condition caused by high-energy trauma that is often accompanied by multiple injuries. It accounts for ~3% of all fracture injuries (1). Patients with pelvic fractures have an overall high injury severity score, which indicates the serious injury (2–4). Due to rapid bleeding and difficulty in stopping the bleeding, the mortality rates are high, reaching up to 30% in hemodynamically unstable pelvic fracture patients. In addition, the severity of the injury, the complexity of the fracture, and the surrounding neurovascular anatomical structure result in very high perioperative blood loss and allogenenic blood transfusion (ABT) rates in patients with pelvic fractures (5, 6).

Allogeneic red blood cells (RBCs) transfusion may increase the risk of complications during surgery and cause serious adverse reactions (7). A recent study reported that 166 patients who received ABT had serious complications, and 26 of them died (8). ABT is an independent risk factor for perioperative morbidity and mortality (9, 10). However, during the initial stages of trauma and preoperative blood preparation, it is difficult to predict the perioperative requirement for RBCs transfusion in patients with pelvic fracture. RBCs transfusion is currently primarily based on the surgeons' experience and on hemoglobin (Hb) concentration (11). As RBCs transfusion solely based on Hb levels is regarded as one-sided and incorrect, accurate method is needed to assist perioperative blood management (PBM) in patients with pelvic fracture. This method should reduce the wasting of blood resources, reduce the morbidity of transfusion-related adverse reactions, and improve patient prognosis. To the best of our knowledge, no reports to date have described a method that can accurately predict the risk and scope of RBCs transfusion during surgery of pelvic fracture.

Machine learning, an application in artificial intelligence, is a scientific discipline that studies the regularities of related data through computer learning. Machine learning has been widely used in multiple fields, such as computer vision, language recognition, and robot control (12). Research and practice in biomedicine have also benefited from machine learning (13–17). For example, an extreme gradient boosting (XGBoost) algorithm, a scalable machine learning system for tree boosting, has particular advantages in machine learning methods. This algorithm has shown an ability to process missing values, utilize data scaling, thus, successfully processing computationally valid variants (18–20).

In this study, an XGBoost-based machine learning model was constructed using clinical and laboratory data from multiple Chinese centers to accurately predict the need (no-transfusion, less-transfusion or more-transfusion) for perioperative RBCs transfusion in patients with pelvic fracture.

## MATERIALS AND METHODS

### Trial Design and Participants

This study was conducted at the six following centers in China between September 2012 and June 2019: the Third Xiangya Hospital of Central South University, the Second Xiangya Hospital of Central South University, Zhejiang Provincial People's Hospital, Affiliated Hospital of Southwest Medical University, Beijing SHIJITAN Hospital, and Aerospace Center Hospital. The subjects were patients who underwent surgery for pelvic fractures in these centers. Patients aged <18 years, patients who refused transfusion, and patients with pathologic pelvic fracture were excluded. We finally included 510 cases with complete data (**Figure 1**). The perioperative period was defined as 7 days before surgery to 7 days after surgery.

The study protocol was approved by the Institutional Review Board of the Third Xiangya Hospital of Central South University (NO: 2019-S009) and was registered at www.ClinicalTrials.gov (NCT03855644).

Data of pelvic fracture surgery patients who underwent surgery in the Third Xiangya Hospital of Central South University between May 1st 2021, and May 20th 2021 were prospectively collected to further validate the model.

### Data Collection

All the variables in this study were retrospectively collected from the electronic medical recording system of each center. A total of 107 variables were collected; variables that were missing for more than 20% of patients were not analyzed. Forty-four variables were included in the correlation analysis, and variables with correlation coefficients >0.5 were not further analyzed according to feature important score (FIS). The correlation coefficient refers to an association between variables. The Pearson correlation coefficient was typically used to compare normally distributed data. For continuous data with non-normal distribution, for ordinal data, or data with relevant outliers, a Spearman rank correlation was used to measure the association. FIS is the feature importance evaluation that comes with XGBoost. The FIC weighs the average importance of each feature at the model level. A total of 17 variables were analyzed, including demographic and clinical characteristics such as cause of fracture (traffic, grind, fall, and others), type of fracture (Tile type), site of fracture (pubic, sacrum, ankle joint, acetabular, iliac ring), Injury Severe Score (ISS score), the

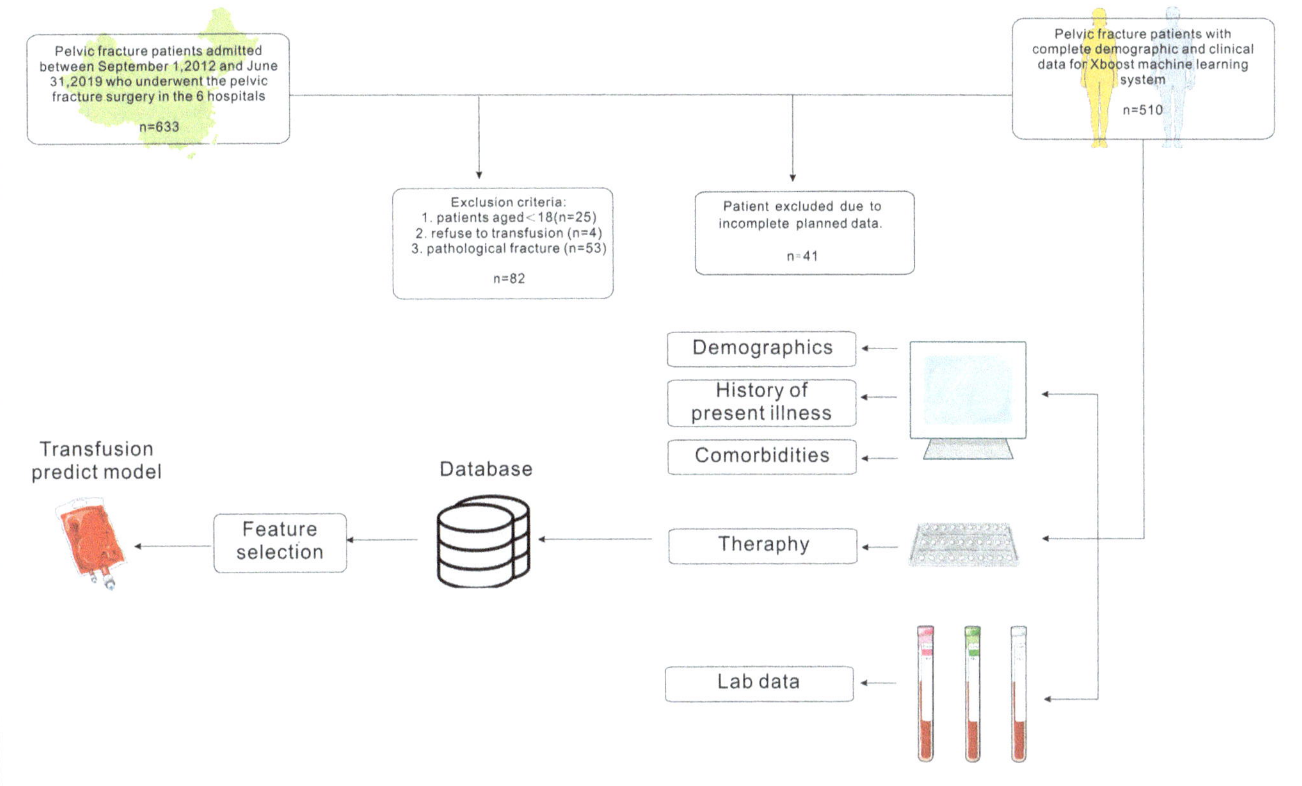


**FIGURE 1** | Flow chart showing the inclusion and exclusion criteria of patients and model-making process for the study.

occurrence of hemorrhagic shock, volume replacement therapy (hydroxyethyl starch injection, HES injection), iron therapy and hemostasis. Laboratory variables included hematocrit (HCT, %) and preoperative Hb concentration (g/L), preoperative mean arterial pressure (MAP, mmHg), total serum protein (U/L), aspartate transaminase (AST, U/L), and partial pressure of carbon dioxide ($PaCO_2$, mmHg). Surgical variables included time from injury to the first operation (TIFO, day), and intraoperative cell salvage (ml). Other factors included organ damage.

Hemostasis treatment was defined as perioperative treatment with tranexamic acid or white eyebrow venom hemagglutinin. Iron therapy was defined as perioperative intravenous injection of ferrous sulfate or iron sucrose or oral administration of ferrous succinate. Hemorrhagic shock was defined as blood pressure below 90/60 mmHg caused by blood loosed. Intraoperative cell salvage was defined as patients who received the blood transfusion from the same patient's blood loss by anticoagulation, salvage, filtration, and washing. MAP = (systolic blood pressure + 2 * diastolic blood pressure)/3; TIFO was defined as the time from the trauma that caused the fracture to the first operation.

## Data Set Processing

Patients were divided into three categories according to the different RBCs transfusion strategies. The no-transfusion group included patients who did not receive perioperative transfusions of allogeneic RBCs; the less-transfusion group included patients who were received with allogeneic RBCs < 4U; and the more-transfusion group included patients who were received with allogeneic RBCs ≥ 4U.

The patients were randomly divided into a training subset, which included 80% of patients, and a test subset, which included the remaining 20%, such that three classifications were maintained across both the training and test subsets. We used the XGBoost algorithm to find the relationship between variables and outcome. Five-fold cross-validation was performed taking into consideration the limited sample size (21), randomly splitting the dataset into 5 subsets, and using them in each iteration, four of them to train the models and the last one for validation. After five iterations, each subset was validated and the validation results were combined to robustly assess the model performance.

## Statistical Analysis

The machine learning based on XGBoost algorithms was compared with blood preparation based on surgeons experience and other predictive models, including random forest, gradient boosting decision tree, K-nearest neighbor, logistic regression, and Gaussian naïve Bayes classifier models using index accuracy, Youden index, Kappa coefficient, the area under the receiver operating characteristic curve (AUC) and the associated 95% confidence interval (CI). Feature ranking was obtained by computing Shapley Additive Explanation values (SHAP values) (22). Accuracy was calculated as the total number of categories

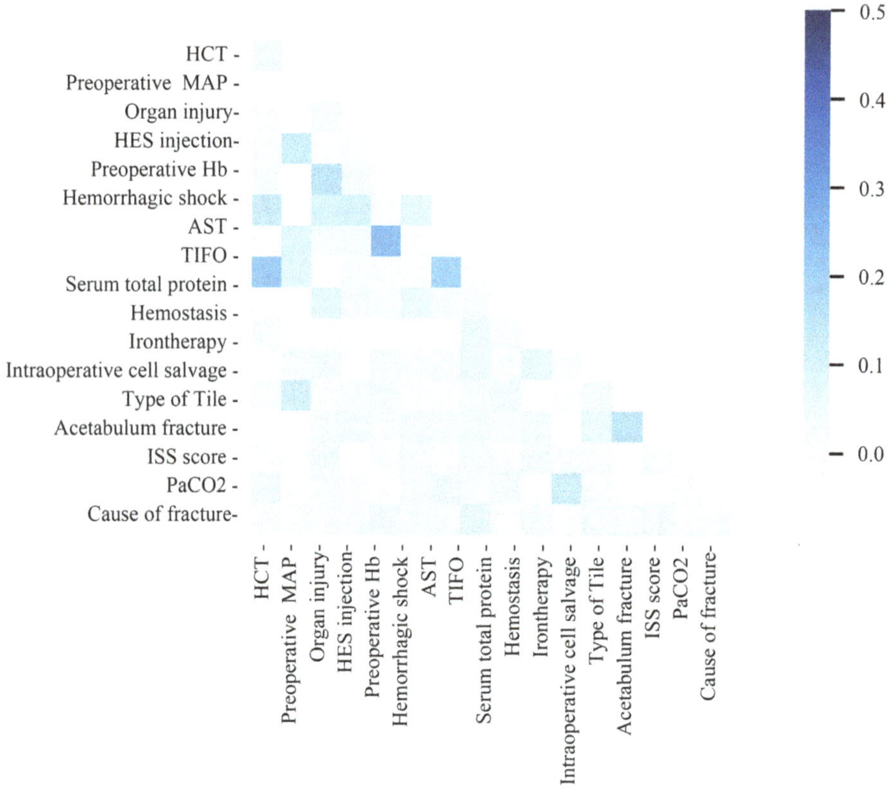


**FIGURE 2 |** Correlation matrix of features included within machine learning algorithms in transfusion predictive model. MAP, preoperative mean arterial pressure; TIFO, time from the injury and the first operation; AST, aspartate transaminase; HCT, hematocrit; ISS, injury severe score; $PaCO_2$, partial pressure of carbon dioxide; HES, hydroxyethyl starch.

predicted correctly divided by the total number of test set samples (Accuracy = the number of samples whose class was predicted correctly/the total number of samples). The Youden index was a type of index measure that combined sensitivity and specificity to evaluate the authenticity of a predictive model. The Youden index was defined as J(t) = sensitivity (t) + specificity (t) −1. The AUC was the area under the receiver operating characteristic (ROC) curve that assessed the accuracy of the model. The Kappa coefficient was a measure of the consistency between a predicted category and an actual category, based on linear weighting; the formula was as follows.

The kappa coefficient is a function of two quantities: the observed percent agreement.

$$P_o = \sum_{i=1}^{k} p_{ii}$$

$$P_e = \sum_{i=1}^{k} p_i + p_{+i,}$$

which is the value of the observed percent agreement under statistical independence of the classifications. The observed percent agreement is generally considered artificially high. It is often assumed that it overestimates the actual agreement since some agreement may simply occur due to chance. The kappa coefficient is given by,

$$k = \frac{P_o - P_e}{1 - P_e}$$

Continuous variables were expressed as the mean with range or median with interquartile range (IQR), compared by ANOVA, while categorical variables as counts (percentages) and by the Pearson $\chi^2$ test. Data that could not be analyzed by these methods were evaluated by Kruskal–Wallis analysis. A $p$-value $<0.05$ was considered statistically significant. Interaction analysis was performed to assess the effects of different variables on changes in transfusion risk.

# RESULTS

## Numbers Analyzed

The study cohort consisted of 510 patients, 408 allocated to the training set and 102 to the test set (**Figure 1**). Seventeen variables were included in the optimization model, with correlation analyses between variables performed to determine the independence of each variable (**Figure 2**). **Table 1** shows

**TABLE 1** | Clinical characteristics of the variables in transfusion predictive model and key features.

| Variable | No-transfusion ($n$ = 192) | Less-transfusion ($n$ = 127) | More-transfusion ($n$ = 191) | $p$-value |
|---|---|---|---|---|
| Age, yr [median, (IQR)] | 54.00 (44.00–73.00) | 60.50 (44.50–60.5) | 50.00 (39.25–60.00) | <0.001‡ |
| Cause of fracture ($n$, %) | | | | <0.001† |
| Traffic | 65 (33.85) | 50 (39.37) | 77 (40.31) | |
| Grind | 18 (9.38) | 8 (6.30) | 12 (6.28) | |
| Fall | 26 (13.54) | 16 (12.60) | 59 (30.89) | |
| Other | 83 (43.23) | 53 (41.73) | 43 (22.51) | |
| Type of tile ($n$, %) | | | | <0.001† |
| **A** | | | | |
| A1 | 58 (30.21) | 14 (11.02) | 20 (10.47) | |
| A2 | 54 (28.13) | 39 (30.71) | 47 (24.61) | |
| **B** | | | | |
| B1 | 4 (2.08) | 7 (5.51) | 15 (7.85) | |
| B2 | 35 (18.23) | 27 (21.26) | 26 (13.61) | |
| B3 | 5 (2.60) | 8 (6.30) | 14 (7.33) | |
| **C** | | | | |
| C1 | 14 (7.29) | 5 (3.94) | 15 (7.85) | |
| C2 | 5 (2.60) | 7 (5.51) | 7 (3.66) | |
| C3 | 17 (8.85) | 20 (15.75) | 47 (24.61) | |
| Site of fracture ($n$, %) | | | | 0.06† |
| Pubis | 80 (41.67) | 37 (29.13) | 76 (39.79) | |
| Ilium | 43 (22.40) | 29 (22.83) | 92 (48.17) | |
| Ischium | 19 (9.90) | 12 (9.45) | 29 (15.18) | |
| Sacrum | 37 (19.27) | 31 (24.41) | 47 (24.61) | |
| Synchondroses pubis | 3 (1.56) | 1 (0.79) | 6 (3.14) | |
| Acetabulum | 21 (10.94) | 30 (23.62) | 65 (32.46) | |
| ASA score ($n$, %) | | | | 0.02† |
| 1 | 66 (34.38) | 34 (26.77) | 57 (29.84) | |
| 2 | 74 (38.54) | 60 (47.24) | 86 (45.03) | |
| 3 | 48 (25.00) | 32 (25.20) | 41 (21.47) | |
| 4 | 3 (1.56) | 0 (0.00) | 6 (3.14) | |
| 5 | 1 (0.52) | 1 (0.79) | 1 (0.52) | |
| Comorbidities ($n$, %) | | | | 0.182† |
| Diabetes | 15 (7.81) | 15 (11.81) | 15 (7.85) | |
| Hypertension | 46 (23.96) | 31 (24.41) | 29 (15.18) | |
| Other | 142 (73.96) | 91 (71.65) | 154 (80.63) | |
| Hemorrhagic shock ($n$, %) | 8 (4.17) | 7 (5.51) | 37 (19.37) | <0.001† |
| Organs injury ($n$, %) | 42 (21.88) | 39 (30.71) | 88 (46.07) | <0.001† |
| TIFO [median, (IQR)] | 4.00 (0.004–40.000) | 5.833 (0.01–210.000) | 7.000 (0.125–69.000) | 0.096‡ |
| **Therapy** | | | | |
| Irontherapy ($n$, %) | 15 (7.89) | 23 (18.11) | 38 (19.90) | <0.001† |
| Hemostasis ($n$, %) | 31 (16.16) | 22 (17.32) | 61 (31.94) | <0.001† |
| Intraoperative cell salvage ($n$, %) | 1 (0.5) | 5 (3.9) | 14 (7.3) | 0.003† |
| Delta Hb [mean, (range)] | 4.00 (−26–34) | 4.86 (−42–41) | 8.02 (−65–62) | 0.314* |
| Preoperative SBP [mean, (range)] | 127.20 (90–193) | 131.82 (90–180) | 122.80 (72–180) | 0.005* |
| Preoperative DBP [mean, (range)] | 72.73 (42–115) | 72.36 (52–101) | 73.31 (40–140) | 0.733* |
| **Data of Lab** | | | | |
| HCT [median, (95% CI)] | 0.31 (0.29–0.37) | 0.31 (0.30–0.33) | 0.28 (0.26–0.28) | <0.001‡ |
| Leukocyte [median, (IQR)] | 8.96 (6.47–11.74) | 8.56 (7.30–10.44) | 9.15 (6.74–13.03) | 0.046‡ |
| PLT [median, (IQR)] | 179.00 (137.50–261.50) | 158.00 (126.50–213.00) | 157.00 (97.25–219.25) | 0.021‡ |
| Neutrophil [median, (IQR)] | 6.94 (5.12–9.67) | 6.80 (5.28–9.01) | 7.48 (5.30–11.33) | 0.024‡ |

*(Continued)*

**TABLE 1** | Continued

| Variable | No-transfusion ($n$ = 192) | Less-transfusion ($n$ = 127) | More-transfusion ($n$ = 191) | $p$-value |
|---|---|---|---|---|
| Lymphocyte [median, (IQR)] | 1.02 (0.75–1.41) | 1.06 (0.74–1.53) | 1.00 (0.72–1.49) | 0.576[‡] |
| Creatinine [median, (IQR)] | 61.15 (53.45–76.05) | 71.35 (58.88–93.78) | 70.8 (54.20–94.50) | 0.003[‡] |
| Urea [median, (IQR)] | 5.84 (4.29–8.03) | 6.60 (5.16–8.69) | 6.27 (4.56–8.33) | 0.015[‡] |
| Serum calcium [median, (IQR)] | 2.00 (1.19–2.12) | 2.00 (1.72–2.13) | 1.98 (1.72–2.14) | 0.947[‡] |
| INR [median, (95% CI)] | 1.18 (1.03–1.32) | 2.24 (−0.07–4.55) | 1.27 (1.17–1.38) | <0.001[‡] |

*TIFO, time from the injury and the first operation; SBP, systolic blood pressure; DBP, diastolic blood pressure; HCT, hematocrit; PLT, platelet; INR, international normalized ratio; ASA score, the American Society of Anesthesiologists score. Delta Hb: surgical variables included change in Hb concentration from before to after surgery.*
**ANOVA analysis.*
*[†]Pearson $\chi^2$.*
*[‡]Kruskal-Wallis.*

the 17 model variables in the patients with pelvic fractures. Of the 510 patients, 192 (37.6%) have not received any RBCs transfusions, 127 (24.9%) received <4U of RBCs, and 191 (37.5%) received ≥4U of RBCs transfusion during the perioperative period, which was classified in no-transfusion group, less transfusion group, and more transfusion group, respectively. Using traditional statistical analyses, we found that some of the variables significantly differed across three groups ($p < 0.05$) (**Table 1**).

## Outcomes and Estimation

The XGBoost machine learning system continued to train the model until errors were minimized and accuracy was maximized, followed by the construction of an accurate RBCs predictive transfusion model. The characteristics are ordered by importance in **Figure 3** with preoperative Hb, TIFO, and preoperative MAP weighted for highest importance in the final accurate transfusion predictive model.

In order to further explore the variable weight in the machine learning model of each group, the characteristics were further analyzed by determining their SHAP values (**Figure 4**). SHAP values provided consistent and locally accurate attribution values for each feature within prediction mode. This is a unified approach for explaining the outcomes of any machine learning model. SHAP values evaluated the importance of the output resulting from the inclusion of feature A for all combinations of features other than A. The XGBoost algorithm based on the tree model has a unique optimization method for calculating A to increase the calculation rate. Preoperative Hb, preoperative MAP, and ISS score were the most predictive values in the machine learning model of no-transfusion, with the risk of transfusion being much lower when preoperative Hb was low (blue points), preoperative MAP was high (red points), and ISS score was low (blue points) (**Figure 4A**). Interestingly, in the machine learning model of less-transfusion or more-transfusion, the most predictive features were different. They were preoperative Hb, TIFO, total serum protein in the less-transfusion predictive model and TIFO, total serum protein, AST in the more-transfusion predictive model, respectively. With a high level of preoperative Hb (red points), short TIFO (blue points), and high serum total protein (red points), the risk of less-transfusion was higher (**Figure 4B**). Meanwhile, the long TIFO (red points), low level of serum total protein (blue points), and high level of AST (red points) were likely to be associated with more-transfusion (**Figure 4C**).

Performance metrics for the model based on XGBoost machine learning are presented in **Table 2**. The ability of this model in accurately predicting the need for perioperative RBCs transfusion (ternary classifications) in patients with pelvic fractures was compared with other transfusion predictive models and with blood preparation based on surgeons' experience. We found that the accuracy of our model was 83.34%, with a Kappa coefficient of 0.7967. This model showed the best performance relative to the ability of the surgeons to perform blood preparation based on their experience, with an accuracy of 65.94% and a Kappa coefficient of 0.5704; the random forest method had an accuracy of 82.35% and a Kappa coefficient of 0.7858; the gradient boosting decision tree method had an accuracy of 79.41% and a Kappa coefficient of 0.7742; the K-nearest neighbor method had an accuracy of 53.92% and a Kappa coefficient of 0.3341. In order to evaluate the prediction performance of XGBoost machine learning more intuitively, we have used the confusion matrix in **Figures 5A,B**. When using the XGBoost machine learning prediction model, the total prediction accuracy was 83.33%; the prediction accuracy was highest for No-Transfusion (96.97%) and lowest for Less-Transfusion (71.88%).

## Prospective Validation

Data of 33 patients were prospectively collected for validation, of which 11 patients transfused RBCs > 4U, 10 patients received RBCs < 4U, and 12 patients did not receive any RBCs preoperatively. The total prediction accuracy of our model was 81.82% (**Figures 5C,D**).

## Ancillary Analyses

If the model was used to carry out a fuzzy prediction, a binary classifications model predicting whether patients did or did not require transfusions revealed that the accuracy of XGBoost was 95.13%, with an AUC of 0.99 [95% CI, 0.97–0.99], and a Youden index of 0.90. The accuracy and AUC of this model were much

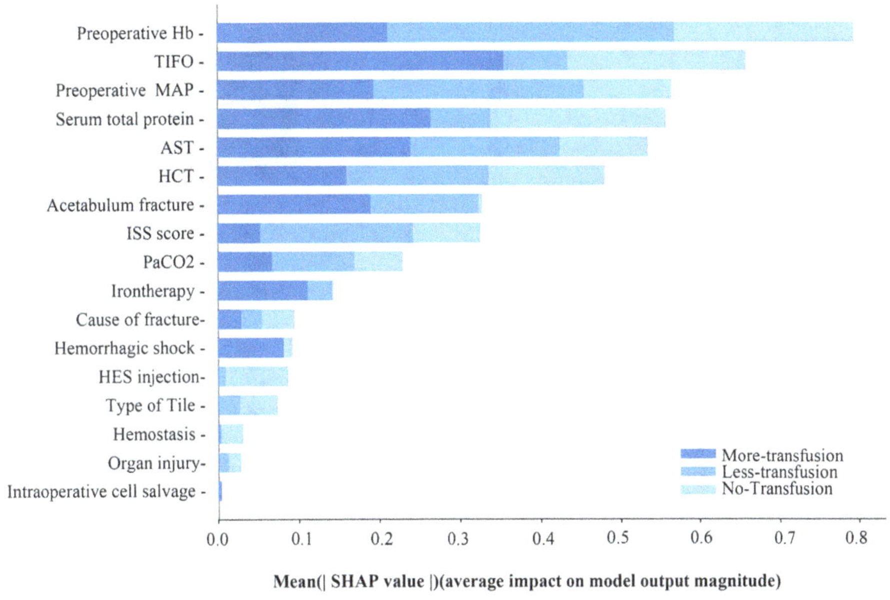


**FIGURE 3 |** The mean SHAP value of variables in RBCs transfusion predictive model of ternary classifications. MAP, preoperative mean arterial pressure; TIFO, time from the injury and the first operation; AST, aspartate transaminase; HCT, hematocrit; ISS, injury severe score; $PaCO_2$, partial pressure of carbon dioxide; HES, hydroxyethyl starch.

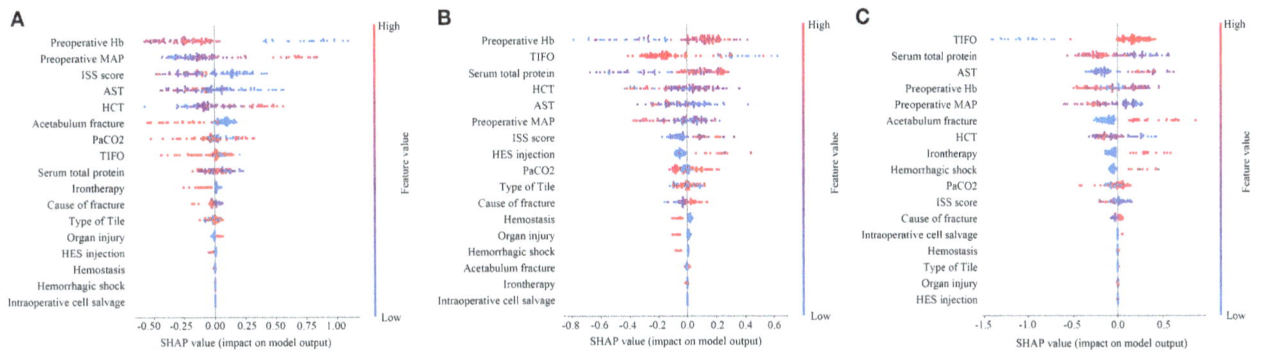


**FIGURE 4 |** Feature importance plot for the **(A)** machine learning predictive model whether RBCs transfusion or not; **(B)** machine learning model to predict whether less RBCs transfusion (<4U) or not and **(C)** machine learning model to predict whether more RBCs transfusion (≥4U) or not. The blue and red points in each row represent participants having low to high values of the specific variable, while the x-axis gives the SHAP value, which gives the impact on the model. SHAP, Shapley Additive Explanation values; MAP, preoperative mean arterial pressure; TIFO, time from the injury and the first operation; AST, aspartate transaminase; HCT, hematocrit; ISS, injury severe score; $PaCO_2$, partial pressure of carbon dioxide; HES, hydroxyethyl starch.

**TABLE 2 |** The ability of different model and surgeons experience to predict the need for perioperative red blood cells transfusion in test subset (ternary classifications).

| | XGBOOST model | Surgeons experience | Random forest model | Gradient-boosting trees model | K-nearest neighbors model |
|---|---|---|---|---|---|
| Accuracy (%) | 83.34 | 65.94 | 82.35 | 79.41 | 53.92 |
| Kappa coefficient | 0.7967 | 0.5704 | 0.7858 | 0.7742 | 0.3341 |

higher than those of other predictive models such as logistic regression, with an accuracy of 77.45%, an AUC of 0.85 (95% CI, 0.76–0.92), and Youden index of 0.53; Gaussian naïve Bayes classifier, with an accuracy of 62.75%, an AUC of 0.72 (95% CI, 0.65–0.79) and Youden index of 0.20; K-nearest neighbor, with an accuracy of 68.63%, an AUC of 0.71 (95% CI, 0.62–0.78) and Youden index of 0.35. Importantly, our model was better at predicting the need for transfusion than a model that was

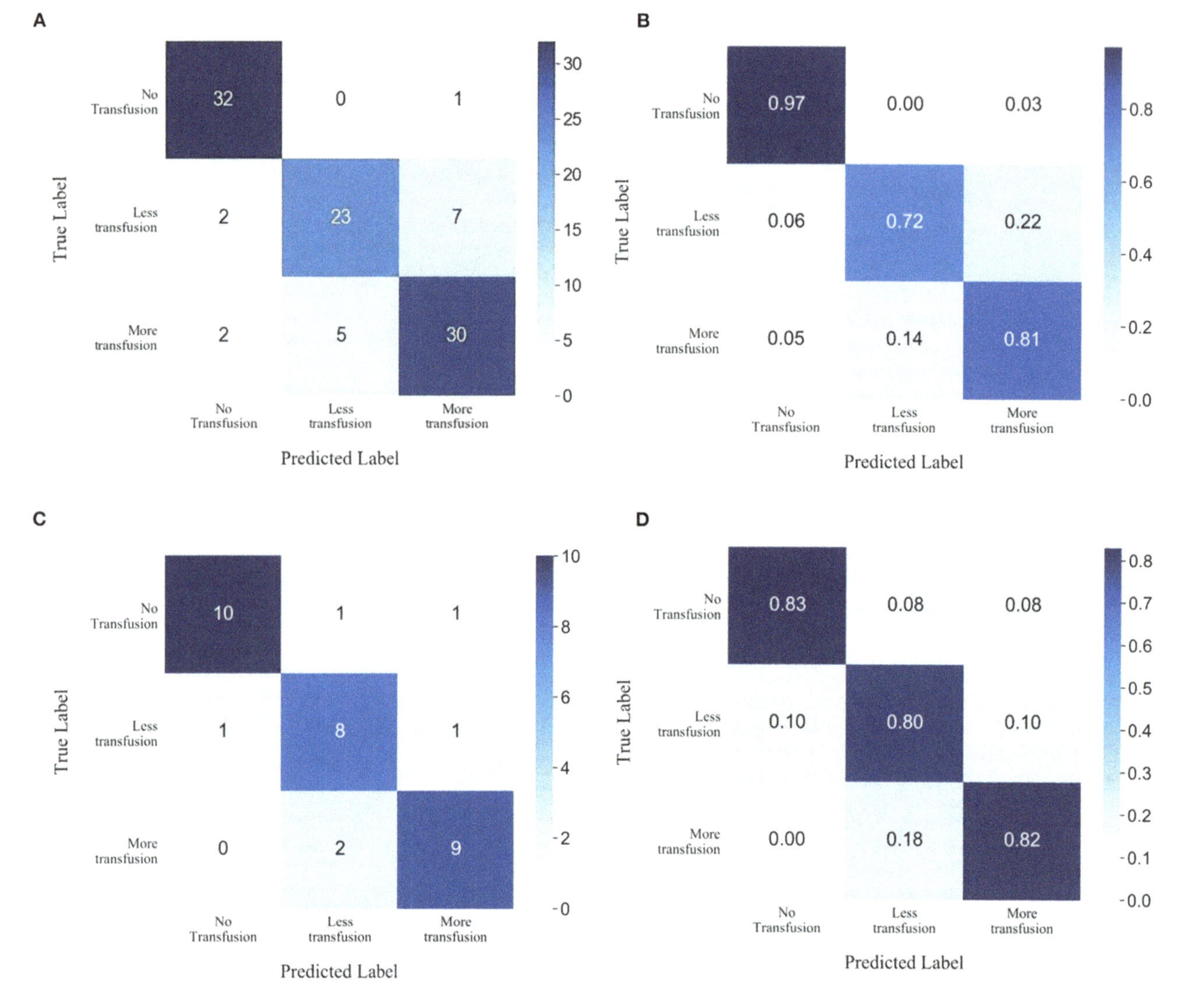


**FIGURE 5 |** Confusion matrix showing the prediction results of XGBoost machine learning in **(A,B)** test subset and **(C,D)** prospective subset.

based on surgeons' experience that had an accuracy of 89.96% and Youden index of 0.72 (**Table 3** and **Figure 6**).

## DISCUSSION

### Generalizability

This multicenter retrospective cohort study was designed to construct a model predicting the need for perioperative RBCs transfusion in patients with pelvic fractures. The RBCs transfusion predictive model constructed by the XGBoost ensemble method achieved an accuracy of 83.34% and a Kappa coefficient of 0.7967, which represent an outstanding predictive power. To the best of our knowledge, this is the first study that used a machine learning method based on an XGBoost algorithm to accurately predict the need for RBCs transfusion (ternary classification).

### Interpretation

Although, this study attempted to make extremely accurate predictions of perioperative RBCs transfusion in patients with pelvic fractures, the outcomes of the general accuracy were not satisfactory, which may be due to the insufficient amount of data and the differences between various centers, such as the differences in surgical approaches and usage of medicines. The average dose of RBCs transfused into these patients in our study was 3.72U. It has been reported that 24% of patients with pelvic fractures require RBCs transfusions, with an average dose of 4.81U per patient (5). We chose 4U RBCs as the cut-off between less-transfusion and more-transfusion groups because a perioperative study of cardiac surgery defined massive red blood cell transfusion (MRT) as receiving at least 4U RBCs (23). The threshold of MRT was based on the increase in mortality and complications when receiving RBCs above 4U.

**TABLE 3 |** The ability of different model and surgeons experience to predict the need for perioperative red blood cells transfusion in test subset (binary classifications).

| | XGBOOST model | Surgeons experience | Logistic regression model | Gaussian naïve bayes classifier | K-nearest neighbors model |
|---|---|---|---|---|---|
| Accuracy (%) | 95.13 | 86.96 | 77.45 | 62.75 | 68.63 |
| Youden index | 0.90 | 0.72 | 0.53 | 0.20 | 0.35 |
| AUC | 0.99 | / | 0.85 | 0.72 | 0.71 |
| AUC 95% CI | 0.97–0.99 | / | 0.76–0.92 | 0.65–0.79 | 0.62–0.78 |
| Sensitivity | 0.93 | 0.89 | 0.87 | 0.93 | 0.84 |
| Specificity | 0.97 | 0.83 | 0.66 | 0.28 | 0.51 |

*AUC, the area under the receiver operating characteristic curve.*

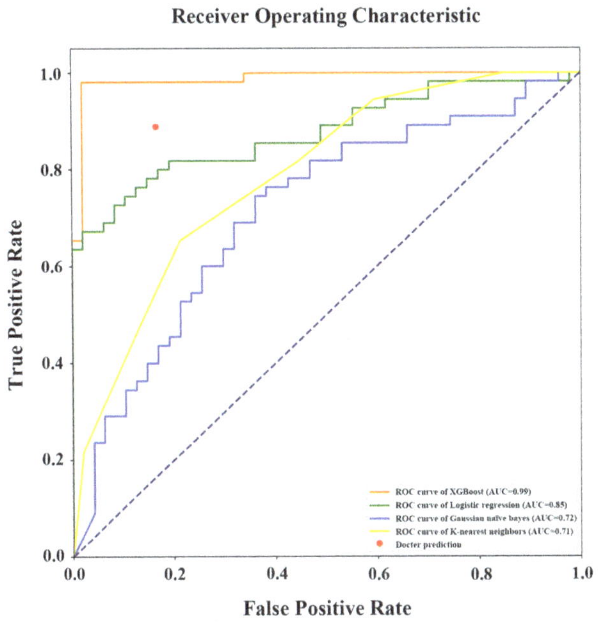


**FIGURE 6 |** Receiver operating characteristic (ROC) curve with area under curve calculation (legend) of the different models in prediction of RBCs transfusion (binary classifications). AUC, the area under the receiver operating characteristic curve.

As there is no guideline-based definition for MRT during the perioperative period, this study adopted the statement of "more-transfusion" and "less-transfusion." Therefore, this study set the cut-off at 4 U to classify the transfusion strategy into three groups: those requiring transfusions of 0U, <4U, and ≥4U of RBCs. Although, the model in this study could not precisely predict RBCs' dose in patients with pelvic fractures, the model could accurately guide clinicians and anesthesiologists. Nonetheless, increasing the amount of data and improving its quality may result in a more precise RBCs transfusion model for patients based on the machine learning algorithm of this study.

XGBoost, the method this study used, is an ensemble method based on gradient boosted trees that have been shown to have good performance in machine learning. This method can analyze large amounts of data quickly, efficiently, and accurately, avoiding over-provisioning. Due to its outstanding advantages, it has received attention in research fields such as biomedicine (24), network security (25), and engineering (15, 16, 26–28). XGBoost has been widely accepted as the one of the models with the most impressive predictive accuracy (29). Moreover, because XGBoost used parallelism, it has been known for its ability to learn quickly and scale appropriately to the problem (30). XGBoost could provide both performance and speed, which was significant and necessary for perioperative blood transfusion. It was why we chose XGBoost instead of other algorithm. In this study, this ensemble method also showed to have a good performance in the construction of RBCs transfusion predictive model, with higher accuracy than other machine learning decision models such as random forest, gradient boosting decision tree, and K-nearest neighbor models. Sun et al. (31) predicted RBCs consumption and demand based on the XGBoost model to increase the safety of inventory management. Feng et al. (32) predicted the RBC demand in trauma patient-based XGBoost (AUC 0.71) and other decision trees. Liu et al. (33) predicted the blood transfusion after liver transplantation surgery based XGBoost (AUC 0.813). Our model showed advantages with a good balance between sensitivity and specificity in the binary prediction of perioperative transfusion risk, (whether or not transfusion is needed) in patients with pelvic fracture, as shown by its accuracy (95.1%), Youden index (0.90) and AUC (0.99). Furthermore, our research innovatively achieved ternary classification prediction and made the foundation for precise prediction of blood transfusion in the future.

The variables included in this model are easy to obtain, with preoperative Hb being the most important variable. We found that the high level of preoperative Hb was associated with a high risk of transfusion, which was not consistent with other studies. Ogbemudia et al. (34) reported that a preoperative Hb <120 g/L was associated with a 10-fold increase in transfusion requirement in patients with rheumatoid arthritis who underwent either total hip or knee arthroplasty. A retrospective study reported that preoperative lower Hb level was the independent risk factor for transfusion in total hip arthroplasty (35). These differences may be due to the longer TIFO and heavier condition (high ISS) in patients from less or more transfusion group, so they underwent a number of treatments for improving the level of Hb before the perioperative period, such as blood transfusion, iron supplementation, etc., which caused the high level of preoperative Hb in these patients. However, due to the seriousness of patients' conditions and the difficulty of operation, the blood loss during operation might be substantial, leading to the high risk of perioperative blood transfusion rate. These results suggested that even if the level of preoperative Hb was high, it was not appropriate to simply speculate the dose of transfusion during the perioperative period, but other factors needed to be considered too.

Timeliness is very important in first aid of traumatology orthopedics, where TIFO represents the time from the first trauma to surgery for patients with pelvic fractures. In our research, we suggested that the longer TIFO was strongly associated with the more transfusion, where the dose of transfused RBCs ≥4U. In many perioperative studies, perioperative RBCs transfusion was considered as an important factor causing poor prognosis (36–38). These findings suggested that emergency doctors and surgeons should reduce TIFO as soon as possible, thereby reducing perioperative allogeneic blood transfusion and improving prognosis.

Some published guidelines for patients with pelvic fracture recommend transfusing RBCs when Hb concentration ≥70 g/L (11, 39, 40). However, the modern concept of PBM points out that Hb level cannot be used solely as an RBCs transfusion strategy. This study provided a more scientific predictive model of RBCs transfusion conformed to PBM. Moreover, the remaining variables not only provided suggestions for the dose of perioperative RBCs transfusion but also proposed a way to work out a program to reduce the need for transfusion during the perioperative period for surgeons, such as iron therapy, hemostasis treatment, intraoperative cell salvage, and active first aid measures to reduce trauma-surgery time. This reflected the importance of multidisciplinary cooperation for PBM.

Most RBCs transfusion predictive models are based on traditional statistical methods, with these binary models roughly predicting the risk for transfusion (41–44). In this study, we first used the XGBoost algorithm to predict the need for perioperative RBCs transfusion (ternary classification). XGBoost-based machine learning models have many advantages over RBCs transfusion scores based on traditional statistical methods. XGBoost-based models can automatically process missing data, thus, preventing the need to make subjective assumptions about independent and dependent variables beforehand. Moreover, machine learning is more effective in dealing with complex situations compared to traditional statistical analyses (45 47). Our XGBoost-based machine learning model revealed to have the best predictive ability among all models, including the RBCs preparation according to surgeons' experience.

## Limitations

This study has several limitations. First, this was a retrospective cohort study, with inherent biases such as selection or recall bias. This model should be further used in prospective research to verify its feasibility. It is meaningful that machine learning methods in this study can continuously optimize variables, thus, providing a reliable method for many clinical predictive models. Second, this study included less data than previous studies, making it difficult to construct an extremely accurate predictive model of perioperative RBCs transfused doses in patients with pelvic fracture. Nevertheless, the present study was the first to accurately predict the risk and scope of RBCs transfusion based on the machine learning from multicenter data, which is more instructive for clinical use.

## CONCLUSION

This multicenter retrospective cohort study constructed an accurate model that could predict perioperative RBCs transfusion in patients with pelvic fractures. This model could simply, rapidly, and accurately predict the risk for perioperative RBCs transfusion as well as the scope of RBCs transfused doses in patients with pelvic fracture.

## AUTHOR CONTRIBUTIONS

XH was responsible for writing the paper. YW, BC, YH, XW, and LC was responsible for data collecting. RG and XM was resposible for formulating plans and management. All authors contributed to the article and approved the submitted version.

## ACKNOWLEDGMENTS

We thank all of the staff, doctors, statistician whose data made this work possible in Participating hospitals. We also thank the HealSci Technology Co., Ltd. to provide algorithm technical support.

## REFERENCES

1. Grotz MR, Allami MK, Harwood P, Pape HC, Krettek C, Giannoudis PV. Open pelvic fractures: epidemiology, current concepts of management and outcome. *Injury.* (2005) 36:1–13. doi: 10.1016/j.injury.2004.05.029
2. Magnone S, Coccolini F, Manfredi R, Piazzalunga D, Agazzi R, Arici C, et al. Management of hemodynamically unstable pelvic trauma: results of the first Italian consensus conference (cooperative guidelines of the Italian Society of Surgery, the Italian Association of Hospital Surgeons, the Multi-specialist Italian Society of Young Surgeons, the Italian Society of Emergency Surgery and Trauma, the Italian Society of Anesthesia, Analgesia, Resuscitation and Intensive Care, the Italian Society of Orthopaedics and Traumatology, the Italian Society of Emergency Medicine, the Italian Society of Medical Radiology -Section of Vascular and Interventional Radiology- and the World Society of Emergency Surgery). *World J Emerg Surg.* (2014) 9:18. doi: 10.1186/1749-7922-9-18
3. Perkins ZB, Maytham GD, Koers L, Bates P, Brohi K, Tai NR. Impact on outcome of a targeted performance improvement programme in haemodynamically unstable patients with a pelvic fracture. *Bone Joint J.* (2014) 96-b:1090–7. doi: 10.1302/0301-620X.96B8.33383
4. Costantini TW, Coimbra R, Holcomb JB, Podbielski JM, Catalano RD, Blackburn A, et al. Pelvic fracture pattern predicts the need for hemorrhage

control intervention-Results of an AAST multi-institutional study. *J Trauma Acute Care Surg.* (2017) 82:1030–8. doi: 10.1097/TA.0000000000001465
5. Magnussen RA, Tressler MA, Obremskey WT, Kregor PJ. Predicting blood loss in isolated pelvic and acetabular high-energy trauma. *J Orthopaed Trauma.* (2007) 21:603–7. doi: 10.1097/BOT.0b013e3181599c27
6. Scannell BP, Loeffler BJ, Bosse MJ, Kellam JF, Sims SH. Efficacy of intraoperative red blood cell salvage and autotransfusion in the treatment of acetabular fractures. *J Orthopaed Trauma.* (2009) 23:340–5. doi: 10.1097/BOT.0b013e31819f691d
7. Tsuda Y, Yasunaga H, Horiguchi H, Ogawa S, Kawano H, Tanaka S. Association between dementia and postoperative complications after hip fracture surgery in the elderly: analysis of 87,654 patients using a national administrative database. *Arch Orthop Traum Su.* (2015) 135:1511–7. doi: 10.1007/s00402-015-2321-8
8. Desai N, Schofield N, Richards T. Perioperative patient blood management to improve outcomes. *Anesth Analg.* (2018) 127:1211–20. doi: 10.1213/ANE.0000000000002549
9. Marik PE, Corwin HL. Efficacy of red blood cell transfusion in the critically ill: a systematic review of the literature. *Critic Care Med.* (2008) 36:2667–74. doi: 10.1097/CCM.0b013e3181844677
10. Murphy GJ, Reeves BC, Rogers CA, Rizvi SI, Culliford L, Angelini GD. Increased mortality, postoperative morbidity, and cost after red blood cell transfusion in patients having cardiac surgery. *Circulation.* (2007) 116:2544–52. doi: 10.1161/CIRCULATIONAHA.107.698977
11. Napolitano LM, Kurek S, Luchette FA, Corwin HL, Barie PS, Tisherman SA, et al. Clinical practice guideline: red blood cell transfusion in adult trauma and critical care. *Critic Care Med.* (2009) 37:3124–57. doi: 10.1097/CCM.0b013e3181b39f1b
12. Jordan MI, Mitchell TM. Machine learning: trends, perspectives, and prospects. *Science.* (2015) 349:255–60. doi: 10.1126/science.aaa8415
13. Lip GY, Nieuwlaat R, Pisters R, Lane DA, Crijns HJ. Refining clinical risk stratification for predicting stroke and thromboembolism in atrial fibrillation using a novel risk factor-based approach: the euro heart survey on atrial fibrillation. *Chest.* (2010) 137:263–72. doi: 10.1378/chest.09-1584
14. O'Mahony C, Jichi F, Pavlou M, Monserrat L, Anastasakis A, Rapezzi C, et al. A novel clinical risk prediction model for sudden cardiac death in hypertrophic cardiomyopathy (HCM risk-SCD). *Eur Heart J.* (2014) 35:2010–20. doi: 10.1093/eurheartj/eht439
15. Zhang WG, Li HR, Li YQ, Liu HL, Chen YM, Ding XM. Application of deep learning algorithms in geotechnical engineering: a short critical review. *Artif Intell Rev.* (2021). doi: 10.1007/s10462-021-09967-1. [Epub ahead of print].
16. Zhang WG, Wu CZ, Zhong HY, Li YQ, Wang L. Prediction of undrained shear strength using extreme gradient boosting and random forest based on Bayesian optimization. *Geosci Front.* (2021) 12:469–77. doi: 10.1016/j.gsf.2020.03.007
17. Zhang Z, Liu J, Xi J, Gong Y, Zeng L, Ma P. Derivation and validation of an ensemble model for the prediction of agitation in mechanically ventilated patients maintained under light sedation. *Critic Care Med.* (2021) 49:e279–s90. doi: 10.1097/CCM.0000000000004821
18. Chen TQ, Guestrin C. XGBoost: a scalable tree boosting system. In: *Kdd'16: Proceedings of the 22nd Acm Sigkdd International Conference on Knowledge Discovery and Data Mining.* San Francisco, CA: Association for Computing Machinery (2016). p. 785–94. doi: 10.1145/2939672.2939785
19. Friedman JH. Greedy function approximation: a gradient boosting machine. *Ann Stat.* (2001) 29:1189–232. doi: 10.1214/aos/1013203451
20. Torlay L, Perrone-Bertolotti M, Thomas E, Baciu M. Machine learning–XGBoost analysis of language networks to classify patients with epilepsy. *Brain Informat.* (2017) 4:159–69. doi: 10.1007/s40708-017-0065-7
21. Badillo S, Banfai B, Birzele F, Davydov, II, Hutchinson L, et al. An introduction to machine learning. *Clin Pharmacol Therapeut.* (2020) 107:871–85. doi: 10.1002/cpt.1796
22. Lundberg, S. M., and Lee, S. I. (2017). "A unified approach to interpreting model predictions," in *Advances in Neural Information Processing Systems*, 4765–4774.
23. Huang D, Chen C, Ming Y, Liu J, Zhou L, Zhang F, et al. Risk of massive blood product requirement in cardiac surgery: a large retrospective study from 2 heart centers. *Medicine.* (2019) 98:e14219. doi: 10.1097/MD.0000000000014219
24. Ji X, Tong W, Liu Z, Shi T. Five-feature model for developing the classifier for synergistic vs. antagonistic drug combinations built by XGBoost. *Front Genet.* (2019) 10:600. doi: 10.3389/fgene.2019.00600
25. Dhaliwal SS, Nahid A-A, Abbas R. Effective intrusion detection system using XGBoost. *Information.* (2018) 9:149. doi: 10.3390/info9070149
26. Le LT, Nguyen H, Zhou J, Dou J, Moayedi H. Estimating the heating load of buildings for smart city planning using a novel artificial intelligence technique PSO-XGBoost. *Appl Sci.* (2019) 9:2714. doi: 10.3390/app9132714
27. Wang L, Wu CZ, Gu X, Liu H, Mei GX, Zhang WG. Probabilistic stability analysis of earth dam slope under transient seepage using multivariate adaptive regression splines. *B Eng Geol Environ.* (2020) 79:2763–75. doi: 10.1007/s10064-020-01730-0
28. Zhang WG, Zhang RH, Wu CZ, Goh ATC, Lacasse S, Liu ZQ, et al. State-of-the-art review of soft computing applications in underground excavations. *Geosci Front.* (2020) 11:1095–106. doi: 10.1016/j.gsf.2019.12.003
29. Shimoda A, Li Y, Hayashi H, Kondo N. Dementia risks identified by vocal features *via* telephone conversations: a novel machine learning prediction model. *PLoS ONE.* (2021) 16:e0253988. doi: 10.1371/journal.pone.0253988
30. Khan IU, Aslam N, Aljabri M, Aljameel SS, Kamaleldin MMA, Alshamrani FM, et al. Computational intelligence-based model for mortality rate prediction in COVID-19 patients. *Int J Environ Res Public Health.* (2021) 18:6429. doi: 10.3390/ijerph18126429
31. Sun X, Xu Z, Feng Y, Yang Q, Xie Y, Wang D, et al. RBC inventory-management system based on XGBoost model. *Indian J Hematol Blood Transfus.* (2021) 37:126–33. doi: 10.1007/s12288-020-01333-5
32. Feng YN, Xu ZH, Liu JT, Sun XL, Wang DQ, Yu Y. Intelligent prediction of RBC demand in trauma patients using decision tree methods. *Mil Med Res.* (2021) 8:33. doi: 10.1186/s40779-021-00326-3
33. Liu LP, Zhao QY, Wu J, Luo YW, Dong H, Chen ZW, et al. Machine learning for the prediction of red blood cell transfusion in patients during or after liver transplantation surgery. *Front Med.* (2021) 8:632210. doi: 10.3389/fmed.2021.632210
34. Ogbemudia AE, Yee SY, MacPherson GJ, Manson LM, Breusch SJ. Preoperative predictors for allogenic blood transfusion in hip and knee arthroplasty for rheumatoid arthritis. *Arch Orthop Trauma Surg.* (2013) 133:1315–20. doi: 10.1007/s00402-013-1784-8
35. Song K, Pan P, Yao Y, Jiang T, Jiang Q. The incidence and risk factors for allogenic blood transfusion in total knee and hip arthroplasty. *J Orthop Surg Res.* (2019) 14:273. doi: 10.1186/s13018-019-1329-0
36. Padmanabhan H, Brookes MJ, Nevill AM, Luckraz H. Association between anemia and blood transfusion with long-term mortality after cardiac surgery. *Ann Thorac Surg.* (2019) 108:687–92. doi: 10.1016/j.athoracsur.2019.04.044
37. Mariani P, Buttaro MA, Slullitel PA, Comba FM, Zanotti G, Ali P, et al. Transfusion rate using intravenous tranexamic acid in hip revision surgery. *Hip Int.* (2018) 28:194–9. doi: 10.1177/1120700018768655
38. Nakanishi K, Kanda M, Kodera Y. Long-lasting discussion: adverse effects of intraoperative blood loss and allogeneic transfusion on prognosis of patients with gastric cancer. *World J Gastroenterol.* (2019) 25:2743–51. doi: 10.3748/wjg.v25.i22.2743
39. Padhi S, Kemmis-Betty S, Rajesh S, Hill J, Murphy MF. Blood transfusion: summary of NICE guidance. *BMJ.* (2015) 351:h5832. doi: 10.1136/bmj.h5832
40. Alexander J, Cifu AS. Transfusion of red blood cells. *JAMA.* (2016) 316:2038–9. doi: 10.1001/jama.2016.12870
41. Hourlier H, Reina N, Fennema P. Single dose intravenous tranexamic acid as effective as continuous infusion in primary total knee arthroplasty: a randomised clinical trial. *Arch Orthop Traum Su.* (2015) 135:465–71. doi: 10.1007/s00402-015-2168-z
42. Singh SA, Prakash K, Sharma S, Anil A, Pamecha V, Kumar G, et al. Predicting packed red blood cell transfusion in living donor liver transplantation: a retrospective analysis. *Indian J Anaesth.* (2019) 63:119–25. doi: 10.4103/ija.IJA_401_18
43. Torres-Campos A, Floria-Arnal LJ, Muniesa-Herrero MP, Ranera-Garcia M, Osca-Guadalajara M, Castro-Sauras A. [Initial hemoglobin value as a predictor of allogeneic blood transfusion in hip fracture]. *Acta Ortop Mex.* (2018) 32:347–53. doi: 10.35366/85432
44. Xing Z, He Y, Ji C, Xu C, Zhang W, Li Y, et al. Establishing a perinatal red blood cell transfusion risk evaluation model for obstetric patients: a retrospective cohort study. *Transfusion.* (2019) 59:1667–74. doi: 10.1111/trf.15208

45. Bzdok D, Altman N, Krzywinski M. Statistics versus machine learning. *Nat Methods.* (2018) 15:232–3. doi: 10.1038/nmeth.4642
46. Singal AG, Mukherjee A, Elmunzer BJ, Higgins PDR, Lok AS, Zhu J, et al. Machine learning algorithms outperform conventional regression models in predicting development of hepatocellular carcinoma. *Am J Gastroenterol.* (2013) 108:1723–30. doi: 10.1038/ajg.2013.332
47. Waljee AK, Higgins PDR. Machine learning in medicine: a primer for physicians. *Am J Gastroenterol.* (2010) 105:1224–6. doi: 10.1038/ajg.2010.173

6

# Artificial Intelligence for Clinical Decision Support in Sepsis

*Miao Wu*[1], *Xianjin Du*[2*], *Raymond Gu*[3] *and Jie Wei*[1]

[1] Department of Emergency, Renmin Hospital of Wuhan University, Wuhan, China, [2] Department of Critical Care Medicine, Renmin Hospital of Wuhan University, Wuhan, China, [3] Department of Surgery, State University of New York Upstate Medical University, Syracuse, NY, United States

***Correspondence:**
Xianjin Du
duxianjin@whu.edu.cn

Sepsis is one of the main causes of death in critically ill patients. Despite the continuous development of medical technology in recent years, its morbidity and mortality are still high. This is mainly related to the delay in starting treatment and non-adherence of clinical guidelines. Artificial intelligence (AI) is an evolving field in medicine, which has been used to develop a variety of innovative Clinical Decision Support Systems. It has shown great potential in predicting the clinical condition of patients and assisting in clinical decision-making. AI-derived algorithms can be applied to multiple stages of sepsis, such as early prediction, prognosis assessment, mortality prediction, and optimal management. This review describes the latest literature on AI for clinical decision support in sepsis, and outlines the application of AI in the prediction, diagnosis, subphenotyping, prognosis assessment, and clinical management of sepsis. In addition, we discussed the challenges of implementing and accepting this non-traditional methodology for clinical purposes.

**Keywords: sepsis, artificial intelligence, machine learning, deep learning, early prediction**

## INTRODUCTION

Sepsis is a syndrome in which infection causes host response imbalance. It leads to life-threatening organ damage, and has a high mortality rate. Sepsis not only threatens human health, but also brings a huge economic burden to medical and health care (1). Given that sepsis has a certain morbidity and high mortality, early prediction and intervention of sepsis is of great significance (2). The management of sepsis is a highly complex and challenging problem, and it is still the subject of well-trained and highly skilled experts. More than a quarter century of research has not produced a reliable diagnostic test or a direct treatment for sepsis. The core of this deficiency is that sepsis is still a clinical/physiological diagnosis, representing many molecularly different pathological trajectories. But as the applications of AI in the medical field continue to emerge, some medical decisions will soon be left to so called "intelligence" machines to improve clinical practice and patient prognosis. In fact, many tasks involved in the clinical management of sepsis can be performed individually or optimized through dedicated algorithms, including early prediction, improvement of antibiotic therapy, and hemodynamic optimization (3, 4). At present, thanks to the dissemination of electronic health records (EHR), the application of AI has a good foundation.

## ARTIFICIAL INTELLIGENCE AND SEPSIS

In 1956, a gathering at the Dartmouth Conference proposed the concept of "artificial intelligence," hoping to use recently developed computers to construct complex machines with the same essential characteristics as human intelligence. However, due to constraints in memory and a lack of processing power, developments in AI proceeded slowly. After 2012, thanks to the increase in data volume, computing power, and the development of new machine learning algorithms, AI began to explode, resulting in expansions in expert systems, machine learning, evolutionary computing, computer vision, natural language processing and other data processing technologies (5). Among them, mechanical learning is the most widely used in sepsis.

The most basic method of machine learning uses algorithms to analyze and learn from data, and then uses the results of learning to make decisions and predictions about events in reality. Unlike traditional hard-coded software programs, machine learning uses numerous amounts of data to learn how to out specific tasks from the data using various algorithms (4) (**Figure 1**). Machine learning has appeared in the early stages of AI development. The initial algorithms include decision trees, support vector machine (SVM), clustering and so on. Machine learning can be classified according to different learning methods. The initial algorithms included supervised learning, unsupervised learning, and semi-supervised learning (**Figure 2**). Later, more algorithms such as integrated learning, deep learning, and reinforcement learning were developed. The application of traditional machine learning algorithms in sepsis management has had preliminary results, but every step forward was extremely difficult, until the emergence of deep learning.

At the very beginning, deep learning was not a brand new learning method, but a deep neural network that could be developed using supervised and unsupervised learning methods. However, due to rapid growth in the field of machine learning in recent years, some unique learning methods have been proposed (such as residual networks). As a result, more and more people regard it as a learning method alone. Originally deep learning used deep neural networks to solve feature expression. Deep neural network itself was not a new concept but could be simply understood as a neural network structure containing multiple hidden layers. People could adjust the connection and activation methods of neurons accordingly to improve the training effect of deep neural networks. In fact, there were many such ideas in the early years, but due to insufficient training data and backward calculation ability, the results were not satisfactory. Deep learning has accomplished various tasks in healthcare, including the management of sepsis (6–12), which provides the possibility for its application in clinical practice.

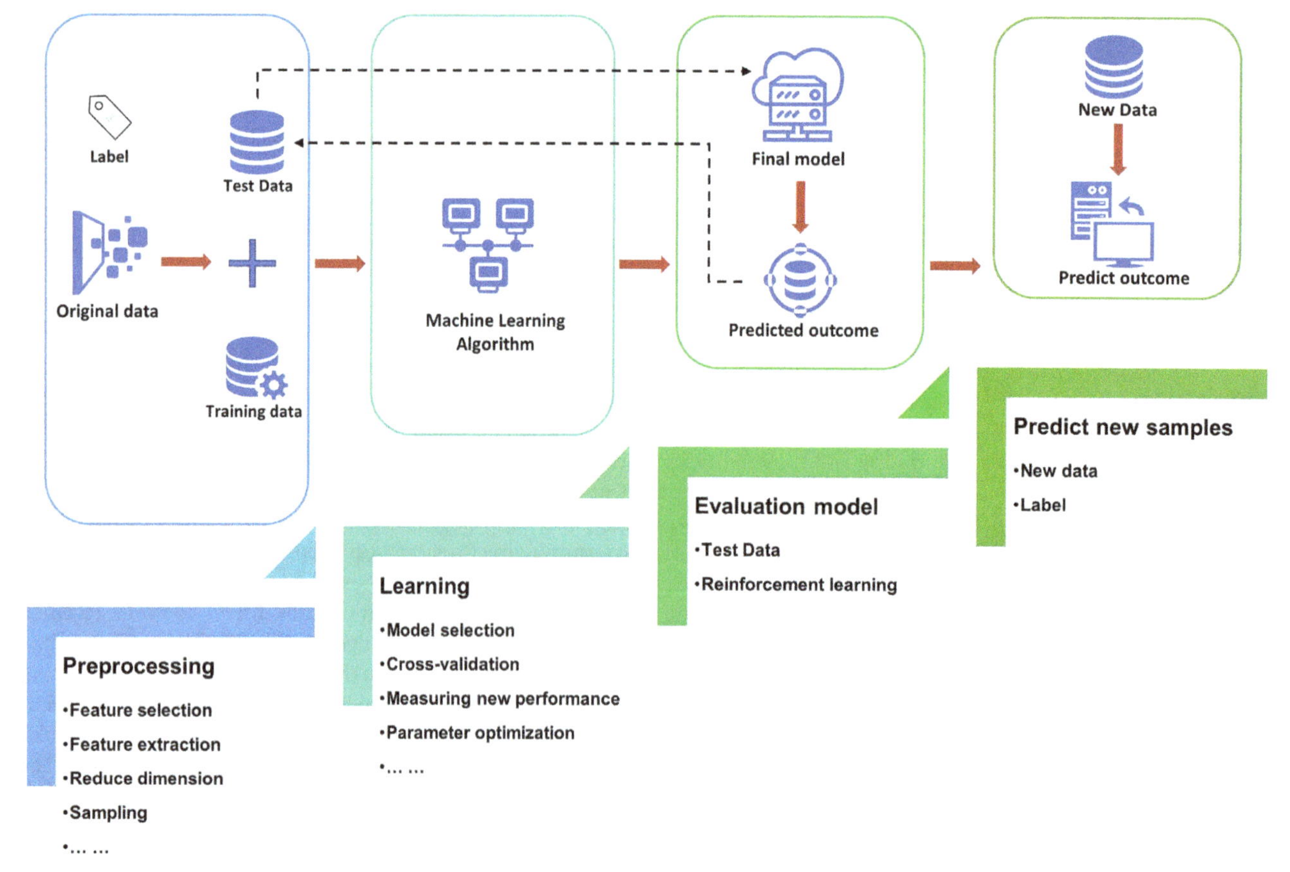


**FIGURE 1** | Roadmap for machine learning systems.

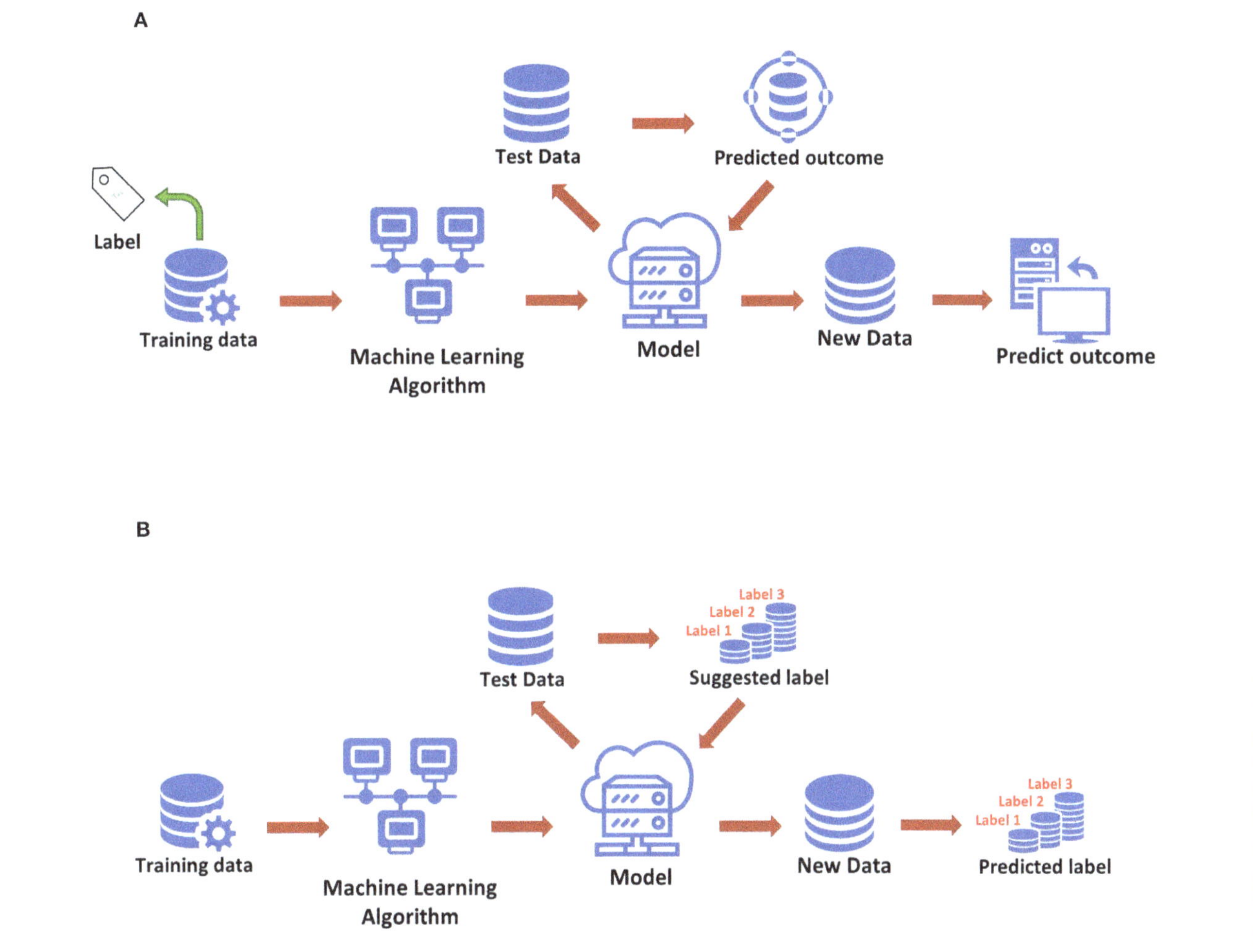


**FIGURE 2** | Two methods of machine learning. **(A)** Supervised learning. **(B)** Unsupervised learning.

## METHODS OF LITERATURE SELECTION

The literature search was conducted in (PubMed). Research papers, systematic reviews, and narrative reviews published prior to January 31, 2021 were included. Abstracts without full text were excluded. The search terms used to find relevant literature included: ("machine learning" OR "deep learning" OR "neural network" OR "artificial intelligence") AND ("sepsis"). A total of 433 papers were initially identified with these search terms, of which 33 abstracts without full text were excluded, leading to a final count of 400. Given the narrative nature of this review, the final cohort of papers was hand-picked to provide the reader with the best general overview of the topic and was not meant to be comprehensive. We selected some research manuscripts and systematic reviews, and referenced a number of narrative reviews. This article is based on previously conducted studies and does not contain any studies with human participants or animals performed by any of the authors.

## APPLICATION OF AI IN THE EARLY PREDICTION AND DIAGNOSIS OF SEPSIS

### Early Prediction of Sepsis

Early intervention of sepsis is the key to treatment, as every hour of delay in treatment increases mortality. If we can predict the occurrence of sepsis early, we can initiate intervention measures as soon as possible. The original sepsis prediction system relies mainly on empirical clinical decision rules (CDR), which usually uses vital signs collected at the bedside. For example, five physiological markers are extracted from the bedside monitor every minute. These data streams include heart rate, respiratory rate, and blood pressure (systolic, diastolic, and mean blood pressure), and then are classified by SVM classifiers (13). The model can accurately predict the incidence of sepsis, with an average detection accuracy of 83.0% and an Area Under Receiving Operator Characteristics (AUROC) of 0.781. This is the minimal AI model developed for early prediction of sepsis. Logistic regression is also used to measure six variables related to sepsis, and a predictive model (automated screening tool) with an AUROC of 0.857 has been developed to help identify patients at risk of sepsis (14). The screening tool can screen all hospitalized patients and pass the results directly to caregivers without any manual intervention.

The main disadvantage of CDR is that when used in a population different from the derived population, there will be generality and performance differences. In addition, it usually takes several years to establish and verify. The growth of deep learning has created more opportunities for the application of AI in sepsis (15–18). Bi-Directional Gated Recurrent Units (GRU) is a deep learning algorithm that uses various parameters related to the vitals, laboratory, and demographics (6). The AUROC of this model is 0.97, which can predict the occurrence of sepsis 6 h in advance. This method is better than the AI models for sepsis prediction found in the current literature. There is also an early warning system for sepsis using deep learning. A new algorithm based on electronic medical record (EMR) was designed, which can detect sepsis 6 h before the occurrence of sepsis, with an AUROC of 0.782 (7). Another sepsis detection system uses a convolutional neural network and a long short-term memory network (12). The quality evaluation of the model is based on standard concepts of accuracy and clinical applicability, and the intervention is evaluated retrospectively by observing intravenous antibiotics and blood cultures before the predicted time. The AUROC at 3 h before the onset of sepsis was 0.856. In the past, due to the delay in sepsis recognition, vast majority of sepsis patients did not start antibiotic treatment or blood culture in time. Therefore, this model can promptly facilitate such interventions through early identification.

With the progress of deep learning, more and more studies have introduced it into clinical decision support for sepsis. In order to evaluate its function, the performance of deep learning was compared to other methods in the early prediction of sepsis, including three machine learning algorithms (random forest, Cox regression and penalized logistic regression) and three scoring screening tools (SIRS, qSOFA and NEWS) (9). Demographics, comorbidities, vital signs, medicines, and test results are all included in the training data set. Multi-output Gaussian process and recurrent neural network (MGP-RNN), a deep learning-based model that can advance the prediction of sepsis by 5 h, performed the best.

In addition to the above-mentioned deep learning, some people have developed an explainable AI model for early prediction of sepsis. They developed a model based on shared ICU public data and verified the challenge score in a completely hidden population (19). The explainable AI model extracts 168 features per hour and is trained to achieve real-time prediction of sepsis. The influence of each feature on the real-time prediction of sepsis is discussed in depth to show its interpretability. This model not only has superior performance in estimating the risk of sepsis in real time, but also provides interpretable information for comprehending the risk of sepsis.

However, traditional supervised models tend to perform better only in certain aspects compared to ensemble learning. Ensemble learning is a comprehensive strongly supervised model, usually composed of multiple weakly supervised models. The potential goal of ensemble learning is that even if one of the weak classifiers makes a prediction error, the other weak classifiers can correct the error. Recently, a study reported a sepsis prediction model based on ensemble learning framework, which combines artificial features extracted from advanced clinical knowledge and deep features based on automatic extraction of long-term and short-term memory (LSTM) neural networks (20). Through ensemble learning, the early prediction of sepsis was achieved 6 h in advance. The results show that the model has a good effect on early detection of sepsis. In particular, ensemble learning is significantly better than other single models in performance (**Table 1**).

## Early Prediction of Septic Shock

The development of decision support systems that relied on advances in machine learning is a field of innovation in healthcare strategies. Predicting the development of septic shock is one of the active areas (27). Many studies have developed intelligent decision support tools related to septic shock to improve clinical results and promote real-time optimization of medical resources. One of the studies compared eight different machine learning algorithms with the goal of developing a predictive model of septic shock, including Random Forest, C5.0, Decision Trees, Boosted Logistic Regression, SVM, Logistic Regression, Regularized Logistic, and Bayes Generalized Linear Model (21). The model using the Random Forest algorithm performed best, with an AUROC of 0.9483, a sensitivity of 83.9%, and a specificity of 88.1%. There are also studies using gradient enhancement algorithms to develop septic shock prediction models, such as XG-Boost, by combining physiological data in EHR with features obtained from natural language processing in clinical medical record data. Among them, the median warning time of the best method is 7.0 h, which is enough to intervene many hours before the onset of septic shock (26).

Transfer learning is a new subfield of machine learning, which allows the promotion of algorithms in various clinical sites. In order to study the effectiveness of AI Sepsis Expert in predicting delayed septic shock in ED, transfer learning was introduced, and the feasibility of improving external effectiveness in the second location was verified (22). The best AUROC of this AI is <0.8, and it has the best performance in predicting delayed septic shock at 8 and 12 h. Transfer learning greatly improves the external validity and generality of the model.

## Improve the Accuracy of Sepsis Diagnosis

Multiple organ failure is a typical manifestation of sepsis and is closely related to the diagnosis of sepsis. However, multiple organ failure itself often has no typical clinical manifestations, which aggravates the complexity of sepsis diagnosis and affects the accuracy of diagnosis. In order to solve the dilemma of the current diagnosis of sepsis, some studies have developed affordable automated diagnostic tools (28). Kok et al. developed a deep temporal convolution network model for sepsis detection, and evaluated it through three verification methods. The final selected model was robust and can be used as an early diagnosis tool for sepsis in the hospital. The accuracy and precision of this diagnostic tool was relatively higher than other

**TABLE 1** | Summary of the results from related works on the prediction of sepsis onset.

| Authorship | Year | Subjects | Features | Techniques | Best model/Algorithms | AUROC | References |
|---|---|---|---|---|---|---|---|
| Misra et al. | 2021 | 45,425 | 15 | • Apache Spark<br>• random under-sampling algorithm<br>• 5-fold cross validation | Random Forest | 0.9483 | (21) |
| Wardi et al. | 2021 | 183,573 | 40 | • transfer learning<br>• a modified Weibull-Cox proportional hazards model<br>• optimized using gradient descent | Artificial Intelligence Sepsis Expert | 0.833 | (22) |
| Wickramaratne et al. | 2020 | 40,336 | 36 | • Recurrent Neural Network Variant<br>• 5% recurrent dropout and early stopping schemes<br>• Nesterov Adam optimizer | Bi-Directional Gated Recurrent Units | 0.97 | (6) |
| Lee et al. | 2020 | 60,000 | 40 | • deep learning-based early warning system<br>• score function used in the Physionet Challenge 2019<br>• Noisy Data Imputation | Graph Convolutional Network | 0.782 | (7) |
| Kok et al. | 2020 | 2,932 | 40 | • Gaussian Process Regression<br>• Radial Basis Function kernel combined with White Noise kernel<br>• 10-fold cross validation | Temporal Convolution Network | 0.98 | (8) |
| Bedoya et al. | 2020 | 42,979 | 86 | • variety of imputation strategies<br>• Internal validation<br>• Temporal validation | Multi-output Gaussian Process and Recurrent Neural Network | 0.88 | (9) |
| Lauritsen et al. | 2020 | 52,229 | 30 | • 5-fold cross validation<br>• Gradient Boosting Classifier<br>• multilayer feedforward neural network | Convolutional Neural Network and Long Short-term Memory Network | 0.856 | (12) |
| Mohammed et al. | 2020 | 5,958 | 5 | • physiological data streams | Support Vector Machine | 0.781 | (13) |
| Cooper et al. | 2020 | 10,792 | 6 | • Logistic regression | Automated Sepsis Screening Tool | 0.857 | (14) |
| Helguera-Repetto et al. | 2020 | 236 | 25 | • SupplementaryMaterial<br>• 5-fold-cross-validation<br>• Internal Validation (Slope and Intercept Test) | Artificial Neural Network | 0.944 | (23) |
| Kaji et al. | 2020 | 56,841 | 119 | • Philippe Re'my's Github repository<br>• a TensorFlow backend<br>• RMSProp optimizer | Long Short-Term Memory Recurrent Neural Network | 0.876 | (16) |
| Yuan et al. | 2020 | 1,588 | 106 | • TED_ICU (continuous data recording)<br>• 5-fold cross-validation<br>• a decision-tree based algorithm | XGBoost | 0.89 | (24) |
| Bloch et al. | 2019 | 4,534 | 4 | • Support Vector Machine with radial basis function<br>• 10-fold cross validation<br>• features which represent the variability in vital signs | Support Vector Machine | 0.8838 | (25) |
| Scherpf et al. | 2019 | 46,520 | 10 | • 4-fold-stratified-cross-validation<br>• Gated recurrent unit<br>• optimized on binary cross-entropy cost function | Recurrent Neural Network | 0.81 | (17) |
| Liu et al. | 2019 | 38,645 | 128 | • Natural Language Processing features<br>• GloVe/GRU-based method<br>• a gradient boosting model | XGBoost | 0.92 | (26) |

algorithms (8). Another study introduced the development of an AI algorithm that can be used for sepsis diagnosis, and compares its performance with the diagnostic method based on SOFA score (24). The algorithm used pre-selected features and prospectively selected 106 clinical features for sepsis diagnosis. The de-identified data was used to develop this AI. The 5-fold cross-validation was applied to assess the performance of several machine learning methods, and finally the best-performing XGBoost based on the decision tree was used in the development of the AI algorithm. The AUROC of the established AI algorithm is about 0.89, while the SOFA score is only 0.596. This AI algorithm was developed through pre-selected features and XGBoost based on data collected by EMR from real cases of sepsis patients. The accuracy of early diagnosis of sepsis exceeds 80%. The timely and accurate response of this AI algorithm can enable clinicians to deploy appropriate treatment methods earlier, which will result in lower medical costs and improved patient prognosis, so the healthcare system, medical staff and patients can all benefit from it.

However, because of the non-specific signs and symptoms, the diagnosis of neonatal sepsis remains a challenge. Traditional scoring systems help distinguish patients with sepsis from those with non-sepsis, but they did not consider the particularity of each patient. There is a neonatal sepsis model based on the training and verification of artificial neural network (ANN) algorithms, mainly for the diagnosis of early-onset and late-onset neonatal sepsis (23). The results show that compared with doctors based on the traditional scoring system, the performance of the model is superior by using the same features. The sensitivity is 93.3%, the specificity is 80.0%, and the AUROC is 94.4%. The 10 most critical factors for the evaluation of neonatal sepsis are maternal age, cervicovaginitis and neonates, fever, apnea, platelet count, gender, bradypnea, band cell, catheter use, and birth weight.

## APPLICATION OF AI IN THE PROGNOSIS AND RISK ASSESSMENT OF SEPSIS

Sepsis is a relatively common cause of death in patients with suspected infection. Its current mortality rate is still high and unacceptable. Appropriate assessment tools that can be used to evaluate the prognosis of sepsis may improve the accuracy of clinical decision-making and reduce mortality (25). A deep neural network (DNN) model developed using LSTM can evaluate the clinical status of patients after treatment in the intensive care unit (ICU), thereby predicting the mortality rate within 96 h after admission. The AUC of the multi-center study was 0.88, and the AUC of the single-center study was 0.85 (10). This LSTM-based model could assist doctors identify patients with poor prognosis early, so as to "re-triage" and adjust treatment plans.

The clinical manifestations and prognosis of sepsis-associated acute kidney injury (AKI) are not all the same. AI can be used to divide them into various sub-phenotypes according to the degree of risk, thereby helping to improve the management of related patients (29). A study used deep learning to determine the subphenotype of sepsis-related AKI and predict the 28-day mortality and dialysis needs of sepsis-related AKI (30). The study utilized the K-means algorithm and used more than 2,500 feature combinations to cluster patients with sepsis-related AKI and identified three subphenotypes. Among them, subtype 1 has the lowest dialysis requirement (4%), and the 28-day mortality rate after AKI is also the lowest (23%). After adjustment, the mortality rate of subtype 3 is 1.9 times that of subtype 1. Similarly, Ibrahim et al. also used AI to stratify the types of organ dysfunction observed in patients with sepsis in the ICU, and identified clinically meaningful sepsis subgroups with different organ dysfunction patterns (31). Random forests, gradient boost trees, and SVMs are used for classification.

Coagulation disorders caused by sepsis have a poor prognosis, and there are currently no definitive tools to predict it. Machine learning technology can be used to create predictive models of coagulopathy progression. According to Japan's Septic Disseminated Intravascular Coagulation (DIC) retrospective research, machine learning algorithms including multiple linear regression (MLR), random forest, SVM and neural network were utilized to estimate the progression of coagulopathy and compare its accuracy with traditional methods (32). In terms of DIC progress, random forest has the highest prediction accuracy rate of 67.0%, and the difference between the ΔDIC predicted by random forest and real ΔDIC is 1.54, which is the smallest.

In order to predict the mortality of patients with suspected infection or sepsis in ED, the performance of AI was also been evaluated. A study compared the effects of several AIs in the classification and mortality prediction of sepsis patients in ED (33). A total of four supervised learning models, random forest, C4.5 decision tree, SVM and ANN were compared. The result is that SVW and ANN using physiological variables have the best discrimination effect. It has good application prospects in assessing the classification and prognosis of sepsis. Convolutional Neural Network plus SoftMax, a deep learning-based algorithm, can also be used to predict the mortality of patients suspected of infection in ED. The results show that compared with other machine learning algorithms and sepsis scoring tools commonly used in clinical practice (SIRS and qSOFA), the accuracy of this deep learning method is significantly superior (34). Deep learning can effectively help identify critically ill patients earlier.

## APPLICATION OF AI IN THE MANAGEMENT OF PATIENTS WITH SEPSIS

Passive leg lift (PLR) can predict fluid responsiveness in sepsis, but the patient's limited mobility usually precludes the use of this hemodynamic challenge. To predict the fluid responsiveness of patients with sepsis or septic shock, machine learning using data from transthoracic echocardiography (TTE) was developed (35). The results show that the partial least-squares regression (PLS) model has an AUC value of 0.97, which was the best model and was comparable to the hemodynamic response of PLR. The key parameters of echocardiography include inferior vena cava collapsibility, velocity-time integral, S-wave, E/Ea ratio, and E-wave. Another study also reported on fluid management strategies for patients with sepsis. Causal inference technology is used to estimate the mortality outcome caused by the "caps" setting of fluid volume administration in the first 24 h in ICU (36). It was found that if the total amount of fluid in these patients is limited to 6–10 L, the 30-day mortality rate may be lower than the mortality rate observed in current practice. The mortality rate of 8 L was found to have the largest decrease.

Sepsis bundles designed to reduce the deleterious effect of sepsis have been recommended for nearly a decade. Despite this, the mortality rate of sepsis is still high, and the compliance of sepsis bundles is still not ideal. A multidisciplinary project used the Model Cell mental model to analyze collected mortality and compliance data, and compared the observed mortality data with predicted data based on comparable acute care facilities (37). The results showed that as the bundle compliance increased, the mortality rate of the entire system decreased significantly. In the linear model, compliance alone can explain nearly two-thirds of the variance. When using only the final 12 months of the project, the median death rate dropped further to 5.3%. The Model Cell intervention successfully improved bundle compliance, thereby reducing mortality. As technology advances, this model can be enhanced and ready for AI to help drive further success.

The etiology of sepsis is also very important for the formulation of treatment strategies. Inflammatix-bacterial-viral-non-infected-version 1 (IMX-BVN-1) is a neural-network classifier that can provide an assessment tool for suspected infected patients on admission (38). It can improve the recognition of bacterial and viral infections, reduce the overuse of antibiotics, block the progression of sepsis, and cut down the healthcare costs.

Critically ill patients in the ICU have an increased risk of infection due to their unique physiological changes, and various special pathogens in the environment can also increase their mortality. Due to various issues, the dosage of antibacterial agents in the ICU may become a tricky matter. These difficulties make the standard antimicrobial dosage regimen unable to achieve the goals related to optimal patient outcomes. In order to explore various ways to optimize the dosage of antibacterial drugs in ICU patients, novel dosing software using AI were developed to assist in the adjustment of antibiotic treatment, one of which was Bayesian forecasting. These plans can use the monitoring results of antibiotic treatment to further personalize the antibacterial program according to the clinical characteristics of each patient (39–42).

## OTHER APPLICATIONS OF AI IN SEPSIS

A study reported the practice results of using AI for quality improvement work. They introduced Sepsis Watch into the routine clinical care process, which is a sepsis detection and management platform based on deep learning (11). The purpose of Sepsis Watch is to improve the prediction and treatment of sepsis. It is formulated based on the quality improvement work report of a multidisciplinary team composed of statisticians, data scientists, data engineers and clinicians. The results show that it is feasible to integrate Sepsis Watch into routine clinical care, and the practice has also improved the implementation of local machine learning projects. Gonçalves et al. also reported the experience of applying AI algorithms in clinical practice, mainly introducing nurses' experience in early identification of sepsis through the use of technical tools developed by AI algorithms and its impact on the nursing work process (43). In the case introduced, the nurses participating in the process of technology integration can make rapid decisions in the early identification of sepsis.

Beginning in 2020, COVID-19 has spread all over the world, and infected patients have severe respiratory symptoms, and may have multiple complications such as severe acute respiratory syndrome, sepsis, septic shock and multiple organ failure. Effective ways to save cost and time are needed to mitigate the burden of disease. In order to seek potential treatments for COVID-19 among all existing drugs, a research combines systems biology and AI-based methods. By using the GUILDify v2.0 Web server as an alternative method, the effects of pirfenidone and melatonin on SARS-CoV-2 infection were confirmed. It also predicts the potential therapeutic effects of combination drugs on respiratory-related pathologies (44).

The pathogenic factors and processes of sepsis are complex and diverse. Its main feature is systemic inflammatory response. Severe Inflammatory Response Syndrome (SIRS) of non-infectious origin also has similar manifestations. Sepsis has a series of pathophysiological and genetic characteristics, which makes it difficult to distinguish from SIRS in clinical practice. This may be related to insufficient research on the key genes or pathways in the process of these diseases. Reasonable use of genetic biomarkers that are convenient for diagnostic tests/testing can make it possible to distinguish sepsis from SIRS. A team used previously published gene expression data sets, using two-tier gene screening, ANN data mining technology, and discovered biomarkers that can be used to identify and verify patients with SIRS, sepsis, and septic shock (45).

Causal AI can also be used to train and validate digital twin models, which can simulate critically ill patients and thus predict the response of sepsis patients to therapeutic interventions (46). The causal relationship between the organ system and a specific treatment is defined using a directed acyclic graph. The therapeutic effects and interactions of major organs at various stages are simulated using a hybrid method of agent-based modeling, discrete event simulation and Bayesian networks, which were visualized using relevant clinical markers. When the expected response simulated by the digital twin was compared with the actual patient response, it was found that the early treatment response of critical illness simulated by the AI model was very consistent with the patient's real response. The existence of a reliable digital twin model will allow clinicians to test the effects of interventions in a virtual environment before using them on real patients.

## THE SAFETY AND CHALLENGES OF USING AI IN SEPSIS

The potential of creating AI-based healthcare applications can match or exceed the ability of clinicians in specific diseases, such as sepsis. However, health care is a complex and ever-changing field with high requirements for safety. Any technical failure may cause harm to patients. When the AI system makes a decision, human clinicians and safety engineers essentially cannot control the process, and it is difficult to fully understand how the AI system accurately makes the decision. Compared with standard clinical practice, AI-based tools lack ethical constraints and safety regulations (47). The clinical setting of sepsis is very complex, and many variables (new therapies, new diagnoses, different intervention times and intervention methods) will affect the results. However, the requirements of all clinical settings shown in the computational model are difficult to achieve in the technical design stage (48). Therefore, the behavior of the software in the system may not adequately reflect appropriate clinical intentions. Currently, this problem is solved by ignoring some aspects of the process, such as by limiting the amount of information input, but it may lead to unintended consequences. One example is the loss of insensible fluid. It cannot be recorded electronically, which may cause the AI to prompt that more fluid needs to be refilled. However, in reality, the clinician sees that the patient has been waterlogged. In addition, when a machine interprets data, it cannot reason on the most important content like a human clinician. For example, clinicians may select to omit highly abnormal test results, which may be due to errors in sampling, testing, or recording.

In addition, there are problems in the AI model itself, for example, many studies have only trained and validated the model in the same patient cohort, but have not yet evaluated its generality to other populations. These models need to undergo further prospective testing to prove their benefits in clinical or other outcomes (49). AI will also face many implementation difficulties when used in clinical practice. Many organizations currently do not have sufficient conditions to implement AI in clinical practice, which requires considerable AI experts and mature information technology or IT capabilities, such as evaluation, merging, continuous monitoring, and recalibration of AI. The security and reliability of the collection and use of digital data also need to be addressed. Furthermore, most healthcare systems worldwide may not have enough capacity to successfully integrate AI into the current workflow. Decision-making and predictive models do not yet match the currently known healthcare systems, and a lot of improvements are needed to successfully integrate these innovations (50).

In short, there is still a big gap between the creation of AI algorithms and their implementation in clinical practice. AI cannot replace the clinical management role of experts in sepsis. AI-based algorithms should always be used as development tools until they can incorporate actions that are compatible with known physiology and prove that the results can be modified prospectively in multiple environments.

## AUTHOR CONTRIBUTIONS

MW, XD, and JW carried out the concepts, design, definition of intellectual content, literature search, data acquisition, and manuscript preparation. MW carried out literature search, data acquisition, and manuscript editing. XD, JW, and RG performed manuscript review, including revision of key technical content and English expression. All authors have read and approved the content of the manuscript.

## REFERENCES

1. Ocampo-Quintero N, Vidal-Cortés P, Del RCL, Fdez-Riverola F, Reboiro-Jato M, Glez-Peña D. Enhancing sepsis management through machine learning techniques: a review. *Med Intensiva.* (2020). doi: 10.1016/j.medin.2020.04.003. [Epub ahead of print].
2. Heming N, Azabou E, Cazaumayou X, Moine P, Annane D. Sepsis in the critically ill patient: current and emerging management strategies. *Expert Rev Anti-Infe.* (2020). doi: 10.1080/14787210.2021.1846522. [Epub ahead of print].
3. Komorowski M. Clinical management of sepsis can be improved by artificial intelligence: yes. *Intensive Care Med.* (2020) 46:375–7. doi: 10.1007/s00134-019-05898-2
4. Peiffer-Smadja N, Rawson TM, Ahmad R, Buchard A, Georgiou P, Lescure FX, et al. Machine learning for clinical decision support in infectious diseases: a narrative review of current applications. *Clin Microbiol Infect.* (2020) 26:584–95. doi: 10.1016/j.cmi.2019.09.009
5. Greco M, Caruso PF, Cecconi M. Artificial intelligence in the intensive care unit. *Semin Resp Crit Care.* (2021) 42:2–9. doi: 10.1055/s-0040-1719037
6. Wickramaratne SD, Shaad MM. Bi-directional gated recurrent unit based ensemble model for the early detection of sepsis. *Annu Int Conf IEEE Eng Med Biol Soc.* (2020) 2020:70–3. doi: 10.1109/EMBC44109.2020.9175223
7. Lee BT, Kwon OY, Park H, Cho KJ, Kwon JM, Lee Y. Graph convolutional networks-based noisy data imputation in electronic health record. *Crit Care Med.* (2020) 48:e1106–11. doi: 10.1097/CCM.0000000000004583
8. Kok C, Jahmunah V, Oh SL, Zhou X, Gururajan R, Tao X, et al. Automated prediction of sepsis using temporal convolutional network. *Comput Biol Med.* (2020) 127:103957. doi: 10.1016/j.compbiomed.2020.103957
9. Bedoya AD, Futoma J, Clement ME, Corey K, Brajer N, Lin A, et al. Machine learning for early detection of sepsis: an internal and temporal validation study. *JAMIA Open.* (2020) 3:252–60. doi: 10.1093/jamiaopen/ooaa006
10. Wernly B, Mamandipoor B, Baldia P, Jung C, Osmani V. Machine learning predicts mortality in septic patients using only routinely available ABG variables: a multi-centre evaluation. *Int J Med Inform.* (2021) 145:104312. doi: 10.1016/j.ijmedinf.2020.104312
11. Sendak MP, Ratliff W, Sarro D, Alderton E, Futoma J, Gao M, et al. Real-world integration of a sepsis deep learning technology into routine clinical care: implementation study. *JMIR Med Inform.* (2020) 8:e15182. doi: 10.2196/15182
12. Lauritsen SM, Kalør ME, Kongsgaard EL, Lauritsen KM, Jørgensen MJ, Lange J, et al. Early detection of sepsis utilizing deep learning on electronic health record event sequences. *Artif Intell Med.* (2020) 104:101820. doi: 10.1016/j.artmed.2020.101820
13. Mohammed A, Van Wyk F, Chinthala LK, Khojandi A, Davis RL, Coopersmith CM, et al. Temporal differential expression of physiomarkers predicts sepsis in critically ill adults. *Shock.* (2020). doi: 10.1097/SHK.0000000000001670. [Epub ahead of print].
14. Cooper PB, Hughes BJ, Verghese GM, Just JS, Markham AJ. Implementation of an automated sepsis screening tool in a community hospital setting. *J Nurs Care Qual.* (2021) 36:132–6. doi: 10.1097/NCQ.0000000000000501
15. Kam HJ, Kim HY. Learning representations for the early detection of sepsis with deep neural networks. *Comput Biol Med.* (2017) 89:248–55. doi: 10.1016/j.compbiomed.2017.08.015
16. Kaji DA, Zech JR, Kim JS, Cho SK, Dangayach NS, Costa AB, et al. An attention based deep learning model of clinical events in the intensive care unit. *PLoS ONE.* (2019) 14:e0211057. doi: 10.1371/journal.pone.0211057
17. Scherpf M, Gräßer F, Malberg H, Zaunseder S. Predicting sepsis with a recurrent neural network using the MIMIC III database. *Comput Biol Med.* (2019) 113:103395. doi: 10.1016/j.compbiomed.2019.103395
18. Saqib M, Sha Y, Wang MD. Early prediction of sepsis in EMR records using traditional ML techniques and deep learning LSTM networks. *Annu Int Conf IEEE Eng Med Biol Soc.* (2018) 2018:4038–41. doi: 10.1109/EMBC.2018.8513254
19. Yang M, Liu C, Wang X, Li Y, Gao H, Liu X, et al. An explainable artificial intelligence predictor for early detection of sepsis. *Crit Care Med.* (2020) 48:e1091–6. doi: 10.1097/CCM.0000000000004550
20. He Z, Du L, Zhang P, Zhao R, Chen X, Fang Z. Early sepsis prediction using ensemble learning with deep features and artificial features extracted from clinical electronic health records. *Crit Care Med.* (2020) 48:e1337–42. doi: 10.1097/CCM.0000000000004644
21. Misra D, Avula V, Wolk DM, Farag HA, Li J, Mehta YB, et al. Early detection of septic shock onset using interpretable machine learners. *J Clin Med.* (2021) 10:301. doi: 10.3390/jcm10020301
22. Wardi G, Carlile M, Holder A, Shashikumar S, Hayden SR, Nemati S. Predicting progression to septic shock in the emergency department using an externally generalizable machine-learning algorithm. *Ann Emerg Med.* (2021) 77:395–406. doi: 10.1101/2020.11.02.20224931

23. Helguera-Repetto AC, Soto-Ramírez MD, Villavicencio-Carrisoza O, Yong-Mendoza S, Yong-Mendoza A, León-Juárez M, et al. Neonatal sepsis diagnosis decision-making based on artificial neural networks. *Front Pediatr.* (2020) 8:525. doi: 10.3389/fped.2020.00525
24. Yuan KC, Tsai LW, Lee KH, Cheng YW, Hsu SC, Lo YS, et al. The development an artificial intelligence algorithm for early sepsis diagnosis in the intensive care unit. *Int J Med Inform.* (2020) 141:104176. doi: 10.1016/j.ijmedinf.2020.104176
25. Bloch E, Rotem T, Cohen J, Singer P, Aperstein Y. Machine learning models for analysis of vital signs dynamics: a case for sepsis onset prediction. *J Healthc Eng.* (2019) 2019:5930379. doi: 10.1155/2019/5930379
26. Liu R, Greenstein JL, Sarma SV, Winslow RL. Natural language processing of clinical notes for improved early prediction of septic shock in the ICU. *Annu Int Conf IEEE Eng Med Biol Soc.* (2019) 2019:6103–8. doi: 10.1109/EMBC.2019.8857819
27. Yee CR, Narain NR, Akmaev VR, Vemulapalli V. A data-driven approach to predicting septic shock in the intensive care unit. *Biomed Inform Insights.* (2019) 11:1178222619885147. doi: 10.1177/1178222619885147
28. Saria S, Henry KE. Too many definitions of sepsis: can machine learning leverage the electronic health record to increase accuracy and bring consensus? *Crit Care Med.* (2020) 48:137–41. doi: 10.1097/CCM.0000000000004144
29. Gunning S, Koyner JL. Not all sepsis-associated acute kidney injury is the same: there may be an app for that. *Clin J Am Soc Nephrol.* (2020) 15:1543–5. doi: 10.2215/CJN.14860920
30. Chaudhary K, Vaid A, Duffy Á, Paranjpe I, Jaladanki S, Paranjpe M, et al. Utilization of deep learning for subphenotype identification in sepsis-associated acute kidney injury. *Clin J Am Soc Nephrol.* (2020) 15:1557–65. doi: 10.2215/CJN.09330819
31. Ibrahim ZM, Wu H, Hamoud A, Stappen L, Dobson R, Agarossi A. On classifying sepsis heterogeneity in the ICU: insight using machine learning. *J Am Med Inform Assoc.* (2020) 27:437–43. doi: 10.1093/jamia/ocz211
32. Hasegawa D, Yamakawa K, Nishida K, Okada N, Murao S, Nishida O. Comparative analysis of three machine-learning techniques and conventional techniques for predicting sepsis-induced coagulopathy progression. *J Clin Med.* (2020) 9:2113. doi: 10.3390/jcm9072113
33. Rodríguez A, Mendoza D, Ascuntar J, Jaimes F. Supervised classification techniques for prediction of mortality in adult patients with sepsis. *Am J Emerg Med.* (2020). doi: 10.1016/j.ajem.2020.09.013. [Epub ahead of print].
34. Perng JW, Kao IH, Kung CT, Hung SC, Lai YH, Su CM. Mortality prediction of septic patients in the emergency department based on machine learning. *J Clin Med.* (2019) 8:1906. doi: 10.3390/jcm8111906
35. Bataille B, de Selle J, Moussot PE, Marty P, Silva S, Cocquet P. Machine learning methods to improve bedside fluid responsiveness prediction in severe sepsis or septic shock: an observational study. *Brit J Anaesth.* (2021) 126:826–34. doi: 10.1016/j.bja.2020.11.039
36. Shahn Z, Shapiro NI, Tyler PD, Talmor D, Lehman LH. Fluid-limiting treatment strategies among sepsis patients in the ICU: a retrospective causal analysis. *Crit Care.* (2020) 24:62. doi: 10.1186/s13054-020-2767-0
37. Delaveris SL, Cichetti JR, Edleblute E. 2019 John M. Eisenberg patient safety and quality awards: a model cell for transformational redesign of sepsis identification and treatment: aligning digital tools with innovative workflows. *Jt Comm J Qual Patient Saf.* (2020) 46:392–9. doi: 10.1016/j.jcjq.2020.04.001
38. Mayhew MB, Buturovic L, Luethy R, Midic U, Moore AR, Roque JA, et al. A generalizable 29-mRNA neural-network classifier for acute bacterial and viral infections. *Nat Commun.* (2020) 11:1177. doi: 10.1038/s41467-020-14975-w
39. Chai MG, Cotta MO, Abdul-Aziz MH, Roberts JA. What are the current approaches to optimising antimicrobial dosing in the intensive care unit? *Pharmaceutics.* (2020) 12:638. doi: 10.3390/pharmaceutics12070638
40. Rawson TM, Hernandez B, Moore L, Herrero P, Charani E, Ming D, et al. A real-world evaluation of a Case-Based Reasoning algorithm to support antimicrobial prescribing decisions in acute care. *Clin Infect Dis.* (2020). doi: 10.1093/cid/ciaa383. [Epub ahead of print].
41. Roggeveen LF, Fleuren LM, Guo T, Thoral P, de Grooth HJ, Swart EL, et al. Right Dose Right Now: bedside data-driven personalized antibiotic dosing in severe sepsis and septic shock - rationale and design of a multicenter randomized controlled superiority trial. *Trials.* (2019) 20:745. doi: 10.1186/s13063-019-3911-5
42. Voermans AM, Mewes JC, Broyles MR, Steuten L. Cost-effectiveness analysis of a procalcitonin-guided decision algorithm for antibiotic stewardship using real-world U.S. hospital data. *Omics.* (2019) 23:508–15. doi: 10.1089/omi.2019.0113
43. Gonçalves LS, Amaro M, Romero A, Schamne FK, Fressatto JL, Bezerra CW. Implementation of an artificial intelligence algorithm for sepsis detection. *Rev Bras Enferm.* (2020) 73:e20180421. doi: 10.1590/0034-7167-2018-0421
44. Artigas L, Coma M, Matos-Filipe P, Aguirre-Plans J, Farrés J, Valls R, et al. In-silico drug repurposing study predicts the combination of pirfenidone and melatonin as a promising candidate therapy to reduce SARS-CoV-2 infection progression and respiratory distress caused by cytokine storm. *PLoS ONE.* (2020) 15:e0240149. doi: 10.1371/journal.pone.0240149
45. Tong DL, Kempsell KE, Szakmany T, Ball G. Development of a bioinformatics framework for identification and validation of genomic biomarkers and key immunopathology processes and controllers in infectious and non-infectious severe inflammatory response syndrome. *Front Immunol.* (2020) 11:380. doi: 10.3389/fimmu.2020.00380
46. Lal A, Li G, Cubro E, Chalmers S, Li H, Herasevich V, et al. Development and verification of a digital twin patient model to predict specific treatment response during the first 24 hours of sepsis. *Crit Care Explor.* (2020) 2:e0249. doi: 10.1097/CCE.0000000000000249
47. Habli I, Lawton T, Porter Z. Artificial intelligence in health care: accountability and safety. *Bull World Health Organ.* (2020) 98:251–6. doi: 10.2471/BLT.19.237487
48. Garnacho-Montero J, Martín-Loeches I. Clinical management of sepsis can be improved by artificial intelligence: no. *Intensive Care Med.* (2020) 46:378–80. doi: 10.1007/s00134-020-05947-1
49. Schinkel M, Paranjape K, Nannan PR, Skyttberg N, Nanayakkara P. Clinical applications of artificial intelligence in sepsis: a narrative review. *Comput Biol Med.* (2019) 115:103488. doi: 10.1016/j.compbiomed.2019.103488
50. Mlodzinski E, Stone DJ, Celi LA. Machine learning for pulmonary and critical care medicine: a narrative review. *Pulm Ther.* (2020) 6:67–77. doi: 10.1007/s41030-020-00110-z

# 7

# A Machine-Learning Approach for Dynamic Prediction of Sepsis-Induced Coagulopathy in Critically Ill Patients with Sepsis

*Qin-Yu Zhao [1,2†], Le-Ping Liu [1†], Jing-Chao Luo [3†], Yan-Wei Luo [1], Huan Wang [3], Yi-Jie Zhang [3], Rong Gui [1*], Guo-Wei Tu [3*] and Zhe Luo [3,4*]*

*[1] Department of Blood Transfusion, The Third Xiangya Hospital of Central South University, Changsha, China, [2] College of Engineering and Computer Science, Australian National University, Canberra, ACT, Australia, [3] Department of Critical Care Medicine, Zhongshan Hospital, Fudan University, Shanghai, China, [4] Department of Critical Care Medicine, Xiamen Branch, Zhongshan Hospital, Fudan University, Xiamen, China*

***Correspondence:**
*Rong Gui*
*aguirong@163.com*
*Guo-Wei Tu*
*tu.guowei@zs-hospital.sh.cn*
*Zhe Luo*
*luo.zhe@zs-hospital.sh.cn*

*† These authors have contributed equally to this work and share first authorship*

**Background:** Sepsis-induced coagulopathy (SIC) denotes an increased mortality rate and poorer prognosis in septic patients.

**Objectives:** Our study aimed to develop and validate machine-learning models to dynamically predict the risk of SIC in critically ill patients with sepsis.

**Methods:** Machine-learning models were developed and validated based on two public databases named Medical Information Mart for Intensive Care (MIMIC)-IV and the eICU Collaborative Research Database (eICU-CRD). Dynamic prediction of SIC involved an evaluation of the risk of SIC each day after the diagnosis of sepsis using 15 predictive models. The best model was selected based on its accuracy and area under the receiver operating characteristic curve (AUC), followed by fine-grained hyperparameter adjustment using the Bayesian Optimization Algorithm. A compact model was developed, based on 15 features selected according to their importance and clinical availability. These two models were compared with Logistic Regression and SIC scores in terms of SIC prediction.

**Results:** Of 11,362 patients in MIMIC-IV included in the final cohort, a total of 6,744 (59%) patients developed SIC during sepsis. The model named Categorical Boosting (CatBoost) had the greatest AUC in our study (0.869; 95% CI: 0.850–0.886). Coagulation profile and renal function indicators were the most important features for predicting SIC. A compact model was developed with an AUC of 0.854 (95% CI: 0.832–0.872), while the AUCs of Logistic Regression and SIC scores were 0.746 (95% CI: 0.735–0.755) and 0.709 (95% CI: 0.687–0.733), respectively. A cohort of 35,252 septic patients in eICU-CRD was analyzed. The AUCs of the full and the compact models in the external validation were 0.842 (95% CI: 0.837–0.846) and 0.803 (95% CI: 0.798–0.809), respectively, which were still larger than those of Logistic Regression (0.660; 95% CI: 0.653–0.667) and SIC scores (0.752; 95% CI: 0.747–0.757). Prediction results were illustrated by SHapley Additive exPlanations (SHAP) values, which made our models clinically interpretable.

**Conclusions:** We developed two models which were able to dynamically predict the risk of SIC in septic patients better than conventional Logistic Regression and SIC scores.

**Keywords: sepsis-induced coagulopathy, dynamic prediction, machine learning, Logistic Regression, external validation, model interpretation**

## INTRODUCTION

Sepsis, defined as life-threatening organ dysfunction caused by a dysregulated host response to infection, remains the first leading cause of mortality in critically ill patients (1, 2). Coagulopathy is one of the major complications of sepsis, leading to a higher risk of thrombosis, the deterioration of organ failure, and an increased mortality rate (3–6). However, the usefulness of anticoagulant therapies has not been confirmed in septic patients (7, 8). Recent observational studies and subgroup analyses of large-scale randomized controlled trials revealed that anticoagulant therapies might result in a significant reduction in mortality risk and improved outcome in septic patients with coagulopathy (9–12). In contrast, anticoagulant therapies in patients without coagulopathy should be avoided due to the increased risk of bleeding with no survival benefit (11, 13). Furthermore, some drugs commonly administered in septic patients, such as linezolid and vancomycin, may alter coagulation function through various mechanisms and should be used with caution in patients with a high risk of coagulopathy (14). These study results have heightened the need for early identification of coagulopathy in septic patients in a timely way.

Sepsis-induced coagulopathy (SIC) criteria were developed by members of the Scientific and Standardization Committee (SSC) on Disseminated Intravascular Coagulation (DIC) of the International Society of Thrombosis and Haemostasis (ISTH) in 2017 (15) (**Supplementary Table 1**). The criteria are a scoring system designed to identify patients with "sepsis and coagulation disorders." SIC is defined as a score $\geq$ 4. It was found that the mortality rate increased as the SIC score rose and exceeded 30% at a score of 4 (15). Compared with DIC, SIC is more relevant for the updated Sepsis-3 criteria (1, 16). In addition, observational evidence has shown that SIC preceded DIC in most cases (17, 18). As a result, the new guideline in 2019 recommended that septic patients with thrombocytopenia (platelet count $< 150 \times 10^9$/L) should be screened, first using SIC diagnostic criteria and then using ISTH DIC diagnostic criteria (16). However, the SIC score mainly serves as a diagnostic system; there is still a lack of reliable predictive tools for SIC in clinical practice.

In recent years, the emergence of new machine-learning algorithms has enabled us to predict disease events dynamically based on huge and complicated clinical information. Advanced machine-learning models can fit high-order relationships between covariates and outcomes, and therefore, they excel in the analysis of complex signals in data-rich environments (19–22). The aims of this study were to develop and validate to develop and validate machine-learning models for the early dynamic prediction of SIC, and to assess the risk features by interpreting the final model.

## MATERIALS AND METHODS

### Source of Data

We conducted this retrospective study based on two sizeable critical care databases the Medical Information Mart for Intensive Care (MIMIC)-IV (23) and the eICU Collaborative Research Database (eICU-CRD) (24). The MIMIC-IV database is an updated version of MIMIC-III and currently contains comprehensive and high-quality data of patients admitted to intensive care units (ICUs) at the Beth Israel Deaconess Medical Center between 2008 and 2019. The other database, eICU-CRD, is a multicenter database comprising de-identified health data associated with over 200,000 admissions to ICUs across the United States between 2014 and 2015. One author (QZ) obtained access to both databases and was responsible for data extraction. The study was reported according to the recommendations of the Transparent Reporting of a multivariable prediction model for Individual Prognosis Or Diagnosis (TRIPOD) statement (25).

### Selection of Participants

In MIMIC-IV, patients who fulfilled the definition of sepsis between 2008 and 2019 were included. According to the Sepsis-3 criteria, sepsis was defined as a suspected infection combined with an acute increase in Sequential Organ Failure Assessment (SOFA) score $\geq$ 2 (1). Patients with prescriptions of antibiotics and sampling of bodily fluids for microbiological culture were considered to have suspected infection. In line with previous research, when the antibiotic was given first, the microbiological sample must have been collected within 24 h; when the microbiological sampling occurred first, the antibiotic must have been administered within 72 h (26). Hourly SOFA was evaluated based on the clinical and laboratory data. In eICU-CRD, microbiology data were not well populated due to the limited availability of microbiology interfaces; instead, infection was identified according to documented diagnosis.

Only patients who were older than 18 years and stayed in the ICU for more than 24 h were included. No patients were excluded due to missing values. We made no attempt to estimate the sample size of the study; instead, all eligible patients in MIMIC-IV and eICU-CRD were included to maximize the statistical power of the predictive model.

### Outcome (SIC)

We annotated patients' every day when the sepsis definition was fulfilled with their current coagulation state according to the SIC criteria, as recommended (16). Specifically, the worst daily values of SIC-related indicators were extracted. Then daily repeated scoring was performed. A patient was annotated as SIC positive if he or she had a SIC score $\geq 4$ on that day.

## Predictors of SIC

Clinical and laboratory variables were extracted during sepsis. For some variables with multiple measurements, average values were assessed. For the prediction of SIC, 88 variables were collected (**Supplementary Table 2**), including patient characteristics (age, gender, ethnicity, admission type), vital signs (respiratory rate, blood pressure, heart rate, $SpO_2$, and temperature), laboratory data (blood gas, routine blood analysis, liver function, renal function, and coagulation profile), transfusion (red blood cells, platelets, and fresh frozen plasma) and urine output. Comorbidities were also collected based on the recorded International Classification of Diseases (ICD)-9 and ICD-10 codes, including hypertension, diabetes mellitus, chronic obstructive pulmonary disease, congestive heart failure, myocardial infarction, chronic kidney disease, leukemia, stroke, cancer, and liver disease. Lastly, medications such as heparin, antibiotics and vasopressors, continuous renal replacement therapy (CRRT), and mechanical ventilation (MV) were collected.

## Statistical Analysis

Baseline characteristics on the first sepsis day were compared between SIC and non-SIC groups in MIMIC-IV. Values are presented as the means [standard deviations] (if normal) or medians [interquartile ranges] (if non-normal) for continuous variables, and total numbers [percentages] for categorical variables. Comparisons were made using the Student *t*-test or rank-sum test for continuous variables, and the Chi-square test or Fisher's exact test for categorical variables, as appropriate.

As shown in **Figure 1A**, our model generated a continuous prediction score based on the above-mentioned 88 variables on each day when patients were diagnosed with sepsis. The scores assessed the risk of SIC in the following day. Prediction was not performed if SIC criteria were already fulfilled on that day; when the patients recovered from SIC, our model then restarted to predict if they still had sepsis. None of the imputation methods were used for advanced boosting machine-learning methods as they automatically handle missing values; in contrast, missing values were imputed using the median values for continuous variables or mode values for categorical values when training other models. As shown in **Figure 1B**, we preliminarily compared the prediction performance of 15

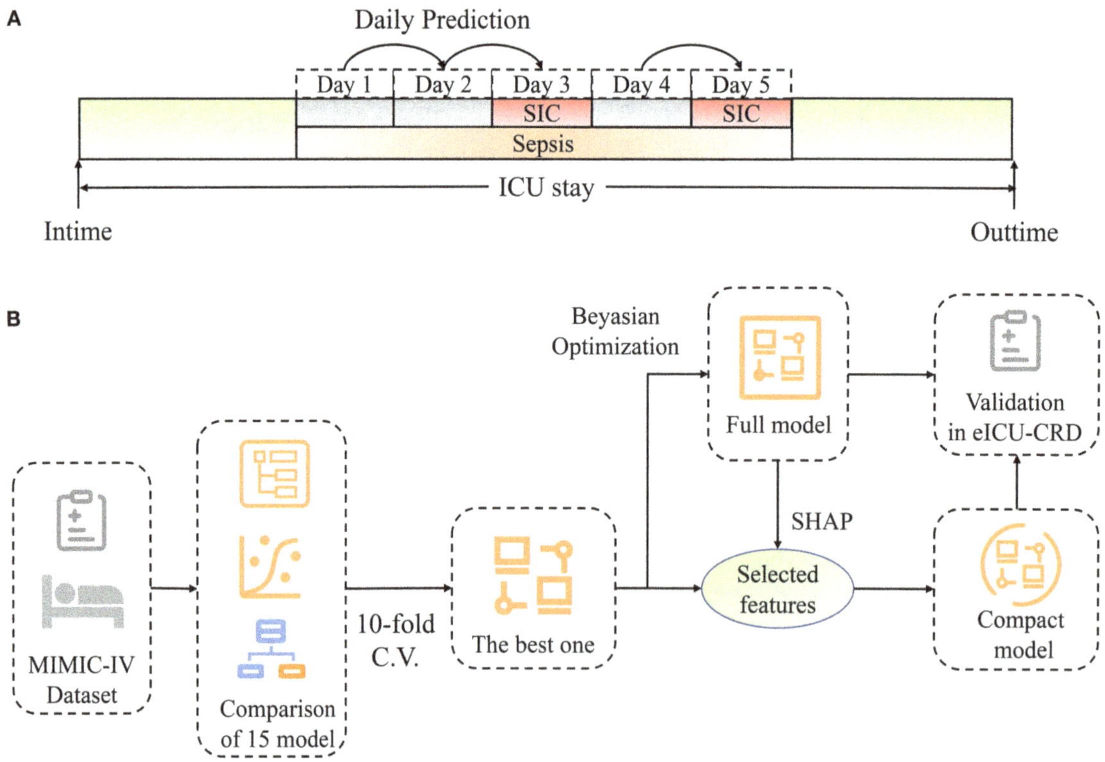


**FIGURE 1 |** Schematic illustration of the study design. **(A)** Design of dynamic prediction in our study. Daily assessment was performed from the time when sepsis was diagnosed. If SIC criteria were not fulfilled, the risk of SIC the next day was predicted by our model. Prediction stopped when SIC was diagnosed, and restarted when patients recovered from SIC. **(B)** Schematic illustration of model development. We compared the discrimination of 15 machine-learning models using 10-fold cross-validation. The model with the best accuracy and greatest AUC was chosen. Fine-grained hyperparameter adjustment was performed using Bayesian Optimization. Fifteen features were selected according to their SHAP values and clinical availability. A compact model was developed based on the selected features. Lastly, these two models were validated in eICU-CRD. ICU, intensive care unit; SIC, sepsis-induced coagulopathy; SHAP, SHapley Additive exPlanations; MIMIC-IV, Medical Information Mart for Intensive Care-IV; C.V., cross-validation; eICU-CRD, the eICU Collaborative Research Database.

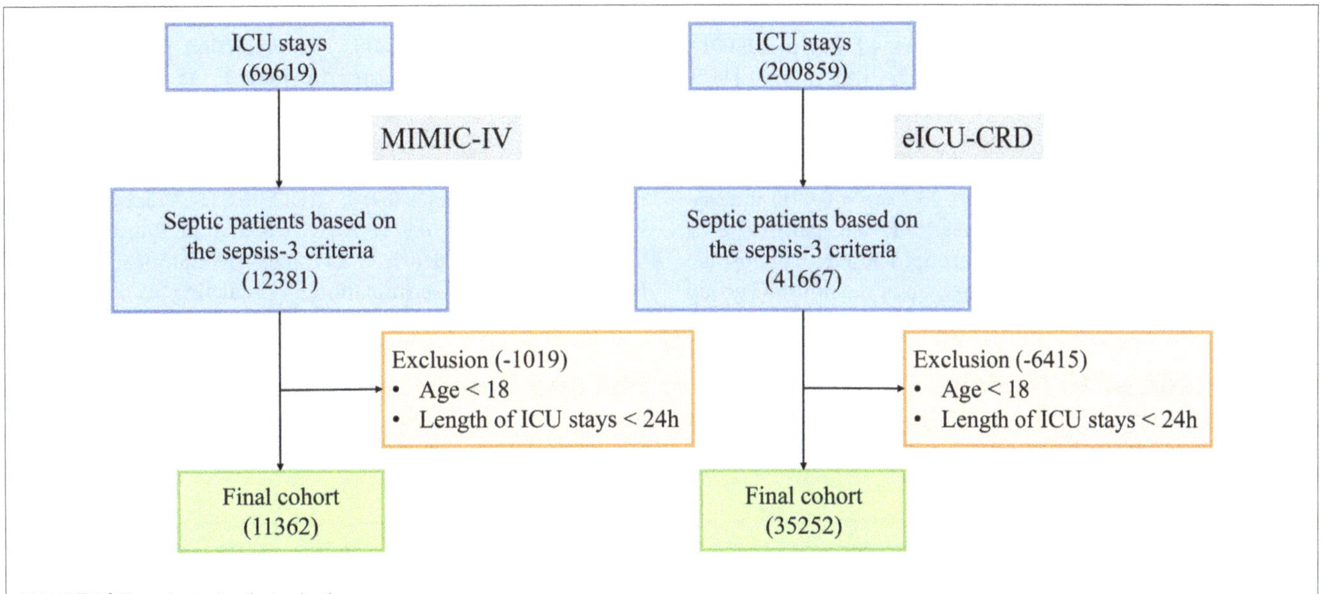


**FIGURE 2** | Flow chart of patient selection.

algorithms using the *PyCaret* Python package (version 1.0.0), an open-sourced, automated machine-learning workflow. The assessment process was performed using 10-fold cross-validation. Accuracy and area under the receiver operating characteristic curve (AUC) were calculated on each fold and pooled to evaluate each model. The algorithm with the highest accuracy and the largest AUC was selected. Then, we performed fine-grained hyperparameter adjustment for the potential model using the Bayesian Optimization Algorithm. This algorithm is an efficient constrained global optimization tool, which was performed using the functions of the *bayes_opt* Python package (version 1.2.0) (27). The optimized model was the best model for SIC prediction in this study and was defined as the full model.

The effects of features on prediction scores were measured using the functions of the *SHapley Additive exPlanations (SHAP)* Python package (version 0.32.1), which assessed the importance of each feature using a game-theoretic approach based on the validation set (28). We selected 15 features which had great importance and were as easy as possible to collect in the clinical setting (**Supplementary Table 2**). A compact model was then trained for SIC prediction based on the selected features. Although this model was not as accurate as the full model, it might be more practical in clinical settings.

External validation of the full and compact models was performed in eICU-CRD. The median and 95% confidence intervals of AUC were calculated using the Bootstrap Resampling technique with 1,000 iterations. Conventional Logistic Regression and the SIC scoring system were assessed to predict the risk of SIC and were compared with our models in both internal and external validations.

All analyses were performed using Python (version 3.7.6), and $p < 0.01$ was considered statistically significant.

**TABLE 1** | Performance of different models in internal validation.

| | Model | Accuracy | AUC |
|---|---|---|---|
| 1 | CatBoost Classifier | 0.913 (±0.004) | 0.841 (±0.025) |
| 2 | Light Gradient Boosting | 0.912 (±0.005) | 0.835 (±0.024) |
| 3 | Extreme Gradient Boosting | 0.912 (±0.004) | 0.837 (±0.025) |
| 4 | Gradient Boosting Classifier | 0.911 (±0.005) | 0.832 (±0.023) |
| 5 | Extra Trees Classifier | 0.911 (±0.002) | 0.819 (±0.032) |
| 6 | Random Forest Classifier | 0.909 (±0.002) | 0.760 (±0.022) |
| 7 | Ridge Classifier | 0.908 (±0.003) | 0.753 (±0.031) |
| 8 | Logistic Regression | 0.908 (±0.002) | 0.746 (±0.030) |
| 9 | K Neighbors Classifier | 0.904 (±0.001) | 0.611 (±0.040) |
| 10 | Ada Boost Classifier | 0.902 (±0.003) | 0.804 (±0.029) |
| 11 | Linear Discriminant Analysis | 0.902 (±0.003) | 0.796 (±0.027) |
| 12 | Multi-Level Perceptron | 0.883 (±0.004) | 0.754 (±0.022) |
| 13 | Decision Tree Classifier | 0.861 (±0.003) | 0.593 (±0.019) |
| 14 | SVM – RBF Kernel | 0.859 (±0.004) | 0.777 (±0.015) |
| 15 | Naive Bayes | 0.805 (±0.005) | 0.756 (±0.031) |

*Models are ordered according to their accuracy.*
*AUC, area under receiver operating characteristic curve; CatBoost, Categorical Boosting; SVM, support vector machine; RBF, Radial Basis Function.*

# RESULTS

## Baseline Characteristics

As shown in **Figure 2**, of 12,381 septic patients in MIMIC-IV, 11,362 were included in the final cohort. A total of 6,744 patients developed SIC during sepsis, and 4,618 patients did not. A cohort of 35,252 septic patients in eICU-CRD was included as external dataset.

Variable values on the first day of sepsis in MIMIC-IV were analyzed; the differences in characteristics were compared (**Supplementary Table 3**). The SIC group had a higher rate of comorbidities, higher SAPS-II scores (44 [35, 54] vs. 37 [30, 45]; $p < 0.001$), higher SOFA scores (6 [4, 9] vs. 4 [3, 5]; $p < 0.001$), longer prothrombin time (PT) (16.9 [14.3, 21.8] vs. 13.0 [11.9, 14.1]; $p < 0.001$), less urine output (790 [300, 1,545] vs. 1,205 [605, 2,015]; $p < 0.001$), higher rates of linezolid (2.9 vs. 1.7%; $p < 0.001$), vancomycin (55.6 vs. 46.0%; $p < 0.001$), CRRT (5.0 vs. 0.6%; $p < 0.001$), vasopressors (46.8 vs. 23.2%; $p < 0.001$) and MV (50.3 vs. 40.6%; $p < 0.001$), and higher 28-day mortality (27.0 vs. 10.8%; $p < 0.001$) than the non-SIC group. The length of hospital stay was also longer in the SIC group than in the non-SIC group (14.4 [7.9, 26.7] vs. 10.9 [6.5, 19.5], $p < 0.001$).

## Comparison of 15 Models

Daily data were extracted, and 16,183 samples for prediction in MIMIC-IV were created. Of these samples, 1,489 were labeled as positive (SIC the next day), 14,694 were labeled as negative (still non-SIC the next day). The prediction performances of the various models are listed in **Table 1**. As shown, Logistic Regression had an acceptable performance (accuracy: 0.908; AUC: 0.746). Ensemble learning algorithms had better accuracy and larger AUC than others, such as Categorical Boosting (CatBoost) (accuracy: 0.913; AUC: 0.841), Light Gradient Boosting (accuracy: 0.912; AUC: 0.835) and Random Forest Classifier (accuracy: 0.909; AUC: 0.760). The CatBoost model had the most powerful discrimination for predicting SIC risk, and we optimized this model in the next step.

## Full and Compact Models

Fifteen iterations of Bayesian optimization were performed. The hyperparameter search domains and final settings are listed in

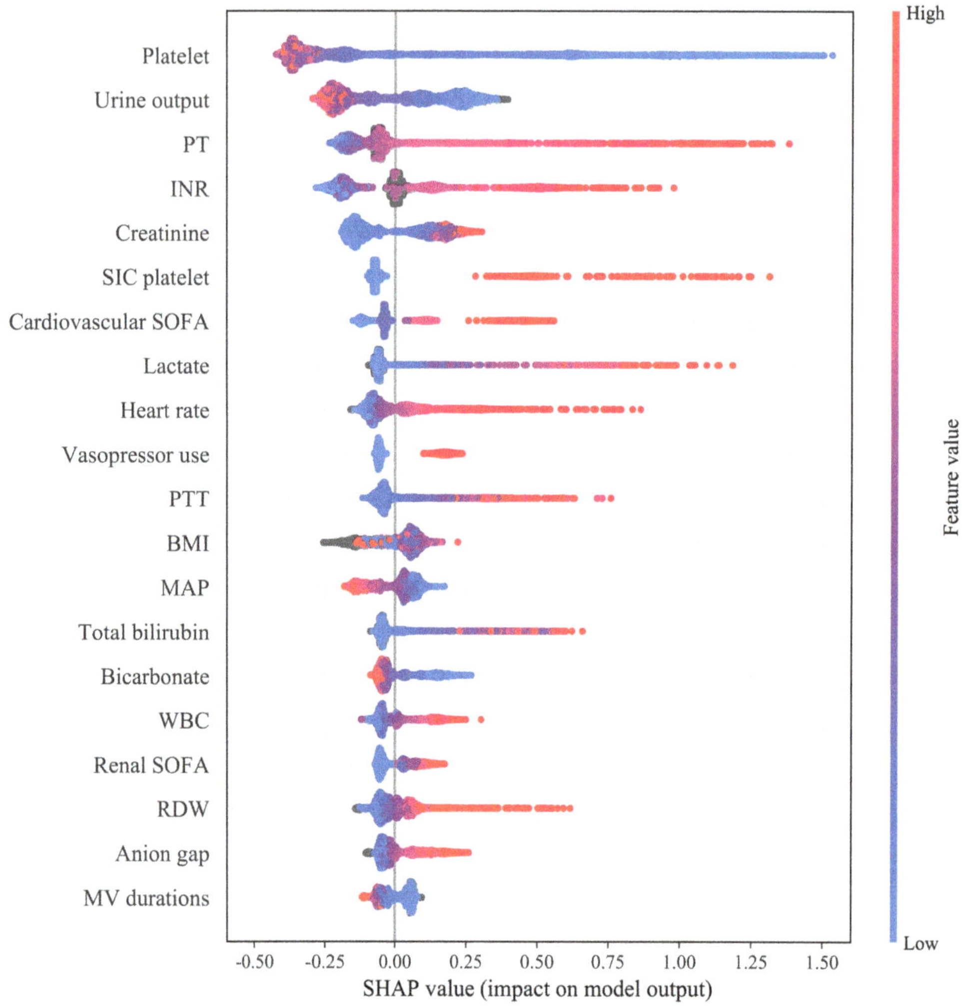


**FIGURE 3 |** Distribution of the impact each feature had on the full model output estimated using the SHapley Additive exPlanations (SHAP) values. The plot sorts features by the sum of SHAP value magnitudes over all samples. The color represents the feature value (red high, blue low). The x axis measures the impact on the model output (right positive, left negative). Taking the feature platelet as an example, red points are on the left whereas blue points are on the right. This means prediction scores will be smaller when patients have a low level of platelets. PT, prothrombin time; INR, international normalized ratio; SIC, sepsis-induced coagulopathy; SIC platelet, platelet term in the SIC score; SOFA, sequential organ failure assessment; PTT, Partial Thromboplastin Time; BMI, body mass index; MAP, mean arterial pressure; WBC, white blood cell count; RDW, red cell distribution width; MV, mechanical ventilation.

**Supplementary Table 4**. The optimized CatBoost model had the greatest AUC in our study (0.869; 95% CI: 0.850–0.886). SHAP values were calculated and are plotted in **Figure 3**. The summary plot sorts features by the sum of SHAP value magnitudes over all samples and shows the distribution of the impact that each feature has on the full model output. As shown, the coagulation profile (platelet, International Normalized Ratio, PT) and renal function indicators (urine output, creatinine) are the most important features for distinguishing the SIC and non-SIC groups. Fifteen features were selected based on their SHAP values and clinical availability. The compact CatBoost model was built based on the selected features. It had a slightly smaller AUC (0.854; 95% CI: 0.832–0.872), but is considered more practical in clinical practice. The medians and 95% confidence intervals of AUCs are plotted in **Figure 4** to compare the discrimination of different methods in MIMIC-IV. As shown, our two models outperformed conventional Logistic Regression (0.746; 95% CI: 0.735–0.755) and the SIC scoring system (0.709; 95% CI: 0.687–0.733) in terms of SIC prediction.

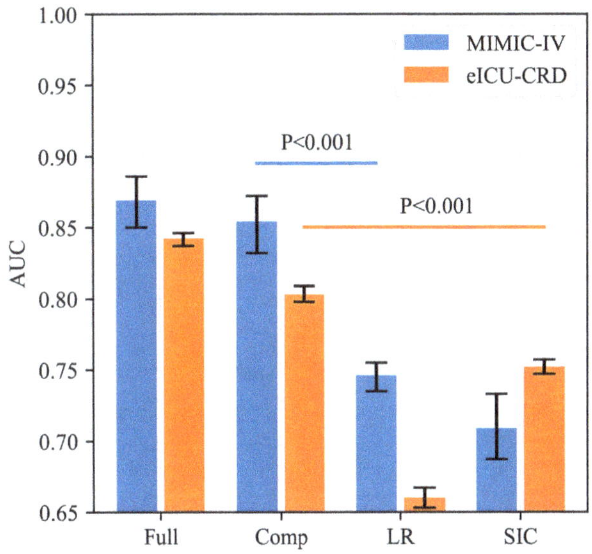


**FIGURE 4** | AUCs of four predictive methods in internal (MIMIC-IV) and external (eICU-CRD) validations. AUCs of our two models, Logistic Regression and SIC scores were assessed using the Bootstrap Resampling technique with 1,000 iterations. The heights of the bars represent the median AUCs, while the error bars represent the 95% confidence intervals. Full, the full model; Comp, the compact model; LR, Logistic Regression; SIC, the sepsis-induced coagulopathy criteria; AUC, area under receiver operating characteristic curve; MIMIC-IV, Medical Information Mart for Intensive Care-IV; eICU-CRD, the eICU Collaborative Research Database.

## Prediction Performance in eICU-CRD

The results of external validation are shown in **Figure 4** ([0.842; 95% CI: 0.837–0.846] for the full model, and [0.803; 95% CI: 0.798–0.809] for the compact model). It can be seen that the SIC scoring system had better predictive power (0.752; 95% CI: 0.747–0.757) than in MIMIC-IV but its AUC was still worse than those of our two models ($p < 0.001$), while Logistic Regression had the poorest generalization ability (0.660; 95% CI: 0.653–0.667). The sensitivity and specificity analysis of the four predictive methods is summarized in **Table 2**.

Model performance in different patient cohorts in eICU-CRD is shown in **Figure 5**. As shown, the two models had the greatest AUC for patients who had APACHE-IV scores between 81 and 100, who were younger than 65 years, or who were admitted to the NICU and SICU. The two models maintained good performance over four regions of the United States. In addition, the two models had better discrimination when sepsis lasted for several days. A similar sub-cohort analysis was also performed in MIMIC-IV (**Supplementary Figure 1**).

## Model Interpretation

The summary plot of SHAP in **Figure 3** provides an overview of the impact of features on the final models. Additionally, the prediction results of two specific instances are explained in **Figure 6**. The bars in red and blue represent risk factors and protective factors, respectively; longer bars represent greater feature importance. For the example in **Figure 6A**, although the patient's coagulation profile was normal, she had a poor circulatory status with a high serum lactate level and the vasopressor administration. The model successfully predicted that she would have SIC the next day. For the example in **Figure 6B**, the patient's condition was more moderate, and our model predicted a low-risk value.

## Website-Based Tool

A website-based tool was established for clinicians to use the compact model, http://www.aimedicallab.com/tool/aiml-sicrisk.html. The SIC risk in the following day can be assessed by using this tool, and interpretation of the prediction result in the instance level will be shown to the user.

## DISCUSSION

To the best of our knowledge, this is first attempt to apply machine-learning models for the dynamic prediction of SIC. Our study developed and validated two variants of dynamic machine-learning models, providing an accurate predictive tool for SIC in sepsis patients.

In this study, we reconfirmed that coagulopathy worsens the clinical outcomes of septic patients (15). As shown in **Supplementary Table 3**, SIC can lead to a higher mortality rate and longer length of hospital/ICU stay. In addition, SIC patients received more advanced antibiotics (linezolid and vancomycin), implying a more severe state of infection. On the other hand, the administration of these drugs may also alter coagulation function through various mechanisms (29, 30). As a result, early identification of septic patients with high coagulopathy risks is of great importance.

Currently, there is a lack of reliable tools for the early prediction of coagulopathy in septic patients. Our study demonstrated that the family of gradient boosting algorithms,

**TABLE 2** | Performance of the final models and SIC scores in internal and external validations.

| | Internal validation (MIMIC-IV) | | | | External validation (eICU-CRD) | | | |
|---|---|---|---|---|---|---|---|---|
| **Model** | **AUC** | **Youden** | **Sensitivity** | **Specificity** | **AUC** | **Youden** | **Sensitivity** | **Specificity** |
| The full model | 0.869 | 0.577 | 0.820 | 0.757 | 0.842 | 0.54 | 0.8 | 0.741 |
| The compact model | 0.854 | 0.564 | 0.848 | 0.716 | 0.803 | 0.477 | 0.745 | 0.732 |
| Logistic Regression | 0.746 | 0.433 | 0.753 | 0.680 | 0.660 | 0.230 | 0.582 | 0.648 |
| SIC scores | 0.709 | 0.368 | 0.707 | 0.661 | 0.752 | 0.448 | 0.655 | 0.793 |

*The discrimination of three models (the full model, the compact model and Logistic Regression) and SIC scores were compared in internal and external validations. The full and the compact models were developed in MIMIC-IV, based on all or selected features, respectively. Logistic Regression was developed based on all features. In addition, the current SIC score was used to predict patient's SIC risk the next day. Youden Index, defined as Sensitivity + Specificity − 1, and AUC assessed the performance of different models. All statistics were the median values in 1,000 iterations of the Bootstrap Resampling technique.*

*SIC, Sepsis-induced coagulopathy; AUC, area under receiver operating characteristic curve; MIMIC, Medical Information Mart for Intensive Care; eICU-CRD, the eICU Collaborative Research Database.*

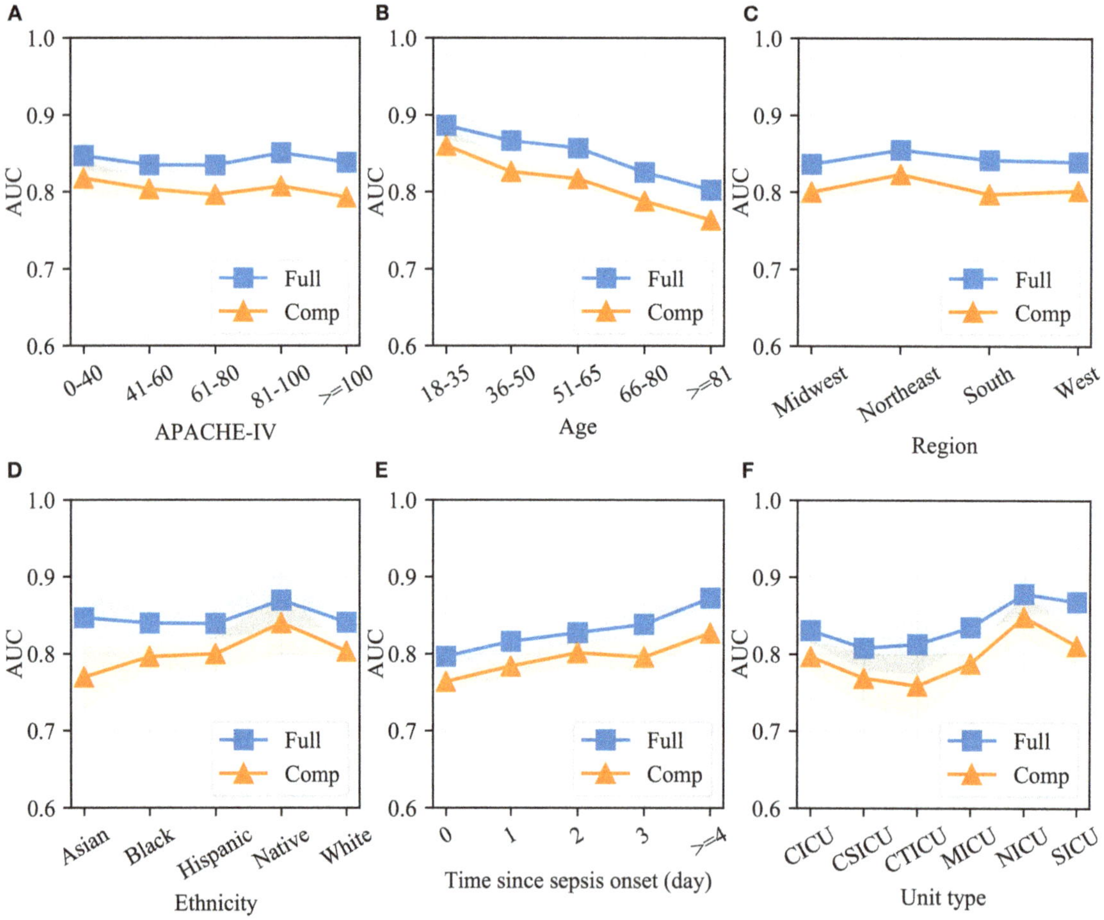


**FIGURE 5** | Model performance in different patient cohorts in eICU-CRD. Different validation sets were derived based on APACHE-IV **(A)**, age **(B)**, region of the United States **(C)**, ethnicity **(D)**, time since sepsis onset **(E)** and unit type **(F)**. AUC of the full and the compact models in each set was measured using the Bootstrap Resampling technique. The colored area represents 95% confidence intervals. Full, the full model; Comp, the compact model; AUC, area under receiver operating characteristic curve; APACHE-IV, Acute Physiology and Chronic Health Evaluation-IV; CICU, cardiac intensive care unit; CSICU, cardiac surgical intensive care unit; CTICU, cardiothoracic intensive care unit; MICU, medical intensive care unit; NICU, neuro intensive care unit; SICU, surgical intensive care unit.

such as CatBoost, Light Gradient Boosting and Extreme Gradient Boosting, can predict SIC with higher accuracy than others. In short, gradient boosting is a powerful machine-learning technique that iteratively trains a weak classifier (e.g., decision tree) to fit residuals of previous models (31). CatBoost, one of gradient boosting algorithms, showed the greatest AUC in our study, partly because it had two main advantages. First, it successfully handles categorical features and deals with them

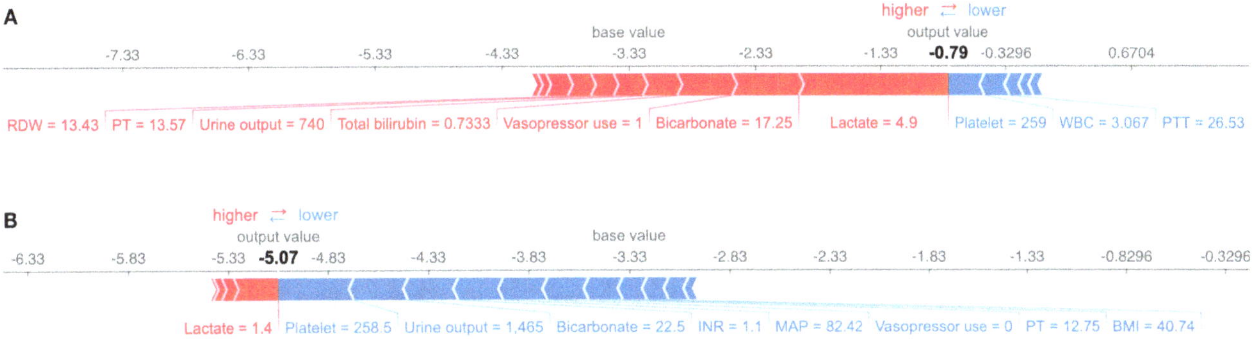


**FIGURE 6 |** Explanation of the prediction results for specific instances. The base value (−3.33) is the average value of the predictive model; the output values are the predicted SIC risks. The bars in red and blue represent risk factors and protective factors, respectively; longer bars mean greater feature importance. Here, these values are the model outputs before the SoftMax layer, and therefore, they are not equal to the final predicted probabilities. This figure shows the explanation for a high-risk instance **(A)** and a low-risk instance **(B)**. RDW, red cell distribution width; PT, prothrombin time; WBC, white blood cell count; PTT, Partial Thromboplastin Time; INR, international normalized ratio; MAP, mean arterial pressure; BMI, body mass index.

during training instead of preprocessing time (32). This means that categorical features no longer need to be encoded, and a CatBoost model can be developed based on raw data. Another advantage of this algorithm is that it uses a new schema to calculate leaf values when selecting the tree structure. The schema helps to reduce overfitting, a major problem that constrains the generalization ability of machine-learning models (32).

In this study, we developed two variants of CatBoost models that can identify patients with a high risk of SIC and provide clinical decision-makers with more information. As shown in **Figure 5**, our models had comparable AUCs in different patient cohorts, demonstrating that machine-learning models based on big data have good generalization capability.

In general, based on more valuable variables, models have better discrimination but worse clinical usability. Therefore, in our study, two model variants were developed for different application scenarios. The full model predicted SIC based on 88 clinical variables and achieved the highest AUC in this study. In the external validation, the full model maintained good discrimination with only a slight reduction in AUC. However, it is difficult to collect 88 variables and apply this model. As a result, the full model is recommended in hospitals with a well-designed clinical data system. By contrast, the compact model was trained based on 15 selected variables. Under the condition of ensuring accuracy, it achieved practicality as far as possible. In addition, a website tool was developed to help clinicians use the compact model in clinical practice. By logging on to the website and entering the values of 15 variables, our compact model will give the prediction result, and interpretation of the prediction result will be shown to the user.

By interpreting the full model, it was found that many clinical variables can help to indicate the risk of SIC. In this study, coagulopathy profile was found to be the most important variable in predicting SIC followed by renal function indicators (urine output and creatinine). As shown in **Figure 3**, patients with poorer renal function (less urine output and higher serum creatinine) tended to have a higher risk of SIC. Also, body mass index (BMI), vital signs (heart rate and mean arterial pressure), laboratory tests (such as lactate and white blood cell count), the use of MV and vasopressors, and SAPS-II scores can help assess the risk of SIC. In addition, prediction results can be illustrated at the instance level, as shown in **Figure 6**, which makes our model clinically interpretable.

Several limitations of this study should be considered. Firstly, only septic adults in ICUs were included, whereas hospitalized sepsis cases were not analyzed. In addition, in consideration of the immaturity of the coagulation system in children, especially newborns, more research is needed on SIC in children with sepsis. Secondly, our models screen out patients with a high risk of SIC but do not indicate who will benefit from anticoagulant therapy. It is still up to clinicians to decide whether to administer anticoagulant agents. However, the process from sepsis to severe coagulopathy is a continuous condition arising from a coagulation disorder. Early and accurate prediction of SIC can provide more time for clinicians to adjust treatment strategies, and study the potential effect of anticoagulant therapy in the early stage. Thirdly, this is a retrospective observational study. Missing data and input errors exist, despite the very high quality of the MIMIC-IV and eICU-CRD databases. Therefore, prospective validation is still required in the future. Compared with septic shock, for which advances have been made in recent years, giving rise to significant survival improvements, there is still a long way to go in the diagnosis and management of sepsis-associated coagulopathy.

## CONCLUSIONS

In conclusion, the present study developed two variants of the CatBoost model, which can discriminate septic patients who would and would not develop SIC.

## ETHICS STATEMENT

The study was an analysis of two third-party anonymized publicly available databases with pre-existing institutional review board (IRB) approval.

## AUTHOR CONTRIBUTIONS

Q-YZ, L-PL, and J-CL: conception and design. RG, G-WT, and ZL: administrative support. Q-YZ: collection and assembly of data. Q-YZ and L-PL: data analysis and interpretation. All authors: manuscript writing and final approval of manuscript.

## ACKNOWLEDGMENTS

We would like to thank the Massachusetts Institute of Technology and the Beth Israel Deaconess Medical Center for the MIMIC project. We also would like to thank the Philips eICU Research Institute and Philips Healthcare for their contribution to the eICU-CRD project.

## REFERENCES

1. Singer M, Deutschman CS, Seymour CW., Shankar-Hari M, Annane D, Bauer M, et al. The third international consensus definitions for sepsis and septic shock (Sepsis-3). *JAMA.* (2016) 315:801–10. doi: 10.1001/jama.201 60287
2. Martin GS, Mannino DM, Eaton S, Moss M. The epidemiology of sepsis in the United States from 1979 through 2000. *N Engl J Med.* (2003) 348:1546–54. doi: 10.1056/NEJMoa022139
3. Lyons PG, Micek ST, Hampton N, Kollef MH. Sepsis-associated coagulopathy severity predicts hospital mortality. *Crit Care Med.* (2018) 46:736–42. doi: 10.1097/CCM0000000000002997
4. Levi M, van der Poll T. Coagulation and sepsis. *Thromb Res.* (2017) 149:38–44. doi: 10.1016/j.thromres.2016.11007
5. Levi M, Ten Cate H. Disseminated intravascular coagulation. *N Engl J Med* (1999) 341:586–92. doi: 10.1056/NEJM199908193410807
6. Zhao H, Cai X, Liu N, Zhang Z. Thromboelastography as a tool for monitoring blood coagulation dysfunction after adequate fluid resuscitation can predict poor outcomes in patients with septic shock. *J Chin Med Assoc.* (2020) 83:674–7. doi: 10.1097/JCMA0000000000000345
7. Allingstrup M, Wetterslev J, Ravn FB, Moller AM, Afshari A. Antithrombin III for critically ill patients. *Cochrane Database Syst Rev.* (2016) 2:CD005370. doi: 10.1002/14651858.CD005370pub3
8. Warren BL, Eid A, Singer P, Pillay SS, Carl P, Novak I, et al. Caring for the critically ill patient. High-dose antithrombin III in severe sepsis: a randomized controlled trial. *JAMA.* (2001) 286:1869–78. doi: 10.1001/jama.286.151869
9. Dhainaut JF, Yan SB, Joyce DE, Pettila V, Basson B, Brandt JT, et al. Treatment effects of drotrecogin alfa (activated) in patients with severe sepsis with or without overt disseminated intravascular coagulation. *J Thromb Haemost* (2004) 2:1924–33. doi: 10.1111/j.1538-7836.2004.00955x
10. Iba T, Gando S, Thachil J. Anticoagulant therapy for sepsis-associated disseminated intravascular coagulation: the view from Japan. *J Thromb Haemost.* (2014) 12:1010–9. doi: 10.1111/jth12596
11. Kienast J, Juers M, Wiedermann CJ, Hoffmann JN, Ostermann H, Strauss R, et al. Treatment effects of high-dose antithrombin without concomitant heparin in patients with severe sepsis with or without disseminated intravascular coagulation. *J Thromb Haemost.* (2006) 4:90–7. doi: 10.1111/j.1538-7836.2005.01697x
12. Umemura Y, Yamakawa K, Ogura H, Yuhara H, Fujimi S. Efficacy and safety of anticoagulant therapy in three specific populations with sepsis: a meta-analysis of randomized controlled trials. *J Thromb Haemost.* (2016) 14:518–30. doi: 10.1111/jth13230
13. Umemura Y, Yamakawa K. Optimal patient selection for anticoagulant therapy in sepsis: an evidence-based proposal from Japan. *J Thromb Haemost.* (2018) 16:462–4. doi: 10.1111/jth13946
14. Aster RH, Bougie DW. Drug-induced immune thrombocytopenia. *N Engl J Med.* (2007) 357:580–7. doi: 10.1056/NEJMra066469
15. Iba T, Nisio MD, Levy JH, Kitamura N, Thachil J. New criteria for sepsis-induced coagulopathy (SIC) following the revised sepsis definition: a retrospective analysis of a nationwide survey. *BMJ Open.* (2017) 7:e017046. doi: 10.1136/bmjopen-2017-017046
16. Iba T, Levy JH, Warkentin TE, Thachil J, van der Poll T, Levi M, et al. Diagnosis and management of sepsis-induced coagulopathy and disseminated intravascular coagulation. *J Thromb Haemost.* (2019) 17:1989–94. doi: 10.1111/jth14578
17. Iba T, Arakawa M, Nisio Di M, Gando S, Anan H, Sato K, et al. Newly proposed Sepsis-induced coagulopathy precedes international society on thrombosis and haemostasis overt-disseminated intravascular coagulation and predicts high mortality. *J Intensive Care Med.* (2020) 35:643–9. doi: 10.1177/0885066618773679
18. Iba T, Arakawa M, Levy JH, Yamakawa K, Koami H, Hifumi T, et al. Sepsis-induced coagulopathy and japanese association for acute medicine DIC in coagulopathic patients with decreased antithrombin and treated by antithrombin. *Clin Appl Thromb Hemost.* (2018) 24:1020–6. doi: 10.1177/1076029618770273
19. Beam AL, Kohane IS. Big data and machine learning in health care. *JAMA.* (2018) 319:1317–8. doi: 10.1001/jama.201718391
20. Zhang Z, Ho KM, Hong Y. Machine learning for the prediction of volume responsiveness in patients with oliguric acute kidney injury in critical care. *Crit Care.* (2019) 23:112. doi: 10.1186/s13054-019-2411-z
21. Zhang Z. Predictive analytics in the era of big data: opportunities and challenges. *Ann Transl Med.* (2020) 8:68. doi: 10.21037/atm.2019.1097
22. Ge H, Pan Q, Zhou Y, Xu P, Zhang L, Zhang J, et al. Lung mechanics of mechanically ventilated patients with COVID-19: analytics with high-granularity ventilator waveform data. *Front Med.* (2020) 7:541. doi: 10.3389/fmed.202000541
23. Goldberger AL, Amaral LA, Glass L, Hausdorff JM, Ivanov PC, Mark RG, et al. PhysioBank, PhysioToolkit, and PhysioNet: components of a new research resource for complex physiologic signals. *Circulation.* (2000) 101:E215–20. doi: 10.1161/01.CIR.101.23e215
24. Pollard TJ, Johnson AEW, Raffa JD, Celi LA, Mark RG, Badawi O. The eICU collaborative research database, a freely available multi-center database for critical care research. *Sci Data.* (2018) 5:180178. doi: 10.1038/sdata.2018178
25. Collins GS, Reitsma JB, Altman DG, Moons KG. Transparent reporting of a multivariable prediction model for individual prognosis or diagnosis (TRIPOD): the TRIPOD statement. *BMC Med.* (2015) 13:1. doi: 10.1186/s12916-014-0241-z
26. Seymour CW, Liu VX, Iwashyna TJ, Brunkhorst FM, Rea TD, Scherag A, et al. Assessment of clinical criteria for Sepsis: for the third international consensus definitions for sepsis and septic shock (Sepsis-3). *JAMA.* (2016) 315:762–74. doi: 10.1001/jama.20160288
27. Wu J, Chen X-Y, Zhang H, Xiong L-D, Lei H, Deng S-H. Hyperparameter optimization for machine learning models based on Bayesian optimization. *J Electron Sci Technol.* (2019) 17:26–40. doi: 10.11989/JEST.1674-862X.80904120
28. Lundberg SM, Erion G, Chen H, DeGrave A, Prutkin JM, Nair B, et al. From local explanations to global understanding with explainable AI for trees. *Nat Mach Intell.* (2020) 2:56–67. doi: 10.1038/s42256-019-0138-9

29. Kishor K, Dhasmana N, Kamble SS, Sahu RK. Linezolid induced adverse drug reactions - an update. *Curr Drug Metab.* (2015) 16:553–9. doi: 10.2174/1389200216666151001121004
30. Mohammadi M, Jahangard-Rafsanjani Z, Sarayani A, Hadjibabaei M, Taghizadeh-Ghehi M. Vancomycin-induced thrombocytopenia: a narrative review. *Drug Saf.* (2017) 40:49–59. doi: 10.1007/s40264-016-0469-y
31. Zhang Z, Zhao Y, Canes A, Steinberg D, Lyashevska O, written on behalf of AMEB-DCTCG. Predictive analytics with gradient boosting in clinical medicine. *Ann Transl Med.* (2019) 7:152. doi: 10.21037/atm.2019.0329
32. Hancock JT, Khoshgoftaar TM. CatBoost for big data: an interdisciplinary review. *J Big Data.* (2020) 7:94. doi: 10.1186/s40537-020-00369-8

8

# Early Prediction of Mortality, Severity and Length of Stay in the Intensive Care Unit of Sepsis Patients Based on Sepsis 3.0 by Machine Learning Models

*Longxiang Su [1†], Zheng Xu [2†], Fengxiang Chang [2†], Yingying Ma [2], Shengjun Liu [1], Huizhen Jiang [3], Hao Wang [1], Dongkai Li [1], Huan Chen [1], Xiang Zhou [1], Na Hong [2*], Weiguo Zhu [3,4*] and Yun Long [1*]*

*[1] Department of Critical Care Medicine, State Key Laboratory of Complex Severe and Rare Diseases, Peking Union Medical College, Peking Union Medical College Hospital, Chinese Academy of Medical Sciences, Beijing, China, [2] Digital Health China Technologies Co., Ltd., Beijing, China, [3] Department of Information Center, State Key Laboratory of Complex Severe and Rare Diseases, Peking Union Medical College, Peking Union Medical College Hospital, Chinese Academy of Medical Sciences, Beijing, China, [4] Department of Primary Care and Family Medicine, State Key Laboratory of Complex Severe and Rare Diseases, Peking Union Medical College, Peking Union Medical College Hospital, Chinese Academy of Medical Sciences, Beijing, China*

***Correspondence:**
*Yun Long*
*ly_icu@aliyun.com*
*Weiguo Zhu*
*zhuwg@pumch.cn*
*Na Hong*
*hongna@dchealth.com*

*† These authors have contributed equally to this work*

**Background:** Early prediction of the clinical outcome of patients with sepsis is of great significance and can guide treatment and reduce the mortality of patients. However, it is clinically difficult for clinicians.

**Methods:** A total of 2,224 patients with sepsis were involved over a 3-year period (2016–2018) in the intensive care unit (ICU) of Peking Union Medical College Hospital. With all the key medical data from the first 6 h in the ICU, three machine learning models, logistic regression, random forest, and XGBoost, were used to predict mortality, severity (sepsis/septic shock), and length of ICU stay (LOS) (>6 days, ≤6 days). Missing data imputation and oversampling were completed on the dataset before introduction into the models.

**Results:** Compared to the mortality and LOS predictions, the severity prediction achieved the best classification results, based on the area under the operating receiver characteristics (AUC), with the random forest classifier (sensitivity = 0.65, specificity = 0.73, F1 score = 0.72, AUC = 0.79). The random forest model also showed the best overall performance (mortality prediction: sensitivity = 0.50, specificity = 0.84, F1 score = 0.66, AUC = 0.74; LOS prediction: sensitivity = 0.79, specificity = 0.66, F1 score = 0.69, AUC = 0.76) among the three models. The predictive ability of the SOFA score itself was inferior to that of the above three models.

**Conclusions:** Using the random forest classifier in the first 6 h of ICU admission can provide a comprehensive early warning of sepsis, which will contribute to the formulation and management of clinical decisions and the allocation and management of resources.

**Keywords: sepsis, prediction, machine learning, outcome, sequential (sepsis-related) organ failure assessment**

## INTRODUCTION

With high morbidity and mortality, sepsis seriously endangers human health and causes a heavy medical burden (1, 2). The understanding of sepsis has evolved from an inflammatory response syndrome caused by infection (sepsis 1.0) to an inflammatory response syndrome with organ dysfunction (sepsis 2.0) to a life-threatening organ disorder caused by the body's uncontrolled response to infection (sepsis 3.0) (3). Employed as the core indicator in sepsis 3.0 diagnosis, the SOFA score was proven to be an accurate and feasible method in the prognosis assessment with its ability to judge the degree of organ failure and assess the severity of patients with sepsis (4, 5). With the establishment of and improvement in critical illness databases and the continuous advancement of machine learning methods, an ever-increasing number of new models are being proposed by researchers. Compared with the SOFA, the Oxford Acute Severity of Illness Score (OASIS) is a scoring system that was constructed by Johnson et al. through machine learning algorithms (6). It contains only 10 variables and no laboratory measure whose diagnostic efficiency is high. Kim et al. (7) also proposed a deep model-based, data-driven early warning score tool, PROMPT, that can predict mortality in critically ill children. With regard to machine learning techniques, Pirracchio et al. proposed that ensemble and neural network models would demonstrate better performance in predicting mortality (8). However, differences exist among the current machine learning models for diagnosis, such as parameter composition, the source population for model construction, and the scope of clinical use. The conclusions obtained by different clinical studies have even been contradictory. This study intends to examine data from the Chinese sepsis patient population under the Chinese medical system and environment using machine learning algorithms to explore a model for predicting the prognosis of sepsis patients, the severity of the disease, and the potential duration of ICU treatment (LOS), which may contribute to understanding sepsis and treating sepsis in the ICU.

## METHODS

### Study Design

This study was conducted in the ICU of Peking Union Medical College Hospital. All electronic medical data from patients diagnosed with sepsis based on sepsis 3.0 were retrospectively gathered from 2016 to 2018 and securely stored in the Peking Union Medical College Hospital Intensive Care Medical Information System and Database (PICMISD). The data consisted of demographic information, ICU length of stay (LOS), medications, and vital signs of the respiratory, cardiovascular, hepatic, coagulation, renal, and neurological systems. As one of the commonly used methods for tracking patient status in the ICU and estimating the risk of mortality due to sepsis, a sequential organ failure assessment (SOFA) was introduced as one of the inclusion criteria and a baseline prediction tool. It was computed from the key measurements from multiple-organ systems.

### Patient Cohort

From 2016 to 2018, a total of 11,512 critically ill patients were admitted and treated in the ICU of Peking Union Medical College Hospital. A total of 2,436 patients with sepsis meeting the following criteria were included in the dataset: SOFA score $\geq 2$; high possibility of infection (pathogenic microbiology examinations obtained) and usage/update of antibiotics; age $\geq$ 18 years. After a thorough examination of the dataset, several constraints were added on some variables to ensure the reliability of the medical data: $0 < P(v\text{-}a)CO_2/C(a\text{-}v)O_2 < 5$; $0 < P(v\text{-}a)CO_2 < 15$; $0 < SO_2 \leq 100$; $0 <$ oxygenation index $\leq 1{,}000$; white blood cell ($\times 10^8$/L) $> 100$; oxygen concentration (%) $\geq 21$; and breath rate (bpm) $> 0$. The number of patients decreased to 2,224 with the extra constraints in place. With reference to the lactic acid values, all patients were labeled as having one of two categories of severity level: sepsis (<2 mmol/L; 1,122 patients) and septic shock ($\geq$2 mmol/L; 1,102 patients). All key measurements of the organs were recorded during the first 6 h after ICU admission. Unlike regular methods of using at least 24 h of measurement in the ICU (9–11), data recorded in the first 6 h can also be sufficiently accurate to assist clinicians in performing early prediction. Informed consent was obtained from all the participants in compliance with the requirements of the Ethics Committee of Peking Union Medical College Hospital.

### Model Development

Regarding the predictor classes, the mortality (survivor, non-survivor) and severity (sepsis, septic shock) predictions depended on the classification model, while patient LOS in the ICU was labeled by dividing patients into two groups: > 6 days and $\leq$ 6 days. The 6-day cut-off point was derived from the quartile values (first quartile: 3 days, second quartile: 6 days, third quartile: 13 days) from the overall patient distribution. The classification model incorporated the following methods: logistic regression (12), random forest (RF) (13), and XGBoost. To select the most relevant features, the least absolute shrinkage and selection operator (LASSO) was applied. All the features were normalized before being introduced into the classification models. The training and testing datasets were randomly split by 70 and 30% of all patients.

K-nearest neighbor (KNN) imputation (14) was utilized to handle the partial missing data. Each entry of missing data was imputed with the average of its five nearest neighbors. The value $k = 5$ in the KNN algorithm was chosen because it achieves the best classification results as supported by validation.

As the dataset is enormously biased toward the survivors, a method of over-sampling [specifically, the synthetic minority oversampling technique (SMOTE) (15)] on the minority class was applied in the training dataset for mortality prediction.

The classification models were assessed with the area under the receiver operating characteristic (AUC) curve, sensitivity (also known as recall), specificity, and F1 score. The foundation of these assessment variables comes from the four possible outcomes (TP = true positive, TN = true negative, FP = false positive, FN = false negative) of the binary classifier. Computed by plotting sensitivity as a function of (1-specificity), the area under the ROC curve is widely used as a performance

**Table 1A** | Subgroups of patients' clinical data for the mortality prediction.

| Variables | Mortality | | |
|---|---|---|---|
| | Survivor (1,809 patients) Mean ± SD | Non-survivor (415 patients) Mean ± SD | *p*-value |
| Age (years) | 58.59 ± 16.82 | 60.58 ± 15.66 | * |
| Perfusion index | 1.72 ± 1.74 | 1.65 ± 1.60 | >0.05 |
| $P(v\text{-}a)CO_2/C(a\text{-}v)O_2$ | 1.62 ± 0.56 | 1.63 ± 0.60 | >0.05 |
| $pCO_2$ (mmHg) | 38.02 ± 8.44 | 38.54 ± 11.53 | >0.05 |
| Noradrenaline dosage (μg/kg/min) | 0.41 ± 0.74 | 0.63 ± 1.61 | ** |
| Adrenaline dosage (μg/kg/min) | 0.16 ± 0.08 | 0.17 ± 0.10 | ** |
| Invasive blood pressure (mmHg) | 92.62 ± 20.50 | 86.36 ± 18.51 | ** |
| Central venous pressure (mmHg) | 9.25 ± 3.10 | 9.88 ± 4.00 | ** |
| $P(v\text{-}a)CO_2$ (mmHg) | 5.49 ± 2.16 | 5.32 ± 2.28 | >0.05 |
| $sO_2$ (%) | 96.51 ± 4.46 | 95.77 ± 4.77 | ** |
| Lactic acid (mmol/l) | 2.74 ± 2.73 | 3.31 ± 3.51 | ** |
| Invasive systolic blood pressure (mmHg) | 139.54 ± 27.81 | 131.40 ± 28.63 | ** |
| Invasive diastolic blood pressure (mmHg) | 69.88 ± 14.93 | 65.40 ± 13.73 | ** |
| Oxygenation index | 311.83 ± 143.35 | 253.27 ± 142.73 | ** |
| White blood cell (×109/l) | 13.83 ± 8.52 | 14.37 ± 9.38 | >0.05 |
| Platelet (×109/l) | 176.83 ± 101.13 | 150.74 ± 105.83 | ** |
| Total bilirubin (μmol/l) | 28.20 ± 47.16 | 43.21 ± 72.54 | ** |
| GCS score | 9.57 ± 4.48 | 8.12 ± 4.60 | ** |
| Creatinine (μmol/L) | 121.11 ± 138.15 | 166.10 ± 156.81 | ** |
| Oxygen concentration (%) | 46.16 ± 16.65 | 56.33 ± 22.98 | ** |
| $SpO_2$ (%) | 97.63 ± 3.58 | 96.49 ± 4.35 | ** |
| $pO_2$ (mmHg) | 108.44 ± 41.27 | 102.08 ± 47.63 | * |
| Heart rate (bpm) | 100.85 ± 21.43 | 107.21 ± 22.16 | ** |
| Body temperature (°C) | 36.83 ± 1.02 | 37.21 ± 1.06 | ** |
| Respiratory rate (bpm) | 20.03 ± 6.31 | 22.79 ± 7.11 | ** |
| SOFA score | 8.82 ± 3.73 | 11.50 ± 4.27 | ** |

**$p < 0.01$, *$p < 0.05$.

measurement for classification problems at various threshold settings. A higher AUC value indicates a better model for distinguishing between classes. In this study, false positives (e.g., a survivor is predicted as a non-survivor) may be overmedicated, while false negatives (e.g., a non-survivor is predicted as a survivor) may not receive any extra actions for early prevention. Both cases should be avoided here. The F1 score, as the harmonic mean of precision and recall, is a better metric for imbalanced classes. Meanwhile, a five-fold cross validation method was applied for all the models in three classification problems to avoid overfitting during the model training.

$$Sensitivity = \frac{TP}{TP + FN}$$

$$Specificity = \frac{TN}{TN + FP}$$

$$F1\ score = \frac{2*TP}{FP + FN + 2*TP}$$

## Statistical Analysis

All continuous variables in the clinical data are presented as the mean value ± standard deviation (SD). The distribution of LOS in the ICU was evaluated through quartile values, and then the second quartile value was chosen as the cut-off point for prediction labeling. $T$-tests with a threshold $p < 0.05$ were performed to determine significant differences between subgroups in each prediction problem. Regarding the mortality prediction, the SOFA score, as a baseline prediction tool, was used to generate an ROC curve for comparison with other machine learning models. The sensitivity and specificity of the SOFA score were estimated on the basis of a preset threshold. All statistical analyses were performed in Python 3.6.

# RESULTS

## General Characteristics of Included Patients

A total of 2,224 patients were included in the analysis. Their average of LOS in the ICU was 10.32 ± 11.84 days. The whole group included 1,292 males and 932 females aged 58.96 ± 16.62 years. Approximately 415 (18.7%) patients with sepsis did not survive in the ICU. A summary of the patients' clinical data for each prediction is presented in **Tables 1A–C**.

**Table 1B** | Subgroups of patients' clinical data for the severity prediction.

| Variables | Severity | | |
|---|---|---|---|
| | Sepsis (1,104 patients) Mean ± SD | Septic shock (1,120 patients) Mean ± SD | *p*-value |
| Age (years) | 60.47 ± 16.60 | 57.48 ± 16.52 | ** |
| Perfusion index | 1.93 ± 1.82 | 1.48 ± 1.56 | ** |
| $P(v\text{-}a)CO_2/C(a\text{-}v)O_2$ | 1.61 ± 0.57 | 1.63 ± 0.56 | >0.05 |
| pCO2 (mmHg) | 38.60 ± 10.27 | 37.64 ± 7.74 | * |
| Noradrenaline dosage (μg/kg/min) | 0.35 ± 0.24 | 0.55 ± 1.34 | ** |
| Adrenaline dosage (μg/kg/min) | 0.16 ± 0.03 | 0.16 ± 0.11 | >0.05 |
| Invasive blood pressure (mmHg) | 91.59 ± 19.89 | 91.31 ± 20.68 | >0.05 |
| Central venous pressure (mmHg) | 9.25 ± 3.03 | 9.48 ± 3.53 | >0.05 |
| $P(v\text{-}a)CO_2$ (mmHg) | 5.34 ± 2.10 | 5.58 ± 2.26 | * |
| $sO_2$ (%) | 96.62 ± 3.47 | 96.12 ± 5.36 | * |
| Lactic acid (mmol/l) | 1.19 ± 0.40 | 4.49 ± 3.34 | ** |
| Invasive systolic blood pressure (mmHg) | 140.04 ± 28.43 | 136.02 ± 27.71 | ** |
| Invasive diastolic blood pressure (mmHg) | 68.29 ± 15.00 | 69.77 ± 14.60 | * |
| Oxygenation index | 298.95 ± 145.17 | 302.74 ± 144.91 | >0.05 |
| White blood cell (×109/l) | 13.40 ± 7.34 | 14.46 ± 9.81 | ** |
| Platelet (×109/l) | 182.86 ± 107.90 | 161.18 ± 95.74 | ** |
| Total bilirubin (μmol/L) | 30.52 ± 52.00 | 31.59 ± 54.29 | >0.05 |
| GCS score | 9.90 ± 4.41 | 8.70 ± 4.59 | ** |
| Creatinine (μmol/L) | 128.75 ± 139.59 | 130.32 ± 146.10 | >0.05 |
| Oxygen concentration (%) | 47.74 ± 17.99 | 48.39 ± 18.86 | >0.05 |
| $SpO_2$ (%) | 97.35 ± 3.77 | 97.48 ± 3.77 | >0.05 |
| $pO_2$ (mmHg) | 103.99 ± 42.34 | 110.46 ± 42.62 | ** |
| Heart rate (bpm) | 99.61 ± 20.96 | 104.44 ± 22.16 | ** |
| Body temperature (°C) | 37.03 ± 1.00 | 36.77 ± 1.07 | ** |
| Respiratory rate (bpm) | 20.56 ± 6.35 | 20.54 ± 6.76 | >0.05 |
| SOFA score | 8.66 ± 3.68 | 9.97 ± 4.14 | ** |

$^{**}p < 0.01$, $^{*}p < 0.05$.

## Mortality Prediction

In the dataset, the number of non-survivors (415 patients) was approximately a quarter of the number of survivors (1,809 patients). The non-survivor group was slightly older than the survivor group. Among the 25 variables in **Table 1A**, only five variables, including perfusion index, $P(v\text{-}a)CO_2/C(a\text{-}v)O_2$, $pCO_2$, $P(v\text{-}a)CO_2$, and white blood cell count, showed no significant difference between the two groups, while the remaining variables did. With regular statistical methods, the SOFA score was used to produce ROC curves individually instead of being included as a feature in the model. It is reasonable that the average SOFA score for the survivor group was significantly lower than that for the non-survivor group.

As presented **Figure 1**, the SMOTE method significantly improved the sensitivity rate (without SMOTE: mean sensitivity = 0.13; with SMOTE: mean sensitivity = 0.49) in all models. Nonetheless, specificity, together with AUC, from all three models was considerably reduced after applying the SMOTE method. RF presented the best classification results (without SMOTE: AUC = 0.77; with SMOTE: AUC = 0.74), regardless of the application of the SMOTE method. All machine learning models demonstrated better prediction results than the SOFA score (AUC = 0.70).

## Severity Prediction

The dataset consisted of 1,104 patients with sepsis and 1,120 patients with septic shock. The subgroup with high severity (age: 57.48 ± 16.52 years) was significantly younger than the other subgroup (age: 60.47 ± 16.60 years). As seen in **Table 1B**, 10 variables related to respiratory [$P(v\text{-}a)CO_2/C(a\text{-}v)O_2$, oxygenation index, oxygen concentration, $SpO_2$], renal (creatinine, adrenaline dosage) and coagulation (invasive blood pressure, central venous pressure, total bilirubin) systems showed no significant differences between the two classes. Among all classifiers, the RF classifier provided the best prediction results for severity (sensitivity = 0.65, specificity = 0.73, F1 score = 0.72, AUC = 0.79) and presented enhanced results compared to the baseline SOFA score (AUC = 0.59) (see **Figure 2**).

## LOS Prediction

The second quartile (6 days) of all LOS data almost equally divided the group into two classes (≤6 days: 1,127 cases, >6 days:

**Table 1C |** Subgroups of patients' clinical data for the LOS prediction.

| Variables | LOS | | |
|---|---|---|---|
| | ≤6 days (988 patients) | >6 days (1,236 patients) | |
| | Mean ± SD | Mean ± SD | *p*-value |
| Age (years) | 57.89 ± 16.61 | 59.82 ± 16.59 | * |
| Perfusion index | 1.74 ± 1.81 | 1.67 ± 1.63 | >0.05 |
| $P(v\text{-}a)CO_2/C(a\text{-}v)O_2$ | 1.64 ± 0.52 | 1.61 ± 0.61 | >0.05 |
| $pCO_2$ (mmHg) | 37.46 ± 8.06 | 38.64 ± 9.82 | ** |
| Noradrenaline dosage (μg/kg/min) | 0.53 ± 1.36 | 0.39 ± 0.45 | ** |
| Adrenaline dosage (μg/kg/min) | 0.17 ± 0.11 | 0.16 ± 0.05 | ** |
| Invasive blood pressure (mmHg) | 94.49 ± 20.91 | 89.02 ± 19.44 | ** |
| Central venous pressure (mmHg) | 9.02 ± 3.16 | 9.64 ± 3.37 | ** |
| $P(v\text{-}a)CO_2$ (mmHg) | 5.62 ± 2.07 | 5.32 ± 2.25 | ** |
| $sO_2$ (%) | 96.67 ± 4.65 | 96.13 ± 4.41 | * |
| Lactic acid (mmol/l) | 2.94 ± 3.11 | 2.77 ± 2.72 | >0.05 |
| Invasive systolic blood pressure (mmHg) | 139.41 ± 28.76 | 136.90 ± 27.59 | * |
| Invasive diastolic blood pressure (mmHg) | 71.59 ± 15.24 | 67.00 ± 14.15 | ** |
| Oxygenation index | 337.15 ± 145.09 | 271.89 ± 138.34 | ** |
| White blood cell (×109/l) | 13.08 ± 8.04 | 14.62 ± 9.12 | ** |
| Platelet (×109/l) | 174.57 ± 98.89 | 169.85 ± 105.31 | >0.05 |
| Total bilirubin (μmol/l) | 33.11 ± 58.50 | 29.33 ± 48.42 | >0.05 |
| GCS score | 10.04 ± 4.48 | 8.71 ± 4.50 | ** |
| Creatinine (μmol/l) | 105.55 ± 119.71 | 148.69 ± 156.39 | ** |
| Oxygen concentration (%) | 44.31 ± 15.79 | 51.06 ± 19.80 | ** |
| $SpO_2$ (%) | 97.85 ± 3.48 | 97.07 ± 3.94 | ** |
| $pO_2$ (mmHg) | 113.13 ± 43.03 | 102.55 ± 41.68 | ** |
| Heart rate (bpm) | 99.68 ± 22.26 | 103.93 ± 21.07 | ** |
| Body temperature (°C) | 36.68 ± 1.00 | 37.08 ± 1.04 | ** |
| Respiratory rate (bpm) | 19.41 ± 5.96 | 21.46 ± 6.86 | ** |
| SOFA score | 8.37 ± 3.89 | 10.08 ± 3.88 | ** |

***p < 0.01, *p < 0.05.*

1,097 cases). The patients with longer ICU stays (>6 days) were older (59.82 ± 16.59 years) than the other patients (age: 57.89 ± 16.61 years). Similar to the previous mortality classes, only five variables [perfusion index, $P(v\text{-}a)CO_2/C(a\text{-}v)O_2$, lactic acid, platelets, and total bilirubin] indicated no significant differences between the LOS subgroups. Meanwhile, the RF model again exhibited the best prediction results for LOS (sensitivity = 0.79, specificity = 0.66, F1 score = 0.69, AUC = 0.76), which was much better than the SOFA score (AUC = 0.62) (see **Figure 3**).

## DISCUSSION

Our study found that this machine learning method using data within the first 6 h of ICU admission can predict sepsis patients' prognosis, the severity of sepsis (i.e., whether there is septic shock), and the length of stay in the ICU (i.e., whether it was longer than 6 days). Furthermore, the RF classifier had stronger diagnostic power for the three predictions, with areas under the ROC curve of 0.74, 0.79, and 0.76, respectively. After the validation set was verified, its effect was significantly better than that of the traditional SOFA score. This implies that the use of RF predictions in the early stages of ICU admission will enable us to know the possibility of ICU patient outcomes earlier, appropriately allocate medical resources, and optimize treatment behavior.

At present, the diagnosis of sepsis is more specific and clearer with the definition of sepsis 3.0 than the previous two versions. More emphasis should be placed on how we can more accurately predict ICU outcomes after the diagnosis of sepsis (16). As mentioned above, the current treatments for sepsis are still not ideal. Early recognition and correct treatment are closely related to improving prognosis (17). Since sepsis is essentially an out-of-control regulation of the systemic immune response, it is not caused by a single factor. The pathophysiological process is complicated, which leads to large differences in clinical manifestations and disease processes across patients (18). A single diagnostic index is obviously difficult to perform. The sepsis scoring system represented by the SOFA score is used in the diagnosis and treatment of sepsis, which is constantly strengthened by an increasing amount of evidence (19). However, it is difficult to balance the massive data and the complexity of the disease in the ICU treatment of sepsis. With the emergence

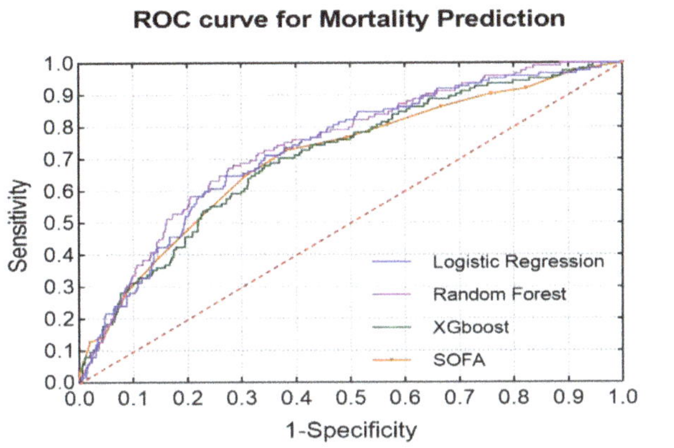


| | Models | Sensitivity | Specificity | F1 score | AUC |
|---|---|---|---|---|---|
| Without SMOTE | Logistic regression | 0.12 | 0.96 | 0.54 | 0.75 |
| | Random Forest | 0.064 | 0.99 | 0.51 | 0.77 |
| | XGboost | 0.21 | 0.94 | 0.58 | 0.73 |
| With SMOTE | Logistic regression | 0.65 | 0.72 | 0.62 | 0.73 |
| | Random Forest | 0.50 | 0.84 | 0.66 | 0.74 |
| | XGboost | 0.33 | 0.89 | 0.62 | 0.71 |

**FIGURE 1 |** ROC curves of each classifier with SMOTE for mortality prediction. Classification results before and after SMOTE are presented in the embedded table.

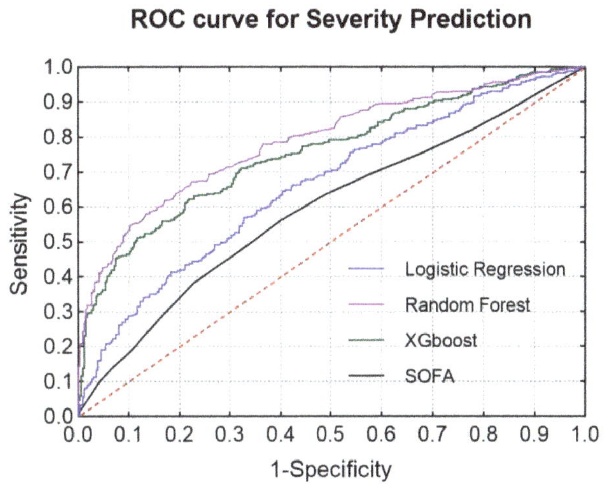


| Model | Sensitivity | Specificity | F1-score | AUC |
|---|---|---|---|---|
| Logistic regression | 0.69 | 0.68 | 0.61 | 0.66 |
| Random Forest | 0.65 | 0.73 | 0.72 | 0.79 |
| XGboost | 0.68 | 0.69 | 0.68 | 0.75 |

**FIGURE 2 |** ROC curves of each classifier for severity prediction and classification results in the table below.

of large electronic databases and the development of advanced algorithms such as machine learning and data mining, new scoring systems will continue to emerge. Our study identified a relatively good machine learning result, suggesting that the RF method can better predict the 28-day prognosis of patients in the first 6 h after ICU admission. Overall, accurate prediction of the prognosis of ICU patients with sepsis is of great clinical significance. It depends on an appropriate prognostic scoring system. However, how to define and select the "appropriate" scoring system requires the comprehensive judgment of multiple studies and multiple evaluation indicators. In the future, with continuous input of multimodal parameters, more machine learning methods are needed to aggregate data and information from all parties and obtain more accurate conclusions to guide clinical practice.

Compared with the previous two versions of the sepsis guidelines, the largest change was the definition of septic shock (3). At present, septic shock is defined as an inability to maintain blood pressure and the need for vasoactive drugs to maintain circulation after sufficient fluid resuscitation; at this time, lactic acid is >2 mmol/L. For this definition, it may be more necessary to understand the patient's situation and have information from multiple dimensions such as whether this patient is sepsis, what the SOFA score is, whether the patient has undergone fluid resuscitation, what the blood pressure is, whether blood pressure medications are currently being used, and what the lactic acid level is. This makes it even more necessary to use computers

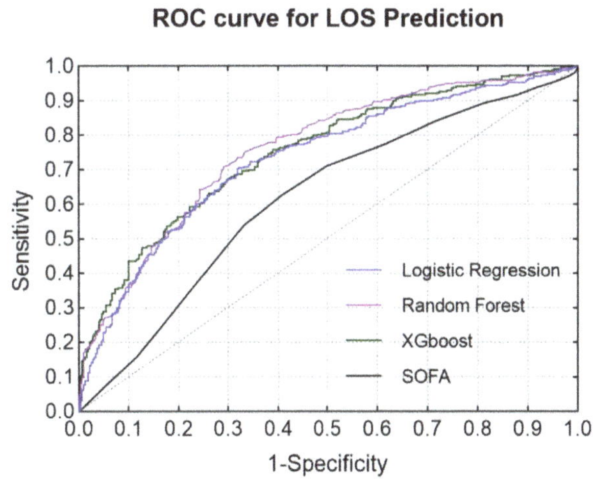


| Models | Sensitivity | Specificity | F1-score | AUC |
|---|---|---|---|---|
| Logistic regression | 0.63 | 0.60 | 0.66 | 0.73 |
| Random Forest | 0.79 | 0.66 | 0.69 | 0.76 |
| XGboost | 0.71 | 0.65 | 0.48 | 0.75 |

**FIGURE 3 |** ROC curves of each classifier for LOS prediction and classification results in the table below.

as an aid to identify and provide an early alert to ICU staff about this severe sepsis situation. This confirmed that the use of clinical information to define septic shock outperformed models developed based on only administrative data (20). Kim et al. (21) demonstrated that ML classifiers significantly outperformed clinical scores in screening septic shock at ED triage. Combined with machine learning methods, we can see that the RF method can accurately predict patients with septic shock for the first time and determine which patients are more severe. This is of great significance for clinical treatment. Another study also supported our conclusion using a RF classifier to predict sepsis and septic shock (13). In addition, we can also predict which sepsis patients needed longer ICU support through the RF method, and the limited ICU resources can be configured and more efficiently better used. Staziaki et al. (22) reported that SVM and ANN models combining CT findings and clinical parameters improved the prediction of length of stay and ICU admission in torso trauma. Castineira et al. (23) added continuous vital sign information to static clinical data to improve the prediction of length of stay after intubation. Even ELM has been used to determine whether the patient can be discharged within 10 days (24). The use of machine learning algorithms is of great significance to patients with sepsis, and it is better than the traditional SOFA score, which is relatively monotonous in the systematic assessment of organ damage.

The algorithms also played an important role in this study. Before inputting data into the model, imputation of the missing data was necessary. In the future, other imputation methods, such as stochastic regression and tree-based models, can be assessed to compete with the only method, "KNN imputation," used in this study. The oversampling method "SMOTE" successfully solved the problem of imbalanced datasets, which often leads to a highly biased prediction result, as the model will place more weight on the majority class. In the meantime, some other methods of oversampling can also be tested to improve the classification results. Certainly, as the core of the prediction problem, choosing the best machine learning model is the most important aspect. Therefore, some additional models from the deep learning field, such as artificial neural networks (ANNs) and convolutional neural networks (CNNs), may be applied in future investigations.

There were also some limitations. Firstly, the research subjects came from a single ICU, and there may be bias caused by regional factors. Whether the research conclusions can be extended to other regions needs further research and testing. Secondly, it is necessary to verify that the next step is to implement forward-looking research based on the current research results to further verify the validity and scalability of the model constructed in this study and provide further improvements. In our study, only three subjects have breath rate below 5 bpm, which is only 0.1% of the whole population. It will not lead to high risk of biased dataset according to the inclusion criteria of breath rate > 0 bpm. In the clinical decision-making, the general cut-off point of LOS is 4–5 days while 6 days was chosen here based on the distribution of LOS.

## CONCLUSION

Machine learning models using the first 6 h of medical data can decently predict mortality, severity, and LOS in the ICU. The overall results demonstrated that the RF model was the best model of classification for all three prediction problems (AUC for all RF models > 0.70) compared to logistic regression and XGBoost models. The prospects of applying machine learning in the ICU are broad, but BCT research is still needed to study the stability of the model and clarify the potential limitations.

## ETHICS STATEMENT

Ethical review and approval was not required for the study on human participants in accordance with the local legislation and institutional requirements. The patients/participants provided their written informed consent to participate in this study.

## AUTHOR CONTRIBUTIONS

YL, WZ, and NH take responsibility for the integrity of the work as a whole, from the inception to the published article. LS, ZX, and FC are responsible for study design and conception. YM, SL, HJ, HW, DL, HC, and XZ are responsible for the data management and statistical analysis. LS drafted the manuscript. All authors revised the manuscript for important intellectual content.

## REFERENCES

1. Dellinger RP, Levy MM, Rhodes A, Annane D, Gerlach H, Opal SM, et al. Surviving sepsis campaign: international guidelines for management of severe sepsis and septic shock: 2012. *Crit Care Med.* (2013) 41:580–637. doi: 10.1097/CCM.0b013e31827e83af
2. Paoli CJ, Reynolds MA, Sinha M, Gitlin M, Crouser E. Epidemiology and costs of sepsis in the United States-an analysis based on timing of diagnosis and severity level. *Crit Care Med.* (2018) 46:1889–97. doi: 10.1097/CCM.0000000000003342
3. Singer M, Deutschman CS, Seymour CW, Shankar-Hari M, Annane D, Bauer M, et al. The third international consensus definitions for sepsis and septic shock (sepsis-3). *JAMA.* (2016) 315:801–10. doi: 10.1001/jama.2016.0287
4. Vincent JL, Moreno R, Takala J, Willatts S, De Mendonca A, Bruining H, et al. The SOFA (sepsis-related organ failure assessment) score to describe organ dysfunction/failure. On behalf of the Working Group on Sepsis-Related Problems of the European Society of Intensive Care Medicine. *Intensive Care Med.* (1996) 22:707–10. doi: 10.1007/BF01709751
5. Vincent JL, de Mendonca A, Cantraine F, Moreno R, Takala J, Suter PM, et al. Use of the SOFA score to assess the incidence of organ dysfunction/failure in intensive care units: results of a multicenter, prospective study. Working group on "sepsis-related problems" of the European Society of Intensive Care Medicine. *Crit Care Med.* (1998) 26:1793–800. doi: 10.1097/00003246-199811000-00016

6. Johnson AE, Kramer AA, Clifford GD. A new severity of illness scale using a subset of acute physiology and chronic health evaluation data elements shows comparable predictive accuracy. *Crit Care Med.* (2013) 41:1711–8. doi: 10.1097/CCM.0b013e31828a24fe
7. Kim SY, Kim S, Cho J, Kim YS, Sol IS, Sung Y, et al. A deep learning model for real-time mortality prediction in critically ill children. *Crit Care.* (2019) 23:279. doi: 10.1186/s13054-019-2561-z
8. Pirracchio R, Petersen ML, Carone M, Rigon MR, Chevret S, van der Laan MJ. Mortality prediction in intensive care units with the Super ICU Learner Algorithm (SICULA): a population-based study. *Lancet Respir Med.* (2015) 3:42–52. doi: 10.1016/S2213-2600(14)70239-5
9. Kramer AA, Zimmerman JE. A predictive model for the early identification of patients at risk for a prolonged intensive care unit length of stay. *BMC Med Inform Decis Mak.* (2010) 10:27. doi: 10.1186/1472-6947-10-27
10. Meadows K, Gibbens R, Gerrard C, Vuylsteke A. Prediction of patient length of stay on the intensive care unit following cardiac surgery: a logistic regression analysis based on the cardiac operative mortality risk calculator, EuroSCORE. *J Cardiothorac Vasc Anesth.* (2018) 32:2676–82. doi: 10.1053/j.jvca.2018.03.007
11. Nielsen AB, Thorsen-Meyer HC, Belling K, Nielsen AP, Thomas CE, Chmura PJ, et al. Survival prediction in intensive-care units based on aggregation of long-term disease history and acute physiology: a retrospective study of the Danish National Patient Registry and electronic patient records. *Lancet Digit Health.* (2019) 1:e78–e89. doi: 10.1016/S2589-7500(19)30024-X
12. Tolles J, Meurer WJ. Logistic regression: relating patient characteristics to outcomes. *JAMA.* (2016) 316:533–4. doi: 10.1001/jama.2016.7653
13. Giannini HM, Ginestra JC, Chivers C, Draugelis M, Hanish A, Schweickert WD, et al. A machine learning algorithm to predict severe sepsis and septic shock: development, implementation, and impact on clinical practice. *Crit Care Med.* (2019) 47:1485–92. doi: 10.1097/CCM.0000000000003891
14. Troyanskaya O, Cantor M, Sherlock G, Brown P, Hastie T, Tibshirani R, et al. Missing value estimation methods for DNA microarrays. *Bioinformatics.* (2001) 17:520–5. doi: 10.1093/bioinformatics/17.6.520
15. Chawla NV, Bowyer KW, Hall LO, Kegelmeyer WP. SMOTE: synthetic minority over-sampling technique. *J Artif Intellig Res.* (2002) 16:321–57. doi: 10.1613/jair.953
16. Power GS, Harrison DA. Why try to predict ICU outcomes? *Curr Opin Crit Care.* (2014) 20:544–9. doi: 10.1097/MCC.0000000000000136
17. Seymour CW, Gesten F, Prescott HC, Friedrich ME, Iwashyna TJ, Phillips GS, et al. Time to treatment and mortality during mandated emergency care for sepsis. *N Engl J Med.* (2017) 376:2235–44. doi: 10.1056/NEJMoa1703058
18. Gotts JE, Matthay MA. Sepsis: pathophysiology and clinical management. *BMJ.* (2016) 353:i1585. doi: 10.1136/bmj.i1585
19. Seymour CW, Liu VX, Iwashyna TJ, Brunkhorst FM, Rea TD, Scherag A, et al. Assessment of clinical criteria for sepsis: for the third international consensus definitions for sepsis and septic shock (sepsis-3). *JAMA.* (2016) 315:762–774. doi: 10.1001/jama.2016.0288
20. Misra D, Avula V, Wolk DM, Farag HA, Li J, Mehta YB, et al. Early detection of septic shock onset using interpretable machine learners. *J Clin Med.* (2021) 10:301. doi: 10.3390/jcm10020301
21. Kim J, Chang H, Kim D, Jang DH, Park I, Kim K. Machine learning for prediction of septic shock at initial triage in emergency department. *J Crit Care.* (2020) 55:163–70. doi: 10.1016/j.jcrc.2019.09.024
22. Staziaki PV, Wu D, Rayan JC, Santo IDO, Nan F, Maybury A, et al. Machine learning combining CT findings and clinical parameters improves prediction of length of stay and ICU admission in torso trauma. *Eur Radiol.* (2021). doi: 10.1007/s00330-020-07534-w. [Epub ahead of print].
23. Castineira D, Schlosser KR, Geva A, Rahmani AR, Fiore G, Walsh BK, et al. Adding continuous vital sign information to static clinical data improves the prediction of length of stay after intubation: a data-driven machine learning approach. *Respir Care.* (2020) 65:1367–77. doi: 10.4187/respcare.07561
24. Ma X, Si Y, Wang Z, Wang Y. Length of stay prediction for ICU patients using individualized single classification algorithm. *Comput Methods Programs Biomed.* (2020) 186:105224. doi: 10.1016/j.cmpb.2019.105224

# 9

# Differing Visual Behavior Between Inexperienced and Experienced Critical Care Nurses While Using a Closed-Loop Ventilation System

*Philipp K. Buehler[1†], Anique Herling[1†], Nadine Bienefeld[2], Stephanie Klinzing[1], Stephan Wegner[3], Pedro David Wendel Garcia[1], Michael Karbach[1], Quentin Lohmeyer[3], Elisabeth Schaubmayr[1], Reto A. Schuepbach[1] and Daniel A. Hofmaenner[1*]*

*[1] Institute of Intensive Care Medicine, University Hospital Zurich, Zurich, Switzerland, [2] Department of Management, Technology, and Economics, Work & Organizational Psychology, ETH Zurich, Zurich, Switzerland, [3] Department of Mechanical and Process Engineering, ETH Zurich, Zurich, Switzerland*

***Correspondence:**
*Daniel A. Hofmaenner*
*danielandrea.hofmaenner@usz.ch*

*[†] These authors share first authorship*

**Introduction:** Closed-loop ventilation modes are increasingly being used in intensive care units to ensure more automaticity. Little is known about the visual behavior of health professionals using these ventilation modes. The aim of this study was to analyze gaze patterns of intensive care nurses while ventilating a patient in the closed-loop mode with Intellivent adaptive support ventilation® (I-ASV) and to compare inexperienced with experienced nurses.

**Materials and Methods:** Intensive care nurses underwent eye-tracking during daily care of a patient ventilated in the closed-loop ventilation mode. Five specific areas of interest were predefined (ventilator settings, ventilation curves, numeric values, oxygenation Intellivent, ventilation Intellivent). The main independent variable and primary outcome was dwell time. Secondary outcomes were revisits, average fixation time, first fixation and fixation count on areas of interest in a targeted tracking-time of 60 min. Gaze patterns were compared between I-ASV inexperienced ($n$ = 12) and experienced ($n$ = 16) nurses.

**Results:** In total, 28 participants were included. Overall, dwell time was longer for ventilator settings and numeric values compared to the other areas of interest. Similar results could be obtained for the secondary outcomes. Visual fixation of oxygenation Intellivent and ventilation Intellivent was low. However, dwell time, average fixation time and first fixation on oxygenation Intellivent were longer in experienced compared to inexperienced intensive care nurses.

**Discussion:** Gaze patterns of intensive care nurses were mainly focused on numeric values and settings. Areas of interest related to traditional mechanical ventilation retain high significance for intensive care nurses, despite use of closed-loop mode. More visual attention to oxygenation Intellivent and ventilation Intellivent in experienced nurses implies more routine and familiarity with closed-loop modes in this group. The findings imply the need for constant training and education with new tools in critical care, especially for inexperienced professionals.

**Keywords: eye-tracking, user interfaces, closed-loop ventilation, monitoring, visual behavior**

## INTRODUCTION

Patients in the intensive care unit (ICU) are particularly vulnerable to harm due to their complex clinical history and critical condition. Owing to a high number of machine user interfaces, challenging and often time-critical processes, the management of critically ill patients involves a high risk of error. Unintentional human errors and lack of situation awareness are among the leading causes of adverse events, not only in the medical setting (1–12). Unintentional errors can be classified into four main sources: slip, lapse, mistake and violations (13). Furthermore, a distinction is made between systemic and individual causes of error (12). Individual causes include distraction, inattention, forgetfulness, motivational deficits, and lack of awareness. Despite decades of research on human factors and sociotechnical system design, in practice the influence of human-environmental interaction (e.g., use of technical devices) is often neglected and could be contributing to individual errors. Increasingly, machines with complex control circuits are challenging human receptiveness. In intensive care medicine, the understanding of human-machine interactions is of particular importance in preventing adverse events (14). Inadequate information processing with respect to monitoring devices may contribute to individual errors leading to impaired patient outcomes. To date, it is largely unclear how user interfaces and specific program modes of technical devices are cognitively processed by specialized ICU nurses, despite some past research on graphical displays and situation awareness (11, 15). More knowledge about human-machine interactions in intensive care medicine is required (9). One example of the emerging role of technical systems in the ICU are closed-loop ventilation modes. In contrast to conventional volume- or pressure-controlled modes, the inherent automaticity of closed-loop modes is reminiscent of autopilot modes in airplanes. Closed-loop ventilation modes operate through an inherent feedback mechanism breath-by-breath. Based on constant measurements (i.e., peripheral oxygen saturation and end-tidal carbon dioxide) and algorithms, these modes automatically adjust the fraction of inhaled oxygen ($FiO_2$), the positive end-expiratory pressure (PEEP) and minute ventilation (16, 17).

When ICU patients are ventilated with closed-loop modes, the specific role allocation and associated tasks of the nurses responsible shift from active, manual machine handling to a rather machine-supervisory role (18). However, it is currently unknown to what extent the transition toward a supervisory role, with its inherent change in the type and assessment of information (19) presented by the new closed-loop ventilation modes, has occurred. Eye-tracking is a tool that enables monitoring of gaze patterns and visual attention. It has been used to analyze various professional scenarios in the medical field, including ICUs (20–32), and might be beneficial in gaining a more profound understanding of the operation of closed-loop ventilation modes.

The aim of this study was thus to analyze gaze patterns of ICU nurses using eye-tracking while ventilating a patient in the closed-loop mode Intellivent adaptive support ventilation (I-ASV)® and to compare the patterns of inexperienced with those of experienced ICU nurses.

## MATERIALS AND METHODS

### Ethics

The Local Ethics Committee (Kantonale Ethikkommission Zurich BASEC ID REQ 2017-00798) approved the study protocol, guaranteeing accordance with the declaration of Helsinki. Written informed consent was given by all participating ICU nurses and the patients involved, or the patients' legal representatives in cases of incapacity of judgement.

### Study Design and Study Population

This was a prospective, observational, real-life eye-tracking study conducted at the ICU of the University Hospital Zurich (Zurich, Switzerland). The interdisciplinary ICU treats about 4,500 patients per year in 64 ICU beds. All specialized ICU nurses working in the ICU were eligible for participation, provided there were no exclusion criteria. Exclusion criteria were visual disturbances (lack of stereoscopic vision, monocular vision and achromatopsia) or withheld informed consent. The respirators used were "Hamilton S1®" respirators (Hamilton Medical Company, Bonaduz, Switzerland). Independently of this study, all nurses underwent a standardized training program in Intellivent adaptive support ventilation (I-ASV, Hamilton Medical Company, Bonaduz, Switzerland) before bedside application of the closed-loop ventilation mode. During the first year of I-ASV application after professional training, the ICU nurses are constantly supervised by senior/teaching nurses while ventilating their patients, whereas after this period they work without supervision. Thus, for the design of this study, nurses who had worked $<1$ year with I-ASV were considered inexperienced, whereas nurses who had worked for more than 1 year with I-ASV were considered experienced. Participation in this study was free of charge and voluntary. If a calibration of the eye-tracker was possible, the participant was included. All recordings were performed in the early afternoon in order to avoid biases due to the regular morning rounds with the treating physicians or due to nightshifts, which might impair standardization of data. Further, all recordings were scheduled in order that they did not coincide with special circumstances such as interventions or patient transports.

For study purposes, participating nurses were responsible for one patient. All patients, with various medical conditions, were invasively mechanically ventilated in I-ASV. Patients were only included if the presumed duration of mechanical ventilation was longer than 24 h. Short-term postoperative patients were not included. Patients with severe acute respiratory distress syndrome (ARDS) were not eligible (in the study center, it is a physician's task to adjust ventilator settings in this patient collective). No patient was intubated only for the purposes of this study. Non-intubated patients were not eligible for participation.

## Study Protocol

Prior to the recordings, demographics and data with possible influence on eye-tracking, such as workload of participants were gathered (33). To avoid biases, no information concerning the aim of the study was provided to the participants. In a questionnaire using validated scales, a participant assessment regarding I-ASV performance and effort expectancy, anxiety, and social influence was collected (34). After a period of habituation to the eye-tracking device lasting 30 min, and a three-point calibration, participants were asked to perform their daily nursing tasks including patient care, handling of perfusors, application of drugs and ventilating the patient in I-ASV, which is the default respiration mode in the ICU. The targeted tracking time was 60 min per nurse. This tracking time was predefined by the study team to maximize the collection of data, while avoiding unnecessary interruptions (e.g., breaks, relatives coming for a visit etc.) or participant fatigue occurring in more prolonged recordings.

To provide a study setting as close to reality as possible, no advise was given to the participants on how to use and handle their respirator. Participants were free to use the respirator in the way they considered useful and to look at the respirator as often as they wanted.

After the eye-tracker recordings, a post-experiment questionnaire was completed. Using validated scales, workload and subjective stress during the tracking were assessed (33). Concerning I-ASV, the questionnaire collected data including the perceived safety of this mode, whether participants had enough specific knowledge about its use, their intention to continue

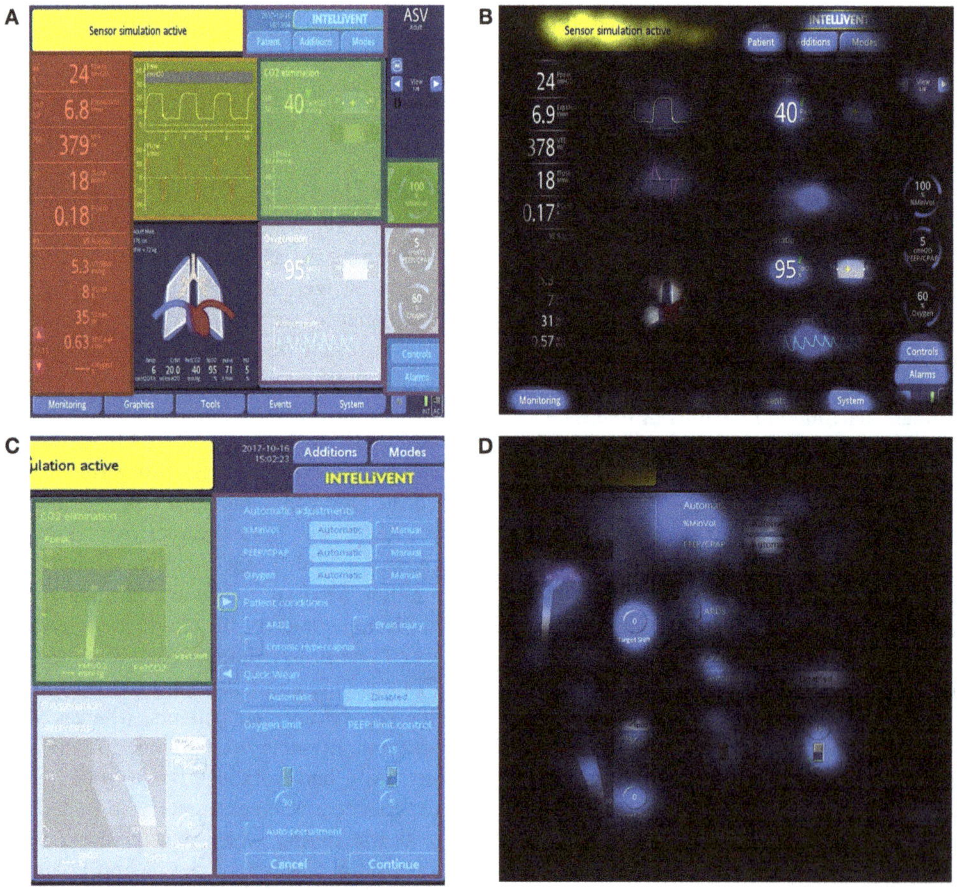


**FIGURE 1 |** Sample screen panels of the Hamilton Medical S1 respirator in closed-loop ventilation mode. The AOIs settings (blue), ventilation curves (yellow), numeric values (red), oxygenation Intellivent (white) and ventilation Intellivent (green) were pre-defined. The AOIs and the standard display of the screen are visualized in **(A,C)**. **(B,D)** depict the integrated focus maps for dwell time of all participants. In focus maps, more/longer fixations lead to a brighter color. Darker areas indicate fewer fixations.

using it in the future and facilitating conditions for future use of I-ASV (34).

## Data Analysis

To address the aim of the study, only gaze patterns relating to the user interface of the respirator and fixations on the ventilator were analyzed (e.g., adjusting the settings, checking values, using touch panels). All other visual fixations (e.g., on the patient, perfusors, other staff, other devices, etc.) were not subject to analysis and thus excluded.

For our analysis, five areas of interest (AOI; i.e., areas on the ventilator's user interface that were important in addressing the aim of the study) were defined by the study team prior to the recordings (**Figures 1A,C**). Three AOIs were not related to the closed-loop system I-ASV and included the conventional ventilator settings (including settings for patient data, ventilation modes, alarms), the classic ventilation curves (pressure-, volume-, flow curves) and numeric values on the displays (including e.g., peak pressure, tidal volume, minute volume, respiratory frequency, end-tidal carbon dioxide CO2). The remaining two AOIs were specifically designed to address the use and the program modes of I-ASV. The AOI "oxygenation Intellivent" combined the oxygenation parameters and controlling oxygenation in I-ASV (including Intellivent oxygenation graphics, positive end-expiratory pressure (PEEP), PEEP limits, fraction of inhaled oxygen (FiO2), target shift for oxygenation). The other AOI "ventilation Intellivent" included ventilation parameters and controlling minute volume in I-ASV (including Intellivent ventilation graphics, %minute-volume, target shift for decarboxylation) (**Figures 1A,C**). All visual fixations on other, irrelevant areas of the respirator (e.g., white space, non-determinable fixations, valves, gauges, tubes) were excluded.

## Primary Outcome

The primary outcome was dwell time (cumulated time spent on an area of interest including fixations, blinks and saccades) for the specific AOIs.

## Secondary Outcomes

Secondary outcomes were revisits (the frequency of revisiting a particular area of interest after gazing at other areas), average fixation time, first fixation (duration of the first fixation of an AOI) and fixation count (the cumulated number of gaze fixations on a particular AOI) to all AOIs.

## Subgroup Analyses

In subgroup analyses, inexperienced nurses (<1 year experience with I-ASV, as described above) were compared with experienced nurses.

## Data Recording

The SMI Eye-tracking Glasses 2 Wireless system (SensoMotoric Instruments, Teltow, Germany) was used. Gaze-tracking was executed at a sampling rate of 60 Hz. Over all distances, the angle of view was measured with an accuracy of 0.5°. The scene video was recorded with a resolution of 960 × 720 pixels at 30 fps. To record audio data, an integrated microphone was used. Eye-tracking data were processed using the SMI BeGaze 3.6 software (SensoMotoric Instruments, Teltow, Germany) and the SMI algorithm for fixation determination. Each ocular fixation during the handling of the respirator was manually assigned to the above-mentioned AOIs.

**TABLE 1** | Baseline characteristics of participants.

| **Baseline characteristics** | | |
|---|---|---|
| Age | Years | 39.5 (29–45.5) |
| Sex | Male | 4 (14.3%) |
| | Female | 24 (85.7%) |
| Vision correction | No | 17 (60.7%) |
| | Yes | 11 (39.3%) |
| Professional experience total | Years | 18 (5.5–25) |
| Professional experience ICU | Years | 11.5 (3–16.5) |
| Being rested* | (Scale 0–10) | 7 (6–8) |
| Mental workload before tracking* | (Scale 0–20) | 12.5 (10–14.8) |
| Physical workload before tracking* | (Scale 0–20) | 10.5 (8–12.5) |
| Mental workload during tracking* | (Scale 0–20) | 12.5 (6.3–14) |
| Physical workload during tracking* | (Scale 0–20) | 7.3 (5.5–11) |
| Subjective stress during tracking* | (Scale 0-10) | 4 (2–5) |

*Data expressed as number (%) or median and interquartile range (IQR). Workload/stress assessed using a numeric scale (where 0 = totally relaxed and 20 = totally stressed). *marks a subjective and self-assessed characteristic.*

## Statistics

No power calculation was performed due to the absence of preliminary tests and partial descriptive statistics. Based on valid data from other eye-tracking studies in the critical care setting (24), a participant number of more than 20 was considered adequate. Data were expressed as the median and interquartile range (25th–75th percentile) for continuous variables or as percentages for categorical variables. Discrete variables were compared using the Chi-square or Fisher exact test, as appropriate. Groups of continuous variables were compared by Mann-Whitney U test, owing to the non-parametric data. For multiple comparisons, Friedman's test with Dunn's correction was used. A $p$-value of $<0.05$ (two-sided p) was considered statistically significant.

Statistical analysis was performed using SPSS Version 23 (SPSS Science, Chicago, IL, USA) and Graphpad prism 7 (San Diego, CA, USA).

# RESULTS

Of a total of 30 ICU nurses assessed, two could not be included owing to exclusion criteria. The remaining 28 agreed to participate in this study and were divided into two groups (inexperienced and experienced groups), with 12 nurses assigned to the inexperienced group and 16 to the experienced group. Median age was 39.5 years; 86% of all participants were female. **Table 1** presents the baseline characteristics of all participants.

The subjective mental and physical workloads assessed by the validated NASA-TLX scale (33) before and during the recordings

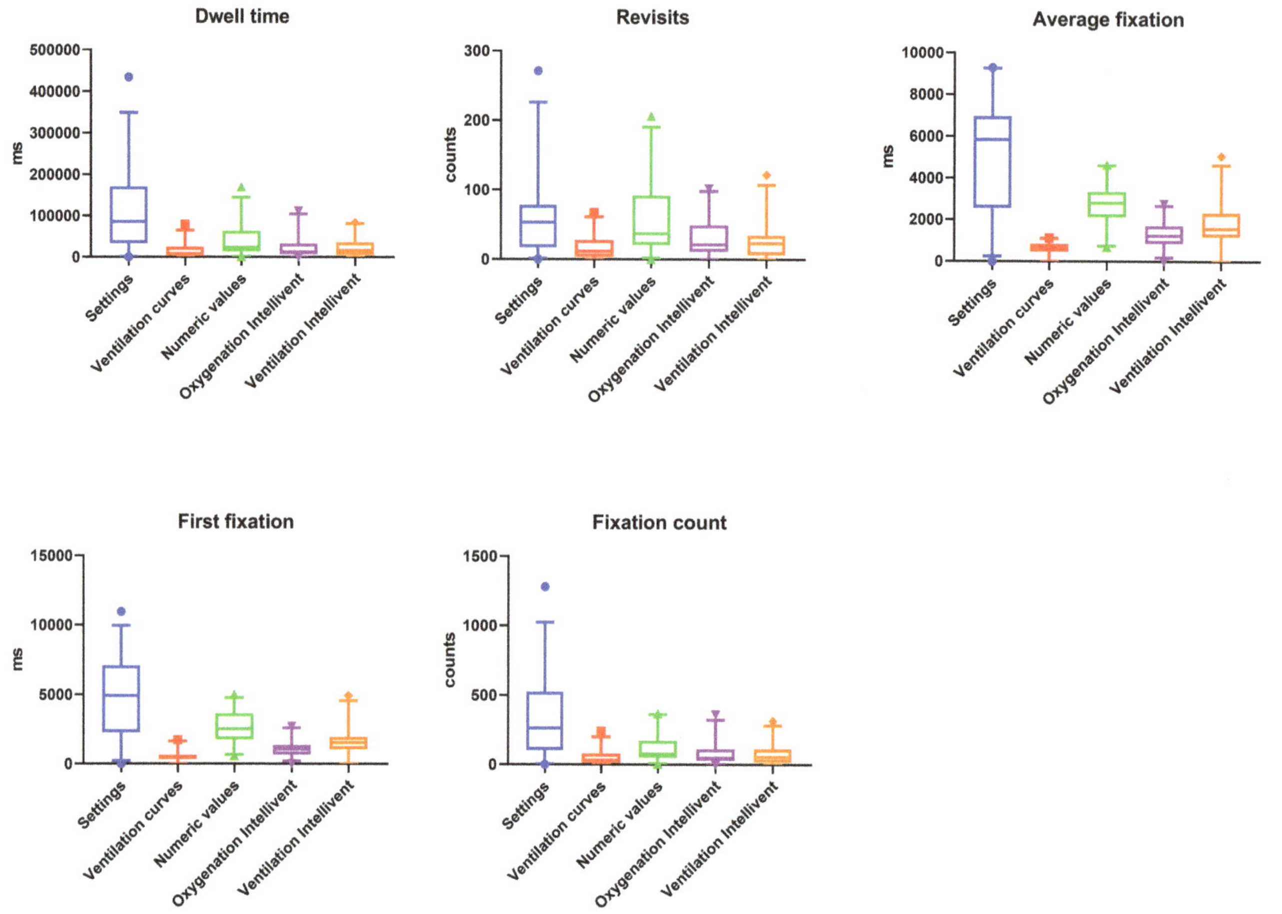


**FIGURE 2 |** Dwell time, Revisits, Average fixation time, First fixation, and Fixation count for all AOIs across the two groups (inexperienced and experienced). Absolute values and *p*-values for multiple comparisons analyzed by Friedman's test are provided in the **Supplementary Tables 1, 2**.

were similar across all participants. Subjective stress during tracking was given a median score of 4 points on a numerical rating scale ranging from 0 to 10 (**Table 1**). No participant was subjectively disturbed by the eye-tracking glasses. No patient emergencies occurred during the recordings and no recordings had to be interrupted or terminated.

Compared to the total tracking time, median fixation of the respirator was 13% and did not differ between the study groups.

Overall, dwell time was significantly prolonged for the settings compared with the other AOIs (**Figures 1B,D, 2**). Similarly, the number of revisits, the average fixation time, first fixation and fixation count were higher for the settings. Furthermore, there was an increased number of revisits, average fixation time and first fixation for the numeric values compared with the other AIOs (**Figure 2**).

Overall, visual attention to the AOIs oxygenation Intellivent and ventilation Intellivent were low for all outcome parameters. Visual attention to the ventilation curves was lowest compared with the other AOIs evaluated. The absolute values for dwell time, revisits, average fixation time, first fixation and fixation count are indicated in **Supplementary Table 1**. *P*-values for multiple comparisons are provided in **Supplementary Table 2**.

**Figure 3** depicts the subgroup analysis for different professional experience.

Dwell time, average fixation time and first fixation on oxygenation Intellivent were significantly higher in experienced participants, and showed a trend toward being elevated for ventilation Intellivent. For the AOI settings, the revisits, average fixation time and first fixation were higher in the experienced group. The *p*-values for all group comparisons are provided in **Supplementary Table 3**.

**Table 2** summarizes data derived from the pre- and post-experiment questionnaires. In particular, it shows that closed loop ventilation is predominantly used on a daily basis. Overall and regardless of previous experience, participants had a positive attitude toward the use of closed-loop ventilation, considered it useful and intended to use it in the future. Subgroup analyses revealed, however, that inexperienced nurses reported significantly higher levels of anxiety toward using I-ASV compared with experienced nurses.

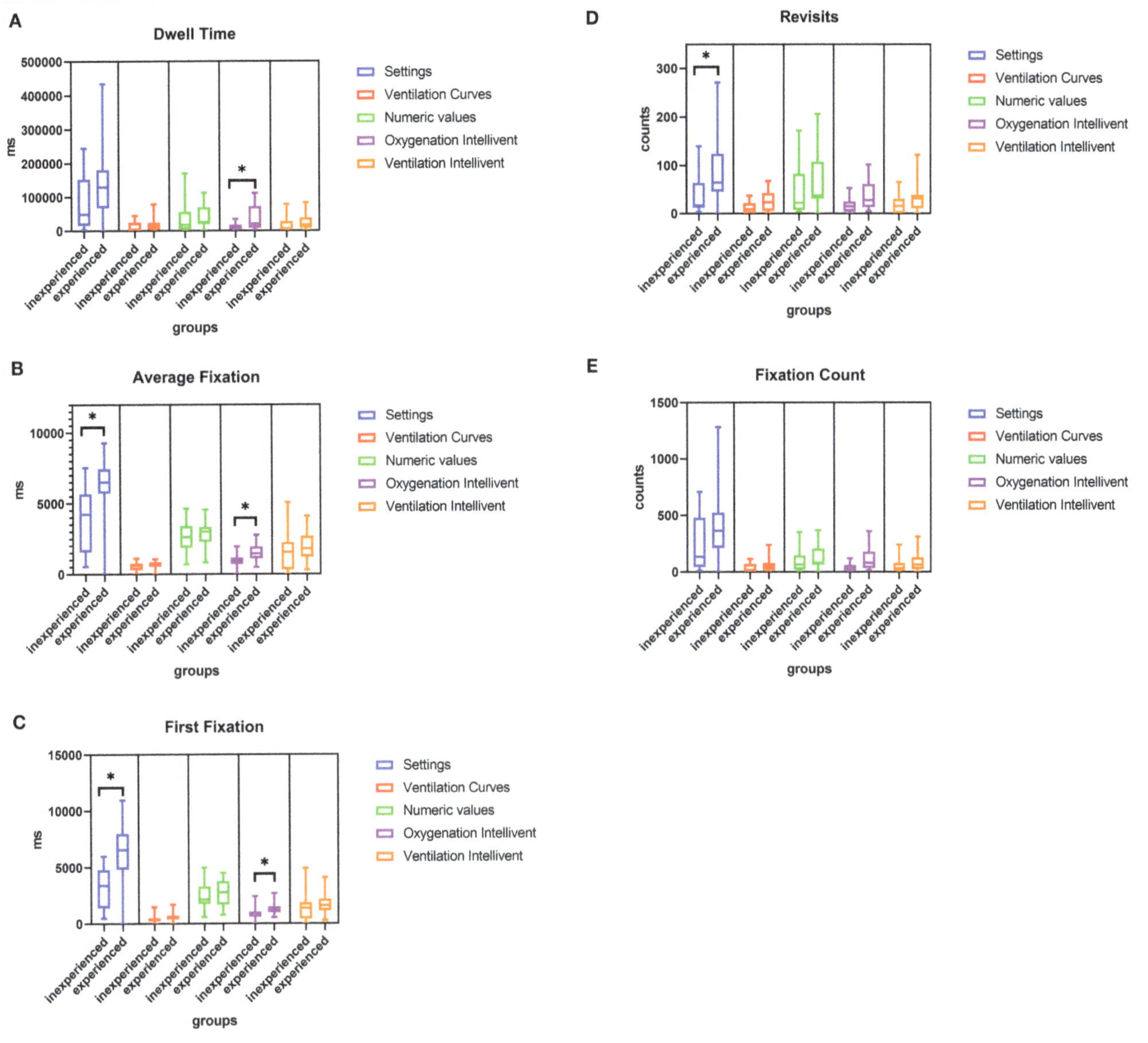


**FIGURE 3 |** Comparison of Dwell time **(A)**, Average fixation time **(B)**, First fixation **(C)**, Revisits **(D)**, and Fixation count **(E)** for all AOIs for inexperienced and experienced participants. $^{*}p < 0.05$. Exact $p$-values for all group comparisons are provided in the **Supplementary Table 3**.

## DISCUSSION

The aim of this study was to analyze gaze patterns of specialized ICU nurses while their patients were undergoing ventilation in the closed-loop mode Intellivent adaptive support ventilation® (I-ASV) and to compare inexperienced with experienced nurses.

The main results of this study imply that, despite the use of a closed-loop ventilation mode, both inexperienced and experienced ICU nurses' gaze patterns were predominantly linked to conventional control and monitor panels (**Figure 2**). As an expression of the nurses' visual attention, the dwell time of the two AOIs settings and numeric values was elevated. The importance of these conventional panels was also mirrored in the significantly higher number of revisits. Moreover, the average fixation time on these AOIs was high as well. This finding suggests that possibly necessary altered visual behavior focusing on new monitoring panels, such as oxygenation and ventilation Intellivent, has not yet been adopted across critical care professionals independent of their experience level and should be specifically trained in the future. As a possible explanation for our findings, relevant visual fixation on numeric values (e.g., peak pressure, tidal volume, respiratory frequency) might represent a high degree of familiarity to ICU nurses. The frequent glances at common numbers reflecting respiratory parameters might mentally be easily linked to ventilation strategies such as protective lung ventilation. As such, it seems plausible that nurses frequently focus on numeric values in order to assure lung protection and anticipate possible ventilation adaptions early.

**TABLE 2** | Pre- and post-experiment questionnaires.

| **Pre-experiment** | **Group** | | |
|---|---|---|---|
| | **Inexperienced (*n* = 12)** | **Experienced (*n* = 16)** | ***p*-value** |
| Professional experience ICU | 7.5 (1–15) | 14.5 (4.5–18) | 0.159 |
| Experience with I-ASV (scale 0–10)* | 1.25 (0.85–3) | 3 (2.75–5) | **0.006** |
| Years using I-ASV (*n*) | 0.9 (0.4–1) | 3 (2.25–4) | **0.001** |
| How often is I-ASV used in everyday practice (scale 0–20) | 15 (5.75–17) | 15.5 (6.5–19) | 0.397 |
| Usefulness of I-ASV (scale 0–7)* | 5 (4.5–6) | 5 (5–6) | 0.478 |
| Productivity with I-ASV (scale 0–7)* | 5 (3–5) | 4 (3–6) | 0.664 |
| Improved patient care with I-ASV (scale 0–7)* | 5 (3.5–6) | 4.5 (4–5.5) | 0.698 |
| Afraid to make mistakes while using I-ASV (scale 0–7)* | 3 (2.5–5) | 1 (1–2) | **0.003** |
| Intimidation caused by I-ASV (scale 0–7)* | 3 (1.5–5) | 1 (1–2) | **0.008** |
| **Post-experiment** I-ASV provided more resources (scale 0–7)* | 5 (5–6) | 4.5 (4–5) | 0.195 |
| Had enough knowledge to use I-ASV (scale 0–7)* | 5 (3–5.5) | 6 (5.5–7) | **0.017** |
| Intention to use I-ASV in the future (scale 0–7)* | 7 (6–7) | 7 (6–7) | 0.837 |
| Use of I-ASV is safe (scale 0–7)* | 3.5 (2–6) | 3 (2–4.5) | 0.568 |

*Data expressed as median and interquartile range (IQR). *marks a subjective and self-assessed characteristic. A higher number represents a higher acceptance of the statement. Groups compared via Mann-Whitney-U test, with < 0.05 considered significant (significant p-values in bold).*

Overall visual attention to oxygenation Intellivent and ventilation Intellivent for the primary and secondary outcomes was markedly lower, despite the use of a closed-loop ventilation mode. Closed-loop ventilation modes such as I-ASV have emerged as new ventilation strategies, but have not been consistently adopted in critical care medicine to date. Our results demonstrate that information displayed by closed-loop ventilation might not be visually presented or mentally processed to a sufficient extent. The frequent visual focus on classic ventilation parameters such as numeric values could also be a sign of a lack of trust in new ventilation modes, especially for less experienced nurses, who reported a significantly higher level of anxiety associated with the use of I-ASV. Furthermore, the question about the subjective safety of I-ASV was answered with a neutral value of 3 on a scale from 1 to 7 (**Table 2**), which might indicate that some degree of skepticism toward modern ventilation modes still remains. However, the use of a single (albeit validated) scale plus one question assessing the subjective safety of I-ASV in the post-experiment questionnaire makes it difficult to draw a conclusive statement. Further trials should compare the visual behavior of ICU nurses between closed-loop and a conventional mode (e.g., pressure-controlled mode).

The sub-analysis of the two professional experience levels revealed that there were differences in gaze behavior between inexperienced and experienced participants. The dwell time and average fixation time on oxygenation Intellivent were significantly longer in experienced nurses. For the AOI settings, the revisits, average fixation time and first fixation were higher. On the one hand, these differences might mirror the greater importance of these AOIs. Research on performing skills among differently trained groups has shown that experts in particular try to focus their attention on critical areas, which is called "target locking" (35, 36). This concept could also be the reason that the dwell time of the experienced nurses was either significantly increased or at least a trend, especially for the settings and the oxygenation and ventilation Intellivent, which are important AOIs in monitoring patients and their clinical condition. In our opinion, the elevated revisits reflect frequent checking glances among the experienced participants. On the other hand, the findings would also support the hypothesis that greater experience might enhance familiarity and routine with the use of closed-loop systems. In line with this postulation, inexperienced nurses might have felt more intimidated by I-ASV and/or were more afraid of making mistakes than experienced nurses, as reflected by the significantly higher levels of anxiety toward the use of I-ASV. Blind faith in the new technology could also have been the reason why the number of revisits and dwell time for the above-mentioned AOIs among novices was reduced. Moreover, in the post-experiment questionnaire, inexperienced nurses reported a lack of knowledge about I-ASV compared with their more experienced counterparts.

One advantage of closed-loop modes could be the enhanced automaticity with less manual adaptation needed to adhere to lung protective ventilation. This implies that frequent visual focus on the conventional AOIs of ventilator curves or numeric values is probably no longer necessary. However, the use of closed-loop systems requires familiarity, ongoing training and a different understanding of one's own supervisory role (18). Nonetheless, the extent to which closed-loop modes under certain specific conditions (e.g., patient-ventilator asynchrony) are superior to the observation of conventional AOIs and the patients themselves is as yet unclear.

Ventilation curves had only low visual importance among the participants in the two groups, probably because ICU nurses are mainly trained to keep an eye on numbers in their professional formation. Another possible reason might be the higher degree of abstraction of ventilation curve shapes, leading to visual disregard. Further, it could be more difficult to cognitively draw conclusions about the patient's respiratory condition by fixating ventilation curves as compared to numeric values or to infer ventilation strategies from the shape of abstract ventilation curves.

This study illustrates that eye-tracking is a useful tool in measuring and quantifying the distribution of visual attention of critical care nurses using a closed-loop system and to reveal differences between inexperienced and experienced participants. Biases due to differences in nurses' workload were minimized, as it proved to be similar among participants.

A main strength of this study is its pragmatic, non-simulated, real-life design. Further, the long tracking time of ~1 h gives a realistic picture of the handling of the respirator, reflecting everyday situations in the ICU. To our knowledge, no comparable real-life studies in an ICU exist. Eye-tracking within such a framework might also assist in designing further novel and innovative studies.

The study has limitations. First, it was a single center study with probable biases due to the specific training of the nurses in I-ASV. Second, the participant number was relatively low. Nevertheless, we found comparable and homogenous distribution of data across dwell time, revisits, average fixation time, first fixation and fixation count among the participants, which adds to the credibility of the data. Third, the patients were from different medical fields, which might mean they had different pulmonary conditions, making distinct ventilation strategies necessary and leading to biases. Moreover, no specific study task was given to the participants, probably making comparisons more difficult. However, the study was explicitly designed to address ICU nurses' everyday behavior in their normal environment and the implementation of a specific task might itself have led to biases (e.g., awareness of the aim of the study). A further limitation of the eye-tracking technology is the difficulty of linking gaze patterns with cognition. Thus, the technology of eye-tracking should be seen as a complementary tool helping to objectively evaluate visual behavior and the visual interaction between humans and machines. This might provide further insights into the significance of visual situation awareness. Further studies with higher participant numbers are needed as well as randomized studies addressing similar questions in nurses with longer professional experience with closed-loop systems. Owing to the probable limitations of classic performance assessment and questionnaire-based human factors analyses in determining individual expertise on ventilation, a neuroscience approach with newer technologies such as eye-tracking could offer more objective and sensitive insights into human factors and human-machine interactions. As a consequence, eye-tracking might also contribute to improved patient safety, enhanced incidence reporting or the detection of factors leading to erroneous behavior in the ICU.

In conclusion, this study demonstrates that the visual fixations of nurses using I-ASV largely remained focused on traditional ventilation parameters. However, experienced nurses fixated AOIs related to the closed-loop system more often than did inexperienced ones, implying the need for constant training and education with new tools in critical care, especially for inexperienced professionals.

## ETHICS STATEMENT

The studies involving human participants were reviewed and approved by Kantonale Ethikkommission Zurich BASEC ID REQ 2017-00798. The patients/participants provided their written informed consent to participate in this study.

## AUTHOR CONTRIBUTIONS

PB, AH, and DH conceived and designed the study, recruited the patients, collected the data, and drafted the report. PB did the ethics submission. PB, AH, NB, SK, SW, PW, MK, QL, ES, RS, and DH analyzed and interpreted the data and contributed to reviewing it. All authors read and approved the final manuscript.

## ACKNOWLEDGMENTS

The authors would like to express their gratitude to all the participants in the study.

## REFERENCES

1. Billings CE, Reynard WD. Human factors in aircraft incidents: results of a 7-year study. *Aviat Space Environ Med.* (1984) 55:960–5.
2. Cooper JB, Newbower RS, Long CD, McPeek B. Preventable anesthesia mishaps: a study of human factors. *Anesthesiology.* (1978) 49:399–406. doi: 10.1097/00000542-197812000-00004
3. Ivatury RR, Guilford K, Malhotra AK, Duane T, Aboutanos M, Martin N. Patient safety in trauma: maximal impact management errors at a level I trauma center. *J Trauma.* (2008) 64:265–70; discussion 70–2. doi: 10.1097/TA.0b013e318163359d
4. Pucher PH, Aggarwal R, Twaij A, Batrick N, Jenkins M, Darzi A. Identifying and addressing preventable process errors in trauma care. *World J Surg.* (2013) 37:752–8. doi: 10.1007/s00268-013-1917-9
5. Shappell SA, Wiegmann DA. U.S. naval aviation mishaps, 1977-92: differences between single- and dual-piloted aircraft. *Aviat Space Environ Med.* (1996) 67:65–9.
6. Vioque SM, Kim PK, McMaster J, Gallagher J, Allen SR, Holena DN, et al. Classifying errors in preventable and potentially preventable trauma deaths: a 9-year review using the Joint Commission's standardized methodology. *Am J Surg.* (2014) 208:187–94. doi: 10.1016/j.amjsurg.2014.02.006
7. Brennan TA, Leape LL, Laird NM, Hebert L, Localio AR, Lawthers AG, et al. Incidence of adverse events and negligence in hospitalized patients. Results of the Harvard Medical practice study I. *N Engl J Med.* (1991) 324:370–6. doi: 10.1056/NEJM199102073240604
8. Carayon P, Wood KE. Patient safety - the role of human factors and systems engineering. *Stud Health Technol Inform.* (2010) 153:23–46. doi: 10.3233/IKS-2009-0134
9. Dominiczak J, Khansa L. Principles of automation for patient safety in intensive care: learning from aviation. *Jt Commiss J Qual Pat Saf.* (2018) 44:366–71. doi: 10.1016/j.jcjq.2017.11.008
10. Endsley MR. From here to autonomy. *Hum Fact.* (2017) 59:5–27. doi: 10.1177/0018720816681350
11. Koch SH, Weir C, Westenskow D, Gondan M, Agutter J, Haar M, et al. Evaluation of the effect of information integration in displays for ICU nurses on situation awareness and task completion time: a prospective randomized controlled study. *Int J Med Inform.* (2013) 82:665–75. doi: 10.1016/j.ijmedinf.2012.10.002
12. Salmon P, Walker G, Stanton N. Pilot error versus sociotechnical systems failure: a distributed situation awareness analysis of air France 447. *Theoret Issues Ergon Sci.* (2015) 17:1–16. doi: 10.1080/1463922X.2015.1106618
13. Reason J, Manstead A, Stradling S, Baxter J, Campbell K. Errors and violations on the roads: a real distinction? *Ergonomics.* (1990) 33:1315–32. doi: 10.1080/00140139008925335
14. Andrade E, Quinlan L, Harte R, Byrne D, Fallon E, Kelly M, et al. Novel interface designs for patient monitoring applications in critical care medicine: human factors review. *JMIR Hum Fact.* (2020) 7:e15052. doi: 10.2196/15052
15. Anders S, Albert R, Miller A, Weinger MB, Doig AK, Behrens M, et al. Evaluation of an integrated graphical display to promote acute change detection in ICU patients. *Int J Med Inform.* (2012) 81:842–51. doi: 10.1016/j.ijmedinf.2012.04.004
16. Platen PV, Pomprapa A, Lachmann B, Leonhardt S. The dawn of physiological closed-loop ventilation-a review. *Crit Care.* (2020) 24:121. doi: 10.1186/s13054-020-2810-1

17. Wendel Garcia PD, Hofmaenner DA, Brugger SD, Acevedo CT, Bartussek J, Camen G, et al. Closed-Loop versus conventional mechanical ventilation in COVID-19 ARDS. *J Intensive Care Med.* (2021). doi: 10.1177/08850666211024139. [Epub ahead of print].
18. Sheridan T. Adaptive automation, level of automation, allocation authority, supervisory control, and adaptive control: distinctions and modes of adaptation. *Syst Man Cybernet Part A Syst Hum IEEE Transac.* (2011) 41:662–7. doi: 10.1109/TSMCA.2010.2093888
19. van Galen LS, Struik PW, Driesen BE, Merten H, Ludikhuize J, van der Spoel JI, et al. Delayed recognition of deterioration of patients in general wards is mostly caused by human related monitoring failures: a root cause analysis of unplanned ICU admissions. *PloS ONE.* (2016) 11:e0161393. doi: 10.1371/journal.pone.0161393
20. Garry J, Casey K, Cole TK, Regensburg A, McElroy C, Schneider E, et al. A pilot study of eye-tracking devices in intensive care. *Surgery.* (2016) 159:938–44. doi: 10.1016/j.surg.2015.08.012
21. Gold JA, Stephenson LE, Gorsuch A, Parthasarathy K, Mohan V. Feasibility of utilizing a commercial eye tracker to assess electronic health record use during patient simulation. *Health Inform J.* (2016) 22:744–57. doi: 10.1177/1460458215590250
22. Grundgeiger T, Klöffel C, Mohme S, Wurmb T, Happel O. An investigation into the effects of real vs. stimulated cases and level of experience on the distribution of visual attention during induction of general anaesthesia. *Anaesthesia.* (2017) 72:624–32. doi: 10.1111/anae.13821
23. Hofmaenner DA, Klinzing S, Brandi G, Hess S, Lohmeyer Q, Enthofer K, et al. The doctor's point of view: eye-tracking as an investigative tool in the extubationprocess in intensive care units. A pilot study. *Minerva Anestesiol.* (2020) 86:1180–9. doi: 10.23736/S0375-9393.20.14468-7
24. Klausen A, Röhrig R, Lipprandt M. Feasibility of eyetracking in critical care environments - a systematic review. *Stud Health Technol Inform.* (2016) 228:604–8. doi: 10.3233/978-1-61499-678-1-604
25. Law BHY, Cheung PY, Wagner M, van Os S, Zheng B, Schmölzer G. Analysis of neonatal resuscitation using eye tracking: a pilot study. *Arch Dis Child Fetal Neonatal Ed.* (2018) 103:F82–4. doi: 10.1136/archdischild-2017-313114
26. Law BHY, Schmölzer GM. Analysis of visual attention and team communications during neonatal endotracheal intubations using eye-tracking: an observational study. *Resuscitation.* (2020) 153:176–82. doi: 10.1016/j.resuscitation.2020.06.019
27. Schulz CM, Schneider E, Fritz L, Vockeroth J, Hapfelmeier A, Brandt T, et al. Visual attention of anaesthetists during simulated critical incidents. *Br J Anaesth.* (2011) 106:807–13. doi: 10.1093/bja/aer087
28. Schulz CM, Schneider E, Fritz L, Vockeroth J, Hapfelmeier A, Wasmaier M, et al. Eye tracking for assessment of workload: a pilot study in an anaesthesia simulator environment. *Br J Anaesth.* (2011) 106:44–50. doi: 10.1093/bja/aeq307
29. Spaeth J, Schweizer T, Schmutz A, Buerkle H, Schumann S. Comparative usability of modern anaesthesia ventilators: a human factors study. *Br J Anaesth.* (2017) 119:1000–8. doi: 10.1093/bja/aex226
30. Tien T, Pucher PH, Sodergren MH, Sriskandarajah K, Yang GZ, Darzi A. Eye tracking for skills assessment and training: a systematic review. *J Surg Res.* (2014) 191:169–78. doi: 10.1016/j.jss.2014.04.032
31. Wagner M, Gröpel P, Bibl K, Olischar M, Auerbach MA, Gross IT. Eye-tracking during simulation-based neonatal airway management. *Pediatr Res.* (2020) 87:518–22. doi: 10.1038/s41390-019-0571-9
32. Hofmaenner DA, Herling A, Klinzing S, Wegner S, Lohmeyer Q, Schuepbach RA, et al. Use of eye tracking in analyzing distribution of visual attention among critical care nurses in daily professional life: an observational study. *J Clin Monitor Comput.* (2020) 9:1–8. doi: 10.1007/s10877-020-00628-2
33. Hart SG, Staveland LE. Development of NASA-TLX (Task Load Index): results of empirical and theoretical research. *Adv Psychol.* (1988) 52:139–83. doi: 10.1016/S0166-4115(08)62386-9
34. Venkatesh V, Morris M, Davis G, Davis F. User acceptance of information technology: toward a unified view. *MIS Q.* (2003) 27:425–78. doi: 10.2307/30036540
35. Causer J, Vickers JN, Snelgrove R, Arsenault G, Harvey A. Performing under pressure: quiet eye training improves surgical knot-tying performance. *Surgery.* (2014) 156:1089–96. doi: 10.1016/j.surg.2014.05.004
36. Wilson MR, Vine SJ, Bright E, Masters RS, Defriend D, McGrath JS. Gaze training enhances laparoscopic technical skill acquisition and multi-tasking performance: a randomized, controlled study. *Surg Endosc.* (2011) 25:3731–9. doi: 10.1007/s00464-011-1802-2

# 10

# Classification of Patients with Sepsis According to Immune Cell Characteristics: A Bioinformatic Analysis of Two Cohort Studies

*Shi Zhang, Zongsheng Wu, Wei Chang, Feng Liu, Jianfeng Xie, Yi Yang and Haibo Qiu**

*Jiangsu Provincial Key Laboratory of Critical Care Medicine, Department of Critical Care Medicine, Zhongda Hospital, School of Medicine, Southeast University, Nanjing, China*

***Correspondence:***
*Haibo Qiu*
*haiboq2000@163.com*

**Background:** Sepsis is well-known to alter innate and adaptive immune responses for sustained periods after initiation by an invading pathogen. Identification of immune cell characteristics may shed light on the immune signature of patients with sepsis and further indicate the appropriate immune-modulatory therapy for distinct populations. Therefore, we aimed to establish an immune model to classify sepsis into different immune endotypes via transcriptomics data analysis of previously published cohort studies.

**Methods:** Datasets from two observational cohort studies that included 585 consecutive sepsis patients admitted to two intensive care units were downloaded as a training cohort and an external validation cohort. We analyzed genome-wide gene expression profiles in blood from these patients by using machine learning and bioinformatics.

**Results:** The training cohort and the validation cohort had 479 and 106 patients, respectively. Principal component analysis indicated that two immune subphenotypes associated with sepsis, designated the immunoparalysis endotype, and immunocompetent endotype, could be distinguished clearly. In the training cohort, a higher cumulative 28-day mortality was found in patients classified as having the immunoparalysis endotype, and the hazard ratio was 2.32 (95% CI: 1.53–3.46 vs. the immunocompetent endotype). External validation further demonstrated that the present model could categorize sepsis into the immunoparalysis and immunocompetent type precisely and efficiently. The percentages of 4 types of immune cells (M0 macrophages, M2 macrophages, naïve B cells, and naïve CD4 T cells) were significantly associated with 28-day cumulative mortality ($P < 0.05$).

**Conclusion:** The present study developed a comprehensive tool to identify the immunoparalysis endotype and immunocompetent status in hospitalized patients with sepsis and provides novel clues for further targeting of therapeutic approaches.

**Keywords: sepsis, immune status, heterogeneity, endotype, immunoparalysis**

## BACKGROUND

Sepsis is a highly heterogeneous syndrome associated with diverse immune status upon pathogen invasion. Normal immune responses can eradicate pathogens, and the pathophysiology of sepsis is caused by the inappropriate regulation of these normal reactions (1, 2). The extent of hyperactivated and hypoactivated immune responses vary among individuals, which results in heterogeneities in immune responses in sepsis (3, 4). It is urgent to clarify the immune status of sepsis to help identify patients who would benefit from immunomodulatory therapies (5–9).

Previous studies attempted to identify diverse immune statuses through clinical features or biomarkers. For example, Seymour et al. classified sepsis patients into four derived phenotypes based on 29 clinical features (temperature, mean arterial pressure, fluid resuscitation response, central venous oxygen saturation, etc.) (10). Using transcriptomic data, researchers identified four subphenotypes of sepsis; among them, one phenotype was associated with higher mortality than the other three phenotypes, which were associated with moderate mortality (11). However, the above described studies of phenotypes were qualitative rather than quantitative, and the immune state level was barely recognized. In addition, the use of one or two biomarkers, such as human leukocyte antigen-DR isotype (HLA-DR) and cytotoxic T lymphocyte-associated antigen-4 (CTLA-4), could not truly represent the global immune status. Moreover, false positive and false negative results might occur for various kinds of patients. Last but not least, routine parameters and biomarkers reflect surface-level phenomena associated with immune cell dysfunction and imbalance and are insufficiently robust to permit an actual intrinsic monitoring of immune status (12–15).

Recently, Newman et al. developed an algorithm to calculate the proportions of 22 types of human immune cells according to the ribonucleic acid (RNA) matrix (16) (using RNAomics or RNA-seq), and the proportions of these 22 human immune cell types have been confirmed to represent the immune status of human beings. Furthermore, it has been demonstrated that the CIBERSORT algorithm has higher accuracy and sensitivity than conventional technologies such as immunohistochemistry and flow cytometry (17, 18). To date, this algorithm has been widely utilized in assessing the immune status of patients with cancer for guiding immunotherapy, but it has never been used in sepsis patients. Thus, with the CIBERSORT approach, we assessed the proportions of 22 types of infiltrating immune cells based on two published cohort studies of sepsis. To analyze and quantitatively measure the patient immune responses to pathogens, an immune model for categorizing the immune endotypes of sepsis was constructed, and the immune cell subsets associated with potential therapeutic targets with prognostic value were also explored simultaneously.

## METHODS

### Data Sources and Study Selection

A public database (GEO database) was searched for all expression microarrays that matched terms associated with sepsis. The datasets were collected from clinical studies investigating sepsis in adults using peripheral blood within 48 h after ICU admission. The exclusion criteria were as follows: (1) datasets that utilized endotoxin or lipopolysaccharide infusion like those used in *in vitro* or animal models of sepsis; (2) clinical gene expression microarray analyses derived from sorted cells; and (3) a sample size <100.

### Data Preprocessing

All datasets were downloaded as.txt files, and the outputs from the mRNA array were normal-exponential background-corrected and then between-array quantile-normalized using the limma R package. To ensure compatibility with the microarray study, expression was normalized using weighted linear regression, and the estimated precision weights of each observation were multiplied by the corresponding log2 value to yield the final gene expression values.

The dataset with the most complete prognostic data and the maximum sample size was used as the training cohort, and another dataset was used as the external validation cohort.

### Cell Type Identification by Estimating the Relative Subset of Known RNA Transcripts (CIBERSORT)

We used the CIBERSORT algorithm for quantification and discrimination of the absolute proportions of 22 human immune cell phenotypes from transcriptomic data, including seven T cell types (CD8 T cells, CD4 naïve T cells, CD4 memory resting T cells, CD4 memory activated T cells, follicular helper T cells, regulatory T cells, and gamma delta T cells), naïve and memory B cells, plasma cells, NK cells, and myeloid subsets. Immune cells are classified as high, median, and low expression according to the high and low interquartile ranges (IQRs). Pearson correlation analyses for various immune cell types were performed to assess the collinearity of the enrolled immune cells.

### Identification of Immune Cells With Prognostic Value and Construction of an Immunity Risk Model

The univariate Cox proportional hazards model with Bonferroni correction for multiple comparisons was used to determine the prognostic signatures with a cut-off value of $P < 0.05$ by using the survival R package. Then, both backward and forward stepwise selection with the Akaike information criterion (AIC) were used to identify the final variables for the multivariable Cox proportional hazards regression models through the survival R package.

The associations of relevant immune cell types with survival were assessed using multivariable Cox proportional hazard regression models. Hazard ratios (HRs) were presented with the 95% CIs. Selected variables were incorporated into the risk model to predict the probability of 28-day mortality using the rms R package. The risk scores for each sample were calculated according to the risk model. The respective medians of two clusters were used as the cut-off values to classify the patients as having either the Immunity-A endotype or the Immunity-B endotype.

## Assessment and Validation of the Immune Model

To multidimensionally evaluate the discrimination ability of the risk model in categorizing sepsis-induced immune dysfunction, we investigated the variation in immune cells, immune molecules, and immunity-related signal transduction pathways between the immunity-A endotype and immunity-B endotype. An empirical Bayesian approach was implemented to estimate immune cell and immune molecule changes using moderated *t*-tests. Gene set enrichment analysis (GSEA) was performed to assess immunity-related pathway activity variation between the Immunity-A and Immunity-B types. A $P < 0.05$ was set as the significance criterion. Kaplan-Meier (KM) curves and principal component analysis (PCA) were performed to evaluate the calibration capability of the risk model. External datasets were utilized for model validation. Perl 64 was used to merge data. Data processing, analysis, and diagram plotting were conducted in R x64 3.6.1.

## Sensitive Analysis

To further evaluate whether the current model could identify the immune status of a pneumonia and non-pneumonia induced sepsis population, the sensitive analyses were conducted to investigate discrimination ability of the current model in pneumonia and non- pneumonia patients respectively.

# RESULTS

## Characteristics of the Datasets and Patients

After the search strategy and inclusion criteria were determined, 2 mRNA datasets from patients with sepsis (GSE65682 and GSE63042) were used to build the mRNA expression profiling datasets. The flow-process diagrams of the process of dataset screening are shown in **Supplementary Figure 1**. The GSE65682 dataset (479 patients with sepsis) was used as the training cohort since the contributors (University Medical Center in Utrecht and the Academic Medical Center in Amsterdam) uploaded relatively complete prognostic data, and this dataset had the maximum sample size. Simultaneously, GSE63042 (106 patients with sepsis) was used as the external validation cohort. All patients were older than 18 years and were diagnosed with sepsis. The septic shock ratios for GSE65682 and GSE63042 were 34.8 and 31.1%, respectively. Details of the demographic and clinical characteristics are shown in **Table 1**.

**TABLE 1** | Demographic and clinical characteristics.

| | GSE65682 (*N* = 479) | GSE63042 (*N* = 106) |
|---|---|---|
| Male sex | 272 (56.8%) | 63 (59.4%) |
| Age | 63 (18–89) | 59 (38–85) |
| Country | Netherlands | USA |
| Pneumonia diagnoses | 183 (38.0%) | 24 (22.6%) |
| Septic shock | 167 (34.8%) | 33 (31.1%) |
| 28 day mortality | 115 (24.0%) | 28 (26.4%) |
| Main study | Classification for sepsis through transcriptomic data | Bioinformatic analysis for host response in sepsis |

*N, number.*

## Construction of the Immunity Risk Model

According to the univariate Cox regression analyses and stepwise selection, the percentages of 4 immune cell types (M0 macrophages, M2 macrophages, naïve B cells, and naïve CD4 T cells) were significantly associated with 28-day cumulative mortality (**Figure 1A**). The 4 identified immune cell types were included in the immunity risk model generated through multivariate Cox regression (**Figure 1B**). Each patient was assigned a risk score through this model. Correlation analyses among various immune cell types to find the links among immune cells was shown in **Figure 1C**.

## Model Assessment

The three-dimensional results (immune cells, immune molecules, and immunity-related pathways) demonstrate that this risk model could stratify sepsis patients with either immunocompetent status or immunoparalysis. Patients with the immunity-B endotype displayed an immunocompetent status, while the immunity-A endotype patients suffered from immunoparalysis (**Figure 2**). At the level of immune cells, differential expression analysis indicated that the percentages of immune-enhancing cells (neutrophils, gamma delta T cells, activated dendritic cells, and activated mast cells) were significantly downregulated in the immunity-A endotype (**Figure 2A**) compared with those in the immunity-B endotype, $P < 0.05$. Moreover, the percentages of immunosuppressive cells (regulatory T cells and M2 macrophages) and naïve immune cells (naïve B cells, naïve CD4 T cells, and M0 macrophages) were obviously upregulated in the immunity-A endotype compared with those in the immunity-B endotype, $P < 0.05$.

On the other hand, immune-enhancing molecules (HLA-DRA, HLA-DRB, IL1B, IFNAR, IFNGR, CD5, and CD86) were significantly downregulated, and immunosuppressive molecules (IL10) were obviously upregulated in the immunity-A endotype compared with those in the immunity-B endotype at the molecular level according to the violin plot (**Figure 2B**), $P < 0.05$.

Finally, at the level of immunity-related signal transduction pathways, GSEA demonstrated that immune enhancement-related pathways were significantly suppressed in the immunity-A endotype in sepsis (**Figure 2C**). In contrast, these pathways were activated in the immunity-B endotype. The summary view of the GSEA results in the training cohort is shown in **Figure 2C**; the details for every pathway are shown in **Supplementary Figures 2–5**. These pathways could be classified as associated with innate immunity (endocytosis and natural killer cell-mediated cytotoxicity), humoral immunity (antigen processing and presentation, B cell receptor signaling pathway, and intestinal immune network for IgA production), cellular immunity (T cell receptor signaling pathway and Toll-like receptor signaling pathway), and the promotion of immunity

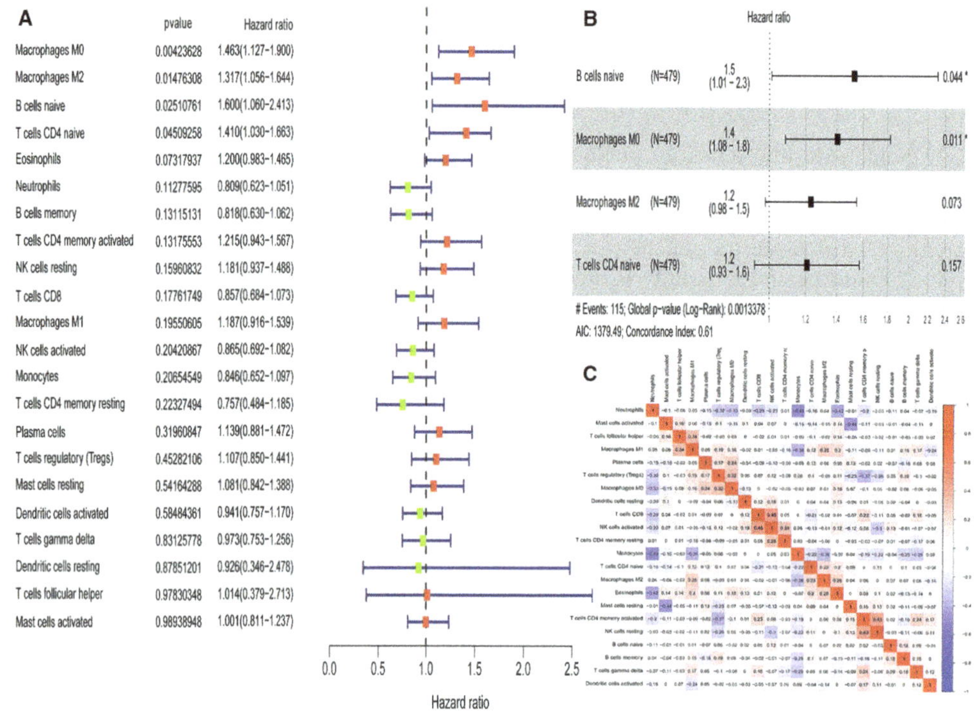


**FIGURE 1 |** Identification of immune cells with prognostic value and construction of an immunity risk model. **(A)** Forest plots of univariate Cox proportional hazard analysis for the identification of prognostic immune cells (red forest plots represent hazard factors, and green forest plots represent protective factors). **(B)** Forest plots of multivariable Cox proportional hazard analysis for the construction of the immunity risk model (AIC, Akaike information criterion), **(C)** Correlation heat map for the assessment of collinearity (numbers in the heatmap represent Pearson correlation coefficients; red represents a positive correlation and blue represents a negative correlation). $^{*}P < 0.05$.

(Fc epsilon RI signaling pathway, chemokine signaling pathway, RIG-I-like receptor signaling pathway, and NOD-like receptor signaling pathway).

The KM curves indicated that the immunity-A endotype was associated with a significantly higher cumulative 28-day mortality rate compared to the immunity-B endotype, with a hazard ratio (95% CI) of 2.32 (1.53–3.46) and a *P*-value of 0.00 (**Figure 3A**). PCA shows an obvious clustering trend for immune status between the Immunity-A and Immunity-B endotypes (**Figure 3B**).

## Sensitivity Analysis

In a sensitivity analysis evaluating the removal of sepsis induced by pneumonia in GSE65682, similar results in the overall population are observed which are shown in **Figures 4**, **5**. However, this sensitivity analysis could not be done in GSE63042, since the original case data of individuals were not provided by researchers.

## External Validation

To validate the model of Immunity-A and Immunity-B, the GSE63042 datasets were set as the external validation cohort. External validation further confirms that the ability of this model to categorize based on immune dysfunction is efficient and precise.

In the external validation cohort, analysis of the levels of immune cells, immune molecules, and immune pathways robustly confirmed that patients in the Immunity-A endotype classified by the current model suffered from immunoparalysis. Conversely, patients in the immunity-B endotype showed immunocompetent status ($P < 0.05$) (**Figure 6**). The details of every pathway are shown in **Supplementary Figures 6–9**.

# DISCUSSION

Accumulating evidence supports the central role of the immune system in the pathogenesis of sepsis, a better insight to uncover the immunological phenotype of sepsis patients is crucial for effective immunomodulatory treatment. The current study is the first to identify two distinct immune endotypes based on the microarray data of sepsis patients by using CIBERSORT analysis and provides novel evidence and clues for further research on the molecular mechanisms of sepsis. In particular, sepsis can be divided into subphenotypes based on infiltrating immune cell characteristics. The immunocompetent subphenotype (immunity-B endotype) is characterized by increased expression levels of immune response-associated molecules, decreases in immature immune cells (naïve B cells, naïve CD4 T cells, and M0 macrophages), and increased activity of immune-enhancing pathways compared to the immunity-A

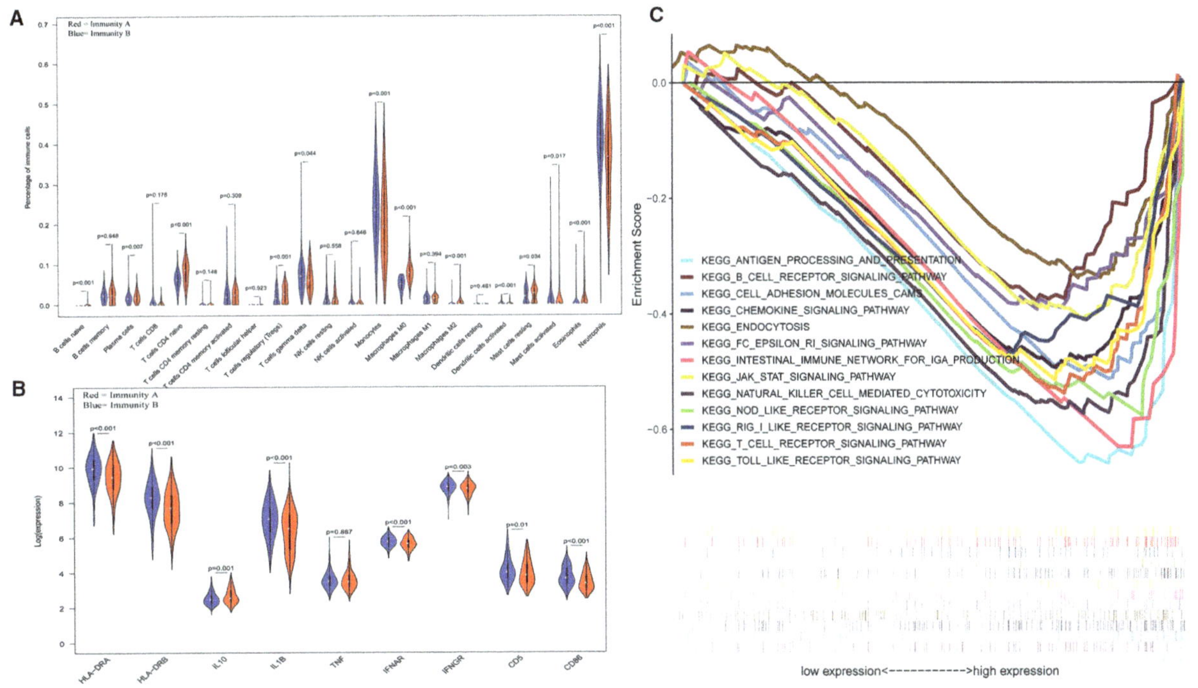


**FIGURE 2 |** Three-dimensional assessments demonstrate that patients with the immunity-A endotype suffer from immune suppression. **(A)** Violin plots of immune cell analyses (medians, quartiles, extremums, data distributions, and *P*-values for the difference analysis are described in the violin plots. The percentages of immune-enhancing cells (neutrophils, gamma delta T cells, activated dendritic cells, and activated mast cells) were significantly decreased in the immunity-A endotype. The percentages of immunosuppressive cells (regulatory T cells, M2 macrophages) and naïve immune cells (naïve B cells, naïve CD4 T cells and M0 macrophages)—were obviously upregulated in the immunity-A endotype. **(B)** Violin plots of the immune molecule difference analysis. The immune-enhancing molecules (HLA-DRA, HLA-DRB, IL1B, IFNAR, IFNGR, CD5, and CD86) were significantly downregulated and an immunosuppressive molecule—IL10—was obviously upregulated in the immunity-A endotype. **(C)** Diagrams of the Gene Set Enrichment Analysis. The innate immunity, humoral immunity, cellular immunity, and promotion of immunity-related pathways were all suppressed in the immunity-A endotype group.

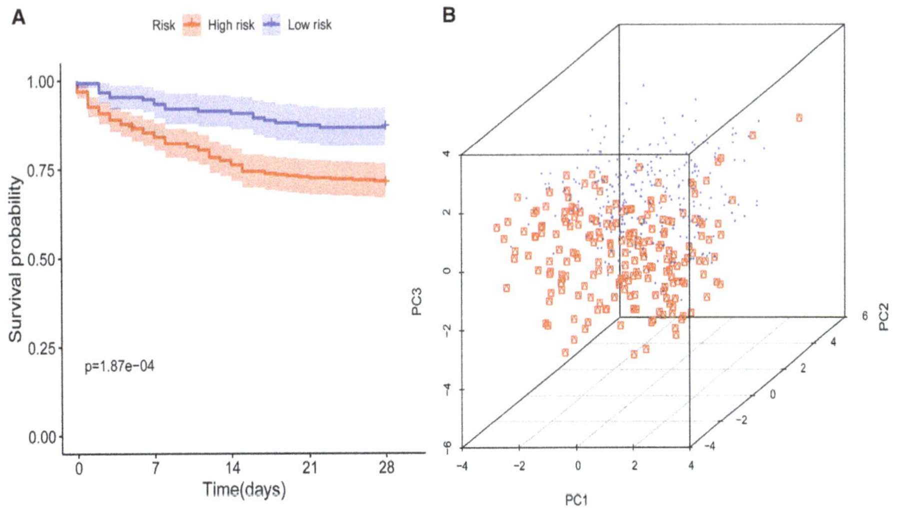


**FIGURE 3 |** Survival curves and principal component analysis for evaluating the calibration ability of the immunity risk model. **(A)** Survival curves of the immunity-A and immunity-B endotypes (Kaplan-Meier curves indicate that the immunity-A endotype was associated with significantly higher mortality than the immunity-B endotype), **(B)** Principal component analysis between the immunity-A and immunity-B endotypes (the red dots represent patients with the immunity-A endotype, and the blue dots represent patients with the immunity-B endotype; an obvious clustering trend can be found).

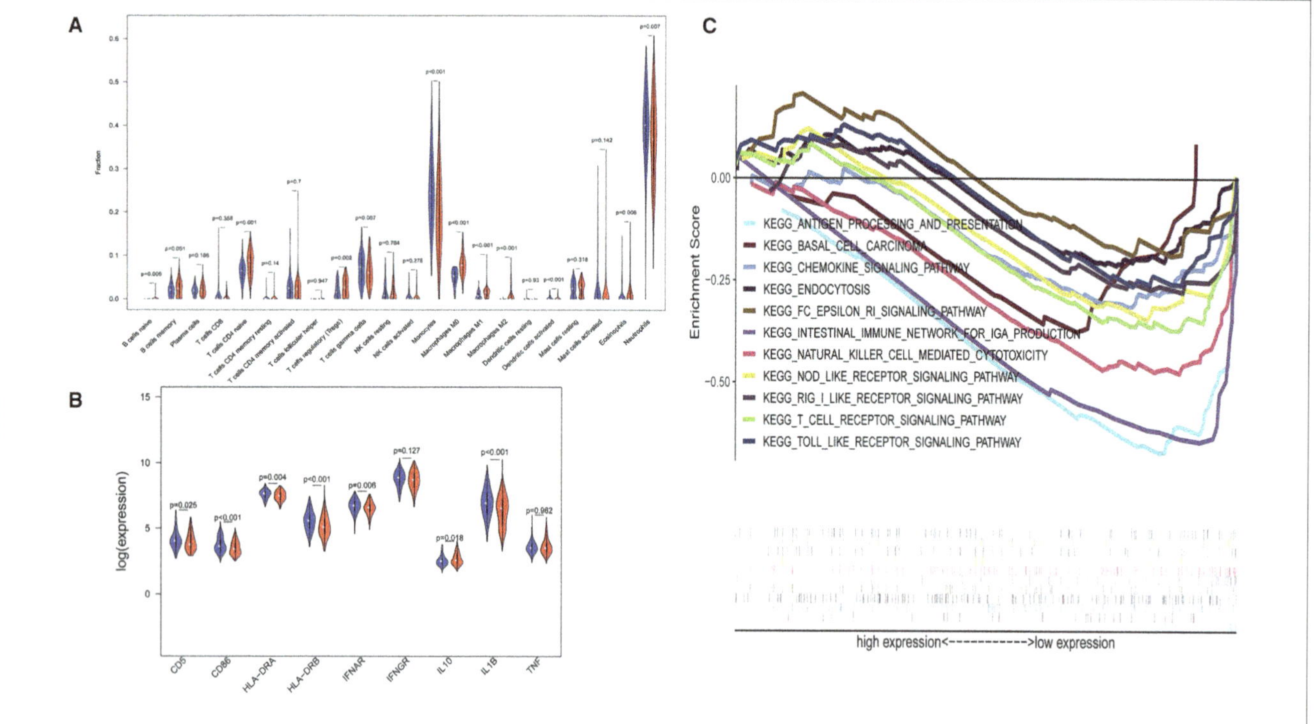


**FIGURE 4** | Subgroup analysis on septic population after removing patients with pneumonia. **(A)** Violin plots of immune cell difference analyses (medians, quartiles, extremums, data distributions, and *P*-values for the difference analysis are described in violin plots. The percentages of immune-enhancing cells (activated neutrophils and dendritic cells) were significantly downregulated in the immunity-A endotype. The percentages of immune suppressive cells (regulatory T cells, and macrophage M2) and naïve immune cells (naïve B cells, naïve CD4 T cells, and M0 macrophages) were obviously upregulated in the immunity-A endotype). **(B)** Violin plots of the immune molecule difference analysis (immune-enhancing molecules—HLA-DRA, HLA-DRB, IL1B, IFNAR, CD5, and CD86—were significantly downregulated and the immunosuppressive molecule IL10 was obviously upregulated in the immunity-A endotype). **(C)** Diagrams of the Gene Set Enrichment Analysis. The innate immunity, humoral immunity, cellular immunity, and promotion of immunity-related pathways were all suppressed in the immunity-A endotype group.

endotype (immunoparalysis). In addition, we also revealed that elevations in M0 macrophages, M2 macrophages, naïve B cells, and naïve CD4 T cells in peripheral blood were independent risk factors for poor prognosis in sepsis at onset. Patients with the immunity-A endotype were confirmed as having immunoparalysis and a higher cumulative 28-day mortality, and patients with the immunity-B endotype seemed to have an immunocompetent status and a higher survival rate. The immune score calculated by this model could represent the severity of immunoparalysis.

Normal immune and physiologic responses eradicate pathogens, and the pathophysiology of sepsis is due to the improper regulation of these normal reactions. Pathogen contact with the inflammatory system should eliminate the microbe and rapidly return the host to homeostasis. The septic response may accelerate due to continued activation of macrophages/monocytes, which play a key role in the regulation of both innate and adaptive immunity. The large contribution to immune suppression of peripheral blood mononuclear cells (including macrophages and T and B lymphocytes) reveal the downregulation of genes involved in the inflammatory response and the increased expression of genes involved in apoptosis. Massive mononuclear cell death leads to naïve cell proliferation in the bone marrow. These findings may explain why immature peripheral blood mononuclear cells were more common in the immune A endotype.

A number of alterations in the expression of distinct cell surface markers, such as HLA-DRA, HLA-DRB, IL1B, IFNAR, IFNGR, CD5, and CD86, have been described in these two endotypes, and these molecules were defined as immunoactivated molecules in previous studies (19, 20). Furthermore, Venet et al. and Carson et al. showed that sepsis induced an increase in the proportion of anti-inflammatory immune cells (such as Tregs) that release anti-inflammatory cytokines (such as IL10), which resulted in epigenetic alterations of naïve immune cells and further suppressed inflammatory activation-related pathways (such as the Toll-like receptor signaling pathway) (21, 22). To date, researchers believe that immunoparalysis is an independent risk factor for poor prognosis in sepsis (19, 20), which was also confirmed in our study. Therefore, it was indicated that an increase in the proportion of naïve immune cells and immunosuppressive cells were the essential characteristics of immunoparalysis in sepsis.

However, previous studies of immunoparalysis in sepsis evaluated only some immune features (single immune cells or immune molecules) and lacked global assessment and validation (19–22). Therefore, the present study attempted to explore immune models appropriate for identifying immunoparalysis

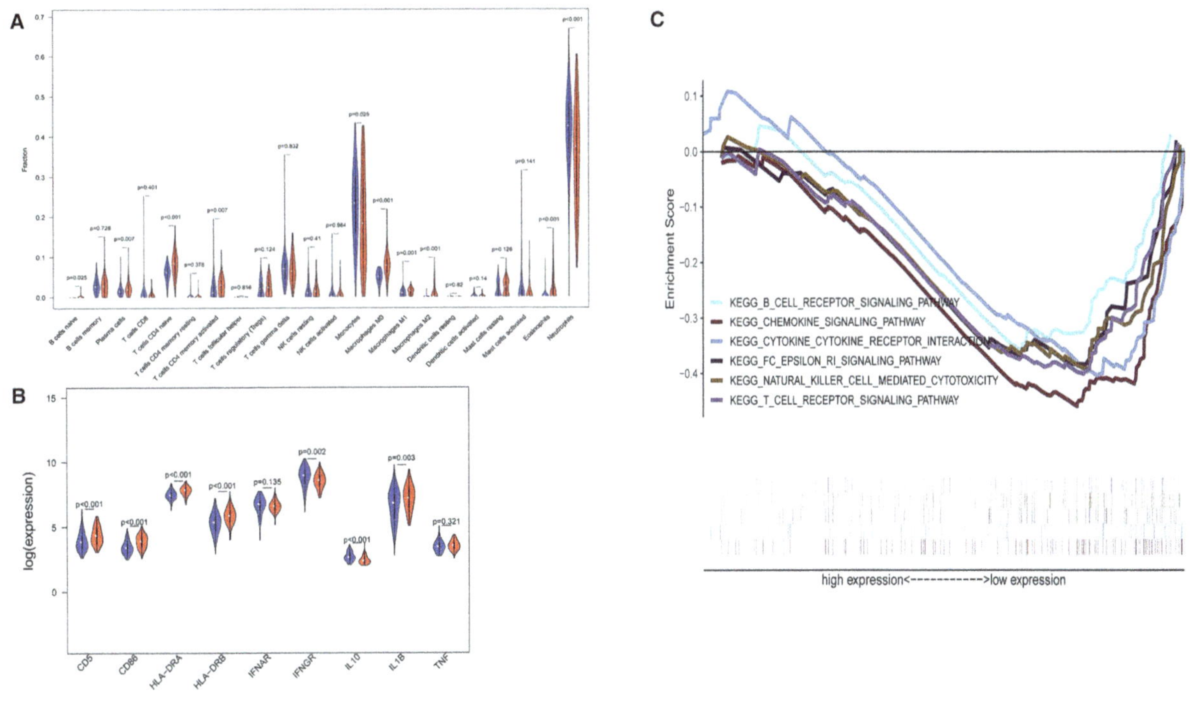


**FIGURE 5 |** Subgroup analysis on septic population with pneumonia. **(A)** Violin plots of immune cell difference analyses (medians, quartiles, extremums, data distributions, and *P*-values for the difference analysis are described in violin plots. The percentages of immune-enhancing cells—activated neutrophils- were significantly downregulated in the immunity-A endotype. The percentages of immune suppressive cells—M2 macrophages—and naïve immune cells (naïve B cells, naïve CD4 T cells, and M0 macrophages) were obviously upregulated in the immunity-A endotype). **(B)** Violin plots of the immune molecule difference analysis. The immune-enhancing molecules—HLA-DRA, IL1B, IFNGR, CD5, and CD86—were significantly downregulated and the immunosuppressive molecule IL10 was obviously upregulated in the immunity-A endotype. **(C)** Diagrams of the Gene Set Enrichment Analysis. The innate immunity, humoral immunity, cellular immunity, and promotion of immunity-related pathways were all suppressed in the immunity-A endotype group.

in sepsis via multiple parameters. Robustly, the discrimination performance of the current model was confirmed according to the assessment of immune cells, immune molecules, immune signal transduction pathways, and survival curves. Differential expression analysis of immune cells demonstrated that patients with the immunity-A endotype suffered from immune paralysis due to decreases in immune-enhancing cells, increases in immunosuppressive cells and increases in naïve immune cells. Poll et al. pointed out that the characteristics of immune suppression in sepsis were the low expression of HLA-DR on blood leucocytes and the high expression of IL-10 (an anti-inflammatory molecule), which could also be found in the immunity-A endotype, as shown by the violin plot of immune molecules (23–25). Furthermore, GSEA suggested that innate immunity-, cellular immunity-, and humoral immunity-related biological pathways were all suppressed in the high-risk group (26–28). In addition, the KM curves obviously suggested that patients in the high group (immunoparalysis) had decreased survival and poor prognosis. The external validation cohorts further demonstrated that the current model could effectively identify patients with the immunity-A endotype (immunoparalysis).

Sepsis 3.0 is defined as a life-threatening condition of organ dysfunction caused by the dysregulation of the host immune response to infection. The most important question is whether therapeutic interventions that target specific immune process mechanisms implicated in the pathophysiological changes of sepsis might further improve the therapeutic effects. It was reported that the number of immunotherapy studies of sepsis is almost 1,000 to date, but none of the results have been used in clinical practice. The primary reason for this is the lack of recognition of patient immune status. In future RCTs, scholars could use this model to categorize sepsis to design more precise immune therapies. In addition, our model could help clinicians identify patients with immunoparalysis. Avoidance of superinfection and the use of immunity enhancement drugs (such as interferon or thymosin) should be considered in these patients. In contrast, corticosteroids could be safely used for patients with low immunity risk scores calculated by this model in consideration of the effects of corticosteroids on improving the cardiovascular response to exogenous catecholamines. Furthermore, the present study demonstrated that naïve immune cells (M0 macrophages, naïve B cells, and naïve T cells) and immunity-regulating cells (Tregs and M2 macrophages) were significantly increased in the poor prognostic group. These results were similar to those of previous studies showing that immunoparalysis is crucially detrimental to sepsis patient survival. Due to the fast development and wide applications of next-generation sequencing (NGS) technologies, genomic sequence information is within reach to aid in the achievement

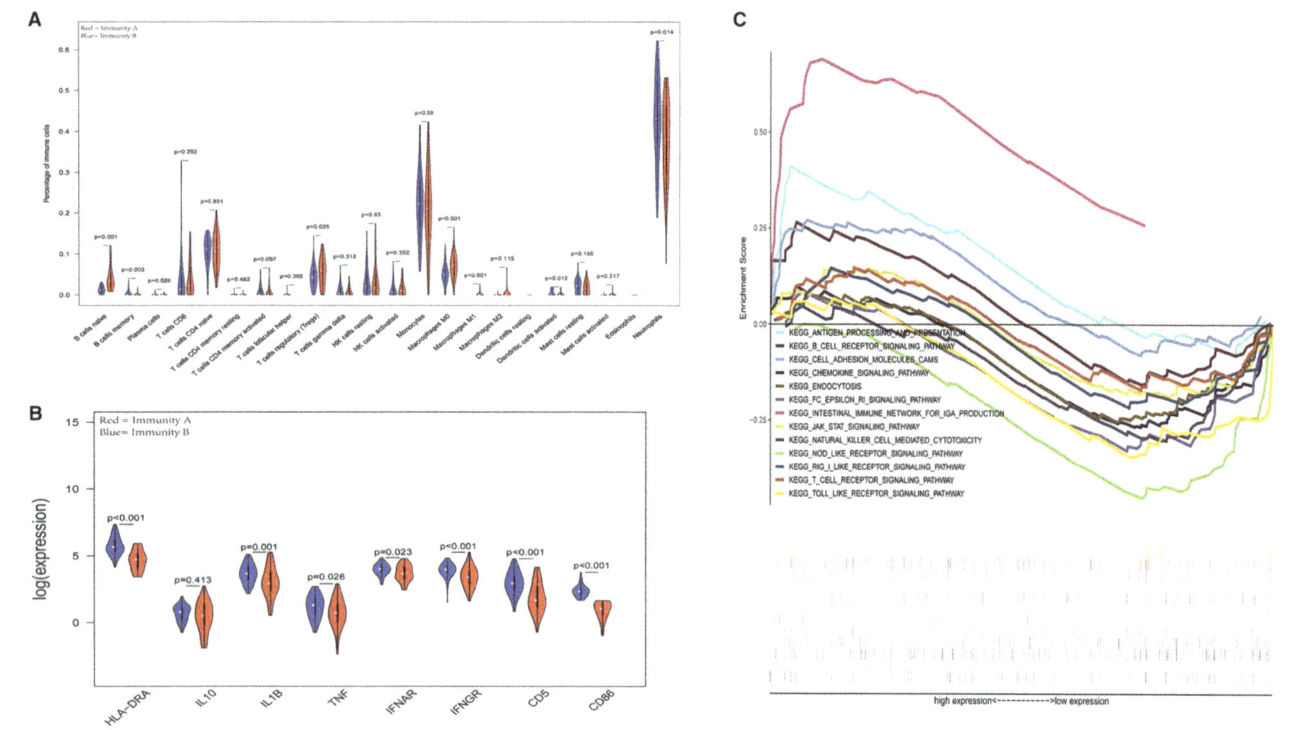


**FIGURE 6 |** External validation further demonstrates that patients in the immunity-A endotype suffer from immune suppression. **(A)** Violin plots of immune cell difference analyses (medians, quartiles, extremums, data distributions, and *P*-values for the difference analysis are described in violin plots. The percentages of immune-enhancing cells (activated neutrophils and dendritic cells) were significantly downregulated in the immunity-A endotype. The percentages of immune suppressive cells (regulatory T cells) and naïve immune cells (naïve B cells, naïve CD4 T cells, and M0 macrophages) were obviously upregulated in the immunity-A endotype). **(B)** Violin plots of the immune molecule difference analysis. The immune-enhancing molecules (HLA-DRA, IL1B, IFNAR, IFNGR, CD5, and CD86) were significantly downregulated and the immunosuppressive molecule IL10 was obviously upregulated in the immunity-A endotype. **(C)** Diagrams of the Gene Set Enrichment Analysis (most immune enhancement-related pathways except humoral immunity-related pathways are significantly suppressed in the immunity-A endotype).

of goals to determine the immune status in patients with sepsis onset and improve the survival of sepsis patients. The alterations of these immune cells could be used as potential therapeutic targets to improve the treatment strategies for sepsis.

There are several limitations to the present study. First, as a retrospective study of primarily publicly available data, the demographics and clinical features such as severity, complications, and individual treatment of each patient for detailed could not be acquired. Thus, the sensitivity and longitudinal analyses cannot be totally completed. This may restrict the generalizability of the present model. Second, despite the use of two external validation cohorts, we do not present the results for any prospective clinical studies using this model. Prospective RCTs will be paramount in translating the results to clinical applications. In addition, despite a seemingly large sample size, we were unable to perform robust subgroup analyses (based on infection site or pathogen type) due to the lack of relevant information in public databases. In addition, this model was not sensitive enough to identify a hyperactivated immune response to sepsis because it was constructed based on naïve immune cells and M2 macrophages (screened by prognostic analysis). The patients with poor prognosis in this database mainly suffered from early immunosuppression (9, 11).

In conclusion, the present study developed a comprehensive tool to identify immunoparalysis endotypes and immunocompetent status in sepsis patients that have been hospitalized, and provides novel clues for further targeting of therapeutic approaches.

## ETHICS STATEMENT

Written informed consent was not obtained from the individual(s) for the publication of any potentially identifiable images or data included in this article.

## AUTHOR CONTRIBUTIONS

SZ had full access to all of the data in the study and took responsibility for the integrity and the accuracy of the data analysis. SZ, WC, and ZW performed the data download, bioinformatic analysis, and preparation of the article for publication. All authors participated in writing the article and preparing the figures.

Discipline (ZDXKA2016025) and Jiangsu Provincial Special Program of Medical Science (BE2018743).

## ACKNOWLEDGMENTS

We would like to thank all of the microarray data contributors of this study and all of the patients and volunteers who participated in this study.

## REFERENCES

1. Reinhart K, Daniels R, Kissoon N, Machado FR, Schachter RD, Finfer S. Recognizing sepsis as a global health priority - A WHO resolution. *N Engl J Med.* (2017) 377:414–7. doi: 10.1056/NEJMp17 07170
2. Fleischmann C, Scherag A, Adhikari NK, Hartog CS, Tsaganos T, Schlattmann P, et al. Assessment of global incidence and mortality of hospital-treated sepsis: current estimates and limitations. *Am J Respir Crit Care Med.* (2016) 193:259–72. doi: 10.1164/rccm.201504-0781OC
3. Davenport EE, Burnham KL, Radhakrishnan J, Humburg P, Hutton P, Mills TC, et al. Genomic landscape of the individual host response and outcomes in sepsis: a prospective cohort study. *Lancet Respir Med.* (2016) 4:259–71. doi: 10.1016/S2213-2600(16)00046-1
4. Kempker JA, Martin GS. Does sepsis case mix heterogeneity prevent outcome comparisons? *Crit Care Med.* (2016) 44:2288–9. doi: 10.1097/CCM.0000000000001933
5. Li J, Li M, Su L, Wang H, Xiao K, Deng J, et al. Alterations of T helper lymphocyte subpopulations in sepsis, severe sepsis, and septic shock: a prospective observational study. *Inflammation.* (2015) 38:995–1002. doi: 10.1007/s10753-014-0063-3
6. Poll T, Veerdonk FL, Scicluna BP, Netea MG. The immunopathology of sepsis and potential therapeutic targets. *Nat Rev Immunuol.* (2017) 17:407–20. doi: 10.1038/nri.2017.36
7. Docke WD, Randow F, Syrbe U, Krausch D, Asadullah K, Reinke P, et al. Monocyte deactivation in septic patients: restoration by IFN-gamma treatment. *Nat Med.* (1997) 3:678–81. doi: 10.1038/nm06 97-678
8. Petit I, Kravitz MS, Nagler A, Lahav M, Peled A, Habler L, et al. G-CSF induces stem cell mobilization by decreasing bone marrow SDF-1 and up-regulating CXCR4. *Nat Immunol.* (2002) 3:687–94. doi: 10.1038/ni813
9. Nelson S, Belknap SM, Carlson RW, Dale D, DeBoisblanc B, Farkas S, et al. A randomized controlled trial of filgrastim as an adjunct to antibiotics for treatment of hospitalized patients with community-acquired pneumonia. CAP Study Group. *J Infect Dis.* (1998) 178:1075–80. doi: 10.1086/515694
10. Seymour CW, Kennedy JN, Wang S, Chang CH, Elliott CF, Xu Z, et al. Derivation, validation, and potential treatment implications of novel clinical phenotypes for sepsis. *JAMA.* (2019) 321:2003–17. doi: 10.1001/jama.2019.5791
11. Scicluna BP, van Vught LA, Zwinderman AH, Wiewel MA, Davenport EE, Burnham KL, et al. Classification of patients with sepsis according to blood genomic endotype: a prospective cohort study. *Lancet Respir Med.* (2017) 5:816–26. doi: 10.1016/S2213-2600(17)30294-1
12. Sweeney TE, Perumal TM, Henao R, Wiewel MA, Davenport E, Burnham KL, et al. A community approach to mortality prediction in sepsis via gene expression analysis. *Nat Commun.* (2018) 9:694. doi: 10.1038/s41467-018-03078-2
13. Wu HP, Chung K, Lin CY, Jiang BY, Chuang DY, Liu YC, et al. Associations of T helper 1, 2, 17 and regulatory T lymphocytes with mortality in severe sepsis. *Inflamm Res.* 62:751–63. doi: 10.1007/s00011-013-0630-3
14. Delano MJ, Ward PA. Sepsis-induced immune dysfunction: can immune therapies reduce mortality? *J Clin Invest.* (2016) 126:23–31. doi: 10.1172/JCI82224
15. Hanahan D, Weinberg RA. Hallmarks of cancer: the next generation. *Cell.* (2011) 144:646–74. doi: 10.1016/j.cell.2011.02.013
16. Newman AM, Liu CL, Green MR, Gentles AJ, Feng W, Xu Y, et al. Robust enumeration of cell subsets from tissue expression profiles. *Nat Methods.* (2015) 12:453–7. doi: 10.1038/nmeth.3337
17. Coussens LM, Zitvogel L, Palucka AK. Neutralizing tumor-promoting chronic inflammation: a magic bullet? *Science.* (2013) 339:286–91. doi: 10.1126/science.1232227
18. Shen-Orr SS, Gaujoux R. Computational deconvolution: extracting cell type-specific information from heterogeneous samples. *Curr Opin Immunol.* (2013) 25:571–8. doi: 10.1016/j.coi.2013.09.015
19. Cazalis MA, Friggeri A, Cave L, Barbalat V, Cerrato E, Lepape A, et al. Decreased HLA-DR antigen-associated invariant chain (CD74) mRNA expression predicts mortality after septic shock. *Crit Care.* (2013) 17:R287. doi: 10.1186/cc13150
20. Cheron A, Floccard B, Allaouchiche B, Guignant C, Poitevin F, Malcus C, et al. Lack of recovery in monocyte human leukocyte antigen-DR expression is independently associated with the development of sepsis after major trauma. *Crit Care.* (2010) 14:R208. doi: 10.1186/cc9331
21. Landelle C, Lepape A, Voirin N, Tognet E, Venet F, Bohé J, et al. Low monocyte human leukocyte antigen-DR is independently associated with nosocomial infections after septic shock. *Intensive Care Med.* (2010) 36:1859–1866. doi: 10.1007/s00134-010-1962-x
22. Carson WF, Cavassani KA, Dou Y, Kunkel SL. Epigenetic regulation of immune cell functions during post-septic immunosuppression. *Epigenetics-US.* (2011) 6:273–83. doi: 10.4161/epi.6.3.14017
23. Pastille E, Didovic S, Brauckmann D, Rani M, Agrawal H, Schade FU, et al. Modulation of dendritic cell differentiation in the bone marrow mediates sustained immunosuppression after polymicrobial sepsis. *J Immunol.* (2011) 186:977–86. doi: 10.4049/jimmunol.1001147
24. Venet F, Pachot A, Debard AL, Bohe J, Bienvenu J, Lepape A, et al. Human CD4+CD25+ regulatory T lymphocytes inhibit lipopolysaccharide-induced monocyte survival through a Fas/Fas ligand-dependent mechanism. *J Immunol.* (2006) 177:6540–7. doi: 10.4049/jimmunol.177.9.6540
25. Nalos M, Santner-Nanan B, Parnell G, Tang B, McLean AS, Nanan R, et al. Immune effects of interferon gamma in persistent staphylococcal sepsis. *Am J Respir Crit Care Med.* (2012) 185:110–2. doi: 10.1164/ajrccm.185.1.110
26. Kawakami T, Galli SJ. Regulation of mast-cell and basophil function and survival by IgE. *Nat Rev Immunol.* (2002) 2:773–86. doi: 10.1038/nri914
27. Yoneyama M, Kikuchi M, Natsukawa T, Shinobu N, Imaizumi T, Miyagishi M, et al. The RNA helicase RIG-I has an essential function in double-stranded RNA-induced innate antiviral responses. *Nat Immunol.* (2004) 5:730–7. doi: 10.1038/ni1087
28. Vandenabeele P, Bertrand MJ. The role of the IAP E3 ubiquitin ligases in regulating pattern-recognition receptor signalling. *Nat Rev Immunol.* (2012) 12:833–44. doi: 10.1038/nri3325

# 11

# Machine Learning for the Prediction of Red Blood Cell Transfusion in Patients During or After Liver Transplantation Surgery

*Le-Ping Liu [1†], Qin-Yu Zhao [1,2†], Jiang Wu [3], Yan-Wei Luo [1], Hang Dong [1], Zi-Wei Chen [4], Rong Gui [1*] and Yong-Jun Wang [5*]*

*[1] Department of Blood Transfusion, The Third Xiangya Hospital of Central South University, Changsha, China, [2] College of Engineering and Computer Science, Australian National University, Canberra, ACT, Australia, [3] Department of Blood Transfusion, Renji Hospital Affiliated to Shanghai Jiao Tong University, Shanghai, China, [4] Department of Laboratory Medicine, The Third Xiangya Hospital of Central South University, Changsha, China, [5] Department of Blood Transfusion, The Second Xiangya Hospital of Central South University, Changsha, China*

***Correspondence:**
*Rong Gui*
*aguirong@163.com*
*Yong-Jun Wang*
*wangyongjun@csu.edu.cn*

*† These authors have contributed equally to this work*

**Aim:** This study aimed to use machine learning algorithms to identify critical preoperative variables and predict the red blood cell (RBC) transfusion during or after liver transplantation surgery.

**Study Design and Methods:** A total of 1,193 patients undergoing liver transplantation in three large tertiary hospitals in China were examined. Twenty-four preoperative variables were collected, including essential population characteristics, diagnosis, symptoms, and laboratory parameters. The cohort was randomly split into a train set (70%) and a validation set (30%). The Recursive Feature Elimination and eXtreme Gradient Boosting algorithms (XGBOOST) were used to select variables and build machine learning prediction models, respectively. Besides, seven other machine learning models and logistic regression were developed. The area under the receiver operating characteristic (AUROC) was used to compare the prediction performance of different models. The SHapley Additive exPlanations package was applied to interpret the XGBOOST model. Data from 31 patients at one of the hospitals were prospectively collected for model validation.

**Results:** In this study, 72.1% of patients in the training set and 73.2% in the validation set underwent RBC transfusion during or after the surgery. Nine vital preoperative variables were finally selected, including the presence of portal hypertension, age, hemoglobin, diagnosis, direct bilirubin, activated partial thromboplastin time, globulin, aspartate aminotransferase, and alanine aminotransferase. The XGBOOST model presented significantly better predictive performance (AUROC: 0.813) than other models and also performed well in the prospective dataset (accuracy: 76.9%).

**Discussion:** A model for predicting RBC transfusion during or after liver transplantation was successfully developed using a machine learning algorithm based on nine preoperative variables, which could guide high-risk patients to take appropriate preventive measures.

**Keywords: liver transplantation, machine learning, prediction model, red blood cell transfusion, SHapley Additive exPlanations**

## INTRODUCTION

Liver transplantation is an effective method for treating end-stage liver disease. Prolonged and complicated surgical procedures may cause bleeding during the perioperative period. Most patients require an infusion of concentrated red blood cells (RBCs) during or after the surgery. Although blood transfusion can increase the patient's oxygen supply and improve tissue perfusion, it is also accompanied by many side effects, such as the increased risk of deep vein thrombosis, increased fibrosis, cancer recurrence, and increased mortality, thus adversely affecting the patient's prognosis (1–5). The methods of reducing blood transfusions include the preoperative use of tranexamic acid, intraoperative blood salvage, and intraoperative autotransfusion. However, these approaches cannot be applied to all patients, considering their risks and the costs (6–8).

It is necessary to predict RBC transfusion before the surgery and provide clinicians with practical clinical decision-making guidance. Clinically, physicians make transfusion decisions primarily based on a patient's hemoglobin level and symptoms of anemia. However, other perioperative indicators should not be ignored, for example, essential patient characteristics such as sex, age, and weight; preoperative symptoms such as the presence of portal hypertension, ascites, and hepatic encephalopathy; and preoperative laboratory parameters such as hemoglobin, creatinine, and transaminases. Meanwhile, data on the transfusion of RBCs before surgery and the clinical significance of intraoperative and postoperative risk factors such as operation time, intraoperative blood loss, and postoperative laboratory indicators are limited. Studies have been conducted to predict blood transfusion in joint surgery, craniofacial surgery, and obstetric surgery by developing clinical prediction models combined with patients' preoperative risk factors (9–11).

Machine learning is a field of artificial intelligence that learns from data based on computational modeling. Cutting-edge machine learning models can fit high-order relationships between covariates and outcomes in a vast amount of data. Therefore, they can be applied to complex medical problems and usually perform better than traditional statistical analysis, especially when analyzing big medical data (12). If the RBC transfusion in liver transplant patients can be predicted before surgery, targeted preventive measures are taken for high-risk patients. Unnecessary costs and side effects can be reduced, which is beneficial to the treatment and prognosis of patients. Most studies on predicting RBC transfusion during liver transplantation are based on traditional linear models and logistic regression (LR). However, no studies have been conducted to predict RBC transfusion in patients during or after liver transplantation using a machine learning model (13, 14). Therefore, this study hypothesized that preoperative data from patients could be used to predict RBC transfusion during or after surgery using machine learning.

The purpose of this study was to determine the preoperative risk factors associated with RBC transfusion in patients undergoing liver transplantation and then develop a machine learning model to predict RBC transfusion during and after surgery.

## MATERIALS AND METHODS

### Study Subjects

The participants were patients aged more than 18 years who underwent liver transplantation, from March 2014 to September 2019, at one of the following three tertiary hospitals: the Second Xiangya Hospital of Central South University, the Third Xiangya Hospital of Central South University, and the Renji Hospital affiliated to Medical College of Shanghai Jiao Tong University. The transplanted livers used in three hospitals were provided free of charge by the Red Cross Society of China. Approval was obtained from the institutional review board for this study (Ref 2019-S007). No written consent was required in view of the purely observational nature of the study. No identifiable data of the donors or live transplant patients were recorded during the whole study.

The commonly used operative methods for liver transplantation currently include the classical liver transplantation (15), piggyback liver transplantation (16), and classical venous bypass liver transplantation (17). Most patients in the three hospitals in our study underwent the piggyback liver transplantation. The major advantage of this method is less intraoperative bleeding (18, 19). Especially for patients with portal hypertension, it can reduce the massive bleeding of posterior peritoneal collateral circulation due to the removal of inferior vena cava (19, 20). Therefore, only patients who underwent the piggyback liver transplantation were included in our study.

Patients who received preoperative blood transfusions and those whose missing rates of data were more than 80% were excluded. Data of patients who underwent liver transplantation from October 2019 to January 2020 were collected prospectively in the Third Xiangya Hospital of Central South University to validate the proposed model further.

### Study Design and Data Collection

A total of 24 preoperative variables were collected within 24 h before the day of surgery. For some variables with multiple measurements, the values closest to the surgery's start time were assessed. The collected preoperative information included patients' demographic characteristics (age and sex), clinical characteristics (weight), diagnosis (cirrhosis, malignant liver tumor, liver failure, alcoholic hepatitis, viral hepatitis, hepatic space-occupying lesions, cholestatic liver disease, or others), preoperative clinical signs (portal hypertension, hepatic encephalopathy, and ascites), and preoperative laboratory indicators (albumin, globulin, and total protein). All variables were obtained from the electronic medical record systems of the three hospitals. Three authors (LL, JW, and YW) had access to the systems and collected the data.

The data collected by different hospitals were converted and unified. For example, 1 mg/dl of creatinine is equal to 88.4 μmol/L. The related variables were combined into one; for example, "hepatocellular carcinoma" and "primary liver cancer" were combined into "malignant liver tumor." The diagnostic variables were transformed into ordinal variables: 1 = cirrhosis; 2 = liver malignant tumor; 3 = liver failure; 4 = alcoholic hepatitis;

5 = viral hepatitis; 6 = hepatic space-occupying lesions; 7 = cholestatic liver disease; and 8 = others.

## Statistical Analysis

The dataset was randomly split into a training set and a validation set. The data of 835 (70%) patients were used to develop our models, while the data of 358 (30%) patients were used as a validation set.

Continuous variables between transfused and nontransfused groups were compared using either the Student *t*-test or rank-sum test as appropriate. The chi-square test or Fisher's exact test was employed to compare the differences in the categorical variables.

The dataset was imputed using multiple imputation. Then, the recursive feature elimination (RFE) algorithm was used to select key variables and develop a machine learning model named eXtreme Gradient Boosting (XGBOOST) (21–23). In short, RFE is a feature selection method that recursively fits a model based on smaller feature sets until a specified termination criterion is reached. In each loop, features are ranked by their importance in the trained model. By recursively eliminating one feature with the lowest importance, RFE attempts to eliminate dependencies and collinearity that may exist in the model. Features were recursively eliminated until the model's AUROC was <0.80. Then, the last eliminated feature was replaced to make the AUROC more than 0.80. At last, the most important features were screened out, and a XGBOOST model was developed based on the feature set. Other features were not added because they only brought a small increment in AUROC but significantly increased the difficulty of model application.

The proposed prediction model was built in the XGBOOST package in Python language, validation was carried out using the five-fold cross-validation method, and then the AUROC of the training set was calculated. After the model was established, the SHapley Additive exPlanations (SHAP) package in Python was used to explain the model by analyzing two cases. The SHAP package interpreted the output of the machine learning model using a game-theoretic approach (24). For each prediction sample, the model connected optimal credit allocation with local explanations.

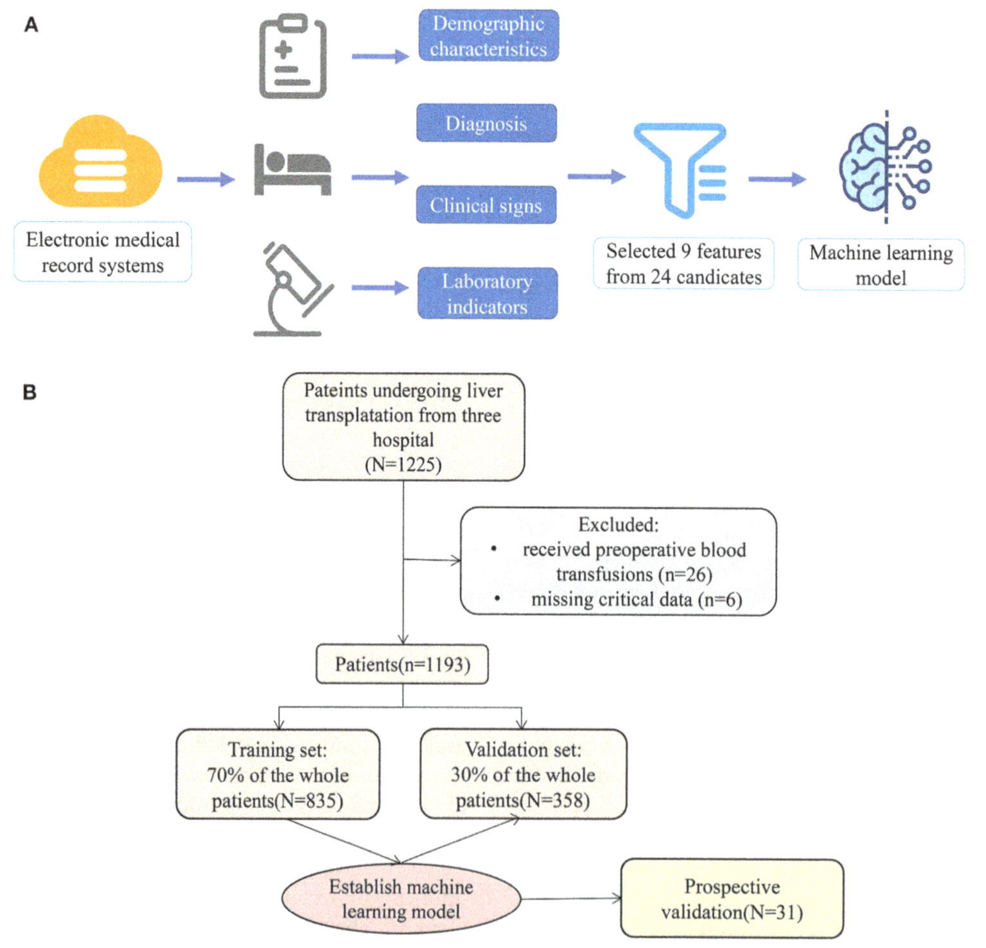


**FIGURE 1 |** Model-making process and flowchart of the study. **(A)** This figure demonstrated that the data were obtained from the electronic medical record systems of the three hospitals, and all variables included demographic characteristics, diagnosis, clinical signs, and laboratory indicators. A total of 24 preoperative variables were collected, and 9 variables were screened. Moreover, the study used the 9 variables to establish a machine learning model. **(B)** The flowchart of our study.

**TABLE 1** | Preoperative information.

| Variable | | All ($n$ = 1,193) | Non-transfusion group ($n$ = 329) | Transfusion group ($n$ = 684) | $p$-value |
|---|---|---|---|---|---|
| Age, mean (SD) | | 46.17 (11.76) | 44.38 (13.95) | 46.86 (10.73) | 0.004 |
| Sex, $n$ (%) | Male | 206 (17.27) | 60 (18.24) | 146 (16.90) | 0.645 |
| | Female | 987 (82.73) | 269 (81.76) | 718 (83.10) | 0.646 |
| Diagnosis, $n$ (%) | Cirrhosis | 150 (17.34) | 43 (24.02) | 107 (15.60) | <0.001 |
| | Liver malignant tumor | 154 (17.80) | 37 (20.67) | 117 (17.06) | <0.002 |
| | Liver failure | 83 (9.60) | 28 (15.64) | 55 (8.02) | <0.003 |
| | Alcoholic hepatitis | 42 (4.86) | 2 (1.12) | 40 (5.83) | <0.004 |
| | Viral hepatitis | 257 (29.71) | 19 (10.61) | 238 (34.69) | <0.005 |
| | Cholestatic liver disease | 24 (2.77) | 5 (2.79) | 19 (2.77) | <0.006 |
| | Others | 155 (17.92) | 45 (25.14) | 110 (16.03) | <0.007 |
| Portal hypertension, $n$ (%) | | 340 (28.50) | 43 (13.07) | 297 (34.38) | <0.002 |
| Hepatic encephalopathy, $n$ (%) | | 136 (11.40) | 201(6.38) | 115 (13.31) | 0.002 |
| Ascites, $n$ (%) | | 390 (32.69) | 64 (19.45) | 326 (37.73) | <0.002 |
| Weight, mean (SD) | | 64.15 (13.22) | 62.94 (16.33) | 64.43 (12.39) | 0.323 |
| ALB, mean (SD) | | 34.76 (6.16) | 35.06 (5.70) | 34.68 (6.27) | 0.476 |
| ALT, median (Q1, Q3) | | 53.60 (26.90, 154.90) | 51.50 (31.10, 100.90) | 54.00 (26.00, 170.00) | 0.609 |
| APTT, mean (SD) | | 51.15 (20.09) | 46.06 (13.00) | 52.32 (21.22) | <0.001 |
| AST, median (Q1, Q3) | | 72.00 (38.80, 197.10) | 76.60 (40.40, 161.60) | 72.00 (38.30, 201.38) | 0.527 |
| CR, median (Q1, Q3) | | 67.00 (55.85, 89.00) | 64.00 (56.08, 78.17) | 67.80 (55.60, 92.00) | 0.035 |
| DBIL, median (Q1, Q3) | | 67.75 (15.83, 230.18) | 29.60 (11.78, 198.00) | 84.45 (17.90, 240.70) | 0.001 |
| GLO, mean (SD) | | 26.94 (8.78) | 29.39 (7.54) | 26.43 (8.94) | <0.001 |
| HB, mean (SD) | | 102.38 (25.19) | 112.30 (29.25) | 99.97 (23.51) | <0.001 |
| INR, median (Q1, Q3) | | 1.63 (1.29, 2.29) | 1.46 (1.17, 1.94) | 1.67 (1.32, 2.37) | <0.001 |
| PLT, median (Q1, Q3) | | 69.00 (42.00, 104.50) | 87.00 (53.00, 123.00) | 66.00 (41.00, 101.00) | <0.001 |
| PT, median (Q1, Q3) | | 18.90 (15.20, 25.20) | 17.20 (14.30, 22.02) | 19.25 (15.40, 26.20) | 0.002 |
| TBIL, median (Q1, Q3) | | 105.20 (33.50, 378.27) | 51.10 (23.40, 298.70) | 135.40 (35.80, 395.80) | 0.001 |
| TP, median (Q1, Q3) | | 61.50 (54.80, 68.25) | 65.00 (59.10, 71.20) | 60.40 (54.35, 67.30) | <0.001 |
| TT, median (Q1, Q3) | | 19.50 (17.40, 22.20) | 17.80 (16.50, 19.75) | 19.80 (17.60, 23.00) | <0.001 |
| UA, median (Q1, Q3) | | 225.90 (135.05, 332.57) | 252.20 (157.12, 339.55) | 220.00 (131.25, 332.00) | 0.093 |
| Urea, median (Q1, Q3) | | 5.45 (3.87, 8.10) | 5.00 (3.68, 6.71) | 5.69 (3.91, 8.50) | 0.009 |
| WBC, median (Q1, Q3) | | 5.21 (3.42, 8.08) | 5.58 (3.51, 7.32) | 5.21 (3.42, 8.23) | 0.972 |

*SD, standard deviation; ALT, alanine aminotransferase; APTT, activated partial thromboplastin time; AST, aspartate aminotransferase; DBil, Direct bilirubin; PLT, platelet; INR, International standard ratio; PT, prothrombin time; TT, thrombin time; TBil, total bilirubin; WBC, white blood cell.*

Besides, eight other models were developed and compared with the proposed machine learning model, including K-Nearest Neighbors, Naïve Bayes, Support Vector Machine, Multi-Layer Perceptron, Random Forest, AdaBoost and Gradient Boosting Decision Tree, and LR. The validation was also carried out using the five-fold cross-validation, and then the AUROCs were calculated. The sensitivity and specificity were also analyzed.

Finally, the proposed model and the other models were applied to prospective validations. Wrongly predicted samples were analyzed by an experienced clinician and a data scientist.

## RESULTS

As shown in **Figure 1**, 1,193 patients were finally included in this study; the preoperative information of the cohort is shown in **Table 1**. The average age of patients was 46.17 years, men accounted for 82.73%, and the average weight was 64.15 kg.

Data of 835 patients were used as the training set for model building, and data of 358 patients were used as the validation set. In the training set, 602 (72.1%) patients received RBC transfusion during or after the surgery, and 233 patients did not receive RBC transfusion. In the validation set, 262 (73.2%) patients received RBC transfusion during or after the surgery, and 96 patients did not receive RBC transfusion.

### Key Variables

The nine preoperative variables, including portal hypertension, age, hemoglobin, diagnosis, direct bilirubin, activated partial thromboplastin time (APTT), globulin, aspartate aminotransferase (AST), and alanine aminotransferase (ALT), were selected as crucial variables using the RFE

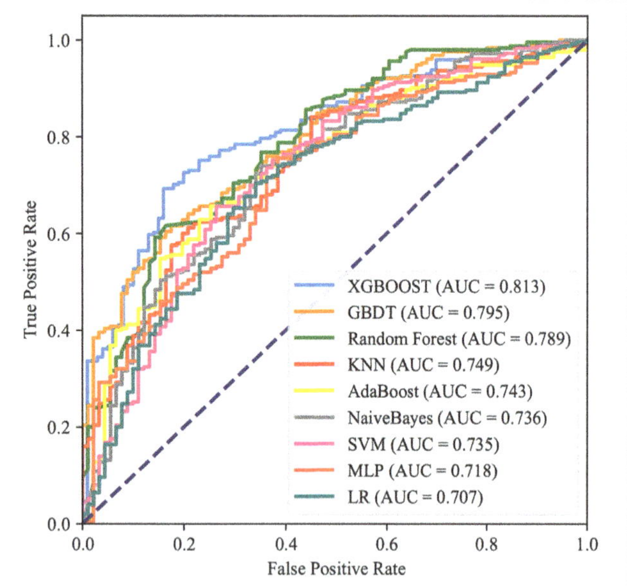


**FIGURE 2 |** Receiver operating characteristic curves for the machine learning model and logistic regression. XGBOOST, eXtremely Gradient Boosting; GBDT, Gradient Boosting Decision Tree; KNN, K-Nearest Neighbor; SVM, Support Vector Machine; MLP, Multi-Layer Perceptron; LR, Logistic Regression.

algorithm. As expected, patients with portal hypertension, older age, lower preoperative hemoglobin and globulin levels, approximately longer preoperative APTT, and higher preoperative direct bilirubin, AST, and ALT were more likely to receive RBC transfusion.

After identifying these nine variables, machine learning was used to predict RBC transfusion during or after liver transplantation. As shown in **Figure 2**, the AUROC of the proposed model was 0.813. The proposed model significantly outperformed the conventional LR (AUROC: 0.707) and seven other machine learning models. According to the Youden Index, defined as sensitivity + specificity - 1, the best cutoff of prediction probabilities of the proposed model was 0.737 (shown in **Table 2**), with a sensitivity and specificity of 66.4 and 85.0%, respectively. The best cutoff of prediction probabilities of LR was 0.626, with a sensitivity and specificity of 70.4 and 65.9%, respectively.

## Application of the Model

The SHAP package analyzed the entire training set, showing the impact of each variable on predicting transfusion (**Figure 3**). The preoperative information of a patient was input into the model: age 56 years, no portal hypertension, diagnosed with viral hepatitis, hemoglobin 65 g/L, direct bilirubin level 158.2 μmol/L, APTT 81.2 s, globulin level 12.3 g/L, ALT 688 U/L, and AST 991 U/L. The model analyzed that the risk of RBC transfusion in this patient was 91.58%, indicating that the probability of RBC transfusion for the patients was high, and RBC transfusion was recommended (**Figure 4A**). The preoperative information of another patient was input into the model: age 23 years, no portal hypertension, diagnosed with other disease, hemoglobin 160 g/L, direct bilirubin 30.5 μmol/L, APTT 44.2 s, globulin 49.2 g/L, ALT 83.3 U/L, and AST 28.2 U/L. The predicted probability of transfusion in this patient was 27.80%, indicating that the patient was at low risk of needing an RBC transfusion (**Figure 4B**). Furthermore, a website was established for clinicians to use the proposed model, http://www.aimedicallab.com/tool/aiml-livertrans.html.

## Prospective Validation

Data of 31 patients were prospectively collected for validation, of which 87% (25) were transfused during or after liver transplantation surgery. The accuracy of the proposed model on the prospective dataset was 76.9%. There was one patient who was transfused but whom the model predicted as negative. He had an accidental intraoperative hemorrhage (about 2,000 ml of blood loss). In the eight patients who were nontransfused but whom the model predicted as positive, two was transfused with a large number of platelets and the others had probabilities (75.41–83.49%) close to the cutoff.

# DISCUSSION

This study was novel in using machine learning algorithms to predict RBC transfusion during or after liver transplantation. A machine learning model was built that could accurately predict RBC transfusion during or after liver transplantation before the surgery, better than other models developed in this study. The model established in this study had great discrimination and showed satisfactory specificity and sensitivity. Therefore, the hypothesis proposed in this study was supported by the results.

Several studies showed that RBC transfusion increased complications and was related to a lower 5-year survival rate (3, 26). In addition, costs associated with transfusing a single unit of blood were significantly high, including the cost of treating any adverse effect of transfusion or the associated increased length of hospital stay. These costs far outweighed the lower cost of the use of tranexamic acid, erythropoietin (EPO), oral treatments of anemia, intravenous iron therapy, and cell salvage utilization. As a result, clinicians have taken many measures to reduce RBC transfusions (25, 27). By predicting RBC transfusion before surgeries, high-risk patients could be identified. The management of patients could be improved, thus improving outcomes and reducing morbidity and cost (4, 28, 29). Therefore, it was of great importance to predict RBC transfusion before surgeries and take corresponding preoperative measures.

In this study, a machine learning model was developed to predict RBC transfusion, which could help clinicians identify high-risk patients. If the model identified patients at low probability of transfusion, potentially unnecessary repeat testing was exempt, such as a complete blood count or further preoperative laboratory testing. Therefore, this model might be a valuable tool to avoid wasteful and unnecessary medical tests. Alternatively, identifying patients at high risk for transfusion might improve the efficiency of perioperative blood management and reduce transfusions. It was suspected that for each transfusion avoided, the patient and financial benefit might be significant due to the large number of

**TABLE 2** | Analysis of sensitivity and specificity.

| Model | Best cutoff | Accuracy | Youden Index | Sensitivity | Specificity | PPV | NPV |
|---|---|---|---|---|---|---|---|
| XGBOOST | 0.737 | 0.718 | 0.514 | 0.664 | 0.850 | 0.914 | 0.512 |
| GBDT | 0.803 | 0.672 | 0.440 | 0.616 | 0.824 | 0.906 | 0.439 |
| Random Forest | 0.790 | 0.674 | 0.451 | 0.616 | 0.835 | 0.911 | 0.442 |
| KNN | 0.763 | 0.660 | 0.403 | 0.612 | 0.791 | 0.890 | 0.426 |
| AdaBoost | 0.507 | 0.680 | 0.403 | 0.656 | 0.747 | 0.877 | 0.442 |
| NaiveBayes | 0.124 | 0.716 | 0.388 | 0.740 | 0.648 | 0.853 | 0.476 |
| SVM | 0.743 | 0.677 | 0.392 | 0.656 | 0.736 | 0.872 | 0.438 |
| MLP | 0.631 | 0.718 | 0.371 | 0.756 | 0.615 | 0.844 | 0.479 |
| LR | 0.626 | 0.692 | 0.363 | 0.704 | 0.659 | 0.850 | 0.448 |

*The best cutoff was determined by Youden index, defined as sensitivity + specificity − 1. XGBOOST, eXtremely Gradient Boosting; GBDT, Gradient Boosting Decision Tree; KNN, K-Nearest Neighbor; SVM, Support Vector Machine; MLP, Multi-Layer Perceptron; LR, Logistic Regression; PPV, Positive Predictive Value; NPV, Negative Predictive Value.*

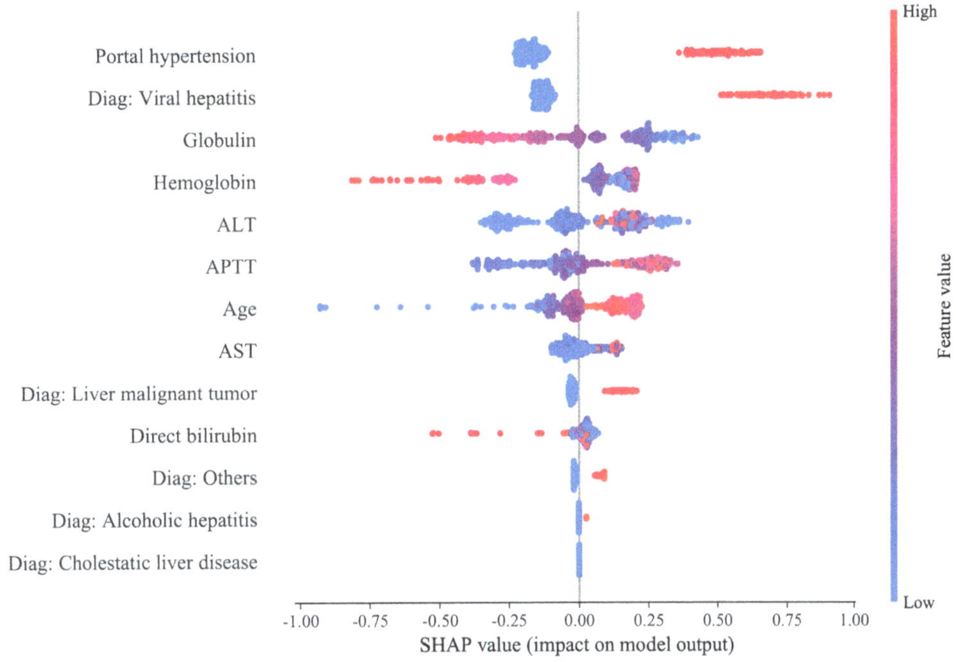


**FIGURE 3** | SHAP analysis of the proposed model on the validation set. This figure described data from the validation set, with each point representing one patient. The color represents the value of the variable; red represents the larger value; blue represents the smaller value. The horizontal coordinates represent a positive or negative correlation with transfusion risk, with a positive value indicating a risk of transfusion and a negative value indicating no need for transfusion. The absolute value of the horizontal coordinate indicates the degree of influence; the greater the absolute value of the horizontal coordinate, the greater the degree of influence.

patients undergoing gynecologic surgery. Future investigations should include measuring the model's impact on patient and cost outcomes.

In addition, two examples were used to visualize how the model could predict RBC transfusion and determine the relative importance of each variable for the clinician. With millions of liver transplants taking place each year, the findings could help surgeons perform liver transplants, while also giving patients information about their probabilities of receiving RBC transfusion before surgery.

Previous studies reported that intraoperative blood loss and postoperative decreased hemoglobin levels were associated with the risk of receiving an RBC transfusion (30–32). However, preoperative information should be used to predict the need for RBC transfusion so as to find other risk features; otherwise, it is too late to take action to determine transfusion risk through intraoperative or postoperative information.

The significance of this study was that it combined preoperative characteristic variables other than hemoglobin to establish a clinical prediction model. Portal hypertension, age, hemoglobin, diagnosis, direct bilirubin, APTT, ALT, AST, and globulin were selected as important variables. Arshad found that portal hypertension was associated with increased blood loss and RBC transfusion in orthotopic liver transplantation (33), which was similar to the result of the present analysis. Fabio Bagante established a nomogram of hepatectomy to predict

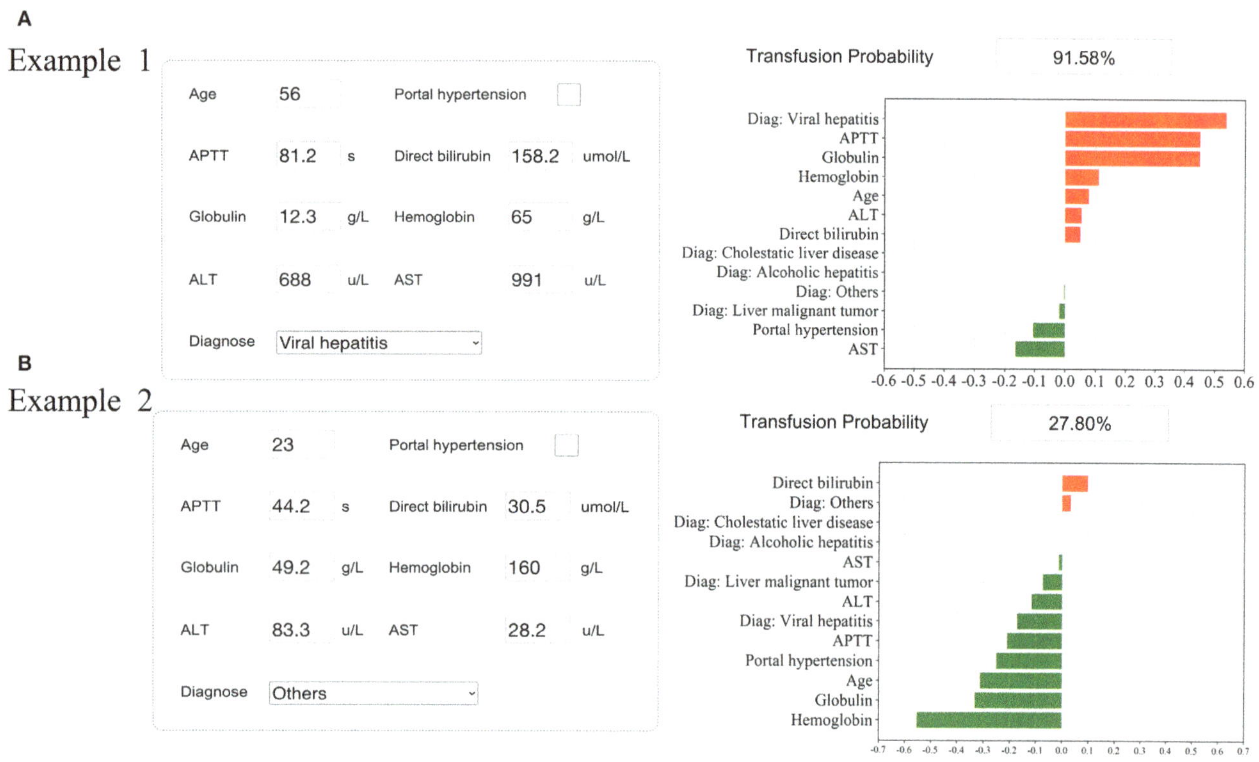


**FIGURE 4 |** Examples of website usage. Entering the input value determined the transfusion requirements and displayed how each value contributed to the prediction. **(A)** Example 1 needs RBC transfusion, and **(B)** Example 2 does not need RBC transfusion.

the risk of transfusion and included total bilirubin among the risk factors for transfusion. However, the present study found that the level of direct bilirubin correlated with the risk of transfusion in patients undergoing liver transplantation (34). Most studies assessing the risk of transfusion also demonstrated a vital role for age and preoperative hemoglobin in predicting transfusion (3, 35, 36). All of the aforementioned studies supported the results of the present study very well. Besides, this study also found other variables that increased the risk of RBC transfusion, including preoperative APTT, AST, ALT, and globulin. APTT reflects the patient's coagulation function; the lower the coagulation function, the greater the likelihood of intraoperative blood loss, thus increasing the risk of RBC transfusion. Therefore, clinical decision-makers should consider using the pro-coagulation treatment and administering drugs that could alter the coagulation state with careful thinking for patients predicted as high-risk groups. An abnormal level of AST, ALT, or globulin reflected the poor state of a patient's liver function, which might indirectly represent a decreased coagulation state and increased risk of transfusion. Focusing solely on hemoglobin to determine whether to transfuse might be of limited utility, and comprehensive inclusion of preoperative patient information could help guide clinical transfusion decisions and more effective blood management. For high-risk patients, clinicians should consider correcting hemoglobin before surgery and provide liver protection treatment to improve liver function, coagulation function, and portal hypertension.

In this study, an RBC transfusion prediction model was developed with great discrimination. This study included multi-center datasets and prospective validation, which was also an advantage compared with other studies; the abundant data allowed rigorous evaluation of the performance of machine learning models. Ultimately, the approach used in the present study can be applied to a variety of problems that arise before and after surgery to make the surgery safe. Furthermore, it can also be applied to other complications and operations, such as sepsis and acute kidney injury (37–41).

This study had several limitations. First, the transfusion criteria were not the same in each institution; therefore, the definition of the transfusion group was different. A vast majority of institutions were based on a restrictive transfusion strategy, where patients were transfused when their hemoglobin was <70 g/L (42, 43). Second, the surgeons at each institution had different surgical plans; other factors might also lead to blood transfusions, thus affecting the results. Third, the training and the validation sets were divided as a 7:3 ratio, and using other external validation sets might yield different results. Therefore, more datasets from other centers were needed for validation. Fourth, patients with missing critical data were excluded, causing selection bias. Fifth, like other retrospective studies, a selection bias might exist without considering unknown confounding factors. Lastly, although SHAP values were used to help interpret our machine learning model, a more interpretable model is still needed in clinical practice (44). As a future work, we planned to develop a Nomogram or machine learning-based automatic clinical scoring system based on our data, in order to provide clinicians a more usable and easy-to-understand tool (45).

## CONCLUSIONS

In this study, a machine learning algorithm was used to develop an RBC transfusion prediction model during and after liver transplantation, which was expedient and had good performance. This model could realize the individualized prediction of RBC transfusion and minimize the cost and risk of various blood transfusion preventive measures. The study recommended using this model to predict RBC transfusion before liver transplantation and instruct high-risk patients to take appropriate preventive measures. A prospective blood management database should be built to minimize selection bias, machine learning models should be developed based on the preoperative characteristics of patients undergoing liver transplantation, and the models should be validated with data from such patients in the future. Finally, a randomized controlled trial should be conducted to evaluate the impact of machine learning models, as decision supporters for clinicians, on clinician behavior, healthcare utilization, and patient outcomes.

## ETHICS STATEMENT

The present study did not intervene in liver transplantation surgeries. That means the study did not decide who and when to undergo surgery, who to be the donors, and when to transfuse RBCs. They were all carried out according to the standard procedure at the three hospitals. Patients' clinical data were collected, and the model was developed. None of their identifiable data were collected. The study was approved by local ethics committees.

## AUTHOR CONTRIBUTIONS

L-PL, Q-YZ, and RG designed and performed the study. L-PL, HD, Z-WC, Y-JW, and JW collected the data. Q-YZ performed the analytic calculations and statistical analysis. L-PL and Q-YZ wrote the manuscript, which was improved under the guidance of Y-WL. All authors provided critical feedback and helped to shape the research, analysis, and manuscript.

## REFERENCES


1. Dai WC, Chok KSH, Sin SL, Chan ACY, Cheung TT, Wong TCL, et al. Impact of intraoperative blood transfusion on long-term outcomes of liver transplantation for hepatocellular carcinoma. *ANZ J Surg.* (2018) 88:E418–23. doi: 10.1111/ans.13815
2. Subramanian V, Bharat A, Vachharajani N, Crippin J, Shenoy S, Mohanakumar T, et al. Perioperative blood transfusion affects hepatitis C virus (HCV)-specific immune responses and outcome following liver transplantation in HCV-infected patients. *HPB.* (2014) 16:282–94. doi: 10.1111/hpb.12128
3. Dejam A, Malley BE, Feng M, Cismondi F, Park S, Samani S, et al. The effect of age and clinical circumstances on the outcome of red blood cell transfusion in critically ill patients. *Crit Care.* (2014) 18:487. doi: 10.1186/s13054-014-0487-z
4. Benson AB, Burton JR Jr, Austin GL, Biggins SW, Zimmerman MA, Kam I, et al. Differential effects of plasma and red blood cell transfusions on acute lung injury and infection risk following liver transplantation. *Liver Transpl.* (2011) 17:149–58. doi: 10.1002/lt.22212
5. Cywinski JB, Alster JM, Miller C, Vogt DP, Parker BM. Prediction of intraoperative transfusion requirements during orthotopic liver transplantation and the influence on postoperative patient survival. *Anesth Analg.* (2014) 118:428–37. doi: 10.1213/ANE.0b013e3182a76f19
6. Badenoch A, Sharma A, Gower S, Selzner M, Srinivas C, Wasowicz M, et al. The effectiveness and safety of tranexamic acid in orthotopic liver transplantation clinical practice: a propensity score matched cohort study. *Transplantation.* (2017) 101:1658–65. doi: 10.1097/TP.0000000000001682
7. Gurusamy KS, Pissanou T, Pikhart H, Vaughan J, Burroughs AK, Davidson BR. Methods to decrease blood loss and transfusion requirements for liver transplantation. *Cochrane Database Syst Rev.* (2011) 7:CD009052. doi: 10.1002/14651858.CD009052
8. Feltracco P, Brezzi M, Barbieri S, Galligioni H, Milevoj M, Carollo C, et al. Blood loss, predictors of bleeding, transfusion practice and strategies of blood cell salvaging during liver transplantation. *World J Hepatol.* (2013) 5:1–15. doi: 10.4254/wjh.v5.i1.1
9. Xing Z, He Y, Ji C, Xu C, Zhang W, Li Y, et al. Establishing a perinatal red blood cell transfusion risk evaluation model for obstetric patients: a retrospective cohort study. *Transfusion.* (2019) 59:1667–74. doi: 10.1111/trf.15208
10. Jalali A, Lonsdale H, Zamora LV, Ahumada L, Nguyen ATH, Rehman M, et al. Machine learning applied to registry data: development of a patient-specific prediction model for blood transfusion requirements during craniofacial surgery using the pediatric craniofacial perioperative registry dataset. *Anesth Analg.* (2020) 132:160–71. doi: 10.1213/ANE.0000000000004988
11. Wang JQ, Chen LY, Jiang BJ, Zhao YM. Development of a nomogram for predicting blood transfusion risk after hemiarthroplasty for femoral neck fractures in elderly patients. *Med Sci Monit.* (2020) 26:e920255. doi: 10.12659/MSM.920255
12. Beam AL, Kohane IS. Big data and machine learning in health care. *JAMA.* (2018) 319:1317–8. doi: 10.1001/jama.2017.18391
13. McCluskey SA, Karkouti K, Wijeysundera DN, Kakizawa K, Ghannam M, Hamdy A, et al. Derivation of a risk index for the prediction of massive blood transfusion in liver transplantation. *Liver Transpl.* (2006) 12:1584–93. doi: 10.1002/lt.20868
14. Pustavoitau A, Lesley M, Ariyo P, Latif A, Villamayor AJ, Frank SM, et al. Predictive modeling of massive transfusion requirements during liver transplantation and its potential to reduce utilization of blood bank resources. *Anesth Analg.* (2017) 124:1644–52. doi: 10.1213/ANE.0000000000001994
15. Starzl TE, Marchioro TL, Porter KA, Brettschneider L. Homotransplantation of the liver. *Transplantation.* (1967) 5:790–803. doi: 10.1097/00007890-196707001-00003
16. Tzakis A, Todo S, Starzl TE. Orthotopic liver transplantation with preservation of the inferior vena cava. *Ann Surg.* (1989) 210:649–52. doi: 10.1097/00000658-198911000-00013
17. Shaw BW Jr, Martin DJ, Marquez JM, Kang YG, Bugbee AC Jr, Iwatsuki S, et al., Venous bypass in clinical liver transplantation. *Ann Surg.* (1984) 200:524–34. doi: 10.1097/00000658-198410000-00013
18. Chan T, DeGirolamo K, Chartier-Plante S, Buczkowski AK. Comparison of three caval reconstruction techniques in orthotopic liver transplantation: a retrospective review. *Am J Surg.* (2017) 213:943–9. doi: 10.1016/j.amjsurg.2017.03.045
19. Sakai T, Matsusaki T, Marsh JW, Hilmi IA, Planinsic RM. Comparison of surgical methods in liver transplantation: retrohepatic caval resection with venovenous bypass (VVB) versus piggyback (PB) with VVB versus PB without VVB. *Transpl Int.* (2010) 23:1247–58. doi: 10.1111/j.1432-2277.2010.01144.x
20. Schmitz V, Schoening W, Jelkmann I, Globke B, Pascher A, Bahra M,

et al. Different cava reconstruction techniques in liver transplantation: piggyback versus cava resection. *Hepatobiliary Pancreat Dis Int.* (2014) 13:242–9. doi: 10.1016/S1499-3872(14)60250-2
21. Zhang Z, Zhao Y, Canes A, Steinberg D, Lyashevska O, written on behalf of AMEB-DCTCG. Predictive analytics with gradient boosting in clinical medicine. *Ann Transl Med.* (2019) 7:152. doi: 10.21037/atm.2019.03.29
22. Fan Y, Li Y, Bao X, Zhu H, Lu L, Yao Y, et al. Development of machine learning models for predicting postoperative delayed remission in patients with cushing's disease. *J Clin Endocrinol Metab.* (2021) 106:e217–31. doi: 10.1210/clinem/dgaa698
23. Zhang Z, Ho KM, Hong Y. Machine learning for the prediction of volume responsiveness in patients with oliguric acute kidney injury in critical care. *Crit Care.* (2019) 23:112. doi: 10.1186/s13054-019-2411-z
24. Lundberg SM, Erion G, Chen H, DeGrave A, Prutkin JM, Nair B, et al. From local explanations to global understanding with explainable ai for trees. *Nat Mach Intell.* (2020) 2:56–67. doi: 10.1038/s42256-019-0138-9
25. Ickx BE, van der Linden PJ, Melot C, Wijns W, de Pauw L, Vandestadt J, et al. Comparison of the effects of aprotinin and tranexamic acid on blood loss and red blood cell transfusion requirements during the late stages of liver transplantation. *Transfusion.* (2006) 46:595–605. doi: 10.1111/j.1537-2995.2006.00770.x
26. Lagarto F, Gomes B, Couto PS, Correia de Barros F, Moreira Z, Branco T, et al. Perioperative predictors of survival after liver transplantation for familial amyloid polyneuropathy in a portuguese center. *Transplant Proc.* (2016) 48:2098–101. doi: 10.1016/j.transproceed.2016.04.020
27. Corwin HL, Gettinger A, Pearl RG, Fink MP, Levy MM, Shapiro MJ, et al. Efficacy of recombinant human erythropoietin in critically ill patients: a randomized controlled trial. *JAMA.* (2002) 288:2827–35. doi: 10.1001/jama.288.22.2827
28. Massicotte L, Sassine MP, Lenis S, Seal RF, Roy A. Survival rate changes with transfusion of blood products during liver transplantation. *Can J Anaesth.* (2005) 52:148–55. doi: 10.1007/BF03027720
29. Ramos E, Dalmau A, Sabate A, Lama C, Llado L, Figueras J, et al. Intraoperative red blood cell transfusion in liver transplantation: influence on patient outcome, prediction of requirements, and measures to reduce them. *Liver Transpl.* (2003) 9:1320–7. doi: 10.1016/jlts.2003.50204
30. Will ND, Kor DJ, Frank RD, Passe MA, Weister TJ, Zielinski MD, et al. Initial postoperative hemoglobin values and clinical outcomes in transfused patients undergoing noncardiac surgery. *Anesth Analg.* (2019) 129:819–29. doi: 10.1213/ANE.0000000000004287
31. McCaughan GW, Herkes R, Powers B, Rickard K, Gallagher ND, Thompson JF, et al. Thrombocytopenia post liver transplantation. Correlations with pre-operative platelet count, blood transfusion requirements, allograft function and outcome. *J Hepatol.* (1992) 16:16–22. doi: 10.1016/S0168-8278(05)80089-3
32. Real C, Sobreira Fernandes D, Sa Couto P, Correia de Barros F, Esteves S, Aragao I, et al. Survival predictors in liver transplantation: time-varying effect of red blood cell transfusion. *Transplant Proc.* (2016) 48:3303–6. doi: 10.1016/j.transproceed.2016.08.045
33. Arshad F, Lisman T, Porte RJ. Blood markers of portal hypertension are associated with blood loss and transfusion requirements during orthotopic liver transplantation. *Semin Thromb Hemost.* (2020) 46:751–6. doi: 10.1055/s-0040-1714202
34. Bagante F, Spolverato G, Ruzzenente A, Wilson A, Gani F, Conci S, et al. Validation of a nomogram to predict the risk of perioperative blood transfusion for liver resection. *World J Surg.* (2016) 40:2481–9. doi: 10.1007/s00268-016-3544-8
35. Steib A, Freys G, Lehmann C, Meyer C, Mahoudeau G. Intraoperative blood losses and transfusion requirements during adult liver transplantation remain difficult to predict. *Can J Anaesth.* (2001) 48:1075–9. doi: 10.1007/BF03020372
36. Araujo T, Cordeiro A, Proenca P, Perdigoto R, Martins A, Barroso E. Predictive variables affecting transfusion requirements in orthotopic liver transplantation. *Transplant Proc.* (2010) 42:1758–9. doi: 10.1016/j.transproceed.2009.10.007
37. Li X, Xu X, Xie F, Xu X, Sun Y, Liu X, et al. A time-phased machine learning model for real-time prediction of sepsis in critical care. *Crit Care Med.* (2020) 48:e884–8. doi: 10.1097/CCM.0000000000004494
38. Legrand M, Pirracchio R, Rosa A, Petersen ML, Van der Laan M, Fabiani JN, et al. Incidence, risk factors and prediction of post-operative acute kidney injury following cardiac surgery for active infective endocarditis: an observational study. *Crit Care.* (2013) 17:R220. doi: 10.1186/cc13041
39. Bunn C, Kulshrestha S, Boyda J, Balasubramanian N, Birch S, Karabayir I, et al. Application of machine learning to the prediction of postoperative sepsis after appendectomy. *Surgery.* (2020) 169:671–7. doi: 10.1016/j.surg.2020.07.045
40. Koyner JL, Carey KA, Edelson DP, Churpek MM. The development of a machine learning inpatient acute kidney injury prediction model. *Crit Care Med.* (2018) 46:1070–7. doi: 10.1097/CCM.0000000000003123
41. Lee HC, Yoon SB, Yang SM, Kim WH, Ryu HG, Jung CW, et al. Prediction of acute kidney injury after liver transplantation: machine learning approaches vs. logistic regression model. *J Clin Med.* (2018) 7:428. doi: 10.3390/jcm7110428
42. Carrier FM, Chasse M, Wang HT, Aslanian P, Iorio S, Bilodeau M, et al. Restrictive fluid management strategies and outcomes in liver transplantation: a systematic review. *Can J Anaesth.* (2020) 67:109–27. doi: 10.1007/s12630-019-01480-y
43. Donohue CI, Mallett SV. Reducing transfusion requirements in liver transplantation. *World J Transplant.* (2015) 5:165–82. doi: 10.5500/wjt.v5.i4.165
44. Rudin C. Stop explaining black box machine learning models for high stakes decisions and use interpretable models instead. *Nat Mach Intell.* (2019) 1:206–15. doi: 10.1038/s42256-019-0048-x
45. Xie F, Chakraborty B, Ong MEH, Goldstein BA, Liu N. AutoScore: a machine learning-based automatic clinical score generator and its application to mortality prediction using electronic health records. *JMIR Med Inform.* (2020) 8:e21798. doi: 10.2196/21798

# 12

# Machine Learning Prediction Models for Mechanically Ventilated Patients: Analyses of the MIMIC-III Database

*Yibing Zhu [1,2†], Jin Zhang [3†], Guowei Wang [4†], Renqi Yao [5,6], Chao Ren [6], Ge Chen [1], Xin Jin [7], Junyang Guo [8], Shi Liu [9], Hua Zheng [10], Yan Chen [10], Qianqian Guo [11], Lin Li [4], Bin Du [10], Xiuming Xi [12], Wei Li [1*], Huibin Huang [13*], Yang Li [14*] and Qian Yu [14*]*

*[1] Medical Research and Biometrics Center, National Center for Cardiovascular Diseases, Fuwai Hospital, Chinese Academy of Medical Sciences and Peking Union Medical College, Beijing, China, [2] Department of Emergency, Guang'anmen Hospital, China Academy of Chinese Medical Sciences, Beijing, China, [3] School of Economics and Management, Beijing Institute of Technology, Beijing, China, [4] School of Computer Science and Technology, Wuhan University of Technology, Wuhan, China, [5] Department of Burn Surgery, The First Affiliated Hospital of Naval Medical University, Shanghai, China, [6] Translational Medicine Research Center, Fourth Medical Center and Medical Innovation Research Division of the Chinese People's Liberation Army (PLA) General Hospital, Beijing, China, [7] Yidu Cloud Technology Inc., Beijing, China, [8] Beijing Big Eye Xing Tu Culture Media Co., Ltd., Beijing, China, [9] School of Information Science and Engineering, Hebei North University, Shijiazhuang, China, [10] Medical ICU, Peking Union Medical College Hospital, Peking Union Medical College and Chinese Academy of Medical Sciences, Beijing, China, [11] Department of Anesthesiology, Peking University Shougang Hospital, Beijing, China, [12] Department of Critical Care Medicine, Fuxing Hospital, Capital Medical University, Beijing, China, [13] Department of Critical Care Medicine, Beijing Tsinghua Changgung Hospital, School of Clinical Medicine, Tsinghua University, Beijing, China, [14] Academy for Advanced Interdisciplinary Studies, Peking University, Beijing, China*

***Correspondence:**
Wei Li
liwei@mrbc-nccd.com
Huibin Huang
hhba02922@btch.edu.cn
Yang Li
1801213970@pku.edu.cn
Qian Yu
yuq18@pku.edu.cn

*† These authors have contributed equally to this work*

**Background:** Mechanically ventilated patients in the intensive care unit (ICU) have high mortality rates. There are multiple prediction scores, such as the Simplified Acute Physiology Score II (SAPS II), Oxford Acute Severity of Illness Score (OASIS), and Sequential Organ Failure Assessment (SOFA), widely used in the general ICU population. We aimed to establish prediction scores on mechanically ventilated patients with the combination of these disease severity scores and other features available on the first day of admission.

**Methods:** A retrospective administrative database study from the Medical Information Mart for Intensive Care (MIMIC-III) database was conducted. The exposures of interest consisted of the demographics, pre-ICU comorbidity, ICU diagnosis, disease severity scores, vital signs, and laboratory test results on the first day of ICU admission. Hospital mortality was used as the outcome. We used the machine learning methods of *k*-nearest neighbors (KNN), logistic regression, bagging, decision tree, random forest, Extreme Gradient Boosting (XGBoost), and neural network for model establishment. A sample of 70% of the cohort was used for the training set; the remaining 30% was applied for testing. Areas under the receiver operating characteristic curves (AUCs) and calibration plots would be constructed for the evaluation and comparison of the models' performance. The significance of the risk factors was identified through models and the top factors were reported.

**Results:** A total of 28,530 subjects were enrolled through the screening of the MIMIC-III database. After data preprocessing, 25,659 adult patients with 66 predictors were included in the model analyses. With the training set, the models of KNN, logistic regression, decision tree, random forest, neural network, bagging, and XGBoost were established and the testing set obtained AUCs of 0.806, 0.818, 0.743, 0.819, 0.780, 0.803, and 0.821, respectively. The calibration curves of all the models, except for the neural network, performed well. The XGBoost model performed best among the seven models. The top five predictors were age, respiratory dysfunction, SAPS II score, maximum hemoglobin, and minimum lactate.

**Conclusion:** The current study indicates that models with the risk of factors on the first day could be successfully established for predicting mortality in ventilated patients. The XGBoost model performs best among the seven machine learning models.

**Keywords: prediction model, machine learning, mechanical ventilation, intensive care unit, death**

## INTRODUCTION

Mechanically ventilated patients account for more than a quarter in the intensive care unit (ICU) (1). Invasive mechanical ventilation is associated with multiple complications and high mortality (2). The mechanical ventilation ratio has been increasing in the ICU in recent years due to the aging population, more survivors with cancers and comorbidities, and the advancements in treatment (3, 4).

Prediction models are useful tools to unearth underlying causes and provide assistance for clinical practice (5). Establishing a death prediction model of mechanically ventilated patients using their early-stage, easily obtained, and well-generalized features might be helpful for ICU physicians for early alerting and judgment.

With the development of machine learning algorithms, modeling methods are more diversified (6, 7). Extreme Gradient Boosting (XGBoost) has been widely recognized and highly praised in a number of data mining challenges (8–10). With its notable advantages, we hypothesized that the XGBoost model would perform better than other models. We planned to develop and validate multiple machine learning models using the data available in the early stages to predict hospital mortality and identify risk factors in mechanically ventilated ICU patients.

## METHODS

### Database and Study Design

The Medical Information Mart for Intensive Care (MIMIC-III) database was used as the data resource (11). MIMIC-III is a single-center database covering 38,597 distinct adult patients admitted to the ICU in the Beth Israel Deaconess Medical Center in Boston from 2001 to 2012. MIMIC-III integrates comprehensive clinical data and makes them accessible to researchers worldwide under data use agreement. We have obtained permission after application and completion of the course and test (record IDs: 32994435 and 32450965). We established and validated the prediction models using the retrospectively extracted data in MIMIC-III. This study was performed based on the transparent reporting of a multivariable prediction model for individual prognosis or diagnosis (TRIPOD) guideline (12).

### Subjects, Variables, and the Outcome Extraction

Adult ICU patients treated with invasive mechanical ventilation during ICU stay were included. Subjects aged younger than 18 years or older than 90 years or who lack information on the outcome measure were excluded. Hospital mortality was used as the outcome measure.

The subject IDs were used to identify distinct adult patients. The predictors included: (a) demographic information: age and gender; (b) medical history: uncomplicated hypertension (defined as hypertension without complication), complicated hypertension (defined as hypertension with complication),

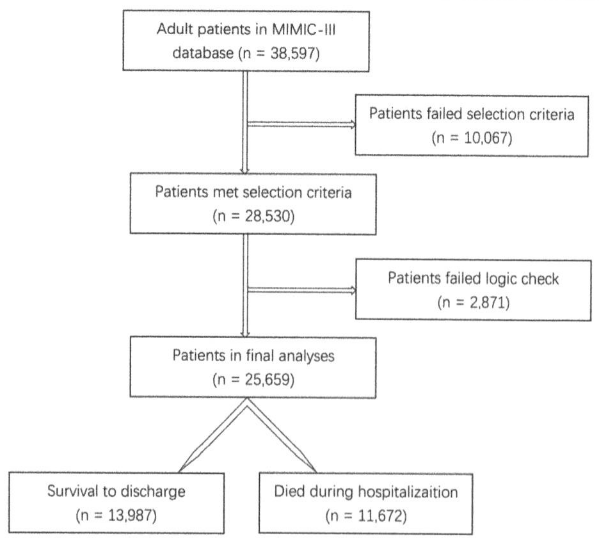


**FIGURE 1** | Flow diagram of the selection process of patients.

**Abbreviations:** AUCs, areas under the receiver operating characteristic curves; DBP, diastolic blood pressure; HR, heart rate; ICU, intensive care unit; KNN, *k*-nearest neighbors; MAP, mean arterial pressure; MIMIC-III, Medical Information Mart for Intensive Care; OASIS, Oxford Acute Severity of Illness Score; ROC, receiver operating characteristic; RRT, renal replacement therapy; SAPS II, Simplified Acute Physiology Score II; SHAP, Shapley additive explanation; SBP, systolic blood pressure; SGB, stochastic gradient boosting; SOFA, Sequential Organ Failure Assessment; SQL, Structured Query Language; WBC, white blood cell; XGBoost, Extreme Gradient Boosting.

**TABLE 1** | Characteristics between survivors and non-survivors.

| | Survivors ($N = 13{,}987$) | Non-survivors ($N = 11{,}672$) | *p*-value |
|---|---|---|---|
| **Demographic** | | | |
| Age (years) | 61.0 (21.9) | 70.3 (20.4) | <0.0001 |
| Gender (male) | 8,681 (62.1) | 6,728 (57.6) | <0.0001 |
| **Medical history** | | | |
| Uncomplicated hypertension | 6,888 (49.3) | 4,346 (37.2) | <0.0001 |
| Complicated hypertension | 1,098 (7.9) | 1,655 (14.2) | <0.0001 |
| Uncomplicated diabetes | 2,938 (21.0) | 2,557 (21.9) | 0.0815 |
| Complicated diabetes | 730 (5.2) | 908 (7.8) | <0.0001 |
| Malignancy | 894 (6.4) | 2,167 (18.6) | <0.0001 |
| Hematologic disease | 1,296 (9.3) | 1,884 (16.1) | <0.0001 |
| Metastasis | 1,142 (8.2) | 1,762 (15.1) | <0.0001 |
| Peripheral vascular disease | 1,225 (8.8) | 1,142 (9.8) | 0.0049 |
| Hypothyroidism | 1,217 (8.7) | 1,172 (10.0) | 0.0002 |
| Chronic heart failure | 744 (5.3) | 780 (6.7) | <0.0001 |
| Stroke | 731 (5.2) | 725 (6.2) | 0.0007 |
| Liver disease | 616 (4.4) | 919 (7.9) | <0.0001 |
| **Disease severity** | | | |
| SAPS II | 32.0 (16.0) | 43.0 (19.0) | <0.0001 |
| SOFA | 4.0 (4.0) | 5.0 (5.0) | <0.0001 |
| OASIS | 33.0 (10.0) | 37.0 (12.0) | <0.0001 |
| **Diagnosis** | | | |
| Sepsis | 1,617 (11.6) | 3,375 (28.9) | <0.0001 |
| Any organ failure | 8,150 (58.3) | 9,920 (85.0) | <0.0001 |
| Severe respiratory failure | 659 (5.7) | 966 (10.9) | <0.0001 |
| Severe coagulation failure | 27 (0.2) | 149 (1.3) | <0.0001 |
| Severe liver failure | 101 (2.0) | 323 (5.2) | <0.0001 |
| Severe cardiovascular failure | 1,070 (7.7) | 2,116 (18.3) | <0.0001 |
| Severe central nervous system failure | 711 (5.1) | 608 (5.3) | <0.0001 |
| Severe renal failure | 398 (2.9) | 1,178 (10.1) | <0.0001 |
| Respiratory dysfunction | 6,172 (44.1) | 8,478 (72.6) | <0.0001 |
| Cardiovascular dysfunction | 1,388 (9.9) | 2,687 (23.0) | <0.0001 |
| Renal dysfunction | 2,934 (21.0) | 5,103 (43.7) | <0.0001 |
| Hematologic dysfunction | 1,296 (9.3) | 1,884 (16.1) | <0.0001 |
| Metabolic dysfunction | 1,142 (8.2) | 1,764 (15.1) | <0.0001 |
| Neurologic dysfunction | 1,245 (8.9) | 1,371 (11.8) | <0.0001 |
| **Vital signs** | | | |
| Mean HR (bpm) | 85.7 (17.9) | 86.8 (22.1) | <0.0001 |
| Minimum HR (bpm) | 71.0 (18.0) | 71.0 (21.0) | <0.0001 |
| Maximum HR (bpm) | 103.0 (25.0) | 106.0 (29.0) | <0.0001 |
| Mean MAP (mmHg) | 76.7 (11.9) | 75.1 (13.9) | <0.0001 |
| Minimum MAP (mmHg) | 59.0 (12.0) | 55.7 (15.0) | <0.0001 |
| Maximum MAP (mmHg) | 101.7 (22.0) | 102.0 (25.0) | <0.0001 |
| Mean systolic pressure (mmHg) | 115.0 (17.9) | 113.9 (22.5) | <0.0001 |
| Minimum systolic pressure (mmHg) | 89.0 (18.0) | 86.0 (22.0) | <0.0001 |
| Maximum systolic pressure (mmHg) | 148.0 (28.0) | 149.0 (33.0) | <0.0001 |
| Mean diastolic pressure (mmHg) | 59.9 (11.6) | 57.5 (13.2) | <0.0001 |
| Minimum diastolic pressure (mmHg) | 45.0 (12.0) | 41.0 (15.0) | <0.0001 |
| Maximum diastolic pressure (mmHg) | 80.0 (19.0) | 80.0 (22.0) | 0.0636 |
| Mean temperature (°C) | 37.0 (0.8) | 36.8 (0.9) | <0.0001 |
| Minimum temperature (°C) | 36.1 (1.0) | 36.1 (1.0) | <0.0001 |
| Maximum temperature (°C) | 37.7 (1.0) | 37.6 (1.1) | <0.0001 |

*(Continued)*

**TABLE 1** | Continued

| | Survivors (*N* = 13,987) | Non-survivors (*N* = 11,672) | *p*-value |
|---|---|---|---|
| **Laboratory results** | | | |
| Mean lactate (mmol/L) | 1.9 (1.2) | 2.0 (1.9) | <0.0001 |
| Minimum lactate (mmol/L) | 1.3 (0.8) | 1.5 (1.2) | <0.0001 |
| Maximum lactate (mmol/L) | 2.4 (2.0) | 2.4 (2.8) | <0.0001 |
| Mean pH | 7.4 (0.1) | 7.4 (0.1) | <0.0001 |
| Minimum pH | 7.3 (0.1) | 7.3 (0.2) | <0.0001 |
| Maximum pH | 7.4 (0.1) | 7.4 (0.1) | <0.0001 |
| Mean glucose (mg/dL) | 128.6 (32.1) | 136.7 (50.2) | <0.0001 |
| Minimum glucose (mg/dL) | 96.0 (35.0) | 104.0 (44.0) | <0.0001 |
| Maximum glucose (mg/dL) | 169.0 (60.0) | 174.0 (86.0) | <0.0001 |
| Mean WBC ($\times 10^9$/L) | 11.7 (5.9) | 11.8 (7.6) | <0.0001 |
| Minimum WBC ($\times 10^9$/L) | 9.8 (5.5) | 10.1 (6.9) | <0.0001 |
| Maximum WBC ($\times 10^9$/L) | 13.4 (7.3) | 13.4 (8.9) | <0.0001 |
| Mean BUN (mg/dl) | 15.5 (10.3) | 24.5 (24.0) | <0.0001 |
| Minimum BUN (mg/dl) | 14.0 (9.0) | 23.0 (22.0) | <0.0001 |
| Maximum BUN (mg/dl) | 17.0 (11.0) | 26.0 (25.0) | <0.0001 |
| Mean creatinine (mg/dl) | 0.9 (0.4) | 1.1 (1.0) | <0.0001 |
| Minimum creatinine (mg/dl) | 0.8 (0.4) | 1.0 (0.9) | <0.0001 |
| Maximum creatinine (mg/dl) | 0.9 (0.5) | 1.2 (1.2) | <0.0001 |
| Mean hemoglobin (g/dl) | 10.6 (2.5) | 10.3 (2.3) | <0.0001 |
| Minimum hemoglobin (g/dl) | 9.5 (3.0) | 9.4 (2.6) | <0.0001 |
| Maximum hemoglobin (g/dl) | 12.4 (2.6) | 11.3 (2.6) | <0.0001 |
| **Treatment** | | | |
| Ventilation duration (h) | 15.0 (45.9) | 46.0 (122.6) | <0.0001 |
| RRT | 654 (4.7) | 1,628 (14.0) | <0.0001 |

*Continuous variables are presented as the median and interquartile range (IQR). Counting data are presented as numbers and percentages.*
*Complicated or uncomplicated hypertension refers to hypertension with or without complication. Complicated or uncomplicated diabetes refers to diabetes with or without complication. Severe respiratory failure, severe coagulation failure, severe liver failure, severe cardiovascular failure, severe central nervous failure, and severe renal failure refer to the scores of the specific organ or system that reaches 4 in the SOFA score. The definition of the medical condition was referred to the ICD-9 code. A mean, minimum, or maximum parameter refers to the mean, the highest, or the lowest level of the parameter on the first day of ICU admission.*
*HR, heart rate; MAP, mean arterial pressure; OASIS, Oxford Acute Severity of Illness Score; RRT, renal replacement therapy; SAPS II, Simplified Acute Physiology Score II; SOFA, Sequential Organ Failure Assessment; WBC, white blood cell.*

uncomplicated diabetes (defined as diabetes without complication), complicated diabetes (defined as diabetes with complication), malignancy, hematologic disease, metastasis, peripheral vascular disease, hypothyroidism, chronic heart failure, stroke, and liver disease; (c) disease severity score: Simplified Acute Physiology Score II (SAPS II), Sequential Organ Failure Assessment (SOFA), and Oxford Acute Severity of Illness Score (OASIS); (d) diagnosis: sepsis, any organ failure, severity of respiratory failure, severity of coagulation failure, severity of liver failure, severity of cardiovascular failure, severity of central nervous system failure, severity of renal failure, respiratory dysfunction, cardiovascular dysfunction, renal dysfunction, hematologic dysfunction, metabolic dysfunction, and neurologic dysfunction; (e) vital signs on the first day of ICU admission: the highest, lowest, and mean levels of heart rate (HR), mean arterial pressure (MAP), systolic blood pressure (SBP), diastolic blood pressure (DBP), and temperature; and (f) laboratory results of the first day of ICU admission: the highest, lowest, and mean levels of lactate, pH, glucose, white blood cell (WBC), blood urea nitrogen (BUN), creatinine, and hemoglobin. Treatment information on renal replacement therapy (RRT) and the duration of mechanical ventilation were extracted to present the characteristics of the included subjects; they were not analyzed as predictors since we included only early-stage predictors, which can be obtained on the first day of ICU admission in this prediction model. The lengths of stay in hospital of survivors and non-survivors were reported. The target subjects together with all the predefined predictors, subject ID, characteristic variables, and the outcome measure were extracted using a Structured Query Language (SQL) script. The definition of the medical condition was referred to the ICD-9 code (13) and derived from the GitHub (https://github.com/MIT-LCP/mimic-code). The severity of respiratory, coagulation, liver, cardiovascular, central nervous system, or renal failure referred to the SOFA score of the specific organ (scores 0–4). The first day indicates the first 24 h of ICU admission. The SOFA, SAPS II, and OASIS scores refer to the first scores after ICU admission. After the extraction of the data, subjects who met the exclusion criteria were excluded. Then, the extreme and error values failing the logic check were censored. We excluded variables with missing values accounting for more than 30% of the sample size (14). Otherwise, we used the mean imputation method to deal with missing values. Thus, the subset was established for the final analyses.

## Statistical Analysis

The characteristics of the included patients were compared between survivors and non-survivors. The continuous variables are presented as the median and interquartile range (IQR) and compared using the *t*-test. The counting data are presented as numbers and percentages and compared using the chi-square test.

We employed seven machine learning methods—*k*-nearest neighbors (KNN), logistic regression, bagging, decision tree, random forest, XGBoost, and neural network—for model establishment. A sample of 70% of the cohort generated randomly using a seed was applied for the training set; the remaining 30% was used for testing. Areas under the receiver operating characteristic curves (AUCs) were used to evaluate the performance of the models. Calibration plots were drawn to visualize the prediction abilities of the models. For the best-performing model, the significance of the model parameters was identified and reported; the Shapley additive explanation (SHAP) plot was drawn. SAS software (version 9.4), R software (version 3.6.1), and Python software (version 3.4.3) were used for statistical analyses.

# RESULTS

## Participants

Among the 38,597 adult patients in the MIMIC-III database, 28,530 subjects met our selection criteria. After the logic check, 25,659 patients were included in the final analyses (**Figure 1**). Sixty-seven predictors were extracted from the database. After data cleaning, the predictor severe liver failure was excluded because of more than 30% of missing data; 66 predictors were included in the model. The mortality rate of the cohort was 45.5% (13,987 survivors and 11,672 non-survivors). The median length of stay in hospital of survivors was 9.2 days (IQR = 11.1) and that of non-survivors was 11.1 days (IQR = 15.3, $p < 0.0001$). The comparison of characteristics between the survivors and the non-survivors is reported in **Table 1**. Non-survivors were older and had higher SAPS II, SOFA, and OASIS scores; more medical history of hypertension with complication, diabetes with complication, malignancy, hematologic disease, peripheral vascular disease, hypothyroidism, chronic heart failure, stroke, and liver disease; more diagnosis of sepsis, any organ failure, severe respiratory failure, severe coagulation failure, severe liver failure, severe cardiovascular failure, severe central nervous system failure, severe renal failure, respiratory dysfunction, cardiovascular dysfunction, renal dysfunction, hematologic dysfunction, metabolic dysfunction, and neurologic dysfunction; had higher mean HR, maximum HR, maximum MAP, maximum SBP, mean lactate, minimum lactate, mean

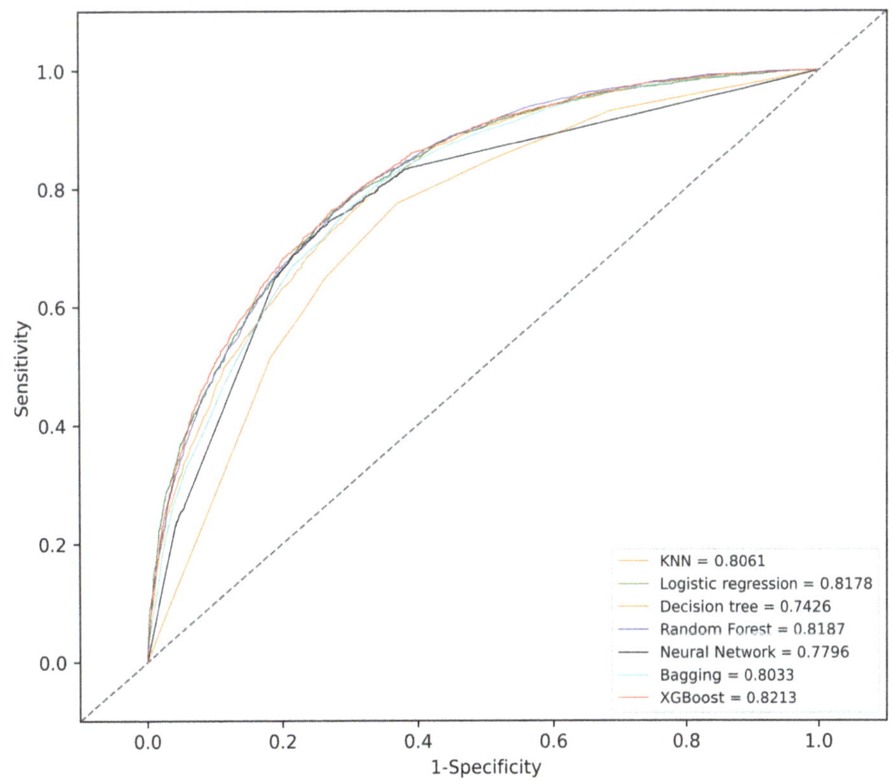


**FIGURE 2** | Receiver operating characteristic (ROC) curves of the seven models. KNN, k-nearest neighbors; XGBoost, Extreme Gradient Boosting.

glucose, minimum glucose, maximum glucose, mean WBC, minimum WBC, maximum WBC, mean creatinine, minimum creatinine, and maximum creatinine; and had longer duration of mechanical ventilation and more RRTs ($p < 0.05$), while they had a lower male ratio, hypertension without complication, mean MAP, minimum MAP, mean SBP, minimum SBP, mean DBP, minimum DBP, mean temperature, maximum temperature, mean hemoglobin, minimum hemoglobin, and maximum hemoglobin ($p < 0.05$). There were no significant differences in diabetes without complication ($p = 0.0815$) and maximum DBP ($p = 0.0636$) between the two groups.

## Models

With the training set, the KNN, logistic regression, decision tree, random forest, neural network, bagging, and XGBoost models were established and the testing set obtained AUCs of 0.806, 0.818, 0.743, 0.819, 0.780, 0.803, and 0.821, respectively.

The KNN, logistic regression, decision tree, random forest, neural network, bagging, and XGBoost models were established with the training set; the AUCs of the testing set were 0.806, 0.818, 0.743, 0.819, 0.780, 0.803, and 0.821, respectively (**Figure 2**). The calibration plots of the seven models are presented in **Figure 3**. The calibration curves of all the models, except that of the neural network, performed well. Among the seven models, XGBoost performed best, with the highest receiver operating characteristic (ROC) and the best calibration curve. The hyperparameters applied in the final XGBoost model were as follows: learning rates = 0.008, number of estimators = 800, maximum depth of a tree = 6, $\alpha = 0$, $\lambda = 0$. The significance of the predictors in the XGBoost model is presented in **Figure 4**. In the SHAP methodology, the top five predictors were age, respiratory dysfunction, SAPS II score, maximum hemoglobin, and minimum lactate (the importance values were 0.410, 0.309, 0.302, 0.209, and 0.194, respectively). The confusion matrix of the XGBoost model is presented in **Table 2**. The SHAP plot and a decision tree of the XGBoost model are in the **Supplementary Material**.

## DISCUSSION

This study identified various clinical features associated with increased hospital mortality among mechanically ventilated ICU patients. Through sophisticated machine learning methods, we determined that age, respiratory dysfunction, SAPS II score, maximum hemoglobin, and minimum lactate were most associated with hospital death. Among the seven models, XGBoost revealed the best performance in discrimination.

Our results showed that more than half of the ICU patients were under mechanical ventilation; the mortality of the mechanically ventilated patients was high (45.5%). The requirement for mechanical ventilation has increased in recent

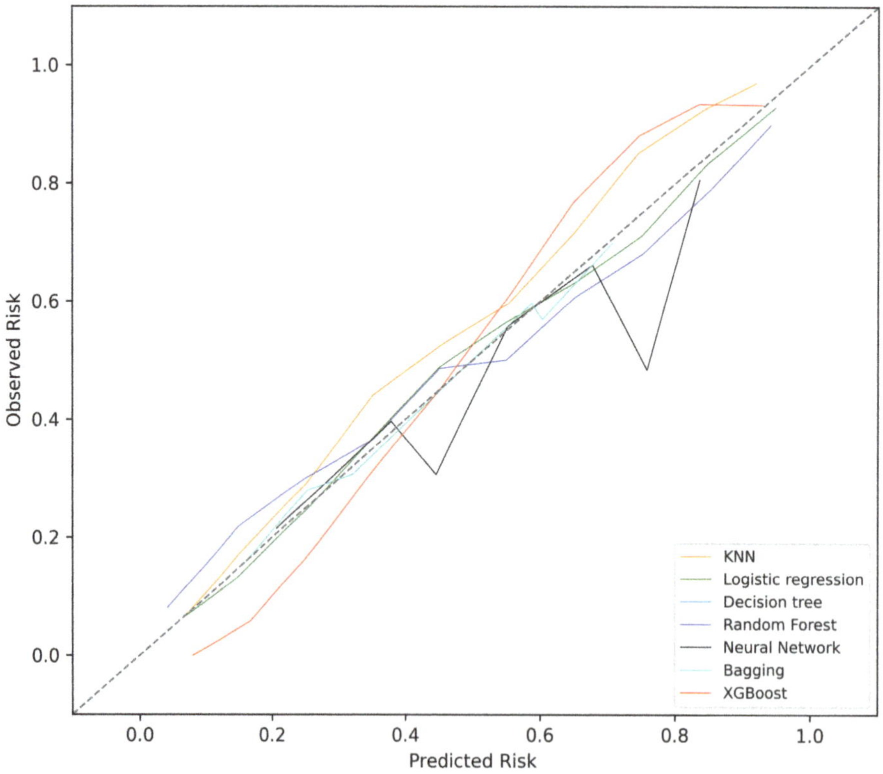


**FIGURE 3** | Calibration plots of the seven models. KNN, k-nearest neighbors; XGBoost, Extreme Gradient Boosting.

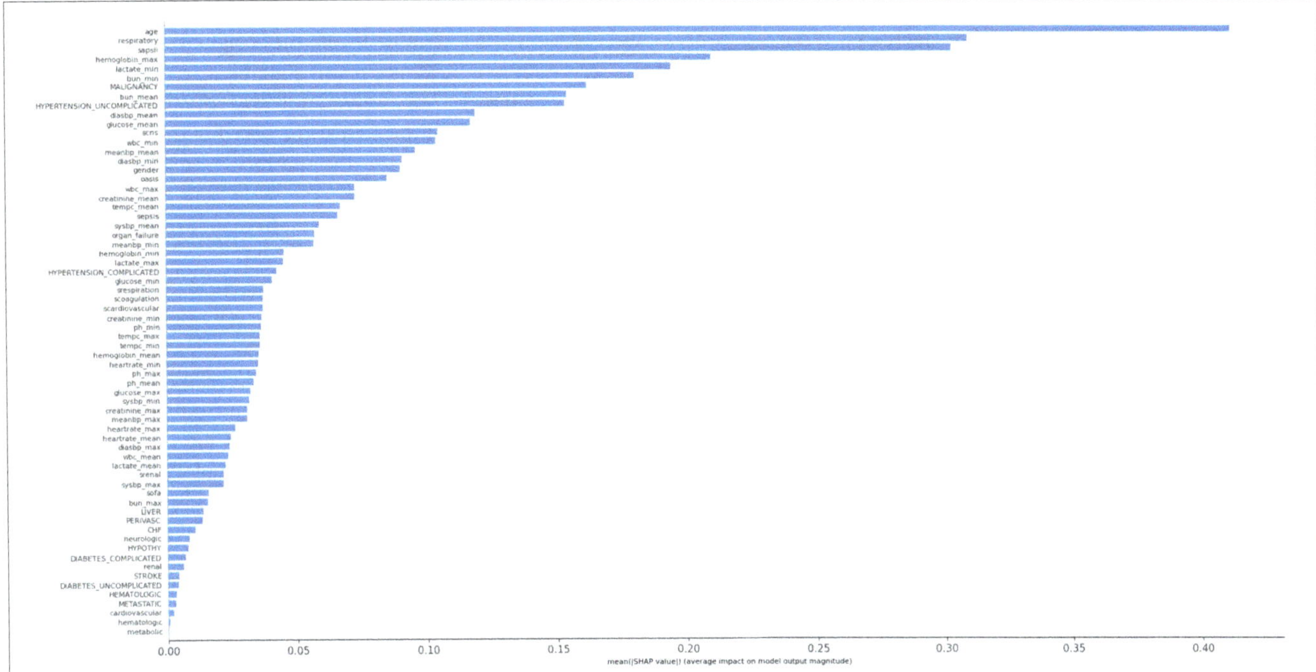


**FIGURE 4 |** Significance of the predictors in the XGBoost model. CHF, chronic heart failure; Diabetes_complicated, diabetes with complication; Diabetes_uncomplicated, diabetes without complication; Diasbp, diastolic blood pressure; Hypertension_complicated, hypertension with complication; Hypertension_uncomplicated, hypertension without complication; OASIS, Oxford Acute Severity of Illness Score; Organ_failure, any organ failure; Perivasc, perivascular disease; SAPS II, Simplified Acute Physiology Score II; sCardiovascular, severe cardiovascular failure; sCNS, severe central nervous system failure; sCoagulation, severe coagulation failure; SOFA, Sequential Organ Failure Assessment; sRenal, severe renal failure; sRespiration, severe respiratory failure; Sysbp, systolic blood pressure; Tempc, temperature; WBC, white blood cell.

**TABLE 2 |** Confusion matrix of the XGBoost model.

| | Precision | Recall | F1 score |
|---|---|---|---|
| Survival | 0.87 | 0.81 | 0.84 |
| Death | 0.66 | 0.74 | 0.70 |

years (1). Therefore, it is of great importance to recognize early the patients at high risk of death with early-stage, well-generalized, and easily obtained features (15). With the development of machine learning algorithms, the magnitude of predictors that can be processed has mainly been largely enriched. Thus, advanced machine learning techniques allow researchers to establish more optimal models in comparison with conventional models (16). With such models, ICU physicians could be alerted early when patients become complicated and have deteriorated with mechanical ventilation.

A previous study conducted by Yao et al. (16) explored the death prediction model in postoperative septic patients using the MIMIC-III database. Similar to our results, they also found that the XGBoost model performed better in predicting hospital mortality than the other models. However, due to the different patient types and the various features included, the feature importance rankings were quite different (their top five predictors: fluid–electrolyte disturbance, coagulopathy, RRT, urine output, and cardiovascular surgery). Another study (5) used information from the first 24 h after admission to the ICU to build a 1-year death prediction model in septic patients based on the stochastic gradient boosting (SGB) methodology. The AUC of the SGB model was 0.8039, similar to the performance of XGBoost in our study. Both the SGB and XGBoost models belong to gradient boosting algorithms. Similar to our results, age ranked first in the feature importance (their top five predictors: age, urine output, maximum BUN, metastatic cancer, and maximum temperature).

There are strengths of our study. Firstly, this is the first study that established several advanced machine learning death prediction models focused on mechanically ventilated ICU patients. Secondly, we used MIMI-III, a high-quality database with a large sample size and comprehensive clinical information. Thirdly, we utilized advanced statistical methods, including seven machine learning models, with the 30% subset used for internal validation and the ROCs and calibration plots to evaluate the models (17).

There are limitations to our study. Firstly, our models were retrospectively established based on a single-center database. Thus, further prospective studies are needed to evaluate the generalization of our models and predictors. Secondly, there were missing data in our research. There was also a potential confounding variable that we were unable to assess because its missing data exceeded the predesigned limit. Thirdly, external validation has not been employed in this study; hence, the significance and evidence level were decreased. Fourthly, our study only focused on hospital mortality, while other important outcome measures such as ventilator-free days within 28 days and long-term mortalities still needed further investigation. Lastly, we did not exclude patients who were withdrawn from care, which may also provide bias.

## CONCLUSION

Our results suggest that age, respiratory dysfunction, SAPS II score, maximum hemoglobin, and minimum lactate might be closely associated with hospital mortality in mechanically ventilated ICU patients. The XGBoost model performs better than the KNN, logistic regression, bagging, decision tree, random forest, and neural network models in our study. Further external validations are needed to test the generalization of our models and predictors.

## ETHICS STATEMENT

The establishment of this database was approved by the Massachusetts Institute of Technology (Cambridge, MA) and Beth Israel Deaconess Medical Center (Boston, MA), and consent was obtained for the original data collection. Therefore, the ethical approval statement and the need for informed consent were waived for this manuscript. Written informed consent for participation was not required for this study in accordance with the national legislation and the institutional requirements.

## AUTHOR CONTRIBUTIONS

YZ and HH conceptualized the research aims, planned the analyses, and guided the literature review. YL and QY extracted the data from the MIMIC-III database. JZ, GW, GC, SL, XJ, and JG participated in processing the data and doing the statistical analysis. YZ wrote the first draft of the paper. RY, CR, HZ, YC, QG, LL, BD, XX, WL, and HH provided comments and approved the final manuscript. All authors read and approved the final manuscript.

## ACKNOWLEDGMENTS

The abstract of this work was reported on the 43th Annual Conference on Shock (June 6–9, 2020, Toronto) and published on Shock 2020; 53(1S):P14.

## REFERENCES

1. Wunsch H, Wagner J, Herlim M, Chong DH, Kramer AA, Halpern SD. ICU occupancy and mechanical ventilator use in the United States. *Crit Care Med.* (2013) 41:2712–9. doi: 10.1097/CCM.0b013e318298a139
2. Hung YS, Lee SH, Hung CY, Chao-Hui Wang, Chen-Yi Kao, Hung-Ming Wang, et al. Clinical characteristics and survival outcomes of terminally ill patients undergoing withdrawal of mechanical ventilation. *J Formos Med Assoc.* (2018) 117:798–805. doi: 10.1016/j.jfma.2017.09.014
3. Herring AA, Ginde AA, Fahimi J, Alter HJ, Maselli JH, Espinola JA, et al. Increasing critical care admissions from U.S. emergency departments, 2001-2009. *Crit Care Med.* (2013) 41:1197–204. doi: 10.1097/CCM.0b013e31827c086f
4. Al-Omari A, Abdelwahed HS, Alansari, MA. Critical care service in Saudi Arabia. *Saudi Med J.* (2015) 36:759–61. doi: 10.15537/smj.2015.6.11204
5. García-Gallo JE, Fonseca-Ruiz NJ, Celi LA, Duitama-Muñoz JF. A machine learning-based model for 1-year mortality prediction in patients admitted to an Intensive Care Unit with a diagnosis of sepsis. *Med Intensiva.* (2020) 44:160–70. doi: 10.1016/j.medine.2018.07.019
6. Komorowski M, Celi LA, Badawi O, Gordon AC, Faisal AA. The Artificial Intelligence Clinician learns optimal treatment strategies for sepsis in intensive care. *Nat Med.* (2018) 24:1716–20. doi: 10.1038/s41591-018-0213-5
7. Yuan KC, Tsai LW, Lee KH, Cheng YW, Hsu SC, Lo YS, et al. The development an artificial intelligence algorithm for early sepsis diagnosis in the intensive care unit. *Int J Med Inform.* (2020) 141:104176. doi: 10.1016/j.ijmedinf.2020.104176
8. Bighamian R, Soleymani S, Reisner AT, Seri I, Hahn JO. Prediction of hemodynamic response to epinephrine *via* model-based system identification. *IEEE J Biomed Health Inform.* (2016) 20:416–23. doi: 10.1109/JBHI.2014.2371533
9. Raffort J, Adam C, Carrier M, Ballaith A, Coscas R, Jean-Baptiste E, et al. Artificial intelligence in abdominal aortic aneurysm. *J Vasc Surg.* (2020) 72:321–33.e1. doi: 10.1016/j.jvs.2019.12.026
10. Hou N, Li M, He L, Xie B, Wang L, Zhang R, et al. Predicting 30-days mortality for MIMIC-III patients with sepsis-3: a machine learning approach using XGboost. *J Transl Med.* (2020) 18:462. doi: 10.1186/s12967-020-02620-5
11. Johnson AEW, Pollard TJ, Shen L, Lehman L-WH, Feng M, Ghassemi M, et al. MIMIC-III, a freely accessible critical care database. *Sci Data.* (2016) 3:160035. doi: 10.1038/sdata.2016.35
12. Collins GS, Reitsma JB, Altman DG, Moons KGM. Transparent reporting of a multivariable prediction model for individual prognosis or diagnosis (TRIPOD): the TRIPOD statement. *BMJ.* (2015) 350:g7594. doi: 10.1136/bmj.g7594
13. Quan H, Sundararajan V, Halfon P, Fong A, Burnand B, Luthi J-C, et al. Coding algorithms for defining comorbidities in ICD-9-CM and ICD-10 administrative data. *Med Care.* (2005) 43:1130–9. doi: 10.1097/01.mlr.0000182534.19832.83
14. Rubin DB. Inference and missing data. *Biometrika.* (1976) 63:581–92. doi: 10.1093/biomet/63.3.581
15. Ismaeil T, Almutairi J, Alshaikh R, Althobaiti Z, Ismaeil Y, Othman F. Survival of mechanically ventilated patients admitted to intensive care units. Results from a tertiary care center between 2016-2018. *Saudi Med J.* (2019) 40:781–8. doi: 10.15537/smj.2019.8.24447
16. Yao RQ, Jin X, Wang GW, Yu Y, Wu GS, Zhu YB, et al. A machine learning-based prediction of hospital mortality in patients with postoperative sepsis. *Front Med (Lausanne).* (2020) 7:445. doi: 10.21203/rs.2.24188/v1
17. Van Calster B, McLernon DJ, van Smeden M, Wynants L, Steyerberg EW. Topic Group 'Evaluating diagnostic tests and prediction models' of the STRATOS initiative. Calibration: the Achilles heel of predictive analytics. *BMC Med.* (2019) 17:230. doi: 10.1186/s12916-019-1466-7

13

# Determination of a "Specific Population Who Could Benefit from Rosuvastatin": A Secondary Analysis of a Randomized Controlled Trial to Uncover the Novel Value of Rosuvastatin for the Precise Treatment of ARDS

*Shi Zhang, Zhonghua Lu, Zongsheng Wu, Jianfeng Xie, Yi Yang and Haibo Qiu**

*Jiangsu Provincial Key Laboratory of Critical Care Medicine, Department of Critical Care Medicine, School of Medicine, Nanjing Zhongda Hospital, Southeast University, Nanjing, China*

***Correspondence:***
*Haibo Qiu*
*haiboq2000@163.com*

**Background:** The high heterogeneity of acute respiratory distress syndrome (ARDS) contributes to paradoxical conclusions from previous investigations of rosuvastatin for ARDS. Identification of the population (phenotype) that could benefit from rosuvastatin is a novel exploration for the precise treatment.

**Methods:** The patient population for this analysis consisted of unique patients with ARDS enrolled in the SAILS trial (rosuvastatin vs. placebo). Phenotypes were derived using consensus k-means clustering applied to routinely available clinical variables within 6 h of hospital presentation before the patients received placebo or rosuvastatin. The Kaplan–Meier statistic was used to estimate the 90-day cumulative mortality to screen for a specific population that could benefit from rosuvastatin, with a cutoff $P < 0.05$.

**Results:** The derivation cohort included 585 patients with ARDS. Of the patients with the four derived phenotypes, those with phenotype 3 were classified as the "specific population who could benefit from rosuvastatin" as rosuvastatin resulted in a significant reduction in 90-day cumulative mortality from ARDS [hazard ratio (HR), 0.29; 95% confidence interval (CI), 0.09–0.93; $P = 0.027$]. Additionally, rosuvastatin markedly improved the days free of cardiovascular failure ($10.08 \pm 3.79$ in the rosuvastatin group vs. $7.31 \pm 4.94$ in the placebo group, $P = 0.01$) and coagulation abnormalities ($13.65 \pm 1.33$ vs. $12.15 \pm 3.77$, $P = 0.02$) up to day 14 in the phenotype 3 cohort. Phenotype 3 was summarized as $\text{Platelet}^{\text{high}}$ & $\text{Creat}^{\text{low}}$ phenotype because these patients have a relatively higher platelet count ($390.05 \pm 79.43 \times 10^9$/L) and lower creatinine ($1.42 \pm 1.08$ mg/dL) than do patients classified as other phenotypes. In addition, rosuvastatin seemed to increase 90-day mortality for patients classified as phenotype 4 (HR, 2.76; 95% CI, 0.09–9.93; $P = 0.076$), with an adverse effect on reducing the days free of renal failure up to day 14 ($4.70 \pm 4.99$ vs. $10.17 \pm 4.69$, $P = 0.01$). Patients in phenotype

4 showed relatively severe illness in terms of baseline features, particularly renal failure, with high serum glucose. Therefore, phenotype 4 was defined as $APACHE^{high}$ & Serum $glucose^{high}$ phenotype.

**Conclusions:** This secondary analysis of the SAILS trial identified that rosuvastatin seems to be harmful for patients classified as $APACHE^{high}$ & Serum $glucose^{high}$ phenotype, but benefit patients in $Platelet^{high}$ & $Creat^{low}$ phenotype, thus uncovering the novel value of rosuvastatin for the precise treatment of ARDS.

**Keywords: ARDS, Rosuvastatin, heterogeneity, machine learning, precise treatment**

## BACKGROUND

Acute respiratory distress syndrome (ARDS) is a highly heterogeneous and complicated critical illness. Despite advances in clinical management, the mortality rate of severe ARDS remains as high as 40–46% because of the lack of targeted therapeutic protocols for distinct patients. Categorizing ARDS for further appropriate therapy is a critical unmet need for precise treatment and improvement of the salvage rate of ARDS (1, 2).

In consideration of rosuvastatin's anti-inflammatory effects and pathogenesis of ARDS (inadequate control of inflammatory responses in the lung), rosuvastatin has been utilized in the treatment of ARDS in the last decade (3-7). Previous studies demonstrated that rosuvastatin could improve the outcomes of ARDS in animal models (8–10). Unfortunately, a large multicenter randomized controlled trial conducted in 2014 by Truwit et al. (named the SAILS trial) suggested that rosuvastatin therapy did not improve the clinical outcomes of patients with ARDS (11).

A possible reason for these paradoxical conclusions is the heterogeneity of ARDS. ARDS, as an overly broad definition of a syndrome, encompasses a vast, multidimensional array of clinical and biological features. Markedly different from experimental animals, patients with ARDS actually comprise diverse phenotypes, which appear to have different clinical characteristics, immune statuses, biological processes, and severities. Several investigations successfully classified ARDS into distinct subgroups via biomarkers or clinical features (12, 13) and indicated that appropriate therapies for distinct patients may be a promising strategy for precise treatment in ARDS. Rosuvastatin, as an immunomodulatory intervention to attenuate inflammation, may benefit only some specific populations. Although Sinha et al. (14) conducted a latent class analysis of ARDS subphenotypes in the SAILS trial, the subphenotype that can benefit from rosuvastatin was not identified in their analysis. The reason for this may be that Sinha et al. did not utilize a matched algorithm and appropriate data processing for their data. Obviously, there is a robust need to identify the treatable ARDS phenotype (patients who could benefit from rosuvastatin) through a large number of various algorithms and data analyses.

Fortunately, Truwit et al. (11) uploaded the original data of the SAILS trial to the ARDS-Net database, making it possible for us to perform a secondary analysis to find the specific population that could benefit from rosuvastatin. Thus, we aimed to derive this specific ARDS phenotype by using an unsupervised clustering algorithm to uncover the novel value of rosuvastatin for the precise treatment of ARDS.

## METHODS

This study was reviewed and approved by the Institutional Ethics Committee of Zhongda Hospital. The Institutional Ethics Committee of Zhongda Hospital approved this study, which was conducted under several data use agreements. The data for the ARDSnet project were obtained under a waiver of informed consent and with authorization under the Health Insurance Portability and Accountability Act.

### Patient Population

The patient population for this analysis consisted of unique patients with ARDS enrolled in the SAILS trial (rosuvastatin vs. placebo), which was published in 2014. The diagnostic criterion of ARDS in the SAILS trial referenced the 2012 Berlin definition of ARDS (1, 2). To eliminate the influence of immunosuppression on the evaluation of rosuvastatin for ARDS, the patients were divided into 160 definitely immunosuppressed patients and 585 other patients for the respective analysis. The definitely immunosuppressed patients included ARDS patients with comorbidities such as acquired immune deficiency syndrome, leukemia, and non-Hodgkin lymphoma; patients with cancer receiving chemotherapy; and patients who received immunosuppression therapy in the past 6 months. After excluding the 160 definitely immunosuppressed patients, 585 other patients were enrolled in the derivation cohort for further unsupervised clustering analysis.

### Screening Clinical Features for Phenotyping

Based on the SAILS trial database, we first extracted the available variables within the first 6 h of hospital presentation before the patients received placebo or rosuvastatin and excluded variables with missing rates > 10%. These clinically available characteristics included age, alanine aminotransferase, APACHE III score, aspartate aminotransferase, blood urea nitrogen, C-reactive protein, creatine kinase, creatinine, diastolic blood pressure (BP), Glasgow Coma Scale score, height, heart rate, male sex, $PaCO_2$, $PaO_2$:$FIO_2$, $PaO_2$, platelet count, predicted body weight, respiration rate, serum albumin highest, serum albumin lowest, serum glucose lowest, shock at baseline, systolic BP, temperature, urine output, and weight.

Furthermore, to screen the candidate variables that could identify a "specific population who can benefit from rosuvastatin," we conducted differential analyses by using $t$-tests to compare clinically available variables between the rosuvastatin group and placebo group among surviving patients, and $P < 0.3$ was the threshold value.

## Statistical Methods

To derive the phenotypes, we first assessed the candidate variable distributions, missingness, and correlation. Multiple imputations with chained equations were used to account for missing data (15).

To identify different phenotypes of ARDS, consensus k-means clustering through candidate variables was utilized to perform consistent clustering on 585 patients in the derivation cohort

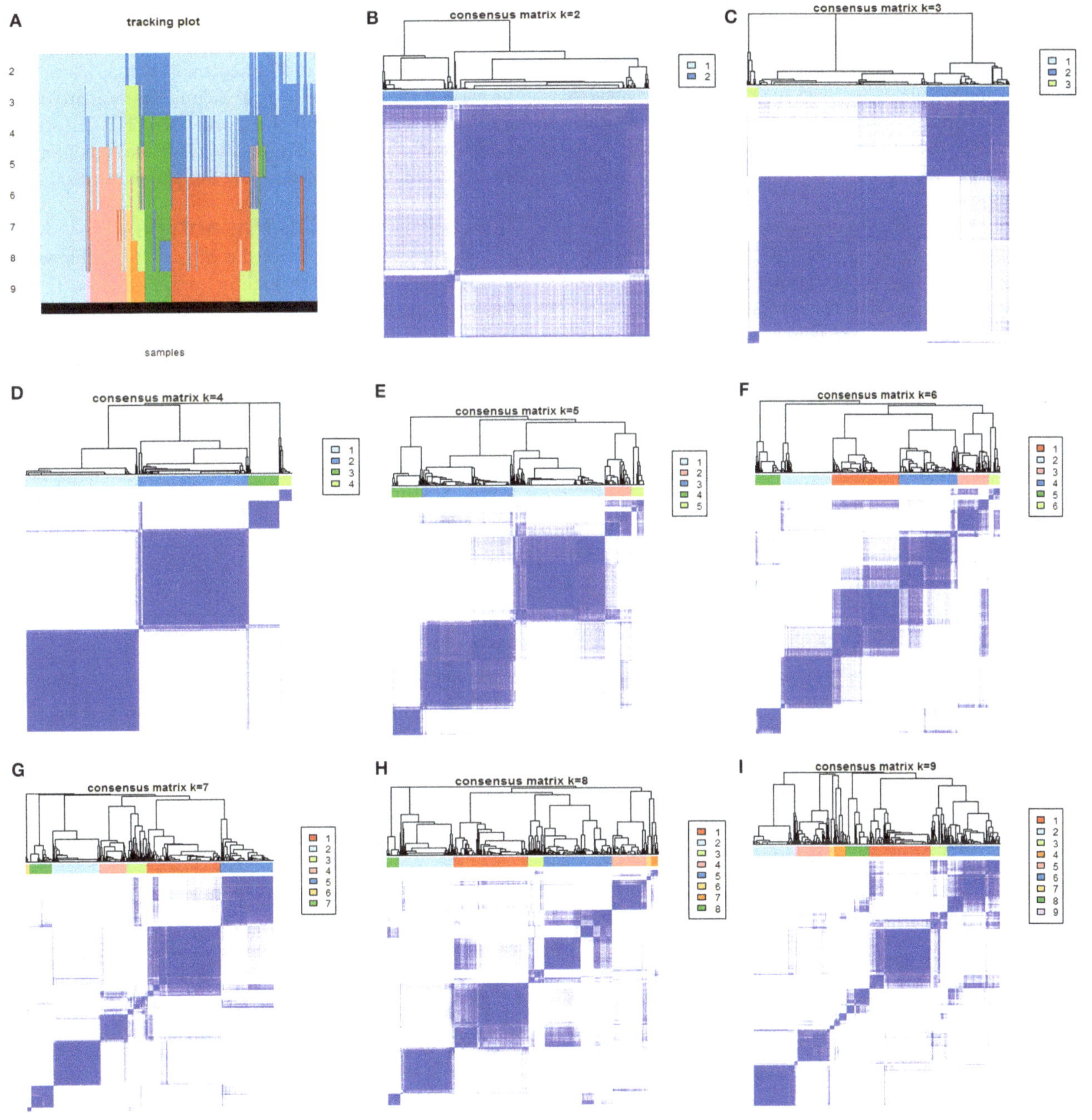


**FIGURE 1 |** The consensus matrix heatmaps of consensus k-means clustering. **(A)** Shows the sample distribution of 4 phenotypes after consensus k-means clustering. **(B–I)** Shows consensus matrix heatmaps of different subgroup numbers ($k$ = 2, 3, 4, 5, 6, 7, 8, and 9). When $k$ = 4, the model exhibited the clearest separation of the consensus matrix heatmap.

(16). Clustering was performed using 100 iterations, with each iteration containing 80% of the samples. The optimal clustering strategy was determined by cumulative distribution function curves of the consensus score, clear separation of the consensus matrix heatmaps, characteristics of the consensus cumulative distribution function plots, and adequate pairwise-consensus values between cluster members.

To evaluate the effect of rosuvastatin on the outcomes of ARDS in different subgroups, Kaplan–Meier statistics were used to estimate 90-day mortality. Organ failure–free days up to day 14 (day), days free of cardiovascular failure up to day 14 (day), days free of coagulation abnormality to up day 14 (day), days free of hepatic failure up to day 14 (day), days free of renal failure up to day 14 (day), intensive care unit–free days to up day 28 (day), and ventilator-free days to up day 28 were analyzed by means of analysis of variance. Twenty-eight-day mortality, 60-day mortality, and 90-day mortality were analyzed by the $\chi^2$ test. $P < 0.05$ was set as the threshold value to screen for significant results.

To observe the clinical feature variations among different phenotypes, the means of analysis of variance and $\chi^2$ tests were utilized to assess continuous variables and dichotomous variables, respectively, with a cutoff value of $P < 0.05$.

Brief flow plots of these analyses are shown in **Supplementary Figure 1**.

## Software and Versions

R × 64 3.6.1 was applied to process the data, analyze the data, and plot diagrams.

# RESULTS

## Patients

A total of 745 patients who met the ARDS criteria were enrolled in the final analysis, with 379 patients in the rosuvastatin group and 366 patients in the placebo group. The age of the investigated patients ranged from 18 to 89 (median, 54), and 51% were male. The mean $PaO_2$:$FIO_2$ level was 143.48 mmHg (standard deviation [SD], 63.57 mmHg), and the mean APACHE III score was 93.42 (SD, 20.15 mmHg). The detailed baseline demographic and clinical characteristics are shown in **Supplementary Tables 1, 2.**

## Derivation of ARDS Phenotypes

After a differential analysis of the clinically available variables, we finally found that the highest serum glucose, C-reactive protein, and platelet count were candidate variables for

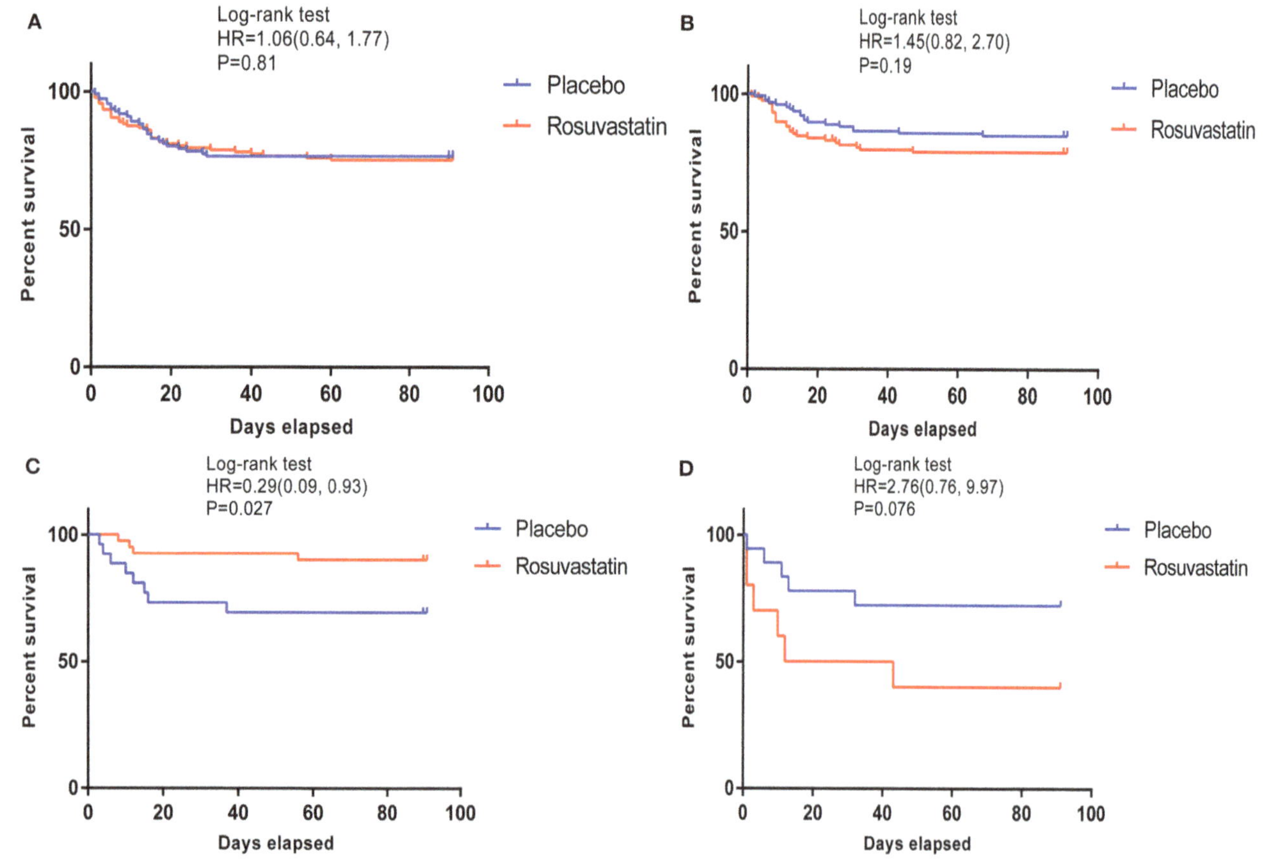


**FIGURE 2** | Kaplan–Meier survival curves of 90-day cumulative mortality for patients receiving rosuvastatin and patients receiving placebo among those with the 4 phenotypes. **(A–D)** shows survival curves of the patients with phenotypes 1–4. In the phenotype 3 cohort, rosuvastatin resulted in a significant reduction in 90-day cumulative mortality [hazard ratio [HR] 0.29 [95% CI 0.09, 0.93]; $P = 0.027$].

further unsupervised clustering analysis, as shown in **Supplementary Table 3**.

After excluding the 160 definitely immunosuppressed patients, 585 patients were enrolled in the derivation cohort. The consensus k-means clustering models suggested that a four-class model was the optimal fit for the four phenotypes, as the clearest separation of the consensus matrix heatmap could be found in the four-class model, as shown in **Figure 1**.

## Patients Classified as Platelet$^{high}$ & Creat$^{low}$ Phenotype Could Benefit From Rosuvastatin

According to Kaplan–Meier statistical analysis, the phenotype 3 cohort was identified as the "specific population who can benefit from rosuvastatin," as shown in **Figure 2**. In the phenotype 3 cohort, rosuvastatin resulted in a significant reduction in cumulative 90-day mortality from ARDS [hazard ratio (HR), 0.29; 95% confidence interval (CI), 0.09–0.93; $P = 0.027$]. Moreover, there were no significant differences in the baseline characteristics between those assigned to rosuvastatin and those assigned to placebo in the phenotype 3 cohort. The baseline characteristics of the patients with the four derived phenotypes are shown in **Supplementary Tables 4–7**.

In the phenotype 3 cohort, the days free of cardiovascular failure and coagulation abnormalities up to day 14 differed significantly between the patients who received rosuvastatin and those who received placebo. Additionally, rosuvastatin resulted in a slight increase in ventilator-free days up to day 28 for patients with ARDS. There were no significant between-group differences in any of the other outcomes. The above results are presented in **Table 1**.

For better insight into the patients who could benefit from rosuvastatin, we compared the clinical characteristics among different phenotypes. Phenotype 3 was summarized as Platelet$^{high}$ & Creat$^{low}$ phenotype because patients in this phenotype have a relatively higher platelet count ($390.05 \pm 79.43 \times 10^9$/L) and lower creatinine ($1.42 \pm 1.08$ mg/dL) than patients classified as other phenotypes. Additionally, the other distinct clinical characteristics of the patients with different phenotypes are described in **Table 2**. Indeed, phenotype 3 could be identified through our four-class model.

## Rosuvastatin Seems to Be Harmful for Patients Classified as APACHE$^{high}$ & Serum Glucose$^{high}$ Phenotype

The survival curves of phenotype 4 illuminated a trend that rosuvastatin resulted in a reduction in the 90-day survival rate of ARDS, despite the less rigorous confidence interval (HR, 2.76; 95% CI, 0.09–9.93; $P = 0.076$). Patients in phenotype 4 showed the early renal failure, with the highest APACHE III score ($110.18 \pm 24.35$), blood urea nitrogen ($38.04 \pm 28.59$ mmol/L), creatinine ($2.25 \pm 1.32$ mg/dL), serum glucose ($484.35 \pm 154.83$ mg/dL), and morbidity of shock at baseline (68%) and the lowest $PaO_2$:$FIO_2$ ($128.61 \pm 76.91$ mmHg) and Glasgow Coma Scale score ($6.46 \pm 3.33$). Therefore, phenotype 4 was summarized as APACHE$^{high}$ & Serum glucose$^{high}$ phenotype.

**TABLE 1** | Outcomes in different phenotypes.

| Outcomes | Placebo | Rosuvastatin | *P* |
|---|---|---|---|
| **28 day mortality (%)** | | | |
| Phenotype 1 | 23% | 21% | 0.70 |
| Phenotype 2 | 12% | 17% | 0.20 |
| Phenotype 3 | 27% | 14% | 0.07 |
| Phenotype 4 | 22% | 50% | 0.28 |
| **60 day mortality (%)** | | | |
| Phenotype 1 | 24% | 25% | 1 |
| Phenotype 2 | 14% | 21% | 0.21 |
| Phenotype 3 | 31% | 10% | 0.07 |
| Phenotype 4 | 28% | 32% | 0.20 |
| **90 day mortality (%)** | | | |
| Phenotype 1 | 24% | 25% | 1 |
| Phenotype 2 | 15% | 21% | 0.28 |
| Phenotype 3 | 31% | 10% | 0.07 |
| Phenotype 4 | 28% | 32% | 0.20 |
| **Organ failure free days to day 14(day)** | | | |
| Phenotype 1 | $6.16 \pm 5.14$ | $6.31 \pm 5.32$ | 0.83 |
| Phenotype 2 | $8.39 \pm 5.04$ | $8.21 \pm 5.16$ | 0.79 |
| Phenotype 3 | $7 \pm 5.23$ | $8.83 \pm 4.62$ | 0.14 |
| Phenotype 4 | $6.72 \pm 5.13$ | $3 \pm 4.62$ | 0.07 |
| **Free of cardiovascular failure to day14 (day)** | | | |
| Phenotype 1 | $10.37 \pm 4.80$ | $10.72 \pm 4.93$ | 0.57 |
| Phenotype 2 | $9.81 \pm 4.44$ | $9.19 \pm 4.67$ | 0.29 |
| Phenotype 3 | $7.31 \pm 4.94$ | $10.08 \pm 3.79$ | 0.01 |
| Phenotype 4 | $7.94 \pm 4.99$ | $6.20 \pm 5.51$ | 0.40 |
| **Free of coagulation abnormality to day14 (day)** | | | |
| Phenotype 1 | $10.83 \pm 5.12$ | $14.93 \pm 9.80$ | 0.38 |
| Phenotype 2 | $13.30 \pm 2.22$ | $12.90 \pm 2.81$ | 0.21 |
| Phenotype 3 | $12.15 \pm 3.77$ | $13.65 \pm 1.33$ | 0.02 |
| Phenotype 4 | $10.67 \pm 5.10$ | $8.10 \pm 6.10$ | 0.24 |
| **Free of hepatic failure to day 14 (day)** | | | |
| Phenotype 1 | $11.06 \pm 4.65$ | $9.89 \pm 5.36$ | 0.07 |
| Phenotype 2 | $13.29 \pm 2.46$ | $12.51 \pm 3.38$ | 0.04 |
| Phenotype 3 | $11.81 \pm 4.17$ | $12.83 \pm 3.01$ | 0.25 |
| Phenotype 4 | $11.50 \pm 4.85$ | $7.70 \pm 6.41$ | 0.09 |
| **Free of renal failure to day 14 (day)** | | | |
| Phenotype 1 | $10.50 \pm 4.88$ | $11.45 \pm 4.25$ | 0.41 |
| Phenotype 2 | $11.74 \pm 4.22$ | $11.44 \pm 4.64$ | 0.60 |
| Phenotype 3 | $10.50 \pm 4.88$ | $11.45 \pm 4.25$ | 0.41 |
| Phenotype 4 | $10.17 \pm 4.69$ | $4.70 \pm 4.99$ | 0.01 |
| **ICU free days to day 28 (day)** | | | |
| Phenotype 1 | $13.82 \pm 9.83$ | $14.93 \pm 9.80$ | 0.38 |
| Phenotype 2 | $17.05 \pm 9.07$ | $15.74 \pm 9.72$ | 0.27 |
| Phenotype 3 | $12.96 \pm 11.38$ | $17.35 \pm 8.59$ | 0.08 |
| Phenotype 4 | $13 \pm 10.45$ | $9 \pm 10.50$ | 0.34 |
| **Ventilator free days to day 28 (day)** | | | |
| Phenotype 1 | $14.17 \pm 10.90$ | $15.43 \pm 10.62$ | 0.36 |
| Phenotype 2 | $18.07 \pm 9.68$ | $17.02 \pm 10.12$ | 0.41 |
| Phenotype 3 | $13.27 \pm 11.90$ | $18.75 \pm 8.93$ | 0.04 |
| Phenotype 4 | $13.67 \pm 11.58$ | $10.1 \pm 11.47$ | 0.44 |

*Organ failure free days to day 14: No. of days without failure of circulatory, coagulation, hepatic, or renal organs from Day 1 to 14.*

**TABLE 2** | Clinical characteristics variations in different phenotypes.

| Characteristics | Phenotype 1 (*n* = 247) | Phenotype 2 (*n* = 244) | Phenotype 3 (*n* = 66) | Phenotype 4 (*n* = 66) | *P* |
|---|---|---|---|---|---|
| Age (year) | 54.07 ± 16.72 | 53.83 ± 16.96 | 54.52 ± 16.64 | 56.79 ± 13.94 | 0.84 |
| Male, No. % | 48% | 51% | 55% | 50% | 0.78 |
| Weight (kg) | 85.94 ± 28.25 | 92.23 ± 34.78 | 92.85 ± 30.63 | 87.36 ± 28.59 | 0.12 |
| Height (kg) | 168.83 ± 10.17 | 168.89 ± 11.41 | 169.46 ± 10.68 | 170.39 ± 13.26 | 0.88 |
| Predicted Body Weight (kg) | 62.74 ± 10.87 | 62.61 ± 11.97 | 63.03 ± 11.18 | 64.11 ± 13.81 | 0.93 |
| APACHE III | 95.47 ± 28.60 | 83.61 ± 24.97 | 87.69 ± 27.28 | 110.18 ± 24.35 | < 0.01 |
| Temperature (°C) | 37.31 ± 0.97 | 37.45 ± 0.98 | 37.52 ± 0.95 | 37.82 ± 0.86 | 0.04 |
| Shock, No. % | 63% | 47% | 55% | 68% | < 0.01 |
| Respiratory rate | 25.10 ± 7.20 | 25.52 ± 7.11 | 24.95 ± 6.03 | 24.64 ± 5.69 | 0.84 |
| $Pao_2$ (mmHg) | 91.21 ± 33.70 | 90.17 ± 31.78 | 95.06 ± 43.23 | 113.64 ± 46.30 | < 0.01 |
| $Paco_2$ (mmHg) | 38.24 ± 9.45 | 41.67 ± 9.99 | 41.29 ± 9.20 | 35.71 ± 9.03 | < 0.01 |
| $Pao_2$:$Fio_2$ (mmHg) | 139.78 ± 61.86 | 148.64 ± 62.31 | 139.27 ± 65.47 | 128.61 ± 76.91 | 0.24 |
| Heart rate (beats/min) | 96.25 ± 19.57 | 95.17 ± 19.05 | 94.97 ± 18.84 | 102 ± 21.06 | 0.34 |
| Systolic BP (mmHg) | 109.77 ± 18.98 | 114.72 ± 18.49 | 115.02 ± 19.37 | 108.11 ± 19.13 | 0.01 |
| Diastolic BP (mmHg) | 60.63 ± 11.76 | 61.37 ± 13.93 | 60.89 ± 14.22 | 55.35 ± 10.30 | 0.14 |
| Glasgow Coma Scale | 7.60 ± 3.24 | 8.24 ± 3.51 | 7.92 ± 3.56 | 6.46 ± 3.33 | 0.03 |
| Alanine aminotransferase (U/liter) | 49.32 ± 8.91 | 47.85 ± 8.83 | 49.03 ± 10.19 | 46.86 ± 10.59 | 0.23 |
| Aspartate aminotransferase (U/liter) | 41.72 ± 4.32 | 42.10 ± 5.20 | 41.29 ± 5.69 | 40.89 ± 5.95 | 0.45 |
| Urine output within 24 h of hospital presentation | 1,457 ± 1,211 | 1,740 ± 1,253 | 1,830 ± 1,380 | 1,456 ± 1,106 | 0.03 |
| Blood urea nitrogen (mmol/L) | 27.40 ± 19.63 | 24.63 ± 17.68 | 24.29 ± 18.11 | 38.04 ± 28.59 | < 0.01 |
| Creatine kinase (U/liter) | 244.63 ± 51.68 | 241.45 ± 53.39 | 233.29 ± 55.59 | 226.5 ± 56.79 | 0.20 |
| Creat (mg/dl) | 1.65 ± 1.28 | 1.47 ± 1.10 | 1.42 ± 1.08 | 2.25 ± 1.32 | < 0.01 |
| Serum Glucose Highest (mg/dL) | 148.36 ± 50.32 | 152.57 ± 49.78 | 157.21 ± 47.07 | 484.35 ± 154.83 | < 0.01 |
| Serum Glucose Lowest (mg/dL) | 114.44 ± 39.74 | 125.02 ± 40.96 | 125.56 ± 39.65 | 186.11 ± 116.62 | < 0.01 |
| Serum Albumin Highest (g/dL) | 2.24 ± 0.74 | 2.43 ± 0.63 | 2.20 ± 0.73 | 2.46 ± 0.88 | < 0.01 |
| Serum Albumin Lowest (g/dL) | 2.18 ± 0.69 | 2.36 ± 0.61 | 2.11 ± 0.70 | 2.36 ± 0.78 | < 0.01 |
| Platelet count ($10^9$/L) | 103.79 ± 39.97 | 222.22 ± 41.66 | 390.05 ± 79.43 | 176.68 ± 94.30 | < 0.01 |
| CRP (µg/L) | 26.04 ± 34.69 | 28.69 ± 27.96 | 20.23 ± 11.99 | 26.25 ± 13.92 | 0.22 |

## Characteristics and Outcomes of Patients With Other Phenotypes

Kaplan–Meier survival analysis indicated that rosuvastatin had no effect on ARDS in the cohorts with the other phenotypes. In the phenotype 2 cohort, rosuvastatin appeared to slightly reduce the days free of hepatic failure up to day 14. In addition, rosuvastatin led to a moderate reduction in the days free of renal failure up to day 14 in the phenotype 4 cohort. More details of the characteristics and outcomes of the patients with other phenotypes are described in **Tables 1, 2.**

The survival curves of the patients with the four phenotypes are shown in **Supplementary Figure 2**, and the survival curves of definitely immunosuppressed patients are shown in **Supplementary Figure 3.**

# DISCUSSION

In this secondary analysis of the SAILS trial, four phenotypes of ARDS were derived through routinely available clinical variables at the time of hospital presentation. These phenotypes were multidimensional, and the patients were heterogeneous in their demographics, clinical characteristics, several laboratory abnormalities, and effects of rosuvastatin therapy; these phenotypes differed from traditional patient classifications such as those based on direct or indirect lung injury, patterns of organ dysfunction, or severity of ARDS. In the phenotype 3 cohort, rosuvastatin exhibited benefits for patients with ARDS compared with placebo. This conclusion highlights the importance of characterizing the heterogeneity of ARDS and early goal-directed therapy.

To the best of our knowledge, the current study is the first to identify a specific population that can benefit from rosuvastatin, which could improve the therapeutic strategies for ARDS and reduce mortality. Furthermore, validation clinical trials are warranted to further assess these factors. These patients exhibited relatively higher platelet counts (390.05 ± 79.43 × $10^9$/L) and lower creatinine (1.42 ± 1.08 mg/dL) levels than other patients with ARDS, thus summarized as Platelet$^{high}$ & Creat$^{low}$ phenotype. These patients probably suffered from a relatively slight infection and might benefit from rosuvastatin because its anti-inflammatory effect could rapidly restore cardiovascular function. Indeed, the current study indicated that rosuvastatin resulted in an obvious improvement in days free of cardiovascular failure up to day 14 (7.31 ± 4.94 in placebo vs. 10.08 ± 3.79 in rosuvastatin, $P = 0.01$). Phenotype 3 could be rapidly identified through our machine learning–constructed four-class model. This model could be utilized to identify specific populations who can benefit from rosuvastatin at the time of patient presentation to the emergency department and thus could be useful with regard to early treatment and enrollment in clinical trials. Only routinely available data were used in the clustering models, and the phenotypes were derived from a large observational cohort to ensure generalizability.

Rosuvastatin may improve inflammatory responses, possibly via modulation of a platelet-dependent mechanism, which might be a potential treatment pathogenesis of rosuvastatin for this novel phenotype for ARDS. It is well-known that platelets play an important role in neutrophil-mediated lung injury (17, 18). The present study indicated that patients classified as phenotype 3 exhibited relatively high platelet counts. Additionally, in these patients, rosuvastatin significantly improved the coagulation abnormalities of ARDS compared with placebo. Therefore, we hypothesized that platelets might be involved in the pharmacological mechanism of rosuvastatin in specific patients with ARDS, and validation experiments are warranted to assess these related mechanisms.

Rosuvastatin might be harmful for patients with definite immunosuppression. Rosuvastatin was previously utilized in patients with ARDS mainly because of rosuvastatin's anti-inflammatory effects. However, infection is the main risk factor for ARDS, and it has been verified that patients with immunosuppression had worse outcomes as their weak immune systems could barely eliminate the pathogens (19, 20). Therefore, the immunosuppressive effect of rosuvastatin could not benefit such patients. This study similarly exhibited a trend that patients with definite immunosuppression probably had a worse outcome when receiving rosuvastatin, as shown in **Figure 1A**.

Rosuvastatin seems to be harmful for patients classified as phenotype 4. The survival curves of phenotype 4 illuminated a trend that rosuvastatin resulted in a reduction in the 90-day survival rate of ARDS, despite the less rigorous confidence interval (HR, 2.76; 95% CI, 0.09–9.93; $P = 0.076$). Furthermore, the current analysis on days free of renal failure up to day 14 suggested that rosuvastatin might aggravate renal damage (10.17 ± 4.69 in the placebo group vs. 4.70 ± 4.99 in the rosuvastatin group, $P = 0.01$). Patients with phenotype 4 showed the highest APACHE III score (110.18 ± 24.35), blood urea nitrogen (38.04 ± 28.59 mmol/L), creatinine (2.25 ± 1.32 mg/dL), serum glucose (484.35 ± 154.83 mg/dL), and morbidity of shock at baseline (68%) and the lowest $PaO_2$:$FIO_2$ (128.61 ± 76.91 mmHg) and Glasgow Coma Scale score (6.46 ± 3.33), as well as other clinical variables. In brief, patients with phenotype 4 showed relatively severe illness according to their baseline features, particularly renal failure, with high serum glucose. Therefore, phenotype 4 was defined as APACHE$^{high}$ & Serum glucose$^{high}$ phenotype.

There are several limitations to the present study. Indeed, the current analysis on treatment × phenotype interactions is largely limited by sample size. Therefore, these novel proof-of-concept ARDS phenotypes should be incorporated prospectively in future study designs that subsequently validate the effect of rosuvastatin on ARDS (21). In addition, for the limitation of clinical correlation analysis, further basic experiments should be conducted to sequentially research the elaborate mechanisms of rosuvastatin for ARDS indicated by our analyses.

## CONCLUSION

This secondary analysis of the SAILS trial identified rosuvastatin seems to be harmful for patients classified as APACHE$^{high}$ & Serum glucose$^{high}$ phenotype, but benefit patients with Platelet$^{high}$ & Creat$^{low}$ phenotype, thus uncovering the novel value of rosuvastatin for the precise treatment of ARDS.

## ETHICS STATEMENT

This study was reviewed and approved by Institutional Ethics Committee of Zhongda Hospital. Institutional Ethics Committee of Zhongda Hospital and conducted under several data use agreements.

## AUTHOR CONTRIBUTIONS

SZ and HQ had full access to all of the data in the study and take responsibility for their integrity and the accuracy of the data analysis. SZ and ZL performed the data process, statistical analysis, and preparation of the article for publication. All authors participated in writing the article and preparing the figures.

## ACKNOWLEDGMENTS

Thanks for Truwit et al. (11) who uploaded the original data. This manuscript has been released as a pre-print at [ResearchSquare] (22).

## REFERENCES

1. Thompson BT, Chambers RC, Liu KD. Acute respiratory distress syndrome. *N Engl J Med.* (2017) 377:1904–5. doi: 10.1056/NEJMra1608077
2. Bellani G, Laffey JG, Pham T, Fan E, Brochard L, Esteban A, et al. Epidemiology, patterns of care, and mortality for patients with acute respiratory distress syndrome in intensive care units in 50 countries. *JAMA.* (2016) 315:788–800. doi: 10.1001/jama.2016.0291
3. Matthay M, Zemans R. The acute respiratory distress syndrome: pathogenesis and treatment. *Annu Rev Pathol.* (2011) 6:147–63. doi: 10.1146/annurev-pathol-011110-130158
4. Caffrey AR, Timbrook TT, Noh E, Sakoulas G, Opal SM, Nizet V, et al. Evidence to support continuation of statin therapy in patients with *Staphylococcus aureus* bacteremia. *Antimicrob Agents Chemother.* (2017) 61:e02228-16. doi: 10.1128/AAC.02228-16
5. Almog Y, Shefer A, Novack V, Maimon N, Barski L, Eizinger M, et al. Prior statin therapy is associated with a decreased rate of severe sepsis. *Circulation.* (2004) 110:880–5. doi: 10.1161/01.CIR.0000138932.17956.F1
6. Fernandez R, De Pedro VJ, Artigas A. Statin therapy prior to ICU admission: protection against infection or a severity marker? *Intensive Care Med.* (2006) 32:160–4. doi: 10.1007/s00134-005-2743-9

7. Kruger P, Fitzsimmons K, Cook D, Jones M, Nimmo G. Statin therapy is associated with fewer deaths in patients with bacteraemia. *Intensive Care Med.* (2006) 32:75–9. doi: 10.1007/s00134-005-2859-y
8. Arnaud C, Braunersreuther V, Mach F. Toward immunomodulatory and anti-inflammatory properties of statins. *Trends Cardiovasc Med.* (2005) 15:202–6. doi: 10.1016/j.tcm.2005.07.002
9. Greenwood J, Mason JC. Statins and the vascular endothelial inflammatory response. *Trends Immunol.* (2007) 28:88–98. doi: 10.1016/j.it.2006.12.003
10. Jacobson JR, Barnard JW, Grigoryev DN, Ma SF, Tuder RM, Garcia JGN. Simvastatin attenuates vascular leak and inflammation in murine inflammatory lung injury. *Am J Physiol Lung Cell Mol Physiol.* (2005) 288:L1026–32. doi: 10.1152/ajplung.00354.2004
11. Truwit D, Bernard R, Steingrub J, Matthay MA, Liu KD, Albertson TE, et al. Rosuvastatin for sepsis-associated acute respiratory distress syndrome. *N Engl J Med.* (2014) 370:2191–200. doi: 10.1056/NEJMoa1401520
12. Bos LD, Scicluna BP, Ong, DY, Cremer O, Poll T, Schultz MJ, et al. Understanding heterogeneity in biological phenotypes of ARDS by leukocyte expression profiles. *Am J Respir Crit Care Med.* (2019) 200:42–50. doi: 10.1164/rccm.201809-1808OC
13. Sinha P, Delucchi KL, McAuley DF, O'Kane CM, Matthay MA, Calfee CS, et al. Development and validation of parsimonious algorithms to classify acute respiratory distress syndrome phenotypes: a secondary analysis of randomised controlled trials. *Lancet Respir Med.* (2020) 8:247–57. doi: 10.1016/S2213-2600(19)30369-8
14. Sinha P, Delucchi KL, Thompson BT. Latent class analysis of ARDS subphenotypes: a secondary analysis of the statins for acutely injured lungs from sepsis (SAILS) study. *Intensive Care Med.* (2018) 44:1859–69. doi: 10.1007/s00134-018-5378-3
15. Newgard CD, Haukoos JS. Advanced statistics: missing data in clinical research—part 2: multiple imputation. *Acad Emerg Med.* (2007) 14:669–78. doi: 10.1111/j.1553-2712.2007.tb01856.x
16. Wilkerson MD, Hayes DN. Consensus cluster plus: a class discovery tool with confidence assessments and item tracking. *Bioinformatics.* (2010) 26:1572–3. doi: 10.1093/bioinformatics/btq170
17. Bozza FA, Shah AM, Weyrich AS, Zimmerman GA. Amicus or adversary: platelets in lung biology, acute injury, and inflammation. *Am J Respir Cell Mol Biol.* (2009) 40:123–34. doi: 10.1165/rcmb.2008-0241TR
18. Looney MR, Nguyen JX, Hu Y, Van Ziffle JA, Lowell CA, Matthay MA. Platelet depletion and aspirin treatment protect mice in a two-event model of transfusion-related acute lung injury. J *Clin Investig.* (2009) 119: 3450–61. doi: 10.1172/JCI38432
19. Fan E, Brodie D, Slutsky AS. Acute respiratory distress syndrome: advances in diagnosis and treatment. *JAMA.* (2018) 319:698–710. doi: 10.1001/jama.2017.21907
20. Zhang S, Wu Z, Xie J, Yi Y, Lei W, Haibo Q. DNA methylation exploration for ARDS: a multi-omics and multi-microarray interrelated analysis. *J Transl Med.* (2019) 17:345. doi: 10.1186/s12967-019-2090-1
21. Seymour CW, Kennedy JN, Wang S, Chang CCH, Elliott CF, Xu Z, et al. Derivation, validation, and potential treatment implications of novel clinical phenotypes for sepsis. *JAMA.* (2019) 321:2003–17. doi: 10.1001/jama.2019.5791
22. Zhang S, Lu Z, Wu Z, Xie J, Yang Y, Qiu H. Derivation of "specific population who could benefit from Rosuvastatin": a secondary analysis on randomised controlled trial to uncover novel value of Rosuvastatin for precise treatment of ARDS. (2020) *[Preprint].* doi: 10.21203/rs.3.rs-35420/v1

# 14

# Explainable Machine Learning to Predict Successful Weaning Among Patients Requiring Prolonged Mechanical Ventilation: A Retrospective Cohort Study in Central Taiwan

*Ming-Yen Lin [1], Chi-Chun Li [1], Pin-Hsiu Lin [1], Jiun-Long Wang [2,3], Ming-Cheng Chan [4,5,6], Chieh-Liang Wu [7,8] and Wen-Cheng Chao [7,8,9]**

*[1] Department of Information Engineering and Computer Science, Feng Chia University, Taichung, Taiwan, [2] Division of Chest Medicine, Department of Internal Medicine, Taichung Veterans General Hospital, Taichung, Taiwan, [3] Department of Life Sciences, National Chung-Hsing University, Taichung, Taiwan, [4] Division of Critical Care and Respiratory Therapy, Department of Internal Medicine, Taichung Veterans General Hospital, Taichung, Taiwan, [5] Central Taiwan University of Science and Technology, Taichung, Taiwan, [6] The College of Science, Tunghai University, Taichung, Taiwan, [7] Department of Critical Care Medicine, Taichung Veterans General Hospital, Taichung, Taiwan, [8] Department of Computer Science, Tunghai University, Taichung, Taiwan, [9] Department of Automatic Control Engineering, Feng Chia University, Taichung, Taiwan*

***Correspondence:**
*Wen-Cheng Chao*
*cwc081@hotmail.com*

**Objective:** The number of patients requiring prolonged mechanical ventilation (PMV) is increasing worldwide, but the weaning outcome prediction model in these patients is still lacking. We hence aimed to develop an explainable machine learning (ML) model to predict successful weaning in patients requiring PMV using a real-world dataset.

**Methods:** This retrospective study used the electronic medical records of patients admitted to a 12-bed respiratory care center in central Taiwan between 2013 and 2018. We used three ML models, namely, extreme gradient boosting (XGBoost), random forest (RF), and logistic regression (LR), to establish the prediction model. We further illustrated the feature importance categorized by clinical domains and provided visualized interpretation by using SHapley Additive exPlanations (SHAP) as well as local interpretable model-agnostic explanations (LIME).

**Results:** The dataset contained data of 963 patients requiring PMV, and 56.0% (539/963) of them were successfully weaned from mechanical ventilation. The XGBoost model (area under the curve [AUC]: 0.908; 95% confidence interval [CI] 0.864–0.943) and RF model (AUC: 0.888; 95% CI 0.844–0.934) outperformed the LR model (AUC: 0.762; 95% CI 0.687–0.830) in predicting successful weaning in patients requiring PMV. To give the physician an intuitive understanding of the model, we stratified the feature importance by clinical domains. The cumulative feature importance in the ventilation domain, fluid domain, physiology domain, and laboratory data domain was 0.310, 0.201, 0.265, and 0.182, respectively. We further used the SHAP plot and partial dependence plot to illustrate associations between features and the weaning outcome at the feature level. Moreover, we used LIME plots to illustrate the prediction model at the individual level. Additionally, we addressed the weekly performance of the three ML models and found that the accuracy of XGBoost/RF was ~0.7 between weeks 4 and week 7 and slightly declined to 0.6 on weeks 8 and 9.

**Conclusion:** We used an ML approach, mainly XGBoost, SHAP plot, and LIME plot to establish an explainable weaning prediction ML model in patients requiring PMV. We believe these approaches should largely mitigate the concern of the black-box issue of artificial intelligence, and future studies are warranted for the landing of the proposed model.

**Keywords: explainable AI, weaning, prediction mode, prolonged mechanical ventilation, machine learning**

## BACKGROUND

Mechanical ventilation (MV) is one of the essential organ support management approaches in critically ill patients, and ~5–10% of patients receiving MV require prolonged MV (PMV), defined as using MV for more than 21 days (1, 2). There is an increasing health burden of PMV globally, and the estimated economic burden in the United States was nearly 25 billion per year (3–5). It has been estimated that merely 50% (95% confidence interval [CI] 47–53%) of patients with PMV can be liberated from MV (6); however, the study to predict weaning outcome in patients under PMV remains scarce despite of an increasing health impact of PMV.

Artificial intelligence (AI) is widely applied in various fields, but the black-box issue remains the main concern for the application of AI in the medical field (7, 8). Recently, explainable AI algorithms, including our recently published research in critically ill influenza patients, have been increasingly applied to interpret the AI model based on *post-hoc* analyses and domain knowledge, and the black-box issue can largely be mitigated (9, 10). Due to the steadily increasing number of patients requiring PMV in Taiwan during the last two decades, a specialized unit, respiratory care center (RCC), has been established to facilitate weaning in patients with PMV (4, 11). In the present study, we aimed to use electronic medical records of an RCC in central Taiwan collected between 2013 and 2018 and an explainable machine learning (ML) approach to establish a weaning prediction model in patients requiring PMV.

## METHODS

### Ethical Approval

This study was approved by the Institutional Review Board of the Taichung Veterans General Hospital (TCVGH: CE19072A). All data were obtained from electronic medical records and anonymized before analyses, and informed consent was hence waived.

### Study Population

This retrospective study was conducted at TCVGH, a tertiary-care referral hospital with ~1,500 beds, six intensive care units (ICUs), and one 12-bed RCC in central Taiwan. All patients who had been admitted to the study RCC for a first attempt at weaning between 2013 and 2018 were enrolled in the study. Liberation from MV for five consecutive days was defined as successful weaning given that one Taiwanese population-based study has shown high durability of weaning success after liberation from the ventilator for 5 days in patients with PMV (12).

### Variables Categorized by Main Clinical Domains

The dataset was established through collecting electronic medical records during the first index admission to RCC, and the first day with MV was defined as day 1 of the index admission. Data were censored after the patient was discharged from RCC, including successful weaning, mortality, or being transferred back to the ICU/ward in ventilator-dependent status. The dataset mainly consisted of five clinical domains: (1) ventilation domain (weekly average fraction of inspired oxygen [$FiO_2$, %], positive end-expiratory pressure [PEEP, $cmH_2O$], peak inspiratory pressure [Ppeak, $cmH_2O$], mean airway pressure [Pmean], tidal volume per predicted body weight [VT/PBW, ml/kg], respiratory rate, and minute ventilation); (2) fluid domain (weekly fluid balance data, including input, feeding amount, urine output, hemodialysis output, and overall fluid balance); (3) physiology domain (weekly average blood pressure, heart rate, body temperature, oxygen saturation [$SaO_2$], and glucose levels); (4) lab domain (main laboratory data, including albumin, white blood cell counts, hemoglobin concentration, platelet counts, liver function tests, and renal function tests); and (5) others, including Acute Physiology and Chronic Health Evaluation (APACHE) II score, comorbidities, and medications.

### Extreme Gradient Boosting (XGBoost)

We used XGBoost to construct a weaning outcome prediction model. Gradient boosting methods including XGBoost employed iterative combinations of ensembles of weak prediction models into one strong learner (13). XGBoost

**Abbreviations:** AI, artificial intelligence; APACHE, Acute Physiology and Chronic Health Evaluation; AUC, area under the curve; CI, confidence interval; DNR, do not resuscitate; $FiO_2$, inspired oxygen; LIME, local interpretable model-agnostic explanations; LR, logistic regression; ML, machine learning; MV, mechanical ventilation; PDP, partial dependence plot; PEEP, positive end-expiratory pressure; Pmean, mean airway pressure; Ppeak, peak inspiratory pressure; PMV, prolonged mechanical ventilation; RCC, respiratory care center; RF, random forest; RIICU, respiratory intermediate intensive care unit; RR, respiratory rate; ROC, receiver operating characteristic; $SaO_2$, oxygen saturation; SHAP, SHapley Additive exPlanations; TCVGH, Taichung Veterans General Hospital; TRL, technology readiness level; VT/PBW, tidal volume per predicted body weight; XGBoost, extreme gradient boosting.

**TABLE 1** | Characteristics of the 963 patients categorized by weaning outcome.

| | All N = 963 | Successful weaning (−) N = 424 | Successful weaning (+) N = 539 | p-value |
|---|---|---|---|---|
| **Demographic data** | | | | |
| Age (years) | 69.3 ± 16.0 | 72.1 ± 14.3 | 67.1 ± 16.8 | <0.01 |
| Sex (female) | 618 (64.2%) | 291 (68.6%) | 327 (60.7%) | 0.01 |
| Body mass index | 22.5 ± 4.5 | 22.6 ± 4.6 | 22.4 ± 4.5 | 0.52 |
| **Comorbidities** | | | | |
| Hypertension | 538 (55.9%) | 236 (55.7%) | 302 (56.0%) | 0.91 |
| Diabetes mellitus | 329 (34.2%) | 152 (35.8%) | 177 (32.8%) | 0.33 |
| Congestive heart failure | 134 (13.9%) | 74 (17.5%) | 60 (11.1%) | <0.01 |
| Atrial fibrillation | 173 (18.0%) | 95 (22.4%) | 78 (14.5%) | <0.01 |
| COPD | 141 (14.6%) | 81 (19.1%) | 60 (11.1%) | <0.01 |
| Asthma | 38 (3.9%) | 17 (4.0%) | 21 (3.9%) | 0.93 |
| End-stage renal disease | 102 (10.6%) | 58 (13.7%) | 44 (8.2%) | <0.01 |
| Liver cirrhosis | 29 (3.0%) | 12 (2.8%) | 17 (3.2%) | 0.77 |
| Cerebral vascular disease | 254 (26.4%) | 122 (28.8%) | 132 (24.5%) | 0.13 |
| Malignancy (inactive) | 77 (8.0%) | 31 (7.3%) | 46 (8.5%) | 0.49 |
| Malignancy (active) | 179 (18.6%) | 100 (23.6%) | 79 (14.7%) | <0.01 |
| **Etiology for mechanical ventilation** | | | | |
| Neurological surgery | 369 (38.4%) | 157 (37.1%) | 55 (10.2%) | <0.01 |
| Medical condition | 594 (61.7%) | 267 (63.0%) | 484 (89.8%) | |
| **Severity scores** | | | | |
| ICU APACHE II | 25.0 ± 6.0 | 25.7 ± 6.1 | 24.5 ± 5.8 | <0.01 |
| RCC APACHE II | 17.8 ± 5.5 | 19.4 ± 5.7 | 16.5 ± 5.1 | <0.01 |
| **Do-not-resuscitate status** | 430 (44.7%) | 250 (59.0%) | 180 (33.4%) | <0.01 |
| **RCC data (day 1)** | | | | |
| White blood cell counts (/ml) | 1,0881.0 ± 5,001.3 | 11,279.6 ± 5,307.1 | 10,567.5 ± 4,728.3 | 0.03 |
| Hematocrit (%) | 29.6 ± 5.2 | 29.0 ± 5.1 | 30.1 ± 5.2 | <0.01 |
| Creatinine (mg/dl) | 1.6 ± 1.8 | 1.7 ± 1.9 | 1.4 ± 1.7 | <0.01 |
| Sodium (mg/dl) | 138.7 ± 6.3 | 139.1 ± 6.9 | 138.3 ± 5.8 | 0.06 |
| Potassium (mg/dl) | 4.3 ± 0.7 | 4.3 ± 0.7 | 4.3 ± 0.6 | 0.25 |
| GCS (eye opening) | 3.0 ± 1.1 | 3.0 ± 1.1 | 3.1 ± 1.0 | 0.37 |
| GCS (motor response) | 4.4 ± 1.7 | 4.2 ± 1.7 | 4.6 ± 1.6 | <0.01 |
| $FiO_2$ (%) | 37 ± 5 | 38 ± 6 | 36 ± 5 | <0.01 |
| Hear rate | 87.8 ± 20.5 | 90.1 ± 20.7 | 85.9 ± 20.2 | <0.01 |
| Respiratory rate | 19.1 ± 5.9 | 19.6 ± 6.1 | 18.7 ± 5.8 | 0.01 |
| Blood pressure (systolic) | 123.3 ± 23.3 | 122.4 ± 24.0 | 124.1 ± 22.7 | 0.24 |
| Blood pressure (diastolic) | 69.0 ± 18.8 | 67.9 ± 19.1 | 69.8 ± 18.5 | 0.12 |
| **Outcome** | | | | |
| ICU day | 23.7 ± 13.1 | 24.4 ± 15.4 | 23.1 ± 10.9 | 0.11 |
| RCC stay | 16.7 ± 9.5 | 19.7 ± 10.7 | 14.3 ± 7.6 | <0.01 |
| Ventilator day | 41.7 ± 17.7 | 50.7 ± 17.9 | 34.6 ± 14.0 | <0.01 |
| Hospital day | 52.6 ± 18.0 | 53.9 ± 18.5 | 51.6 ± 17.6 | 0.05 |
| Mortality | 180 (18.7%) | 164 (38.7%) | 16 (3.0%) | <0.01 |

*Data were presented as mean ± standard deviation and number (percentage).*
*COPD, chronic obstructive pulmonary disease; ICU, intensive care unit; APACHE II, Acute Physiology and Chronic Health Evaluation II; RCC, respiratory care center; GCS, Glasgow Coma Score; $FiO_2$, fraction of inspired oxygen.*

further applies a second-order Taylor series to approximate the value of the loss function and reduces the potential overfitting by application of regularization (14). In the setting of the hyperparameters, the optimal values were identified by a grid search on potential value combinations of the parameters. The key fine-tuned parameters in the present study included the number of trees (n_estimator = 770), learning rate (eta = 0.01), and maximum tree depth (max_depth = 3) (see **Supplementary Table 1** for detailed parameters) (14).

**TABLE 2 |** Weekly ventilatory parameters of the 963 patients categorized by weaning outcome.

| | All<br>$N = 963$ | Successful weaning (–)<br>$N = 424$ | Successful weaning (+)<br>$N = 539$ | $p$-value |
|---|---|---|---|---|
| **$FiO_2$ (%)** | | | | |
| Week 4 | 35.1 ± 5.6 | 36.4 ± 6.1 | 34.1 ± 5.0 | <0.01 |
| Week 5 | 34.9 ± 7.0 | 36.9 ± 8.8 | 33.4 ± 4.7 | <0.01 |
| Week 6 | 35.1 ± 8.6 | 37.6 ± 11.4 | 33.1 ± 4.8 | <0.01 |
| Week 7 | 35.6 ± 10.3 | 38.6 ± 13.4 | 33.2 ± 6.2 | <0.01 |
| Week 8 | 35.8 ± 11.1 | 39.2 ± 14.5 | 33.2 ± 6.3 | <0.01 |
| Week 9 | 36.0 ± 12.0 | 39.7 ± 15.7 | 33.2 ± 6.8 | <0.01 |
| **PEEP ($cmH_2O$)** | | | | |
| Week 4 | 5.8 ± 1.6 | 6.0 ± 1.7 | 5.6 ± 1.5 | <0.01 |
| Week 5 | 5.6 ± 1.4 | 5.9 ± 1.6 | 5.4 ± 1.1 | <0.01 |
| Week 6 | 5.6 ± 1.3 | 5.9 ± 1.5 | 5.3 ± 1.0 | <0.01 |
| Week 7 | 5.5 ± 1.3 | 5.8 ± 1.6 | 5.2 ± 0.9 | <0.01 |
| Week 8 | 5.5 ± 1.3 | 5.8 ± 1.6 | 5.2 ± 0.9 | <0.01 |
| Week 9 | 5.5 ± 1.3 | 5.9 ± 1.6 | 5.2 ± 0.9 | <0.01 |
| **Ppeak ($cmH_2O$)** | | | | |
| Week 4 | 21.7 ± 4.9 | 23.2 ± 4.9 | 20.5 ± 4.5 | <0.01 |
| Week 5 | 20.9 ± 5.6 | 23.2 ± 6.3 | 19.1 ± 4.1 | <0.01 |
| Week 6 | 20.6 ± 5.4 | 23.0 ± 5.8 | 18.6 ± 4.1 | <0.01 |
| Week 7 | 20.6 ± 5.7 | 23.4 ± 6.3 | 18.4 ± 4.1 | <0.01 |
| Week 8 | 20.7 ± 5.79 | 23.7 ± 6.5 | 18.3 ± 4.0 | <0.01 |
| Week 9 | 20.8 ± 6.0 | 24.0 ± 6.6 | 18.3 ± 3.9 | <0.01 |
| **Pmean ($cmH_2O$)** | | | | |
| Week 4 | 10.6 ± 2.4 | 11.3 ± 2.5 | 10.2 ± 2.3 | <0.01 |
| Week 5 | 10.4 ± 2.5 | 11.3 ± 2.9 | 9.6 ± 1.9 | <0.01 |
| Week 6 | 10.3 ± 2.6 | 11.4 ± 3.0 | 9.4 ± 1.9 | <0.01 |
| Week 7 | 10.3 ± 2.7 | 11.5 ± 3.2 | 9.3 ± 1.8 | <0.01 |
| Week 8 | 10.3 ± 2.9 | 11.6 ± 3.4 | 9.2 ± 1.8 | <0.01 |
| Week 9 | 10.3 ± 2.9 | 11.7 ± 3.5 | 9.2 ± 1.7 | <0.01 |
| **VT/PBW (ml/kg)** | | | | |
| Week 4 | 9.0 ± 1.9 | 9.1 ± 1.9 | 8.9 ± 2.0 | 0.12 |
| Week 5 | 8.7 ± 2.0 | 8.9 ± 2.0 | 8.5 ± 2.0 | <0.01 |
| Week 6 | 8.6 ± 2.1 | 8.9 ± 2.0 | 8.3 ± 2.1 | <0.01 |
| Week 7 | 8.6 ± 2.2 | 9.0 ± 2.2 | 8.3 ± 2.1 | <0.01 |
| Week 8 | 8.6 ± 2.2 | 9.0 ± 2.3 | 8.3 ± 2.1 | <0.01 |
| Week 9 | 8.6 ± 2.3 | 9.1 ± 2.4 | 8.3 ± 2.1 | <0.01 |
| **Respiratory rate (/min)** | | | | |
| Week 4 | 18.9 ± 3.2 | 19.0 ± 3.3 | 18.9 ± 3.2 | 0.44 |
| Week 5 | 19.4 ± 3.2 | 19.3 ± 3.4 | 19.4 ± 3.1 | 0.66 |
| Week 6 | 19.6 ± 3.2 | 19.4 ± 3.5 | 19.7 ± 3.0 | 0.26 |
| Week 7 | 19.6 ± 3.3 | 19.5 ± 3.6 | 19.7 ± 3.1 | 0.38 |
| Week 8 | 19.6 ± 3.4 | 19.4 ± 3.7 | 19.7 ± 3.1 | 0.22 |
| Week 9 | 19.5 ± 3.3 | 19.2 ± 3.6 | 19.6 ± 3.0 | 0.07 |
| **Minute ventilation (L/min)** | | | | |
| Week 4 | 9.3 ± 2.5 | 9.6 ± 2.1 | 9.1 ± 2.8 | <0.01 |
| Week 5 | 9.2 ± 2.5 | 9.6 ± 2.4 | 8.8 ± 2.6 | <0.01 |
| Week 6 | 9.1 ± 2.7 | 9.6 ± 2.6 | 8.7 ± 2.7 | <0.01 |
| Week 7 | 9.1 ± 2.9 | 9.6 ± 2.7 | 8.6 ± 2.9 | <0.01 |
| Week 8 | 9.0 ± 2.9 | 9.5 ± 2.9 | 8.6 ± 2.9 | <0.01 |
| Week 9 | 9.0 ± 3.0 | 9.6 ± 3.0 | 8.6 ± 2.9 | <0.01 |

*Data were presented as mean ± standard deviation.*

*$FiO_2$, fraction of inspired oxygen; PEEP, positive end-expiratory pressure; Ppeak, peak inspiratory pressure; Pmean, mean airway pressure; VT/PBW, tidal volume per predicted body weight.*

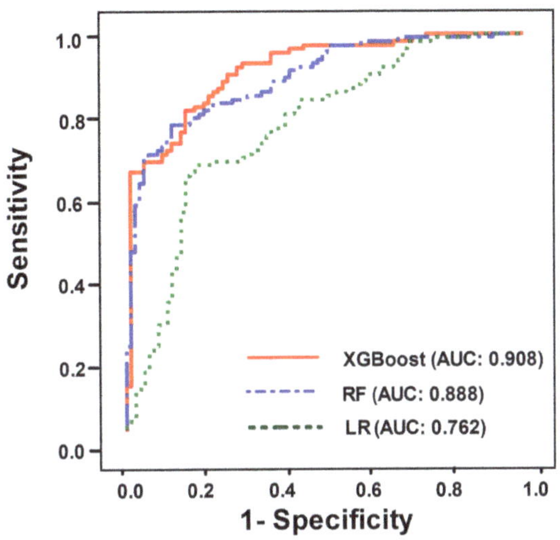


**FIGURE 1 |** ROC curves demonstrating the performance of the XGBoost model (AUC: 0.908, 95% CI 0.864–0.943), RF (AUC: 0.888, 95% CI 0.844–0.934), and LR (AUC 0.762, 95% CI 0.687–0.830) for predicting successful weaning in patients requiring PMV.

## Random Forest (RF)

In addition to XGBoost, we also employed another tree-based classifier, namely, RF. These two ML models have crucial differences in the ensemble method. In brief, XGBoost is based on the ensemble of weak learners, whereas RF is based on fully grown decision trees (13, 15). In RF, n_estimator was 100, max_depth was 4, and default values were applied for the other parameters in RF as well as logistic regression (LR) (see **Supplementary Table 1** for detailed parameters in RF).

## LR

LR is a widely used statistical method in medicine and is frequently used as an ML model for classification tasks. LR mainly based on the assumption that a linear relationship exists between the input variables and the outcomes (16). (see **Supplementary Table 1** for detailed parameters in LR).

## SHapley Additive Explanations (SHAP)

To illustrate the strength and direction of associations between features and the weaning outcome, we implemented SHAP, which is an increasingly used *post-hoc* approach to explain the output of the ML model (17). In brief, SHAP is an additive feature attribution method that gives an explanation of the tree ensemble's overall impact in the format of the contribution of a feature, and the visualized presentation of the SHAP plot is relatively in line with human intuition. Moreover, we also used the partial dependence plot (PDP) to show the marginal effect of features on the predicted outcome.

## Local Interpretable Model-Agnostic Explanations (LIME)

We also used LIME to illustrate the impact of key features at the individual level (18). In brief, LIME provides an explanation of a classifier through approximating the key features by applying a local linear model. The output of LIME is a list of explanations that indicate the contribution of key features to the predicted outcome in an individual patient.

## Statistical Analysis

Categorical data were expressed as frequencies (percentages), and continuous data were presented as means ± standard deviations. Differences between successful weaning and failed weaning were analyzed using Student's *t*-test for continuous variables and Fisher's exact test for categorical variables. Data of 80% of randomly selected patients were used as the training dataset, and the testing set consisted of data of the remaining 20% of the patients (see **Supplementary Figure 1** for the flow diagram of the study). The performance of ML models to predict weaning outcome was determined by using the area under the receiver operating characteristic (ROC) curve (AUC). For the interpretability of the ML models, feature importance was quantified and categorized by clinical domains. In the present study, the score of feature importance was determined by the average gain across all splits of a feature used in the construction of the tree-based model. Furthermore, we used the SHAP summary plot and partial SHAP dependency plot for a visualized interpretation of each feature. We also employed LIME plots for visualized interpretations at the individual level. Python version 3.6 was used in the present study.

# RESULTS

## Demographic and Ventilatory Data

A total of 963 patients requiring PMV were enrolled, and 300 features were used in the present study. The mean age of enrolled patients was 69.3 ± 16.0 years, and 64.2% (618/963) of patients was female. We found that 56.0% (539/963) of patients requiring PMV were weaned from MV. Patients with unsuccessful weaning were more likely to have congestive heart failure (17.5 vs. 11.1%, $p < 0.01$), atrial fibrillation (22.4 vs. 14.5%, $p < 0.01$), chronic obstructive pulmonary disease (19.1 vs. 11.1%, $p < 0.01$), end-stage renal disease (13.7 vs. 8.2%, $p < 0.01$), active malignancy (23.6 vs. 14.7%, $p < 0.01$), and a higher APACHE II score on RCC admission (19.4 ± 5.7 vs. 16.5 ± 5.1, $p < 0.01$) compared with those who were successfully weaned from MV (**Table 1**). **Table 2** summarizes weekly average ventilatory parameters between weeks 4 and 9 at the RCC in patients with PMV. Patients successfully weaned from MV tended to have a lower $FiO_2$, PEEP, Ppeak, Pmean, VT/PBW, and minute ventilation than those who remained ventilator dependent, whereas the respiratory rate was similar between the two groups (**Table 2**).

## Comparisons Among XGBoost, RF, and LR

We then compared the performance of the three ML models to predict successful weaning. Using ROC analysis, we found that the AUC value for predicting successful weaning in the XGBoost was 0.908 (95% CI 0.864–0.943), which was similar

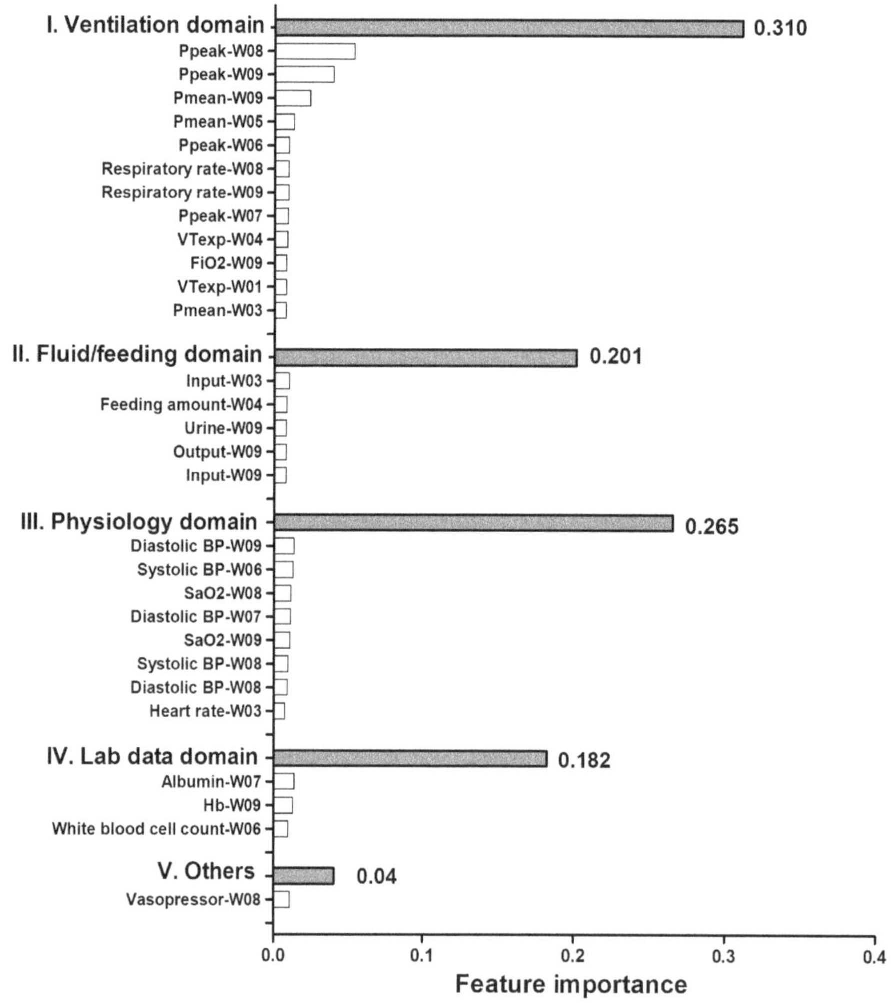


**FIGURE 2** | Relative feature importance of the top 30 features categorized by main clinical domains.

with the accuracy in RF (AUC: 0.888, 95% CI 0.844–0.934) and better than those in LR (AUC: 0.762; 95% CI 0.687–0.830) (**Figure 1**) (see **Supplementary Table 2** for the detailed metric of the performance). Moreover, we also used DeLong's test to determine the difference between two AUCs and confirmed that XGBoost was similar with RF and outperformed LR (XGBoost against RF, $p = 0.36$; XGBoost against LR, $p < 0.01$).

## Explanation of the Model at the Feature Level

To give clinicians an intuitive understanding of the established models, we provided a visualized explanation of the model at the clinical domain level, feature level, and individual level. We categorized the top 30 features by main clinical domains (**Figure 2**). The cumulative feature importance of the ventilatory domain, fluid domain, physiology domain, laboratory data domain, and other domains was 0.310, 0.201, 0.265, 0.182, and 0.04, respectively. Moreover, to enable the visualized interpretation of key features of the model, we used a SHAP plot to illustrate how these features affect weaning outcome (**Figure 3**). Therefore, the strength and direction of each feature were clearly illustrated in the SHAP plot. For example, a lower Ppeak on week 9 was associated with a higher probability of successful weaning. In addition to using a SHAP plot to demonstrate the direction of the impact of key features, we also used PDP to illustrate how each feature affects the model. As shown in **Figure 4**, a Ppeak higher than ~20 $cmH_2O$ was inversely correlated with successful weaning, and such associations were consistent in distinct weeks (**Figure 4**). Taken together, these visualized interpretations provide explanations of the established model at the clinical domain level and feature level.

## Explanation of the Model at the Individual Level

We next used LIME to illustrate the impacts of key features on the weaning prediction model in individual patients. As shown in **Figure 5**, the overall predicted probability of successful weaning (top), true values of the five main features (right), and the classification details (left) of two representative patients were illustrated in the LIME plot. For example, in patient 381, the predicted probability for successful weaning was low (0.20) due to a number of negative conditions, consisting of a high Ppeak (34 $cmH_2O$, >24 $cmH_2O$), a do-not-resuscitate (DNR) status, a low systolic blood pressure (100 mmHg, <112 mmHg), and a high APACHE II score (17, >16), although there was a good feeding amount (1,864 $cm^3$/day, >1,325 $cm^3$/day). In contrast, the weaning probability in patient 459 was high (0.83) due to positive conditions, including a low Ppeak (16 $cmH_2O$, ≤16 $cmH_2O$), a high feeding amount (1,864 $cm^3$/day, >1,325 $cm^3$/day), a high respiratory rate (RR) (19/min, >18/min), and absence of a DNR status, despite a slightly high APACHE II (17, >16). These explanations at the individual level were consistent with the aforementioned explanations at the feature level and should further mitigate the black-box concern.

## Accuracy of the Weekly Weaning Prediction Model

To test the performance of real-time prediction with a 7-day prediction window in the proposed weaning outcome prediction model, we analyzed the accuracy of the weekly prediction model (19). In brief, we measured the performance of the three ML models to predict successful weaning on one selected week using data prior to this selected week. In line with the aforementioned findings (**Figure 1**), the performance was similar between XGBoost and RF, and a lower accuracy was found in the LR model than that in XGBoost/RF (**Figure 6**). The accuracy of XGBoost and RF was ~0.7 between weeks 4 and 7 and slightly declined to 0.6 on weeks 8 and 9. The domain-based distribution of feature importance and the SHAP plot of the weekly prediction model were also compatible with those in the aforementioned prediction model (**Supplementary Figure 2**, **Figures 3, 4**). Collectively, these data demonstrated the feasibility of integrating the proposed ML model into clinical practice in RCC to timely predict the probability of successful weaning.

## DISCUSSION

This study aimed to establish the outcome prediction model in patients requiring PMV through using the explainable ML approach. We found that the accuracy of the XGBoost and RF in predicting successful weaning was high, whereas a relatively low accuracy was found in the LR model. Feature importance analyses illustrated the substantial features based on clinical domains, and SHAP and PDP plots further demonstrated the expected distribution of the impact of each feature in the XGBoost. In addition to the aforementioned interpretability at the feature level, we further used LIME for individual-level interpretability. Furthermore, we addressed the accuracy of the weekly prediction model and found a modest high accuracy to predict successful weaning between weeks 4 and 7. Our findings suggest a practical application of using inherently interpretable ML models to establish a decision support system, particularly in making a high-stake medical decision, given that directly explaining the black-box model remains a niche (20).

Patients requiring PMV is currently a growing issue in Taiwan as well as the world. The advance of critical care has led to

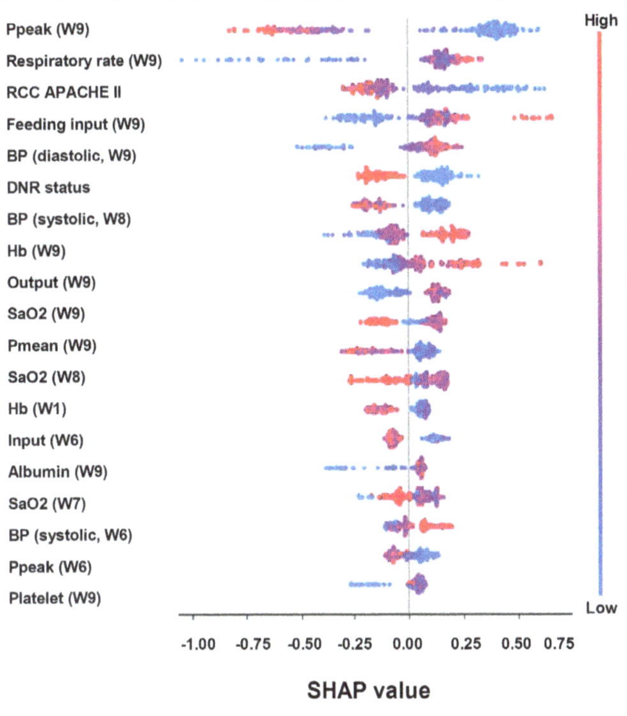


**FIGURE 3 |** SHAP to illustrate successful weaning prediction model in the feature level.

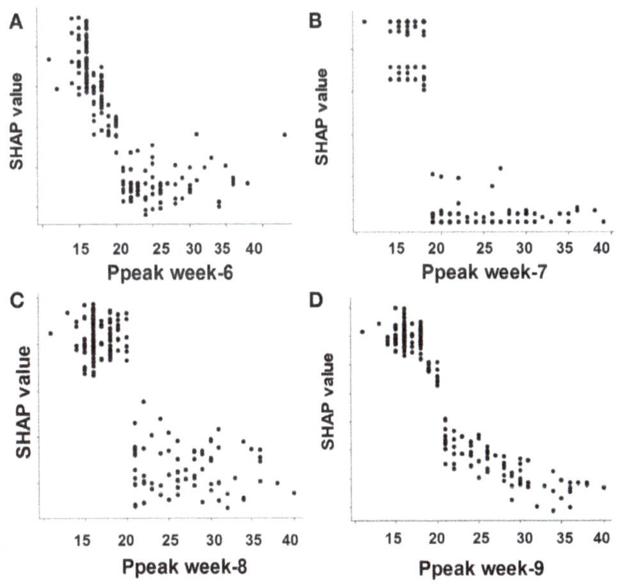


**FIGURE 4 |** Partial dependence plot by the SHAP value of the weekly Ppeak in predicting successful weaning. **(A)** Week-6, **(B)** week-7, **(C)** week-8, **(D)** week-9.

not only a steady decrease of the mortality rate among critically ill patients in the past two decades but also an unexpected increase in the number of patients requiring PMV (21, 22). Hill et al., conducting a Canadian population-based cohort study through investigating 213,680 patients who received MV between 2002 and 2013, reported that 5.4% (11,594) of these patients required PMV (23). Furthermore, Damuth et al., conducting a meta-analysis consisting of 39 studies, reported that the pooled proportion of weaning from MV in patients requiring PMV was 50% (6). Lai et al., investigating 27,654 patients receiving MV in southern Taiwan between 2006 and 2014, found that 6.58% (1,821) of them required PMV, and the hospital mortality in those requiring PMV was 17.6% (24). In the present study, the overall weaning rate and hospital mortality rate in patients requiring PMV were 56 and 18.7%, respectively, and these data were consistent with the aforementioned studies in Taiwan as well as the world. These pieces of evidence highlight an increasing burden of patients requiring PMV worldwide and the crucial need to establish the weaning outcome prediction model in patients with PMV.

Indeed, patients with PMV have distinct ventilatory and physiological alternations from those in the acute status of critical illness; therefore, evidence derived from studies conducted in ICUs, focusing on acute resuscitation-relevant characteristics, is unlikely to be extended to those with PMV (25). Notably, unlike the high weaning rate of up to nearly 85% in patients with acute illness (26, 27), the weaning rate in patients requiring PMV was merely 50% (6). Thus, there is an essential need to establish a PMV-specific weaning outcome prediction decision support system (28). Given the distinct physiological characteristics in patients with PMV, a specialized weaning unit, including respiratory intermediate ICUs (RIICUs) and RCC, is required to facilitate weaning in patients with PMV through a team approach, including respiratory therapists, nutritionists, psychologists, and speech and occupational therapists (29). We believe that the established explainable ML model using multidomain real-world data in the specialized weaning unit should be a practical weaning prediction model to facilitate weaning in patients requiring PMV. Weaning success has been defined as consecutive ventilator-free days for 1–7 days in studies regarding weaning. Ruan et al., using a Taiwanese population-based database in one governmental project aiming to investigate MV use in Taiwan, found that the probabilities

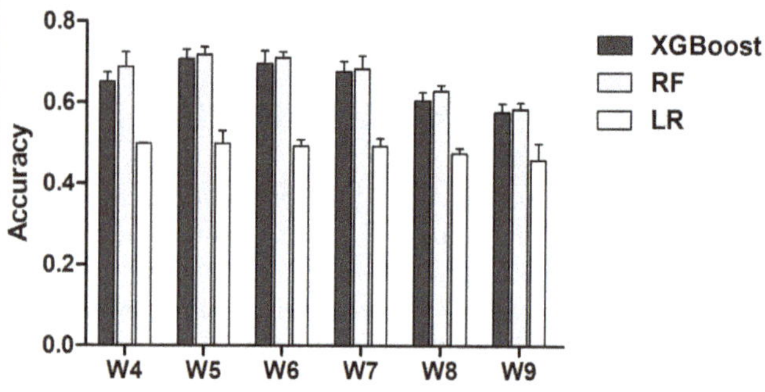


**FIGURE 6 |** Weekly performance to predict weaning outcome among distinct machine learning models.

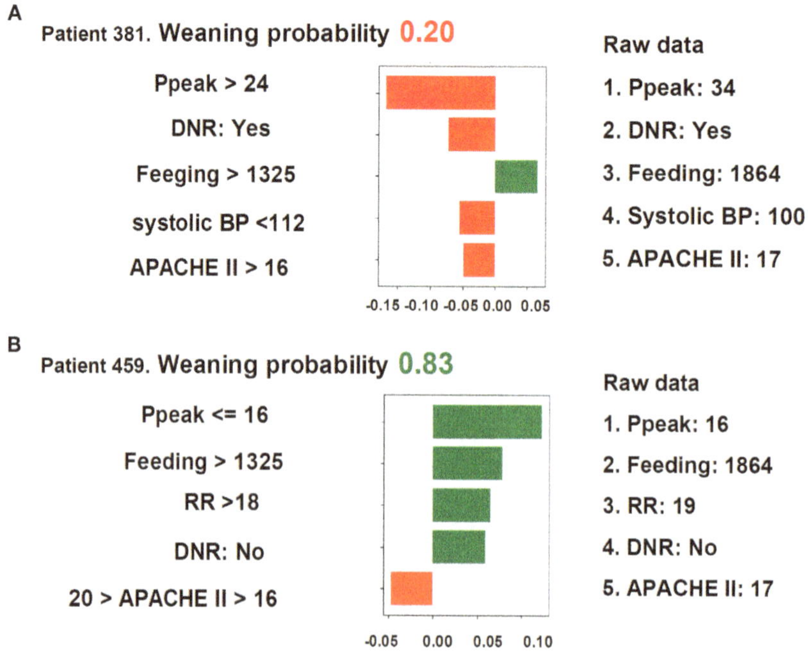


**FIGURE 5 |** LIME plots of two representative individuals. **(A)** Patient 381, **(B)** patient 459.

of the reinstitution of MV for the initial 7 days after ventilator liberation were 25, 8, 3, 3, 2, 1, and 1% in the PMV cohort (12). Therefore, we used liberation from MV for five consecutive days to define a successful weaning success in this study conducted in central Taiwan.

In this study, we identified a similar test accuracy between XGBoost (AUC: 0.908) and RF (AUC: 0.888), whereas the accuracy of LR was relatively low (AUC: 0.762) (**Figure 1**). The LR model is based on assumptions including the independence between input variables and a linear correlation between input and output variables; therefore, the real-world dataset in medical practice may not meet the assumptions of LR. Instead, tree-based classifiers, including XGBoost and RF, based on homogeneity, should be more likely to meet the characteristics of the dataset in the present study. Given that similar performances were found between RF and XGBoost, we think that the use of regularization, applying the Taylor expansion to approximate the loss function, and high flexibility for fine-tuning might enable XGBoost to perform slightly better than RF.

Although AI technologies have achieved extraordinary advancement in a number of fields, the adoption of AI algorithms with the black-box issue in health care remains uncommon mainly due to physicians tending to take action only after realizing the rationale behind the results (30, 31). Given that an incorrect medical decision can lead to catastrophic effects, particularly in critical care medicine, the black-box aspect somehow leads physicians to distrust the AI model when there is no rationale given behind it (7). Clearly, physicians should reserve their judgements in decision making, and we think the interpreted models, including neural networks, which predict patient outcomes (e.g., patient unlikely to liberate MV due to a high Ppeak and low blood pressure) in accordance with the workflow of physicians' daily practice, should be a crucial supporting element in the overall decision process of physicians (32). Therefore, explainable AI algorithms have been increasingly developed for health care applications, aiming not only to establish a predictive model but also to provide justifications for the prediction in a format that physicians can understand (32, 33). In line with our study, Xie et al. recently proposed a framework of automatic clinical score creation to develop 9–12 variables with the interpretability mortality prediction ML model in critically ill patients through using data of the Medical Information Mart for Intensive Care (MIMIC) III database, a widely used critical care database (34). The aforementioned study conducted by Xie et al. and also our study highlight the use of a reasonable number of features to establish a practical model, given that a high number of features may lead to not only the complexity of the model but also to the difficulty in practical landing (34). Similarly, Roimi et al. recently used 50 key features from 7,000 features in two critical care databases to establish a prediction model for bloodstream infections in critically ill patients (35). Indeed, the black-box issue could not be fully clarified; therefore, the *post-hoc* interpretability should at least mimic the real-world behavior of physicians, rather than merely providing explanations of the logical concepts behind the black box. The LIME method offers an interpretable representation with local fidelity. Notably, LIME is model-agnostic and has been increasingly adopted for interpretable data representation (18). Given that the glass-box model is employed in LIME to approximate the black-box model, the quality of the local fit of the glass-box model to the data could not be controlled and objectively assessed (36).

In addition to weaning, end-of-life care is also a crucial issue in patients requiring PMV, particularly those with difficulty weaning in RCC/RIICU given that prolonged use of ventilator with a low possibility of weaning might lead to medical futility (37). Early integrated palliative care has been found to improve quality of life, to reduce intensive life-sustaining treatments, and to improve caregivers' psychological symptoms (38). We found a declining accuracy in predicting successful weaning in weeks 4–7 (**Figure 6**); we hence established the mortality prediction model using the same dataset and explainable ML approach. We found that the accuracy to predict mortality was higher than that to predict successful weaning (**Supplementary Figure 5**). Notably, the high-ranking features to predict mortality appeared to be distinct from that used to predict successful weaning. We found that the DNR status had the highest feature importance in the mortality prediction model, whereas the DNR status was the sixth highest feature importance in the weaning prediction model (**Supplementary Figure 6**, **Figure 3**). Indeed, the consensus for DNR is an essential issue among patients requiring PMV, particularly those with a low possibility of weaning. Nava et al., investigating 6,008 patients in European respiratory intermediate care units and high-dependency units, found that merely 21% of patients received end-of-life decision, including withholding of treatment, DNR/do-not-intubate orders, and non-invasive MV (37). Furthermore, studies have shown that timely communication with families and the interprofessional collaboration for individualized balance between aggressiveness and responsiveness of care, which was recently reported by Rak et al. through conducting a large and delicate ethnographic study in eight long-term acute care hospitals, are crucial in the end-of-life care among patients requiring PMV (39, 40). Therefore, we think that the mortality prediction model and the illustration of main features attributed to high mortality in patients with PMV might indicate the need for timely communication regarding end-of-life issues.

There are limitations in this study. First, this study is a single-center study, and external validation is hence needed. However, the overall weaning and mortality rates were similar to those of previous studies, and the used data were routinely collected data in a real-world setting; the concern with regard to generalization should be largely mitigated. Second, some weaning-relevant data, such as rehabilitation programs, were not included in the dataset. We think the accuracy of the model could be further improved after including the aforementioned data; however, the structured data in a real-world setting remain fundamental in the practical landing of the proposed ML mode. Third, the technology readiness level (TRL) of the proposed explainable ML model should merely be TRL-4 (41); however, we believe that the feasibility of practical use with optimal user interface (TRL-5) should be high given that the variables used in this study were obtained from structured electronic medical records of real-world practice at an RCC. Fourth, the number of subjects was relatively small. Given that merely 5–10% of patients receiving MV require PMV, the sample size in studies focusing on PMV is generally small (1, 2). To mitigate the issue of a small sample size, we have performed a grid search for optimal parameters of XGBoost, RF, and LR and have provided metrics of performance in an independent test cohort (80/20 splitting) to show the acceptable accuracy, Brier score, precision, recall, and F1 score in XGBoost/RF (**Supplementary Table 2**, **Supplementary Figure 1**). Moreover, the observational nature of this study and the medical decision made by the senior attending physician could potentially introduce a confounding effect. Although the individual decision for weaning was made by the attending physician, the weaning protocol and overall weaning process have been certified by the regular external audit at the RCC in Taiwan. Additionally, patients who were transferred from another hospital may be a concern due to data integrity, but we ascertain the ventilatory data of these patients given that the Taiwanese National Health Insurance, a compulsory population-based insurance in Taiwan, has implemented the nationwide Integrated Prospective Payment (IPP) program on patients with PMV since 2000 (12, 42); therefore, in the present study, we used the registered ventilatory data of these patients in the IPP program although the data might be incomplete.

## CONCLUSION

In conclusion, using a real-world dataset in patients requiring PMV, we found that XGBoost/RF outperformed LR for predicting weaning outcome in patients requiring PMV. We used domain-based cumulative feature importance, SHAP plots, and PDP plots for visualized interpretations at the feature level and LIME plots to illustrate key determinants at the individual level. We believe these approaches should largely mitigate the black-box issue. Future prospective research is warranted for the landing of the proposed model and to translate the advantages of ML models into clinical outcomes of patients requiring PMV.

## ETHICS STATEMENT

The studies involving human participants were reviewed and approved by Institutional Review Board of the Taichung Veterans General Hospital (TCVGH: CE19072A). Written informed consent for participation was not required for this study in accordance with the national legislation and the institutional requirements.

## AUTHOR CONTRIBUTIONS

M-YL, J-LW, M-CC, C-LW, and W-CC: study concept and design. M-YL, C-CL, P-HL, and W-CC: acquisition of data and analysis and interpretation of data. M-YL and W-CC: drafting the manuscript. All authors: contributed to the article and approved the submitted version.

## REFERENCES

1. MacIntyre NR, Epstein SK, Carson S, Scheinhorn D, Christopher K, Muldoon S, et al. Management of patients requiring prolonged mechanical ventilation: report of a NAMDRC consensus conference. *Chest.* (2005) 128:3937–54. doi: 10.1378/chest.128.6.3937
2. Lamas D. Chronic critical illness. *N Engl J Med.* (2014) 370:175–7. doi: 10.1056/NEJMms1310675
3. Iwashyna TJ, Hodgson CL, Pilcher D, Bailey M, van Lint A, Chavan S, et al. Timing of onset and burden of persistent critical illness in Australia and New Zealand: a retrospective, population-based, observational study. *Lancet Respir Med.* (2016) 4:566–73. doi: 10.1016/S2213-2600(16)30098-4
4. Shih CY, Hung MC, Lu HM, Chen L, Huang SJ, Wang JD. Incidence, life expectancy and prognostic factors in cancer patients under prolonged mechanical ventilation: a nationwide analysis of 5,138 cases during 1998-2007. *Critical Care.* (2013) 17:R144. doi: 10.1186/cc12823
5. Kahn JM, Le T, Angus DC, Cox CE, Hough CL, White DB, et al. The epidemiology of chronic critical illness in the United States*. *Crit Care Med.* (2015) 43:282–7. doi: 10.1097/CCM.0000000000000710
6. Damuth E, Mitchell JA, Bartock JL, Roberts BW, Trzeciak S. Long-term survival of critically ill patients treated with prolonged mechanical ventilation: a systematic review and meta-analysis. *Lancet Respir Med.* (2015) 3:544–53. doi: 10.1016/S2213-2600(15)00150-2
7. Cabitza F, Rasoini R, Gensini GF. Unintended consequences of machine learning in medicine. *JAMA.* (2017) 318:517–18. doi: 10.1001/jama.2017.7797
8. Topol EJ. High-performance medicine: the convergence of human and artificial intelligence. *Nat Med.* (2019) 25:44–56. doi: 10.1038/s41591-018-0300-7
9. Lauritsen SM, Kristensen M, Olsen MV, Larsen MS, Lauritsen KM, Jorgensen MJ, et al. Explainable artificial intelligence model to predict acute critical illness from electronic health records. *Nat Commun.* (2020) 11:3852. doi: 10.1038/s41467-020-17431-x
10. Hu CA, Chen CM, Fang YC, Liang SJ, Wang HC, Fang WF, et al. Using a machine learning approach to predict mortality in critically ill influenza patients: a cross-sectional retrospective multicentre study in Taiwan. *BMJ Open.* (2020) 10:e033898. doi: 10.1136/bmjopen-2019-033898
11. Lin MS, Yan YH, Wang JD, Lu HM, Chen L, Hung MC, et al. Improved survival for an integrated system of reduced intensive respiratory care for patients requiring prolonged mechanical ventilation. *Respir Care.* (2013) 58:517–24. doi: 10.4187/respcare.01530
12. Ruan SY, Teng NC, Wu HD, Tsai SL, Wang CY, Wu CP, et al. Durability of weaning success for liberation from invasive mechanical ventilation: an analysis of a nationwide database. *Am J Respir Crit Care Med.* (2017) 196:792–95. doi: 10.1164/rccm.201610-2153LE
13. Friedman JH, Popescu BE. Importance sampled learning ensembles. *J Mach Learn Res.* (2003) 4:94305. Available online at: https://statweb.stanford.edu/~jhf/ftp/isle.pdf
14. Chen T, Guestrin C. XGBoost: a scalable tree boosting system. In: *Proceedings of the 22nd ACM SIGKDD International Conference on Knowledge Discovery and Data Mining.* New York, NY: ACM (2016). p. 785–94. doi: 10.1145/2939672.2939785
15. Bryll R, Gutierrez-Osuna R, Quek F. Attribute bagging: improving accuracy of classifier ensembles by using random feature subsets. *Pattern Recogn.* (2003) 36:1291–302. doi: 10.1016/S0031-3203(02)00121-8
16. Dreiseitl S, Ohno-Machado L. Logistic regression and artificial neural network classification models: a methodology review. *J Biomed Inform.* (2002) 35:352–9. doi: 10.1016/S1532-0464(03)00034-0
17. Scott Lunberg, Lee S-I. A unified approach to interpreting model predictions.

*arXiv:170507874v2.* (2018) 1–10.

18. Pedersen TL, Benesty M. *Lime: Local Interpretable Model-Agnostic Explanations.* R package version 0.4.1. (2018). Available online at: https://CRAN.R-project.org/package=lime
19. Fleuren LM, Klausch TLT, Zwager CL, Schoonmade LJ, Guo T, Roggeveen LF, et al. Machine learning for the prediction of sepsis: a systematic review and meta-analysis of diagnostic test accuracy. *Intensive Care Med.* (2020) 46:383–400. doi: 10.1007/s00134-019-05872-y
20. Rudin C. Stop explaining black box machine learning models for high stakes decisions and use interpretable models instead. *Nat Machine Intelligence.* (2019) 1:206–15. doi: 10.1038/s42256-019-0048-x
21. Sakusic A, Gajic O. Chronic critical illness: unintended consequence of intensive care medicine. *Lancet Respir Med.* (2016) 4:531–32. doi: 10.1016/S2213-2600(16)30066-2
22. Villalba D, Gil Rossetti G, Scrigna M, Collins J, Rocco A, Matesa A, et al. Prevalence of and risk factors for mechanical ventilation reinstitution in patients weaned from prolonged mechanical ventilation. *Respir Care.* (2020) 65:210–16. doi: 10.4187/respcare.06807
23. Hill AD, Fowler RA, Burns KE, Rose L, Pinto RL, Scales DC. Long-term outcomes and health care utilization after prolonged mechanical ventilation. *Ann Am Thorac Soc.* (2017) 14:355–62. doi: 10.1513/AnnalsATS.201610-792OC
24. Lai CC, Shieh JM, Chiang SR, Chiang KH, Weng SF, Ho CH, et al. The outcomes and prognostic factors of patients requiring prolonged mechanical ventilation. *Sci Rep.* (2016) 6:28034. doi: 10.1038/srep28034
25. Demoule A, Molinari N, Jung B, Prodanovic H, Chanques G, Matecki S, et al. Patterns of diaphragm function in critically ill patients receiving prolonged mechanical ventilation: a prospective longitudinal study. *Ann Intensive Care.* (2016) 6:75. doi: 10.1186/s13613-016-0179-8
26. Penuelas O, Frutos-Vivar F, Fernandez C, Anzueto A, Epstein SK, Apezteguia C, et al. Characteristics and outcomes of ventilated patients according to time to liberation from mechanical ventilation. *Am J Respir Crit Care Med.* (2011) 184:430–7. doi: 10.1164/rccm.201011-1887OC
27. Subira C, Hernandez G, Vazquez A, Rodriguez-Garcia R, Gonzalez-Castro A, Garcia C, et al. Effect of pressure support vs t-piece ventilation strategies during spontaneous breathing trials on successful extubation among patients receiving mechanical ventilation: a randomized clinical trial. *JAMA.* (2019) 321:2175–82. doi: 10.1001/jama.2019.7234
28. Kahn JM, Carson SS. Generating evidence on best practice in long-term acute care hospitals. *JAMA.* (2013) 309:719–20. doi: 10.1001/jama.2013.848
29. Carpene N, Vagheggini G, Panait E, Gabbrielli L, Ambrosino N. A proposal of a new model for long-term weaning: respiratory intensive care unit and weaning center. *Respir Med.* (2010) 104:1505–11. doi: 10.1016/j.rmed.2010.05.012
30. Chen JH, Asch SM. Machine learning and prediction in medicine - beyond the peak of inflated expectations. *N Engl J Med.* (2017) 376:2507–09. doi: 10.1056/NEJMp1702071
31. Guidotti R, Monreale A, Turini F, Pedreschi D, Giannotti F. A survey of methods for explaining black box models. *arXiv:180201933v3.* (2018) 1–45.
32. Zhang Z, Beck MW, Winkler DA, Huang B, Sibanda W, Goyal H, et al. Opening the black box of neural networks: methods for interpreting neural network models in clinical applications. *Ann Transl Med.* (2018) 6:216. doi: 10.21037/atm.2018.05.32
33. Petkovic D, Kobzik L, Re C. Machine learning and deep analytics for biocomputing: call for better explainability. *Pac Symp Biocomput.* (2018) 23:623–27. doi: 10.1142/9789813235533_0058
34. Xie F, Chakraborty B, Ong MEH, Goldstein BA, Liu N. AutoScore: a machine learning-based automatic clinical score generator and its application to mortality prediction using electronic health records. *JMIR Med Inform.* (2020) 8:e21798. doi: 10.2196/21798
35. Roimi M, Neuberger A, Shrot A, Paul M, Geffen Y, Bar-Lavie Y. Early diagnosis of bloodstream infections in the intensive care unit using machine-learning algorithms. *Intensive Care Med.* (2020) 46:454–62. doi: 10.1007/s00134-019-05876-8
36. Ribeiro MT, Singh S, Guestrin C. "Why Should I Trust You?": explaining the predictions of any classifier. In: *Proceedings of the 22nd ACM SIGKDD International Conference on Knowledge Discovery and Data Mining.* San Francisco, CA: ACM (2016). p. 1135–44. doi: 10.1145/2939672.2939778
37. Nava S, Sturani C, Hartl S, Magni G, Ciontu M, Corrado A, et al. End-of-life decision-making in respiratory intermediate care units: a European survey. *Eur Respir J.* (2007) 30:156–64. doi: 10.1183/09031936.00128306
38. Detering KM, Hancock AD, Reade MC, Silvester W. The impact of advance care planning on end of life care in elderly patients: randomised controlled trial. *BMJ.* (2010) 340:c1345. doi: 10.1136/bmj.c1345
39. Ouyang DJ, Lief L, Russell D, Xu J, Berlin DA, Gentzler E, et al. Timing is everything: early do-not-resuscitate orders in the intensive care unit and patient outcomes. *PLoS ONE.* (2020) 15:e0227971. doi: 10.1371/journal.pone.0227971
40. Rak KJ, Ashcraft LE, Kuza CC, Fleck JC, DePaoli LC, Angus DC, et al. Effective care practices in patients receiving prolonged mechanical ventilation. an ethnographic study. *Am J Respir Crit Care Med.* (2020) 201:823–31. doi: 10.1164/rccm.201910-2006OC
41. Fleuren LM, Thoral P, Shillan D, Ercole A, Elbers PWG, Right Data Right Now C. Machine learning in intensive care medicine: ready for take-off? *Intensive Care Med.* (2020) 46:1486–8. doi: 10.1007/s00134-020-06045-y
42. Liu CJ, Chu CC, Chen W, Cheng WE, Shih CM, Tsai YS, et al. Impact of Taiwan's integrated prospective payment program on prolonged mechanical ventilation: a 6-year nationwide study. *Respir Care.* (2013) 58:676–82. doi: 10.4187/respcare.01242

15

# Development and Validation of a Sepsis Mortality Risk Score for Sepsis-3 Patients in Intensive Care Unit

*Kai Zhang*[1†], *Shufang Zhang*[2†], *Wei Cui*[1], *Yucai Hong*[3], *Gensheng Zhang*[1*] and *Zhongheng Zhang*[3*]

[1] *Department of Critical Care Medicine, Second Affiliated Hospital, Zhejiang University School of Medicine, Hangzhou, China,*
[2] *Department of Cardiology, Second Affiliated Hospital, Zhejiang University School of Medicine, Hangzhou, China,*
[3] *Department of Emergency Medicine, Sir Run-Run Shaw Hospital, Zhejiang University School of Medicine, Hangzhou, China*

***Correspondence:***
*Zhongheng Zhang*
*zh_zhang1984@zju.edu.cn*
*Gensheng Zhang*
*genshengzhang@zju.edu.cn*

*† These authors have contributed equally to this work*

**Background:** Many severity scores are widely used for clinical outcome prediction for critically ill patients in the intensive care unit (ICU). However, for patients identified by sepsis-3 criteria, none of these have been developed. This study aimed to develop and validate a risk stratification score for mortality prediction in sepsis-3 patients.

**Methods:** In this retrospective cohort study, we employed the Medical Information Mart for Intensive Care III (MIMIC III) database for model development and the eICU database for external validation. We identified septic patients by sepsis-3 criteria on day 1 of ICU entry. The Least Absolute Shrinkage and Selection Operator (LASSO) technique was performed to select predictive variables. We also developed a sepsis mortality prediction model and associated risk stratification score. We then compared model discrimination and calibration with other traditional severity scores.

**Results:** For model development, we enrolled a total of 5,443 patients fulfilling the sepsis-3 criteria. The 30-day mortality was 16.7%. With 5,658 septic patients in the validation set, there were 1,135 deaths (mortality 20.1%). The score had good discrimination in development and validation sets (area under curve: 0.789 and 0.765). In the validation set, the calibration slope was 0.862, and the Brier value was 0.140. In the development dataset, the score divided patients according to mortality risk of low (3.2%), moderate (12.4%), high (30.7%), and very high (68.1%). The corresponding mortality in the validation dataset was 2.8, 10.5, 21.1, and 51.2%. As shown by the decision curve analysis, the score always had a positive net benefit.

**Conclusion:** We observed moderate discrimination and calibration for the score termed Sepsis Mortality Risk Score (SMRS), allowing stratification of patients according to mortality risk. However, we still require further modification and external validation.

**Keywords: sepsis-3.0, critical care, intensive care unit (ICU), machine learning, mortality prediction model, severity score system**

## INTRODUCTION

Being a life-threatening organ dysfunction due to a dysregulated host response to infection, sepsis is considered a major global health problem (1, 2). According to the latest Global Burden of Diseases study, ~48.9 million sepsis cases were reported worldwide in 2017 despite the decline in incidence and mortality. A total of 11.0 million patients died from sepsis and its complications, which accounted for 19.7% of deaths worldwide (3). In the intensive care unit (ICU), sepsis remains a significant cause of morbidity and mortality. According to the ICON study, 29.5% of the patients suffered from sepsis during their ICU stay. The ICU mortality rate was significantly higher in septic patients (25.8%) than the whole population (16.2%) (4). Since rapid treatment could improve the outcomes in septic patients, early identification, and risk assessment are of vital importance (5, 6). A pragmatic scoring system could help clinicians make decisions by identifying high-risk patients and providing the probability of death.

To characterize disease severity and predict its outcome, various severity scores have been widely used in the ICU (7). However, in septic patients, the clinical application remains limited because sepsis's pathogenesis is complicated, and no single score has been developed. For example, the Acute Physiology and Chronic Health Evaluation II (APACHE II) score underestimated the risk of death for septic patients in the ICU (8). Similarly, the Simplified Acute Physiology Score II (SAPS II) showed poor calibration in external validation studies (9, 10). Besides the traditional ICU scoring systems, sepsis mortality prediction models based on machine learning algorithms have been published by some researchers. These models, derived from big medical datasets, could accurately predict mortality with good discrimination for septic patients (11–14). However, most of the models were designed for patients with severe sepsis or septic shock, and none of these were developed from the sepsis-3 patient population. Johnson et al. compared five different methods for screening patients with sepsis, and showed that sepsis-3 criteria provided temporal context, possessed high construct validity and were less influenced by coding changes (15). Therefore, screening patients with sepsis by using the sepsis-3 criteria was considered an optimal method in the electronic database.

Based on sepsis-3 criteria and the Medical Information Mart for Intensive Care III (MIMIC III) database, we aimed to develop a Sepsis Mortality Risk Score (SMRS) by Least Absolute Shrinkage and Selection Operator (LASSO) technique, assess its predictive ability, and compare it with traditional severity scores in the validation dataset from the eICU Collaborative Research Database (eICU). In addition, we built four machine learning models to predict 30-day mortality for sepsis-3 patients.

**Abbreviations:** ICU, Intensive care unit; MIMIC III, Medical Information Mart for Intensive Care III; LASSO, Least Absolute Shrinkage and Selection Operator; SMRS, Sepsis Mortality Risk Score; APACHE II, Acute Physiology and Chronic Health Evaluation II; SAPS II, Simplified Acute Physiology Score II; SOFA, Sequential Organ Failure Assessment; APS III, Acute Physiological Score III; LODS, Logistic Organ Dysfunction System; OASIS, Oxford Acute Severity of Illness Score; SIRS, System Inflammatory Reaction Syndrome; qSOFA, quick SOFA; VIF, variance inflation factor; AUC, Area Under the Curve; DCA, decision curve analysis; MARS, multivariate adaptive regression splines; XGBoost, eXtreme Gradient Boosting; ED, emergency department.

## MATERIALS AND METHODS

### Data Source and Participants

We extracted data from the MIMIC III (16) and eICU database (17), respectively. We included adult patients admitted to the ICU with sepsis. Sepsis was identified based on sepsis-3 criteria, which included suspected infection and a Sequential Organ Failure Assessment (SOFA) score $\geq$ 2 (1). For sepsis patient selection, a previous study was referred for identifying the sepsis-3 cohort from MIMIC III (15). We excluded the following patients: (1) non-adults (<16 years old), (2) multiple admissions, (3) receiving cardiothoracic surgical service (their postoperative physiologic derangements or not translating to the same mortality risk as others), (4) with metastatic cancer (inflammatory and immune response different from others); (5) with suspected infection more than 24 h before or after ICU admission (patients admitted to ICU with sepsis), and (6) missing important data (demographics, variables for calculating traditional severity scores).

### Data Extraction

From the MIMIC III and eICU database, we extracted the following information: (1) demographic information; (2) ICU details including vital sign data, laboratory data, respiratory support, renal replacement therapy; and (3) traditional severity scores including SAPS II, Acute Physiological Score III (APS III), Logistic Organ Dysfunction System (LODS), Oxford Acute Severity of Illness Score (OASIS), SOFA, System Inflammatory Reaction Syndrome (SIRS), and quick SOFA (qSOFA). During the first 24 h of ICU admission, all variables were recorded.

### Outcome and Sample Size

Patients who died within 30 days inside or outside the hospital were considered as primary outcome events. We based our sample size calculation on the primary outcome. The sample size was defined as having at least 10 outcome events per variable (EPV) per estimated parameter according to a previous study (18). Our sample and the number of events exceeded that determined by the EPV approach.

### Missing Data

For the development dataset from the MIMIC III database, we handled variables with missing values <20% by a mean value imputation method. Since serum lactate was considered an important predictor, if lactate data on day 1 was missing, the available data on day 2 or day 3 was used. If there was no lactate value in the first 3 days, we used regression imputation to handle the missing data. To calculate severity scores in the eICU database, patients with missing parameters were excluded from this analysis.

### Statistical Analysis

Continuous variables were reported as median and interquartile range, and two groups were compared by the Mann–Whitney

**TABLE 1** | Baseline characteristics of participants in development set.

| Variables | All ($n$ = 5,443) | Survivors ($n$ = 4,536) | Non-survivors ($n$ = 907) | *P*-value |
|---|---|---|---|---|
| **Age, years** | 67.0 (54.0–80.0) | 66.0 (53.0–78.0) | 75.0 (61.0–84.0) | <0.001 |
| **Gender, *n*** | | | | 0.182 |
| Male | 3,020 (55.5) | 2,535 (55.9) | 485 (53.5) | |
| Female | 2,423 (44.5) | 2,001 (44.1) | 422 (46.5) | |
| **Ethnicity, *n*** | | | | <0.001 |
| White | 3,945 (72.5) | 3,309 (72.9) | 636 (70.1) | |
| Black | 475 (8.7) | 421 (9.3) | 54 (6.0) | |
| Others | 1,023 (18.8) | 806 (17.8) | 217 (23.9) | |
| **Admission type, *n*** | | | | <0.001 |
| Emergency | 5,061 (93.0) | 4,175 (92.0) | 886 (97.7) | |
| Others | 382 (7.0) | 361 (8.0) | 21 (2.3) | |
| **Comorbidities, *n*** | | | | |
| Heart failure | 957 (17.6) | 742 (16.4) | 215 (23.7) | <0.001 |
| Hypertension | 868 (15.9) | 701 (15.5) | 167 (18.4) | 0.026 |
| COPD | 1,103 (20.3) | 889 (19.6) | 214 (23.6) | 0.006 |
| Diabetes | 1,563 (28.7) | 1,298 (28.6) | 265 (29.2) | 0.715 |
| Renal failure | 1,000 (18.4) | 799 (17.6) | 201 (22.2) | 0.001 |
| Hepatopathy | 544 (10.0) | 429 (9.5) | 115 (12.7) | 0.003 |
| Lymphoma | 95 (1.7) | 74 (1.6) | 21 (2.3) | 0.151 |
| **Need RRT, *n*** | 395 (7.3) | 281 (6.2) | 114 (12.6) | <0.001 |
| **Need mechanical ventilation, *n*** | 2,638 (48.5) | 2,080 (45.9) | 558 (61.5) | <0.001 |
| **Severity score** | | | | |
| SAPS II | 39 (31–50) | 37 (29–46) | 53 (42–65) | <0.001 |
| APS III | 48 (36–63) | 45 (34–57) | 67 (51–87) | <0.001 |
| OASIS | 35 (29–41) | 34 (28–39) | 42 (36–49) | <0.001 |
| LODS | 5 (3–7) | 4 (3–6) | 7 (5–10) | <0.001 |
| SOFA | 5 (3–7) | 5 (3–7) | 7 (5–11) | <0.001 |
| SIRS | 3 (2–4) | 3 (2–4) | 3 (3–4) | <0.001 |
| qSOFA | 2 (2–2) | 2 (2–2) | 2 (2–3) | <0.001 |

*Data are expressed as frequencies (percentage) or median (interquartile range). The results of the comparison between the two groups was analyzed by Mann–Whitney test for continuous variables or the chi-squared test for categorical variables.*

*RRT, Renal Replacement Therapies; COPD, Chronic Obstructive Pulmonary Disease; SAPS II, Simplified Acute Physiological Score II; APS III, Acute Physiological Score III; OASIS, Oxford Acute Severity of Illness Score; SIRS, Systemic Inflammatory Response Syndrome; qSOFA, quick Sequential Organ Failure Assessment; LODS, Logistic Organ Dysfunction System; SOFA, Sequential Organ Failure Assessment.*

*U*-test. Categorical variables were reported as the number and proportion and were compared with the Chi-square test. The variance inflation factor (VIF) was calculated to verify whether multicollinearity existed in the regression model.

In the development set, we used the LASSO method to select the most useful predictive variables (19). We plotted the continuous variables against 30-day mortality and determined the cutoff value based on the Loess smoothing function and the Youden index (20). Continuous variables were made into dichotomous or dummy variables by the cutoff points. Final variables were entered into a logistic regression, and for each risk predictor, the odds ratio was rounded into an integer value to generate the SMRS. The final score was classified into four risk groups: low (<5%), moderate (5–20%), high (20–50%), and very high (>50%). The survival curves of each mortality risk group were depicted by the Kaplan–Meier method and compared by the log-rank test.

The SMRS was validated in the validation set. To assess discrimination, the Area Under the Curve (AUC) for SMRS and other severity scores was calculated. Calibration was assessed by the calibration slope and the Brier value. To determine the clinical usefulness of the SMRS by quantifying the net benefit at different threshold probabilities, we conducted the decision curve analysis (DCA) (21).

Moreover, the discrimination of four machine learning algorithms in predicting mortality for sepsis-3 patients was compared. In the development set, we developed the logistic regression model, the multivariate adaptive regression splines (MARS) model, the random forest model, and the eXtreme Gradient Boosting (XGBoost) model. The discrimination was validated externally by AUC in the eICU database.

We performed all statistical analyzes using software version 3.6.0 (R Foundation for Statistical Computing).

# RESULTS

## Participants

Our study was reported according to the guidelines of the TRIPOD statement (Checklist in **Additional File 1**) (22). The initial research identified 23,620 ICU admissions from the MIMIC III database. A total of 5,443 adult patients meeting the sepsis-3 criteria were analyzed, including 907 non-survivors and 4,536 survivors. The baseline characteristics of all patients, survivors, and non-survivors are described in **Table 1**. While data extraction, we excluded body mass index, albumin, bands, and bilirubin from the analysis because of the large portion of the missing value (>20%). For other variables, the missing value was <10% (**Additional File 2**). We assigned 5,658 septic patients (1,042 deaths, mortality rate 20.1%) from the eICU database with complete data to the validation set. Comparisons of basic characteristics between development and validation sets are recorded in **Additional File 3**.

## Model Development

Based on 5,443 patients in the development set in the LASSO model, 35 features were reduced to 15 potential predictors (**Additional File 4**). After screening, 13 predictors were entered into the LASSO regression model (**Additional File 5**), and the VIF proved there was no significant multicollinearity in the model (VIF < 5). **Additional File 6** shows loess smoothing curves. The SMRS was composed of 13 factors, and the total score range was 0 to 34 (**Table 2**). The relationship between SMRS and the probability of death is shown in **Figure 1**, and there was an increasing risk of death with a higher score. The SMRS had good discrimination (AUC: 0.789) in the development set, which was better than other severity scores (**Figure 2A**). The calibration of SMRS in the development set was shown in **Figure 3A**. The calibration slope was 1.000 and the Brier value was 0.110. Mortality rates of low (3.2%, 0–6 points), moderate (12.4%, 7–11 points), high (30.7%, 12–14 points), and very high (68.1%, ≥15 points) were yielded by the risk groups for the development set.

**TABLE 2** | Sepsis mortality risk score.

| Variables | Cutoff | Score |
|---|---|---|
| Race | Black | 0 |
| | White | 1 |
| | Others | 2 |
| Age (years old) | <45 | 0 |
| | ≥45 and <60 | 2 |
| | ≥60 and <75 | 3 |
| | ≥75 | 5 |
| Need mechanical ventilation | Yes | 2 |
| Lactate (mmol/L) | <4.5 | 0 |
| | ≥4.5 and <8 | 1 |
| | ≥8 | 3 |
| Temperature (°C) | ≥36 and <39 | 0 |
| | ≥39 | 2 |
| | ≥35 and <36 | 2 |
| | <35 | 5 |
| SBP (mm/Hg) | >100 | 0 |
| | ≥90 and <100 | 1 |
| | <90 | 4 |
| $SpO_2$ (%) | ≥90 | 0 |
| | ≥80 and <90 | 1 |
| | <80 | 2 |
| BUN (mg/dL) | <20 | 0 |
| | ≥20 and <30 | 1 |
| | ≥30 | 2 |
| WBC ($10^9$/L) | ≥4 and ≤12 | 0 |
| | <4 | 1 |
| | >12 and ≤20 | 1 |
| | >20 | 2 |
| Ca (mg/dL) | ≥8 and ≤11 | 0 |
| | ≥7 and <8 | 1 |
| | >11 | 1 |
| | <7 | 3 |
| HR ($min^{-1}$) | >100 | 1 |
| RR ($min^{-1}$) | >22 | 2 |
| INR | >1.5 | 1 |
| **Top score** | | 34 |

*SBP, Systolic Blood Pressure; $SpO_2$, Surplus pulse $O_2$; WBC, White Blood cell Count; BUN, Blood Urea Nitrogen; INR, International Normalized Ratio; HR, Heart Rate; RR, Respiratory Rate.*

## Model Performance

In the validation set, we evaluated the discrimination and calibration of SMRS. SMRS was well-discriminated in the external validation set (AUC: 0.765), which was greater than APACHE IV and SAPS II (AUC: APACHE IV 0.754, SAPS II 0.751; **Figure 2B**). However, no statistical significance of AUCs was observed (De Long method, SMRS vs. APACHE IV: *P*-value 0.221; SMRS vs. SAPS II: *P*-value 0.177). Moreover, the calibration slope was 0.862, and the Brier value was 0.140, indicating that the score has a moderate fit (**Figure 3B**). For predicting 30-day mortality, the DCA results of SMRS, SAPS II, SOFA, and APACHE IV were shown in **Figure 4**. A positive net benefit between the threshold probabilities of 10 to 80% was observed through SMRS. The net benefit of SMRS was comparable to SAPS II and APACHE IV and was better than the SOFA in this range.

SMRS accurately stratified patients from the validation set into groups with increased risk of death: low (2.8%), moderate (10.5%), high (21.1%), and very high (51.2%) (**Figure 5**). The detailed mortality rate stratified by SMRS was reported in **Additional File 7**.

All machine learning models, except the logistic regression model, showed good discrimination ability in the development set (AUC > 0.8). In the development and validation sets, the XGBoost algorithm achieved the best performance among the four models (**Figure 6**).

# DISCUSSION

We used the LASSO method in this study to select the most useful predictive features from the primary sepsis-3 data set, which is

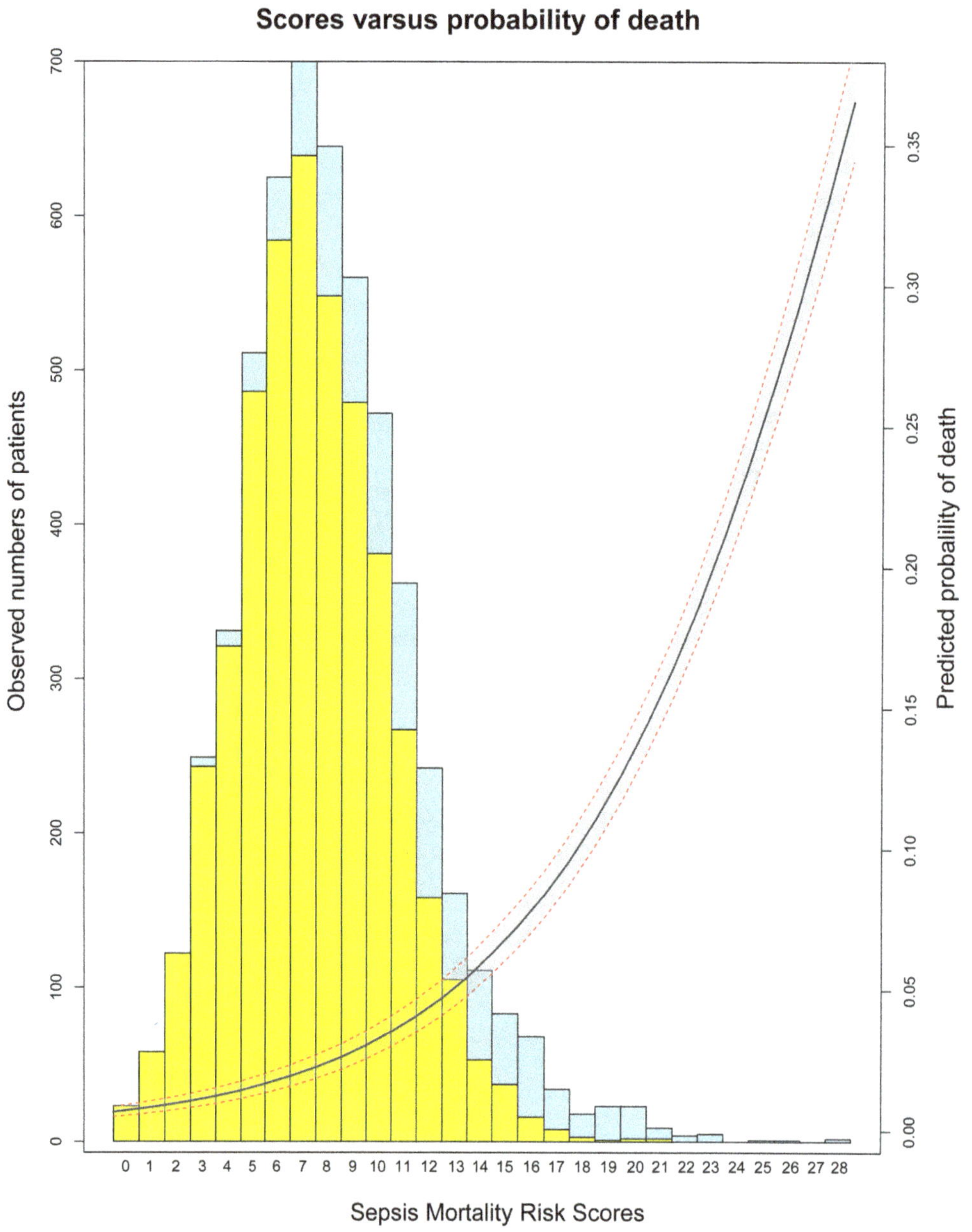


**FIGURE 1** | The relationship between SMRS and probability of death in development set.

suitable for the regression of high-dimensional data (23, 24). Then, we developed a new scoring system, the SMRS. It showed a moderate performance in predicting 30-day mortality and risk-stratifying specifically for ICU patients with sepsis. To identify septic patients, an important strength of our study was the use of new sepsis-3 criteria, and this method would overcome some inherent weaknesses of using hospital discharge data (13, 15). The SMRS contains only 13 simple variables recorded in clinical routines. Therefore, if implemented, the SMRS will not require manual input of additional variables as the model is based on variables routinely collected [the frequently used SAPS II and APACHE IV scores for mortality prediction in the ICU required manually adding additional data (25)]. In the validation set, the discrimination of SMRS was comparable to APACHE IV and SAPS II and was significantly better than the SOFA.

For many years, various scoring systems have been widely used in the ICU, but the ability of general ICU severity scores is insufficient in accurately and reliably predicting mortality in the sepsis patient population. Arabi et al. evaluated four scoring systems in ICU patients with sepsis, reporting poor calibration for all four scores (10). Specifically, the SOFA score was proposed for the sepsis population, and a greater SOFA score was associated with a higher mortality rate (26). However, the SOFA score has several limitations, such as low mortality discrimination power

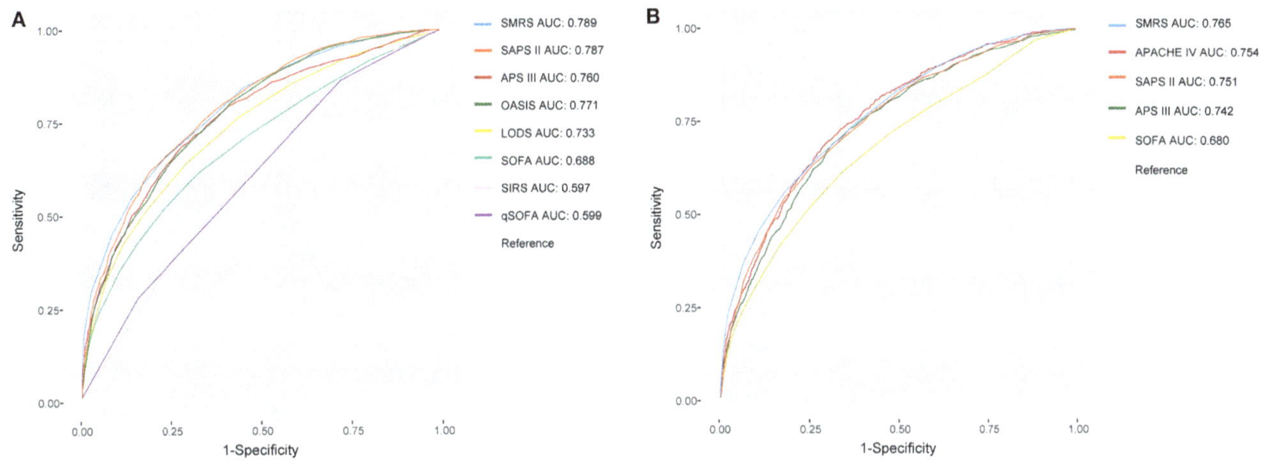


**FIGURE 2** | The ROC curves of SMRS and other severity scores. **(A)** Development set; **(B)** Validation set.

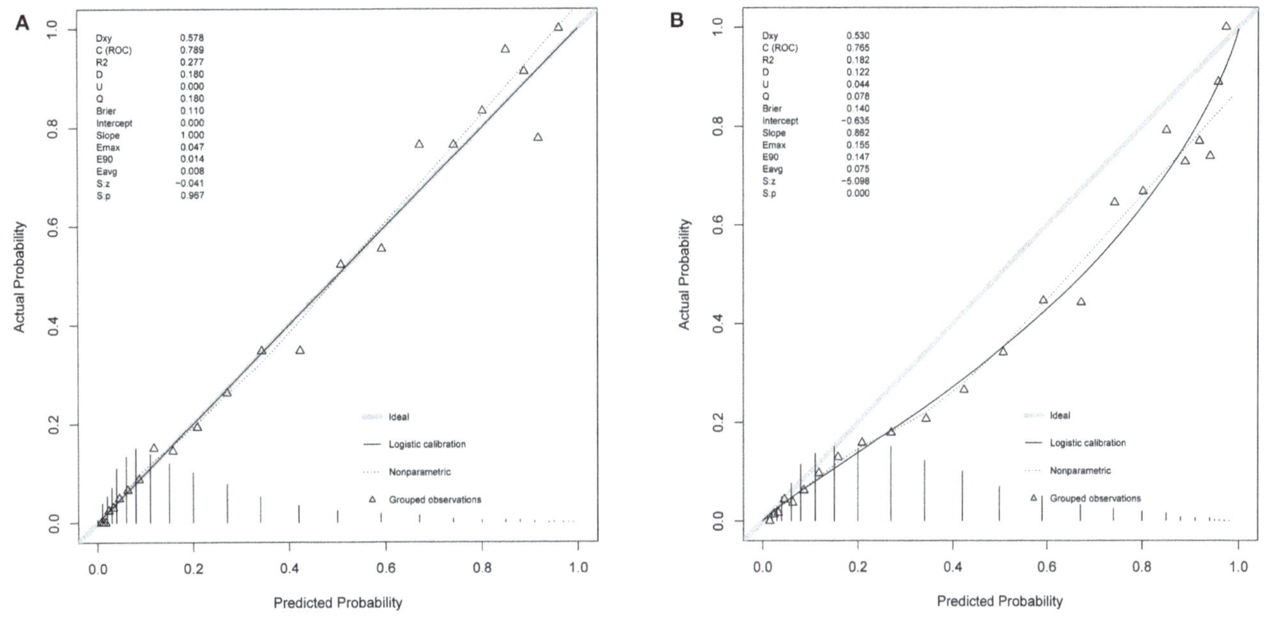


**FIGURE 3** | Calibration of SMRS. **(A)** Development set; **(B)** Validation set.

and limited number of variables (27). For predicting mortality in septic patients, the reported AUC of the initial SOFA score ranged from 0.69 to 0.83(28, 29). In our study, for predicting 30-day mortality, the SOFA score had a low discriminatory power (AUC: 0.69). Unlike other ICU severity scores, the SOFA score was developed to describe organ dysfunction and morbidity instead of mortality prediction, and some strong predictors for mortality were not included.

Therefore, specifically for the sepsis-3 population, we aimed at constructing a mortality risk score. For the 35 clinical features, 13 useful predictive features were finally identified using the LASSO method by examining the predictor–outcome association. A two-fold increase in the odds of death was observed in our model in patients requiring mechanical ventilation within the first 24 h of admission. This was because mechanical ventilation among septic patients was typically due to the concomitant acute respiratory distress syndrome, an early sign of poor clinical outcome in sepsis (6). Similarly, many studies have indicated that a strong predictor of mortality for septic patients is serum lactate (30, 31), which, however, was not included in existing risk scores. Since lactate measurement has become a clinical routine, we assigned three or six points to lactate in the final risk score. In our study and previous research, other variables such as hypothermia, hypotension, and advanced age were found to be associated with increased mortality (11, 13, 14, 32, 33).

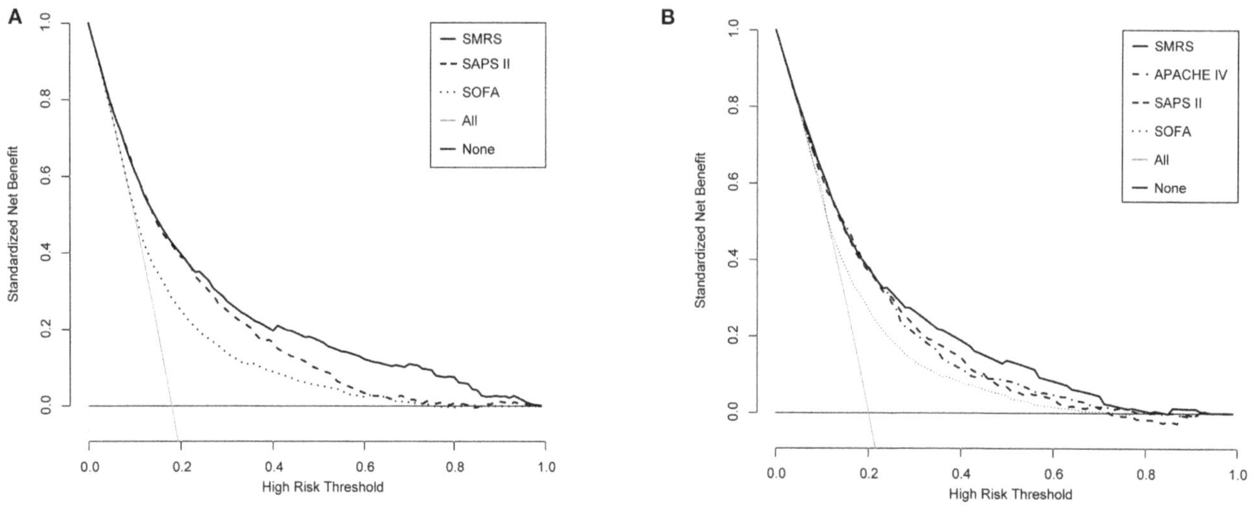


**FIGURE 4 |** Decision curve analysis of SMRS, SAPS II, SOFA, and APACHE IV. **(A)** Development set; **(B)** Validation set.

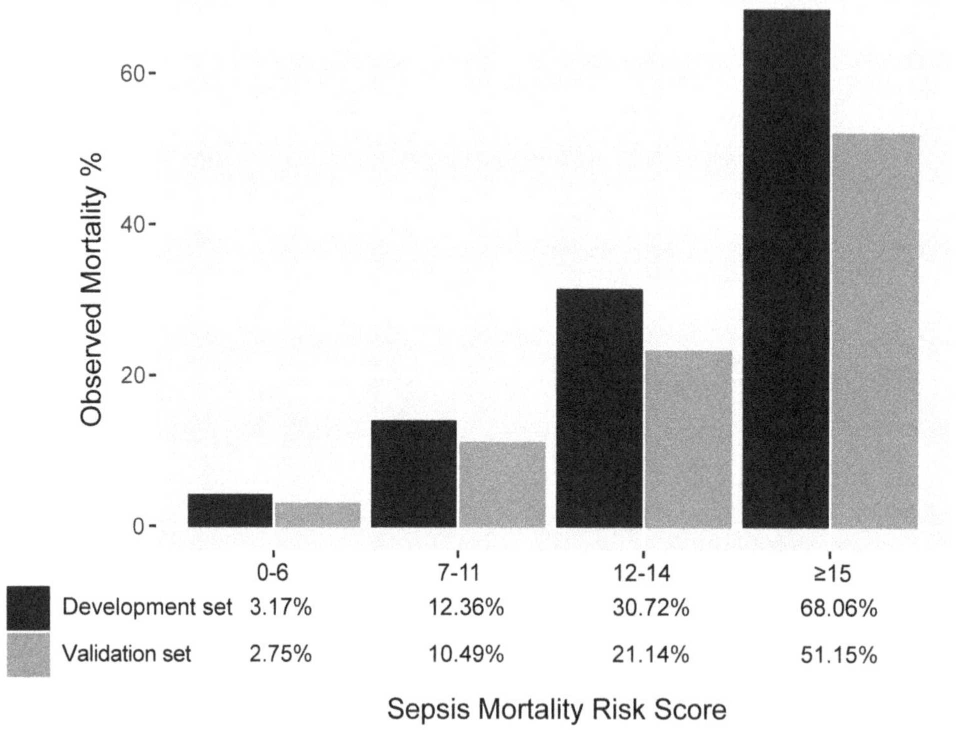


**FIGURE 5 |** Mortality risk groups according to SMRS.

The SMRS is simple for calculation and easy to use, and has robust discrimination and calibration. When we used SMRS to evaluate patients, DCA results indicated that 80% probability could be considered sufficient to assess mortality risk accurately. To predict the mortality risk of patients with sepsis, ICU physicians could use the SMRS and improve clinical decision-making at the bedside. Moreover, the predictor variables that we used were quite universally obtained in the emergency department (ED). After further validation and recalibration, the SMRS appeared to have the potential to help ED clinicians triage decisions and ICU placement.

In addition, machine learning techniques showed having high potentials to be used in the sepsis population. For predicting mortality among septic patients, the proposed models, particularly the XGBoost model, outperformed traditional scoring systems, including SAPS II and SOFA. However, even

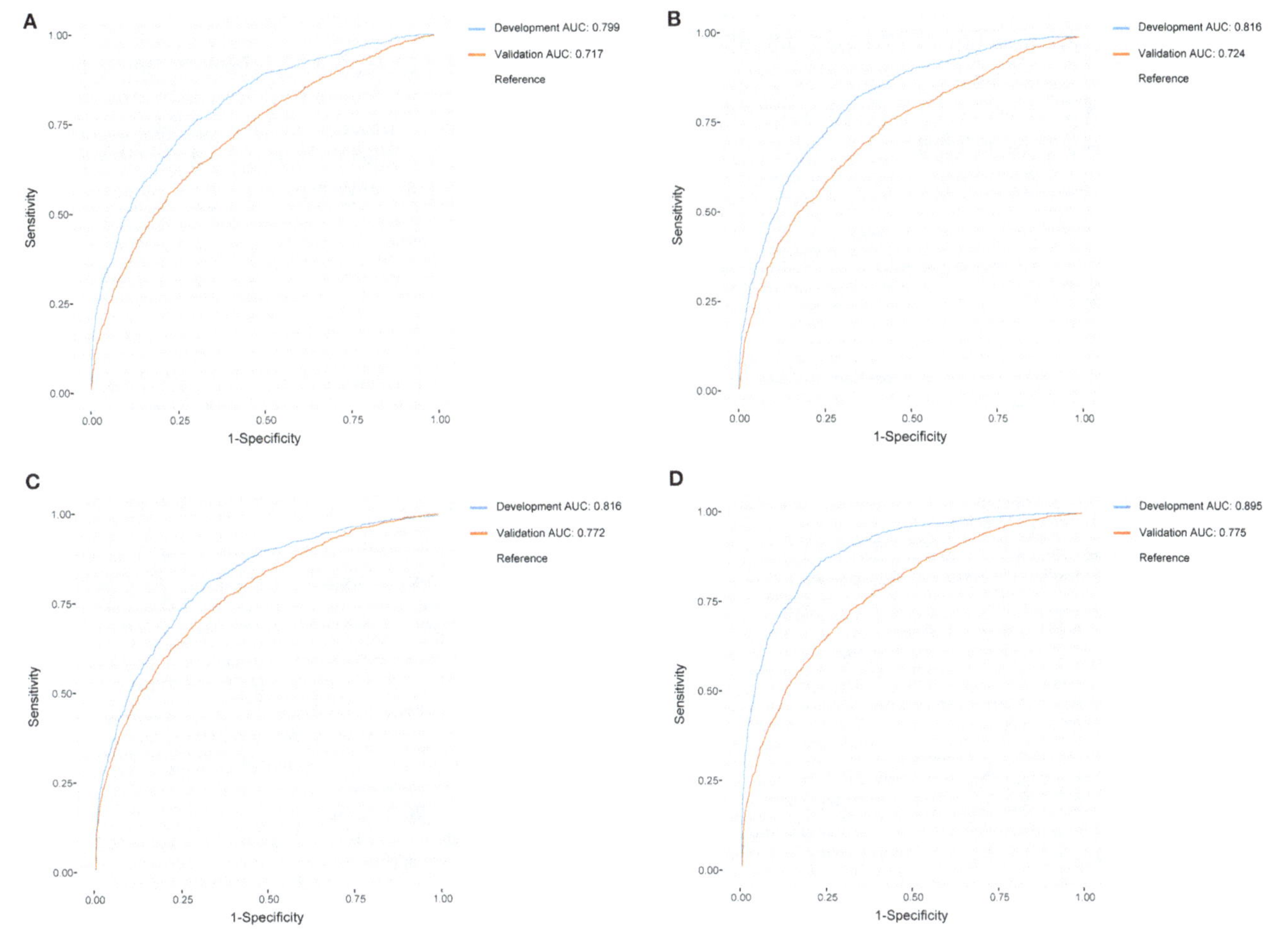


**FIGURE 6 |** The ROC curves of logistic regression model, MARS model, random forest model, XGBoost model. **(A)** Logistic regression model; **(B)** MARS model; **(C)** random forest model; **(D)** XGBoost model.

though machine learning models offer improved performance for predicting 30-day mortality, practical application in clinical practice has not always been straightforward. Among different populations, the applicability of machine learning models might be limited by heterogeneity (34). An external validation study is required to assess performance and ensure generalizability as the clinical implementation of models is currently scarce. Another major issue in the clinical application is the black-box problem (35, 36). Although these models had high accuracy, their utility has been critically limited due to difficulty in interpretation.

## LIMITATIONS

The study has the following limitations. First, we chose to analyze the patients admitted to the ICU with sepsis. There were certainly patients who had been diagnosed with sepsis before or after the ICU admission, but we limited our study population to those who fulfilled sepsis-3 criteria during their first ICU day. Second, we retrospectively identified the septic patient dataset for developing SMRS from a single-center and excluded some patients due to missing data. A few of the variables were also excluded for the same reason, but previous research has shown that they might be associated with septic patients' mortality (e.g., BMI, albumin) (37, 38). Third, in accordance with other severity scores, the timing of variable measurement was determined. If the sampling time was relatively late, the predictive accuracy improved because variables were measured close to the outcome's occurrence, but the timeliness of the prediction was compromised (39). Thus, the use of 24 h after ICU admission was a trade-off between timeliness and prediction accuracy. Furthermore, we conducted an external validation by using the data of 5,658 septic patients from the eICU database, and the results indicated that the calibration of SMRS was relatively poor with an overestimate of 30-day mortality. Finally, we prepared our data set for developing SMRS from 2008 to 2012, and the outcomes of septic patients could have changed over time due to the update of treatment guidclines and advances in treatment and diagnostic technology.

## CONCLUSION

The probability of septic patients' mortality could accurately be estimated by the SMRS, developed on 5,443 septic patients and validated on 5,658 patients. It is a simple score that can be applied in clinical practice. Therefore, further evaluation regarding its clinical application value is required. In the future, prospective validation and refining of our scoring system across diverse patient populations should be included.

## AUTHOR CONTRIBUTIONS

KZ and SZ conceived the idea, performed the analysis, and drafted the manuscript. WC and YH interpreted the results and helped to revise the manuscript. GZ and ZZ helped to frame the idea of the study and helped to analyze the data. All authors read and approved the final manuscript.

## REFERENCES


1. Singer M, Deutschman CS, Seymour CW, Shankar-Hari M, Annane D, Bauer M, et al. The third international consensus definitions for sepsis and septic shock (sepsis-3). *JAMA.* (2016) 315:801–10. doi: 10.1001/jama.2016.0287
2. Fleischmann C, Scherag A, Adhikari NK, Hartog CS, Tsaganos T, Schlattmann P, et al. Assessment of global incidence and mortality of hospital-treated sepsis current estimates and limitations. *Am J Resp Crit Care Med.* (2016) 193:259–72. doi: 10.1164/rccm.201504-0781OC
3. Rudd KE, Johnson SC, Agesa KM, Shackelford KA, Tsoi D, Kievlan DR, et al. Global, regional, and national sepsis incidence and mortality, 1990-2017: analysis for the global burden of disease study. *Lancet.* (2020) 395:200–11. doi: 10.1016/S0140-6736(19)32989-7
4. Vincent JL, Marshall JC, Namendys-Silva SA, Francois B, Martin-Loeches I, Lipman J, et al. Assessment of the worldwide burden of critical illness: the intensive care over nations (ICON) audit. *Lancet Resp Med.* (2014) 2:380–6. doi: 10.1016/S2213-2600(14)70061-X
5. Seymour CW, Gesten F, Prescott HC, Friedrich ME, Iwashyna TJ, Phillips GS, et al. Time to treatment and mortality during mandated emergency care for sepsis. *N Engl J Med.* (2017) 376:2235–44. doi: 10.1056/NEJMoa1703058
6. Rhodes A, Evans LE, Alhazzani W, Levy MM, Antonelli M, Ferrer R, et al. Surviving sepsis campaign: international guidelines for management of sepsis and septic shock: 2016. *Intensive Care Med.* (2017) 43:304–77. doi: 10.1007/s00134-017-4683-6
7. Vincent JL, Moreno R. Clinical review: scoring systems in the critically ill. *Critical Care.* (2010) 14:207. doi: 10.1186/cc8204
8. Huang CT, Ruan SY, Tsai YJ, Ku SC, Yu CJ. Clinical trajectories and causes of death in septic patients with a low apache II score. *J Clin Med.* (2019) 8:1064. doi: 10.3390/jcm8071064
9. Nassar AP Jr, Mocelin AO, Nunes AL, Giannini FP, Brauer L, et al. Caution when using prognostic models: a prospective comparison of 3 recent prognostic models. *J Critical Care.* (2012) 27:423.e421–7. doi: 10.1016/j.jcrc.2011.08.016
10. Arabi Y, Al Shirawi N, Memish Z, Venkatesh S, Al-Shimemeri A. Assessment of six mortality prediction models in patients admitted with severe sepsis and septic shock to the intensive care unit: a prospective cohort study. *Critical Care.* (2003) 7:R116–22. doi: 10.1186/cc2373
11. Phillips GS, Osborn TM, Terry KM, Gesten F, Levy MM, Lemeshow S. The New York sepsis severity score: development of a risk-adjusted severity model for sepsis. *Crit Care Med.* (2018) 46:674–83. doi: 10.1097/CCM.0000000000002824
12. Zhang Z, Hong Y. Development of a novel score for the prediction of hospital mortality in patients with severe sepsis: the use of electronic healthcare records with LASSO regression. *Oncotarget.* (2017) 8:49637–45. doi: 10.18632/oncotarget.17870
13. Ford DW, Goodwin AJ, Simpson AN, Johnson E, Nadig N, Simpson KN. A severe sepsis mortality prediction model and score for use with administrative data. *Crit Care Med.* (2016) 44:319–27. doi: 10.1097/CCM.0000000000001392
14. Osborn TM, Phillips G, Lemeshow S, Townsend S, Schorr CA, Levy MM, et al. Sepsis severity score: an internationally derived scoring system from the surviving sepsis campaign database*. *Crit Care Med.* (2014) 42:1969–76. doi: 10.1097/CCM.0000000000000416
15. Johnson AEW, Aboab J, Raffa JD, Pollard TJ, Deliberato RO, Celi LA, et al. A comparative analysis of sepsis identification methods in an electronic database. *Crit Care Med.* (2018) 46:494–9. doi: 10.1097/CCM.0000000000002965
16. Johnson AE, Pollard TJ, Shen L, Lehman LW, Feng M, Ghassemi M, et al. MIMIC-III, a freely accessible critical care database. *Sci Data.* (2016) 3:160035. doi: 10.1038/sdata.2016.35
17. Pollard TJ, Johnson AEW, Raffa JD, Celi LA, Mark RG, Badawi O. The eICU collaborative research database, a freely available multi-center database for critical care research. *Sci Data.* (2018) 5:180178. doi: 10.1038/sdata.2018.178
18. Austin PC, Steyerberg EW. Events per variable (EPV) and the relative performance of different strategies for estimating the out-of-sample validity of logistic regression models. *Stat Methods Med Res.* (2017) 26:796–808. doi: 10.1177/0962280214558972
19. Tibshirani R. Regression shrinkage selection via the LASSO. *J Royal Statist Soc B.* (1996) 58:267–88. doi: 10.1111/j.2517-6161.1996.tb02080.x
20. Riley RD, Ensor J, Snell KI, Debray TP, Altman DG, Moons KG, et al. External validation of clinical prediction models using big datasets from e-health records or IPD meta-analysis: opportunities and challenges. *BMJ.* (2016) 353:i3140. doi: 10.1136/bmj.i3140
21. Vickers AJ, Elkin EB. Decision curve analysis: a novel method for evaluating prediction models. *Med Decis Making.* (2006) 26:565–74. doi: 10.1177/0272989X06295361
22. Collins GS, Reitsma JB, Altman DG, Moons KG. Transparent reporting of a multivariable prediction model for individual prognosis or diagnosis (TRIPOD): the TRIPOD statement. *BMJ.* (2015) 350:g7594. doi: 10.1136/bmj.g7594
23. Sauerbrei W, Royston P, Binder H. Selection of important variables and determination of functional form for continuous predictors in multivariable model building. *Stat Med.* (2007) 26:5512–28. doi: 10.1002/sim.3148
24. Huang YQ, Liang CH, He L, Tian J, Liang CS, Chen X, et al. Development and validation of a radiomics nomogram for preoperative prediction of lymph node metastasis in colorectal cancer. *J Clin Oncol.* (2016) 34:2157–64. doi: 10.1200/JCO.2015.65.9128
25. Meyer A, Zverinski D, Pfahringer B, Kempfert J, Kuehne T, Sündermann SH, et al. Machine learning for real-time prediction of complications in critical care: a retrospective study. *Lancet Respir Med.* (2018) 6:905–14. doi: 10.1016/S2213-2600(18)30300-X
26. Vincent JL, Moreno R, Takala J, Willatts S, De Mendonca A, Bruining H, et al. The SOFA (Sepsis-related Organ Failure Assessment) score to describe organ dysfunction/failure on behalf of the working group on sepsis-related problems of the European society of intensive care medicine. *Intensive care Med.* (1996) 22:707–10. doi: 10.1007/BF01709751
27. Zygun DA, Laupland KB, Fick GH, Sandham JD, Doig CJ. Limited ability of SOFA and MOD scores to discriminate outcome: a prospective evaluation in 1,436 patients. *Canad J Anaesthesia.* (2005) 52:302–8. doi: 10.1007/BF03016068
28. Cheng B, Li Z, Wang J, Xie G, Liu X, Xu Z, et al. Comparison of the performance between sepsis-1 and sepsis-3 in ICUs in China: a retrospective multicenter study. *Shock.* (2017) 48:301–6. doi: 10.1097/SHK.0000000000000868
29. Khwannimit B, Bhurayanontachai R, Vattanavanit V. Comparison of the performance of SOFA, qSOFA and SIRS for predicting mortality and organ failure among sepsis patients admitted to the intensive care unit in a middle-income country. *J Crit Care.* (2018) 44:156–60. doi: 10.1016/j.jcrc.2017.10.023

30. Houwink AP, Rijkenberg S, Bosman RJ, van der Voort PH. The association between lactate, mean arterial pressure, central venous oxygen saturation and peripheral temperature and mortality in severe sepsis: a retrospective cohort analysis. *Crit Care.* (2016) 20:56. doi: 10.1186/s13054-016-1243-3
31. Liu Z, Meng Z, Li Y, Zhao J, Wu S, Gou S, et al. Prognostic accuracy of the serum lactate level, the SOFA score and the qSOFA score for mortality among adults with Sepsis. *Scand J Trauma Resusc Emerg Med.* (2019) 27:51. doi: 10.1186/s13049-019-0609-3
32. Kushimoto S, Gando S, Saitoh D, Mayumi T, Ogura H, Fujishima S, et al. The impact of body temperature abnormalities on the disease severity and outcome in patients with severe sepsis: an analysis from a multicenter, prospective survey of severe sepsis. *Crit Care.* (2013) 17:R271. doi: 10.1186/cc13106
33. Shapiro NI, Wolfe RE, Moore RB, Smith E, Burdick E, Bates DW. Mortality in Emergency Department Sepsis (MEDS) score: a prospectively derived and validated clinical prediction rule. *Crit Care Med.* (2003) 31:670–5. doi: 10.1097/01.CCM.0000054867.01688.D1
34. Liu VX, Walkey AJ. Machine learning and sepsis: on the road to revolution. *Crit Care Med.* (2017) 45:1946–7. doi: 10.1097/CCM.0000000000002673
35. Cabitza F, Rasoini R, Gensini GF. Unintended consequences of machine learning in medicine. *JAMA.* (2017) 318:517–8. doi: 10.1001/jama.2017.7797
36. Zhang Z, Beck MW, Winkler DA, Huang B, Sibanda W, Goyal H. Opening the black box of neural networks: methods for interpreting neural network models in clinical applications. *Ann Trans Med.* (2018) 6:216. doi: 10.21037/atm.2018.05.32
37. Li S, Hu X, Xu J, Huang F, Guo Z, Tong L, et al. Increased body mass index linked to greater short- and long-term survival in sepsis patients: A retrospective analysis of a large clinical database. *Int J Infect Dis.* (2019) 87:109–16. doi: 10.1016/j.ijid.2019.07.018
38. Shin J, Hwang SY, Jo IJ, Kim WY, Ryoo SM, Kang GH, et al. Prognostic value of the lactate/albumin ratio for predicting 28-day mortality in critically ILL sepsis patients. *Shock.* (2018) 50:545–50. doi: 10.1097/SHK.0000000000001128
39. Nemati S, Holder A, Razmi F, Stanley MD, Clifford GD, Buchman TG. An interpretable machine learning model for accurate prediction of sepsis in the ICU. *Crit Care Med.* (2018) 46:547–53. doi: 10.1097/CCM.0000000000002936

# Development of a Nomogram to Predict 28-Day Mortality of Patients with Sepsis-Induced Coagulopathy: An Analysis of the MIMIC-III Database

*Zongqing Lu*[1,2†], *Jin Zhang*[1,2†], *Jianchao Hong*[1,2], *Jiatian Wu*[1,2], *Yu Liu*[3], *Wenyan Xiao*[1,2], *Tianfeng Hua*[1,2] *and Min Yang*[1,2*]

[1] The 2nd Department of Intensive Care Unit, The Second Affiliated Hospital of Anhui Medical University, Hefei, China, [2] The Laboratory of Cardiopulmonary Resuscitation and Critical Care Medicine, The Second Affiliated Hospital of Anhui Medical University, Hefei, China, [3] Key Laboratory of Intelligent Computing & Signal Processing, Ministry of Education, Anhui University, Hefei, China

***Correspondence:**
Min Yang
512130761@qq.com

† These authors have contributed equally to this work

**Background:** Sepsis-induced coagulopathy (SIC) is a common cause for inducing poor prognosis of critically ill patients in intensive care unit (ICU). However, currently there are no tools specifically designed for assessing short-term mortality in SIC patients. This study aimed to develop a practical nomogram to predict the risk of 28-day mortality in SIC patients.

**Methods:** In this retrospective cohort study, we extracted patients from the Medical Information Mart for Intensive Care III (MIMIC-III) database. Sepsis was defined based on Sepsis 3.0 criteria and SIC based on Toshiaki Iba's criteria. Kaplan–Meier curves were plotted to compare the short survival time between SIC and non-SIC patients. Afterward, only SIC cohort was randomly divided into training or validation set. We employed univariate logistic regression and stepwise multivariate analysis to select predictive features. The proposed nomogram was developed based on multivariate logistic regression model, and the discrimination and calibration were verified by internal validation. We then compared model discrimination with other traditional severity scores and machine learning models.

**Results:** 9432 sepsis patients in MIMIC III were enrolled, in which 3280 (34.8%) patients were diagnosed as SIC during the first ICU admission. SIC was independently associated with the 7- and 28-day mortality of ICU patients. K–M curve indicated a significant difference in 7-day (Log-Rank: $P < 0.001$ and $P = 0.017$) and 28-day survival (Log-Rank: $P < 0.001$ and $P < 0.001$) between SIC and non-SIC groups whether the propensity score match (PSM) was balanced or not. For nomogram development, a total of thirteen variables of 3,280 SIC patients were enrolled. When predicted the risk of 28-day mortality, the nomogram performed a good discrimination in training and validation sets (AUROC: 0.78 and 0.81). The AUROC values were 0.80, 0.81, 0.71, 0.70, 0.74, and 0.60 for random forest, support vector machine, sequential organ failure assessment (SOFA) score, logistic organ dysfunction score (LODS), simplified acute physiology II score (SAPS

II) and SIC score, respectively, in validation set. And the nomogram calibration slope was 0.91, the Brier value was 0.15. As presented by the decision curve analyses, the nomogram always obtained more net benefit when compared with other severity scores.

**Conclusions:** SIC is independently related to the short-term mortality of ICU patients. The nomogram achieved an optimal prediction of 28-day mortality in SIC patient, which can lead to a better prognostics assessment. However, the discriminative ability of the nomogram requires validation in external cohorts to further improve generalizability.

**Keywords: sepsis-induced coagulopathy, logistic regression, short-time mortality, nomogram, MIMIC-III database, prediction of prognosis**

## INTRODUCTION

Sepsis, defined as a dysregulated host response to infection by the Surviving Sepsis Campaign 2016 guideline, remains the leading cause of life-threatening organ dysfunction in the intensive care unit (ICU) (1). Sepsis is rapidly becoming a significant global health burden. The World Health Organization declared that the mortality of hospital-treated adult patients with sepsis is ~189 per 100,000 person-years, and such a rate has been reported in up to 42% or even higher of ICUs depending on its severity in patients (2).

Coagulation abnormalities, as a severe complication, occur in almost all sepsis patients (3). The clinical manifestations of such abnormalities range from thrombocytopenia during the initial phase to advanced disseminated intravascular coagulation, with the latter always leading to multiple organ dysfunction syndromes (MODS) and indicates higher mortality (4). Coagulation abnormality in sepsis patients with a increased international normalized ratio (INR) and reduced platelet count is termed sepsis-induced coagulopathy (SIC) (5). Previous multicenter retrospective observational trials demonstrated that SIC is significantly associated with poor prognosis (6–8). Because SIC is a dynamic process, applying specific interventions based on stratifying SIC patients according to their mortality risks would provide improved strategies to prevent MODS. However, methods to calculate the mortality probability are rarely applied in clinical practice.

Recently, using the logistic regression model, a retrospective analysis of a nationwide study in Japan developed a SIC scoring system in which the platelet count, prothrombin time (PT)-INR and sequential organ failure assessment (SOFA) scores are associated with the 28-day mortality level of sepsis patients (9). Subsequent clinical investigations have shown the value of the SIC score system, for example, with a higher sensitivity (~84.4–96.1) in the prediction of the 28-day mortality of SIC patients compared with the International Society on Thrombosis and Haemostasis (ISTH) scoring system (10). Conversely, another published study demonstrated a smaller area under the curve (AUC) of the SIC system (~0.658) in predicting ICU mortality when compared with the SOFA, Acute Physiologic And Chronic Health Evaluation II (APACHE II) and ISTH scores (11). Therefore, the performances of the SIC scoring system in predicting the prognosis of SIC patients are inconsistent. Furthermore, because the highest total points of the SIC scoring system is six, the correlation between such points and critical patients' outcomes may be ambiguous. Because of the suboptimal performance of existing methods, it is necessary to develop a novel prediction model for the subgroup combined with SIC.

The nomogram as a visualization tool has been widely used in clinical prognosis research on critical patient and cancer patient survival studies (12–14). The primary aim of the present study is to develop a novel prediction nomogram for the 28-day mortality risk in SIC patients. The secondary aim is to explore the differences in the clinical characteristics between SIC and non-SIC patients, and verify whether SIC poses a short-term mortality risk for patients in the ICU.

## METHODS

### Source of Data

An open and free critical care database, which contained comprehensive clinical data of patients admitted to the Beth Israel Deaconess Medical Center in Boston, Massachusetts between June 2001 and October 2012, termed the Medical Information Mart for Intensive Care (MIMIC)-III v 1.4, was retrieved (15). This database was released on 2nd September 2016, in which extensive and de-identified in-hospital information of over 40,000 patients was included. All data were classified into 26 tables, consisting of demographic characteristics, vital signs, laboratory test results, imaging examinations, and a data dictionary. Included patients were assigned a special code on each hospital and ICU admission, thus we could relate each table using these codes to obtain a complete hospitalization record. Hospital staff entered the final precise diagnosis according to the International Classification of Disease 9th Edition code when patients were discharged. In the present study included datasets were extracted by Lu, who had completed the collaborative institution training initiative program course (Record ID: 36763801). Because the present study was conducted using an anonymized public database that satisfied review committee agreements, the requirement for ethical consent was not necessary. Rather, the TRIPOD statement was applied in the present study (16).

## Study Population and Data Extraction

### Sepsis

The following data were extracted from the MIMIC-III database: (1) demographic data; (2) first care unit; (3) outcomes, including ICU stay time, 7-day mortality, 28-day mortality, hospital mortality; (4) severity score, including SOFA and logistic organ dysfunction (LODS) score; (5) mean value of vital signs and the poorest laboratory test value during the first day after ICU admission; (6) infectious sites defined using PgAdmin software (version 4.1, Bedford, MA, USA). We retrieved adult sepsis patients (≥18 years) as defined according to the Sepsis-3.0 criterion: (1) existing evidence of suspected or confirmed infection; (2) SOFA score ≥2 (17). Exclusion criteria were: (1) age <18 years; (2) pregnant women; (3) patients with congenital coagulopathy; (4) the coagulation function was frequently affected by the pathologic states of tumors and the chemotherapy agent used, thus patients with various cancer types were excluded; (5) patients who died or were discharged within 24 h after ICU admission (**Supplementary Figure 1**).

### Sepsis-Induced Coagulopathy

On the basis of all eligible sepsis patients, SIC patients were defined as fulfilling the Toshiaki Iba's criteria, also referred to as the Sepsis-induced coagulopathy scoring system (9). Patients were considered to display SIC when having a total SIC score ≥4 with a total score of PT-INR and platelet count parameters >2 during the first day of ICU admission. Afterwards, the parameters of the eligible SIC patients were applied in the logistic regression to construct the proposed prediction model. The flowchart of study design and data extraction can be found in **Supplementary Figure 1**.

## Statistical Analysis

Normal distributions were confirmed by Agostino tests. Continuous variables are presented as the mean (standard deviation) for parametric variables and as the median (interquartile ranges) for non-parametric variables. Continuous variables were compared by unpaired Student's test or Mann–Whitney *U*-test. Categorical variables were compared using the $\chi^2$-test or Fisher exact test.

Both, the 7- and 28-day survival curves were generated using the Kaplan–Meier method and compared by the log-rank test. To resolve the baseline imbalance problem, the sample was performed using the propensity score match (PSM), and we further explored the difference in short survival time between the SIC and non-SIC patients.

Prior to construction of the nomogram, only SIC patients were randomly assigned to the training or validation cohort based on a ratio of 7:3. In the training cohort, all significant variables associated with the 28-day mortality through univariate logistic regression analysis were candidates for stepwise multivariate analysis. Although these variables were clinically associated with the 28-day mortality, they were not statistically significant; however, they were still included. Besides, those categorical variables in which a set of meaningful values existed were also included. The variance inflation factor (VIF) was calculated to detect the potential collinearity between continuous variables. When the arithmetic square root of the VIF was >2, collinearity was considered to exist and it will be solved by regularization. Stepwise backward regression was conducted according to the Akaike information criterion (AIC), and the best model should achieve a minimum AIC value. Subsequently, the nomogram was plotted using the "rms" package of R software based on the results of multivariate logistic regression. Finally, the predictive performance of the nomogram was evaluated using a calibration with 1,000 bootstrap resampling, and measured using the C-index.

For the clinical use of this model, both receiver operating characteristic (ROC) and decision curve analysis (DCA) were conducted to compare the performance of the SOFA, LODS, SAPS II, and SIC scores with the nomogram. The integrated discrimination improvement (IDI) and net reclassification improvement (NRI) indices of each clinical severity scoring system were also calculated. Furthermore, other common machine-learning models, including random forests (RF) and the support vector machine (SVM), were constructed to compare the generalizability and accuracy of each model.

All statistical analyses were performed using STATA 15.1 (College Station, Texas) and R 3.6.2 (Chicago, Illinois) software. Missing values were handled by the RF method, based on the "randomForest" package of R. However, these variables were omitted when >30% of the values were lacking. $P < 0.05$ was considered to indicate statistical significance.

# RESULTS

## Characteristics of Included Sepsis Participants

A total of 9,432 sepsis patients were included, of whom 34.8% were SIC patients. The baseline characteristics are listed in **Table 1**. The SIC patients with a median age of 67 (54, 79) years were younger than the non-SIC patients of 72 (58, 82) years. Regarding comorbidity, we unexpectedly found that the SIC patients were less likely to suffer from hypertension, chronic obstructive pulmonary disease (COPD), diabetes and myocardial infarction, but not liver disease, when compared with the non-SIC patients. However, the SIC patients displayed higher lactate-max, creatinine-max, and blood urea nitrogen-max levels, INR-max, PT-max, mean corpuscular volume-min (MCV-min), and red cell distribution width-max (RDW-max) and lower platelet levels, $PO_2$-min as well as serum PH-min value in the first 24 h since ICU admission. Additionally, there was a statistical difference in the length of the ICU stay ($P < 0.001$), 7-day ($P < 0.001$), 28-day ($P < 0.001$), and hospital mortalities ($P < 0.001$) between the SIC and non-SIC patients, and the SIC patients had a higher critical illness score, including the SOFA, LODS and SAPS II. Finally, the SIC patients exhibited a higher frequency of epinephrine and/or norepinephrine administration.

## SIC Was Independently Associated With the 7-day and 28-day Mortalities of Sepsis Patients

The result of multivariate logistic regression showed that SIC was an independent risk factor for the 7- and 28-day mortalities of the included patients, with an adjusted odds ratio of 1.52

**TABLE 1** | The characteristics of included patients when first ICU admission.

| Variables | All patients ($n$ = 9432) | Non-SIC patients ($n$ = 6152) | SIC patients ($n$ = 3280) | $p$ |
|---|---|---|---|---|
| **Gender, $n$ (%)** | | | | < 0.001 |
| Male | 5,070 (54) | 3,111 (51) | 1,959 (60) | |
| Female | 4,362 (46) | 3,041 (49) | 1,321 (40) | |
| Age, years | 69.90 (56.38, 80.85) | 71.54 (58.18, 81.86) | 66.93 (53.52, 79.08) | < 0.001 |
| **First care unit, $n$ (%)** | | | | < 0.001 |
| CCU | 1,229 (13) | 914 (15) | 315 (10) | |
| CSRU | 813 (9) | 419 (7) | 394 (12) | |
| MICU | 5,158 (55) | 3,324 (54) | 1,834 (56) | |
| SICU | 1,323 (14) | 885 (14) | 438 (13) | |
| TSICU | 909 (10) | 610 (10) | 299 (9) | |
| **Outcome** | | | | |
| ICU stay time, days | 4.04 (1.92, 9.25) | 3.92 (1.92, 8.92) | 4.21 (1.96, 10.04) | < 0.001 |
| 7-day mortality, $n$ (%) | 1,332 (14) | 756 (12) | 576 (18) | < 0.001 |
| 28-day mortality, $n$ (%) | 2,669 (28) | 1,555 (25) | 1,114 (34) | < 0.001 |
| Hospital mortality, $n$ (%) | 2,452 (26) | 1,380 (22) | 1,072 (33) | < 0.001 |
| **Comorbidity, $n$ (%)** | | | | |
| Hypertension, $n$ (%) | 3,388 (36) | 2,348 (38) | 1,040 (32) | < 0.001 |
| COPD, $n$ (%) | 446 (5) | 376 (6) | 70 (2) | < 0.001 |
| Diabetes, $n$ (%) | 2,819 (30) | 1,949 (32) | 870 (27) | < 0.001 |
| MI, $n$ (%) | 320 (3) | 238 (4) | 82 (2) | < 0.001 |
| CHF, $n$ (%) | 316 (3) | 225 (4) | 91 (3) | 0.027 |
| Cardiac arrhythmias, $n$ (%) | 3,317 (35) | 2,193 (36) | 1,124 (34) | 0.189 |
| Liver disease, $n$ (%) | 1,118 (12) | 338 (5) | 780 (24) | < 0.001 |
| **Severity score** | | | | |
| SOFA | 5.00 (4.00, 8.00) | 5.00 (3.00, 7.00) | 7.00 (5.00, 10.00) | < 0.001 |
| LODS | 5.00 (3.00, 7.00) | 5.00 (3.00, 7.00) | 6.00 (4.00, 8.00) | < 0.001 |
| SAPS II | 42.00 (33.00, 52.00) | 41.00 (32.00, 51.00) | 44.00 (35.00, 55.00) | < 0.001 |
| **Vital signs**[a] | | | | |
| Mean heartrate, ($min^{-1}$) | 87.49 (77.33, 98.93) | 86.82 (76.50, 97.85) | 88.93 (79.08, 101.47) | < 0.001 |
| MAP, (mmHg) | 75.03 (68.81, 81.22) | 75.48 (69.05, 81.83) | 74.18 (68.29, 80.07) | < 0.001 |
| Mean resprate, ($min^{-1}$) | 19.56 (17.10, 22.42) | 19.54 (17.17, 22.29) | 19.62 (16.95, 22.75) | 0.528 |
| Mean temperature, (°C) | 36.86 (36.44, 37.28) | 36.88 (36.47, 37.29) | 36.83 (36.40, 37.25) | < 0.001 |
| **Laboratory tests**[b] | | | | |
| Mean glucose, (mg/dl) | 137.50 (115.00, 161.67) | 138.40 (116.00, 163.50) | 135.27 (112.49, 158.76) | < 0.001 |
| Aniongap_max, | 16.00 (14.00, 19.00) | 16.00 (14.00, 19.00) | 16.00 (14.00, 20.00) | 0.133 |
| Bicarbonate_min, (mEq/L) | 21.00 (18.00, 24.00) | 22.00 (19.00, 25.00) | 20.00 (17.00, 23.00) | < 0.001 |
| Chloride_max, (mEq/L) | 107.00 (103.00, 112.00) | 107.00 (103.00, 111.00) | 109.00 (104.00, 113.00) | < 0.001 |
| Hematocrit_min, (%) | 29.00 (25.30, 33.30) | 30.00 (26.70, 34.10) | 26.80 (23.00, 31.10) | < 0.001 |
| Hemoglobin_min, (g/dL) | 9.80 (8.50, 11.20) | 10.10 (8.90, 11.50) | 9.10 (7.90, 10.60) | < 0.001 |
| Lactate_max, (mmol/L) | 2.63 (1.80, 3.60) | 2.50 (1.70, 3.16) | 3.00 (2.20, 4.80) | < 0.001 |
| Lowest platelet level, (K/uL) | 176.00 (112.00, 247.00) | 221.00 (179.00, 289.00) | 93.00 (60.00, 121.00) | < 0.001 |
| Potassium_max, (K/uL) | 4.50 (4.10, 5.10) | 4.50 (4.10, 5.10) | 4.60 (4.10, 5.30) | < 0.001 |
| PTT_max, (s) | 36.10 (28.90, 48.80) | 33.20 (27.60, 44.00) | 40.70 (32.90, 58.82) | < 0.001 |
| INR_max, | 1.40 (1.20, 1.80) | 1.30 (1.20, 1.60) | 1.64 (1.40, 2.20) | < 0.001 |
| PT_max, (s) | 15.31 (13.70, 18.40) | 14.60 (13.30, 16.80) | 16.90 (15.00, 21.00) | < 0.001 |
| Sodium_min, (mEq/L) | 137.00 (134.00, 140.00) | 137.00 (134.00, 140.00) | 136.00 (133.00, 139.00) | < 0.001 |
| BUN_max, (mg/dL) | 28.00 (18.00, 47.00) | 28.00 (18.00, 45.00) | 30.50 (19.00, 50.00) | < 0.001 |
| WBC_max, (K/uL) | 13.40 (9.40, 18.70) | 14.00 (10.20, 19.30) | 11.90 (7.70, 17.60) | < 0.001 |
| Po2-min, (mmHg) | 89.34 (68.00, 104.06) | 91.00 (70.00, 105.05) | 86.48 (67.00, 102.12) | < 0.001 |
| Pco2-max, (mmHg) | 46.08 (40.00, 51.00) | 46.95 (40.00, 51.11) | 45.45 (39.00, 50.00) | < 0.001 |

*(Continued)*

**TABLE 1** | Continued

| Variables | All patients ($n$ = 9432) | Non-SIC patients ($n$ = 6152) | SIC patients ($n$ = 3280) | $p$ |
|---|---|---|---|---|
| PH-min | 7.31 (7.26, 7.37) | 7.32 (7.27, 7.37) | 7.31 (7.23, 7.36) | < 0.001 |
| MCH_min, (pg) | 30.10 (28.80, 31.50) | 29.90 (28.50, 31.13) | 30.50 (29.30, 32.10) | < 0.001 |
| MCHC_min, (g/L) | 33.30 (32.20, 34.20) | 33.10 (32.10, 34.00) | 33.50 (32.40, 34.50) | < 0.001 |
| RDW_max, (%) | 16.41 (15.32, 17.29) | 15.45 (14.76, 16.77) | 17.41 (16.30, 18.87) | < 0.001 |
| MCV_min, (fL) | 90.00 (86.00, 94.00) | 89.00 (86.00, 93.00) | 90.00 (86.00, 95.00) | < 0.001 |
| Creatinine_max, (μmol/L) | 114.92 (79.56, 194.48) | 114.92 (79.56, 185.64) | 123.76 (88.40, 212.16) | < 0.001 |
| **Infection site, *n* (%)** | | | | |
| Lung, *n* (%) | 3,440 (36) | 2,355 (38) | 1,085 (33) | < 0.001 |
| Urea, *n* (%) | 2,807 (30) | 1,923 (31) | 884 (27) | < 0.001 |
| Catheter, *n* (%) | 240 (3) | 153 (2) | 87 (3) | 0.676 |
| Bacteremia, *n* (%) | 612 (6) | 372 (6) | 240 (7) | 0.019 |
| Septicemic, *n* (%) | 120 (1) | 72 (1) | 48 (1) | 0.266 |
| **Treatment measures** | | | | |
| MV, *n* (%) | 2,493 (26) | 1,639 (27) | 854 (26) | 0.542 |
| Epinephrine, *n* (%) | 329 (3) | 156 (3) | 173 (5) | < 0.001 |
| Norepinephrine, *n* (%) | 2,076 (22) | 1,219 (20) | 857 (26) | < 0.001 |

*Categorical data were presented as frequency (percentage), parametric continuous data were presented as median (interquartile ranges), whereas non-parametric continuous data were presented as median (interquartile ranges).*
[a] *Vital signs were calculated as mean value during the first 24 h since ICU admission of each included patients.*
[b] *The laboratory tests recorded the worest value during the first 24 h since ICU admission of each included patients.*
*CCU, coronary care unit; CSRU, cardiac surgical intensive care unit; MICU, medical intensive care unit; SICU, surgical intensive care unit, TSICU, trauma/surgical intensive care unit; SOFA, Sequential Organ Failure Assessment; LODS, Logistic Organ Dysfunction System; SAPS II, Simplified acute physiology II; SAPS II, Simplified acute physiology; PT, Prothrombin Time; PTT, Partial Thromboplastin Time; INR, International Normalized Ratio; RDW, Red Blood Cell Distribution Widths; MV, Mechanical Ventilation; MAP, Mean arterial pressure.*

[95% confidence interval (CI): 1.35, 1.71] and 1.52 (95% CI: 1.39, 1.67), respectively, after adjusting for baseline characteristics, vital signs, critical illness score, infection sites, and treatment measures. Subsequently, we conducted a PSM between the SIC and non-SIC cohorts according to the differences in the vital signs, critical illness score, infection sites, treatment measures and comorbidities in first 24 h since ICU admission. Kaplan–Meier's survival analysis found significant differences between the SIC and non-SIC patients in the 7- and 28-day survival whether or not a PSM was performed (**Supplementary Figures 2, 3**).

## Development of a Prediction Nomogram

Only 3,280 SIC patients were randomly assigned to the training (2,293 patients) or validation sets (987 patients). The data of non-SIC patients were not suitable for subsequent model development, since the model was designed to predict the short-term death risk in SIC patients. All variables of the included participants in each set are presented in **Supplementary Table 1**. No statistical differences in all the variables were found between the training and validation sets, except for the creatinine-max. The results of the univariate logistic analysis using the training cohort are presented in **Table 2**.

Subsequently, a multivariate logistic regression was performed using variables with $p < 0.05$ in the univariate logistic analysis or those that had clinical significance or these categorical variables in which a set of meaningful values existed. However, the infection site and PH-min were omitted from the model, considering that it was difficult to determine the source of infection in the early stage of ICU admission and the PH value was affected by a variety of factors. Finally, we selected a total of 13 variables based on the AIC. The risk factors independently associated with the 28-day mortality of SIC identified by the multivariable analysis are presented in **Table 3**. Regarding collinearity, the VIF of all continuous variables in **Table 3** was <2, indicating that no collinearity existed in the regression analysis. Next, a model integrating age, combined with liver disease, mean arterial pressure (MAP), mean heart rate, mean respiratory rate, mean temperature, the administration of norepinephrine, lactate-max, PT-max, RDW-max, MCV-min, creatinine-max and lowest platelet level was established using the training set. On the basis of this model, a nomogram was plotted to predict the probability of the 28-day mortality of the SIC patients (**Figure 1**).

## Validation of the Prediction Nomogram

The nomogram demonstrated good accuracy for predicting the 28-day mortality of SIC patients, with an unadjusted C-index of 0.78 (95% CI: 0.76, 0.80). In the validation set, the nomogram displayed an unadjusted C-index of 0.81 (95% CI: 0.78, 0.84). The nomogram when compared with the SOFA, LODS, SAPS II, and SIC scores displayed an area under the receiver operating characteristic (AUROC) that was significantly higher in both sets. Furthermore, the RF and SVM models showed an excellent ability to distinguish the SIC patients who died during the 28 days since admission in the training cohort, but it declined sharply in the validation cohort (**Figure 2**).

The calibration curve was described using the bootstrap method for both, the training and validation sets (**Figure 3**). The

**TABLE 2 |** Factors independently associated with 28-day mortality of patients with SIC by univariate logistic regression analysis in training cohort.

| Variables | OR (95% CI) | *p*-value |
|---|---|---|
| Age, y | 1.01 (1.00, 1.02) | <0.001 |
| Liver-disease, yes vs. no | 1.58 (1.30, 1.93) | <0.001 |
| Cirrhosis, yes vs. no | 1.68 (1.28, 2.20) | <0.001 |
| Mean heart rate (min-1) | 1.02 (1.01, 1.02) | <0.001 |
| MAP (mmHg) | 0.97 (0.96, 0.98) | <0.001 |
| Mean respiratory rate (min$^{-1}$) | 1.08 (1.06, 1.10) | <0.001 |
| Mean temperature (°C) | 0.64 (0.56, 0.72) | <0.001 |
| Norepinephrine, yes vs. no | 2.54 (2.10, 3.08) | <0.001 |
| Lactate (mmol/L) | 1.15 (1.12, 1.19) | <0.001 |
| WBC_max (K/uL) | 1.00 (1.00, 1.01) | <0.001 |
| Potassium_max (K/uL) | 1.12 (1.03, 1.22) | 0.006 |
| INR_max | | |
| 1.2–1.4 vs. ≦1.2 | 0.80 (0.57, 1.11) | 0.176 |
| >1.4 vs. ≦1.2 | 1.47 (1.12, 1.96) | 0.006 |
| PT_max (s) | | |
| 15-18 vs. ≦15 | 0.94 (0.75, 1.20) | 0.641 |
| 18-21 vs. ≦15 | 1.47 (1.12, 1.94) | 0.006 |
| >21 vs. ≦15 | 2.41 (1.89, 3.07) | <0.001 |
| RDW_max (%) | 1.23 (1.19, 1.28) | <0.001 |
| MCV_min (fL) | 1.05 (1.04, 1.06) | <0.001 |
| Creatinine_max (μmol/L) | | |
| 110–170 vs. <110 | 1.43 (1.14, 1.80) | 0.002 |
| 171–299 vs. <110 | 1.89 (1.49, 2.41) | <0.001 |
| 300–440 vs. <110 | 2.94 (2.09, 4.14) | <0.001 |
| >440 vs. <110 | 2.10 (1.52, 2.89) | <0.001 |
| Lowest platelet level (K/uL) | 0.99 (0.98, 0.99) | <0.001 |

*PT, Prothrombin Time; INR, International Normalized Ratio; RDW, Red Blood Cell Distribution Widths; MCV, Mean Corpuscular Volume; MAP, Mean arterial pressure; OR, odds rate; CI, confidence interval.*

**TABLE 3 |** Factors independently associated with 28-day mortality of patients with SIC by multivariate logistic regression analysis in training cohort.

| Variables | $\beta^a$ | OR (95% CI) | *p*-values |
|---|---|---|---|
| Age, y | 0.03 | 1.03 (1.02, 1.04) | <0.001 |
| Liver-disease, yes vs. no | 0.23 | 1.26 (0.96, 1.65) | 0.091 |
| MAP (mmHg) | −0.01 | 0.99 (0.98, 1.00) | 0.033 |
| Mean heart rate (min$^{-1}$) | 0.02 | 1.02 (1.01, 1.03) | <0.001 |
| Mean respiratory rate (min$^{-1}$) | 0.06 | 1.06 (1.04, 1.10) | <0.001 |
| Mean temperature (°C) | −0.33 | 0.72 (0.62, 0.83) | <0.001 |
| Norepinephrine, yes vs. no | 0.73 | 2.07 (1.66, 2.57) | <0.001 |
| Lactate (mmol/L) | 0.08 | 1.11 (1.05, 1.12) | <0.001 |
| PT_max (s) | | | |
| 15-18 vs. ≦15 | −0.27 | 0.76 (0.58, 0.99) | 0.045 |
| 18-21 vs. ≦15 | −0.21 | 0.81 (0.58, 1.11) | 0.189 |
| >21 vs. ≦15 | 0.11 | 1.12 (083, 1.52) | 0.440 |
| RDW_max (%) | 0.16 | 1.18 (1.13, 1.23) | <0.001 |
| MCV_min (fL) | 0.04 | 1.04 (1.03, 1.06) | <0.001 |
| Lowest platelet level (K/uL) | −0.01 | 0.99 (0.98, 0.99) | <0.001 |
| Creatine_max (μmol/L) | | | |
| 110–170 vs. <110 | 0.13 | 1.14 (0.88, 1.48) | 0.312 |
| 171–299 vs. <110 | 0.11 | 1.12 (0.84, 1.48) | 0.453 |
| 300–440 vs. <110 | 0.46 | 1.59 (1.07, 2.35) | 0.022 |
| >440 vs. <110 | 0.41 | 1.50 (1.04, 2.16) | 0.030 |

*PT, Prothrombin Time; RDW, Red Blood Cell Distribution Widths; MCV, Mean Corpuscular Volume; MAP, Mean arterial pressure.*
*[a]Unstandardized β coefficients were calculated from the multivariate logistic regression model.*
*OR, odds rate; CI, confidence interval.*

apparent line and a bias-corrected line only slightly deviated from the ideal line, indicating a good agreement between the prediction and reality. The Brier score of the nomogram was 0.17 and 0.15 in the training and validation sets, respectively. The IDI and NRI indices of the nomogram were also significantly higher than those of the SOFA, LODS, SAPS II, and SIC scores in both sets, as shown in **Table 4**, which indicated that this nomogram had a better prediction probability in 28-day mortality prediction.

## Clinical Use of the Nomogram

The DCA curve was plotted to perform a clinical application of this nomogram, and compared with other clinical severity scoring systems. In the training set, clinical intervention guided by this nomogram provided a greater net benefit when the threshold probability was within 0.1 and 0.9 (**Figure 4A**). In the validation set, the analysis indicated that when the threshold probability was >0.15, using this nomogram to predict the 28-day mortality of SIC patients could provide a greater net benefit than the SOFA, LODS, and SAPS II (**Figure 4B**). However, we found that the SIC score performed the worst. When the threshold probability was >0.45, the DCA curve of the SIC score overlapped with the horizontal line.

On the basis of the DCA, the clinical impact curve for this nomogram is presented (**Supplementary Figure 4**). In both sets, the red solid curve (number of high-risk individuals) represented the number of patients classified as high risk by this nomogram under each risk threshold of 1,000 patients, and the blue dashed curve (number of high-risk individuals with outcome) showed the number of true positive patients under each risk threshold.

## Risk of 28-day Mortality Based on the Nomogram Scores

The results showed that this nomogram is a good predictive model, with high sensitivity, specificity, positive predictive value, and negative predictive value in recognizing whether the patients survived or were deceased after 28 days since ICU admission, with 0.70 (95% CI: 0.67, 0.73), 0.74 (95% CI: 0.71, 0.76), 0.58 (95% CI: 0.55, 0.62) and 0.83 (95% CI: 0.80, 0.84) in the training set, and 0.78 (95% CI: 0.74, 0.83), 0.69 (95% CI: 0.65, 0.72), 0.56 (95% CI: 0.52, 0.63), and 0.86 (95% CI: 0.83, 0.88) in the validation set, respectively (**Supplementary Table 2**).

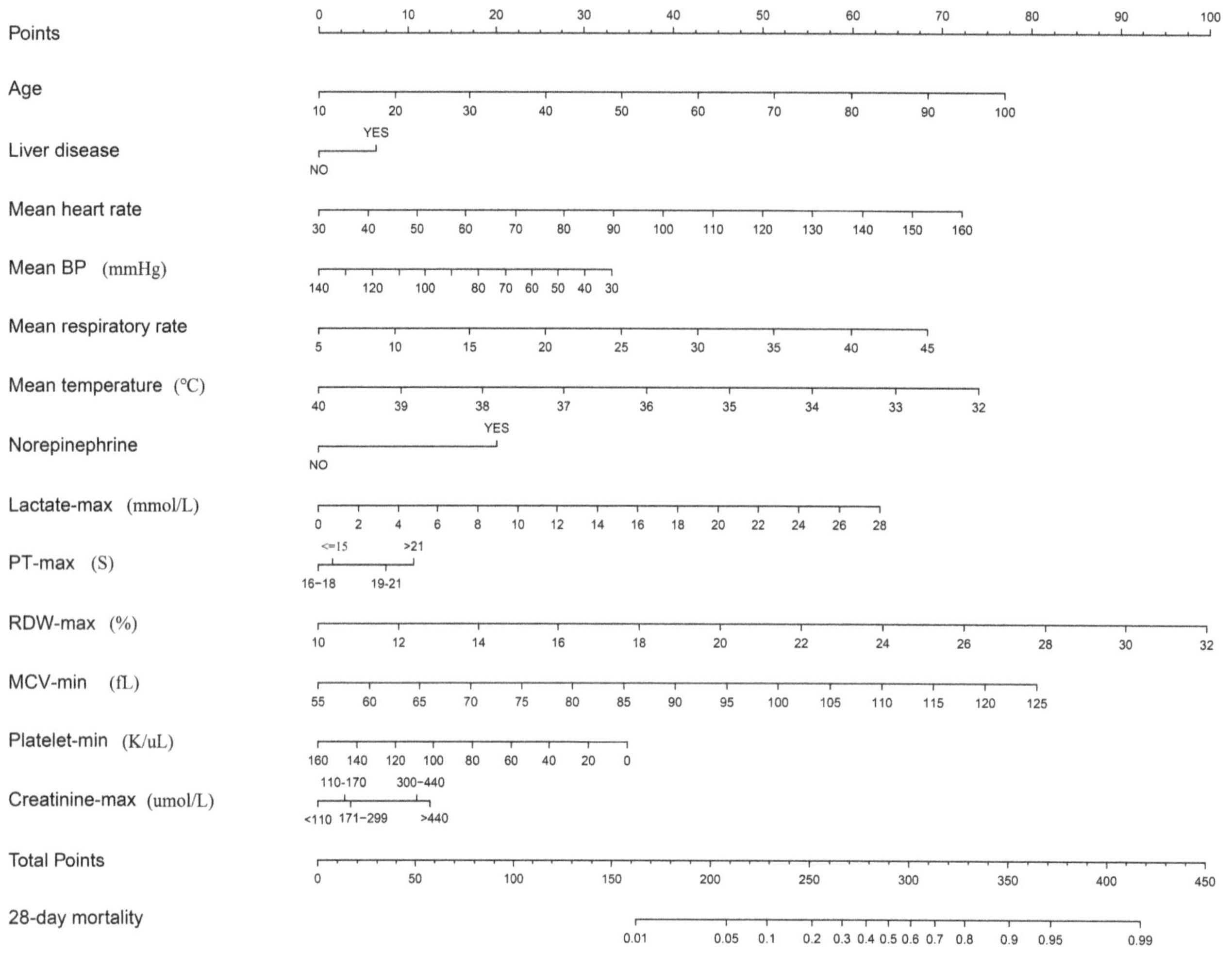


**FIGURE 1 |** Nomogram to predict the risk of 28-day mortality of patients with SIC. When using it, drawing a vertical line from each variable to the points axis for the score, then the points for all the parameters were added, finally, a line from the total points axis was drawn to correspond the risk of 28-day mortality at the bottom.

## DISCUSSION

In this retrospective cohort study of a large open-source database, univariate and multivariate logistic regression analyses were successively applied to identify the independent risk factor associated with the 28-day mortality of SIC patients in the ICU. Finally, a total of 13 clinical variables were recognized and incorporated into a best-fit model, that is, the age, mean heart rate, MAP, mean respiratory rate, mean temperature, lactate-max, PT-max, RDW-max, MCV-min, creatinine-max, lowest level of platelet count, the administration of norepinephrine and combined with liver disease.

The results showed a SIC incidence of 34.8% and a 28-day mortality of 34.0%. These rates were higher than in previous reports (6, 9). Only sepsis patients admitted to the ICU were included in the present study; therefore, population diversity could explain these differences. Most SIC patients were male and commonly found in the medical ICU. Moreover, patients who had SIC displayed a significantly reduction in their short-term survival by the Kaplan–Meier's survival analysis and a prolonged hospitalization time compared with non-SIC patients. These findings were similar to those of Lyons et al. (18). Interestingly, some related comorbidities, including diabetes and COPD, were less prevalent in the SIC cohort. This tendency was also displayed in another study (18).

Among the thirteen included variables, the RDW was a major factor. Indeed, it was the strongest predictor for 28-day mortality in terms of relative contribution. The RDW is a routine parameter in reflecting the heterogeneity of erythrocyte cell size and discriminating anemic types (19). Numerous studies have recently revealed a significant association between the RDW value and increased mortality in sepsis patients (20, 21). A large cohort study that included 11,691 sepsis patients demonstrated that the initial RDW within the first 24 h of admission was an independent risk factor for the 28-day mortality. For every one unit increase in the RDW value, the 28-day mortality increased by 6.86% (20). During the first 72 h of hospitalization, the extent of the rise in the RDW value was also associated with a poorer prognosis of sepsis patients or septic shock patients (21). Although the underlying mechanism was unclear,

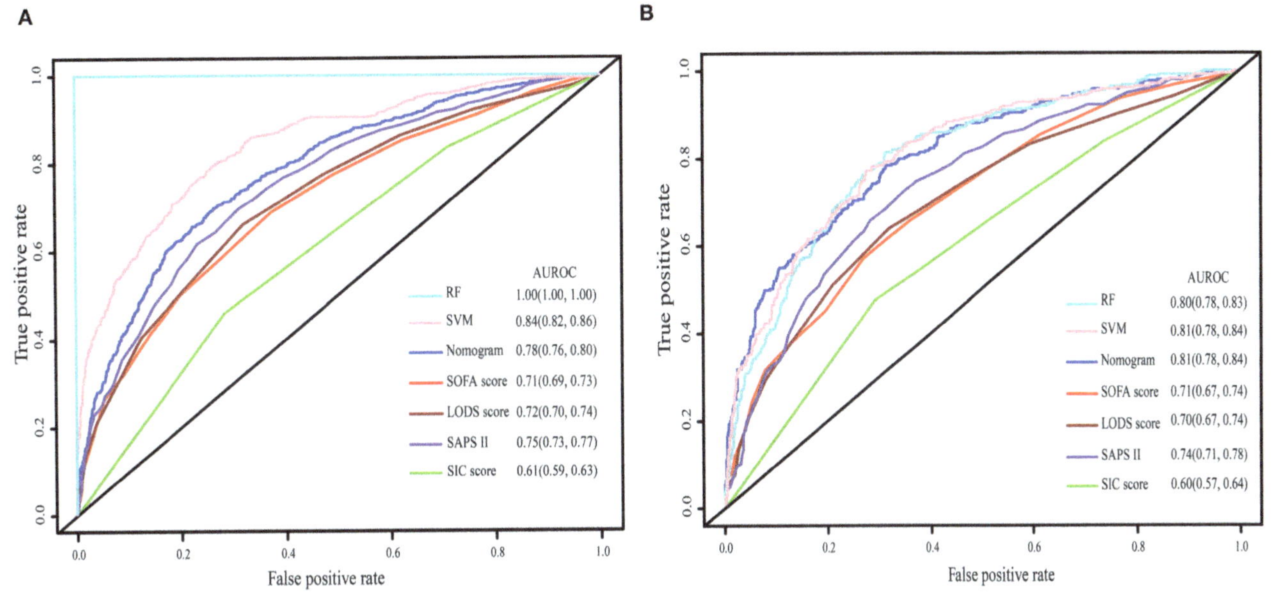


**FIGURE 2 |** The ROC curve of the nomogram, RF model, SVM model, SOFA, LODS, SAPS II and SIC. **(A)** Training set; **(B)** Validation set. The variables entered in nomogram, RF model and SVM model are the same.

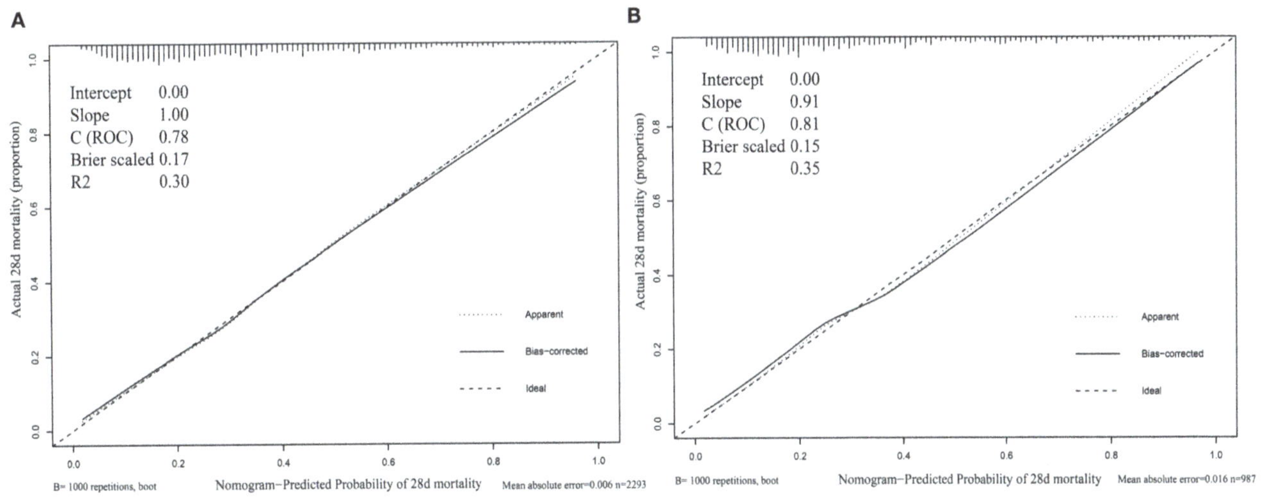


**FIGURE 3 |** Calibration curves of nomogram. **(A)** Training set; **(B)** Validation set.

several possible reasons could explain the correlation between the RDW and sepsis patient mortality. The systemic inflammation response can impact the status of hematopoietic organs. In fluorodeoxyglucose positron emission tomography (FDG-PET) scanning, an association between the RDW and splenic and lumbar bone marrow activation was revealed (22). Furthermore, previous research proved that inflammation could suppress erythrocyte maturation and accelerate reticulocyte transfer into the peripheral circulation (23). Another explanation may be related to high oxidative stress. The excessive expression of reactive oxygen species induced severe cellular dysfunctions or even MODS in sepsis patients (24).

Several other parameters in the nomogram were associated with sepsis or coagulation abnormalities. Epidemiological data demonstrated that age is an independent risk factor for thrombosis and is associated with the 90-day and 1-year mortalities in sepsis patients (25–27). During sepsis, the incidence of liver dysfunction approaches 34–46% (28). When sepsis patients also had a liver disease, including cirrhosis and tumor, the risks for MODS and mortality were

**TABLE 4** | Comparison of models in predicting the 28-day mortality of patients with SIC.

| Predictive model | | AUROC | *P*-value | IDI | *P*-value | NRI | *P*-value |
|---|---|---|---|---|---|---|---|
| **Training set** | Nomogram | 0.78 (0.76, 0.80) | | | | | |
| | SOFA | 0.71 (0.69, 0.73) | <0.001 | 0.09 (0.007, 0.11) | <0.001 | 0.30 (0.20, 0.47) | <0.001 |
| | LODS | 0.72 (0.70, 0.74) | <0.001 | 0.08 (0.06, 0.10) | <0.001 | 0.17 (0.06, 0.29) | <0.001 |
| | SAPS II | 0.75 (0.73, 0.77) | 0.01 | 0.05 (0.03, 0.07) | <0.001 | 0.12 (0.08, 0.22) | <0.001 |
| | SIC score | 0.61 (0.59, 0.63) | <0.001 | 0.12 (0.08, 0.22) | <0.001 | 0.54 (0.39, 0.62) | <0.001 |
| **Validation set** | Nomogram | 0.81 (0.78, 0.84) | | | | | |
| | SOFA | 0.71 (0.67, 0.74) | <0.001 | 0.15 (0.12, 0.18) | <0.001 | 0.40 (0.24, 0.53) | <0.001 |
| | LODS | 0.70 (0.67, 0.74) | <0.001 | 0.16 (0.13, 0.19) | <0.001 | 0.34 (0.23, 0.46) | <0.001 |
| | SAPS II | 0.74 (0.71, 0.78) | <0.001 | 0.12 (0.09, 0.15) | <0.001 | 0.23 (0.17, 0.31) | <0.001 |
| | SIC score | 0.60 (0.57, 0.64) | <0.001 | 0.25 (0.22, 0.28) | <0.001 | 0.58 (0.42, 0.65) | <0.001 |

*The P-value was calculated by comparing the results of nomogram with SOFA or LODS, SAPS II, and SIC score.*
*AUROC, area under the receiver operating characteristic curve; IDI, integrated discrimination improvement; NRI, net reclassification improvement; SOFA, Sequential Organ Failure Assessment; LODS, Logistic Organ Dysfunction System; SAPS II, Simplified acute physiology II.*

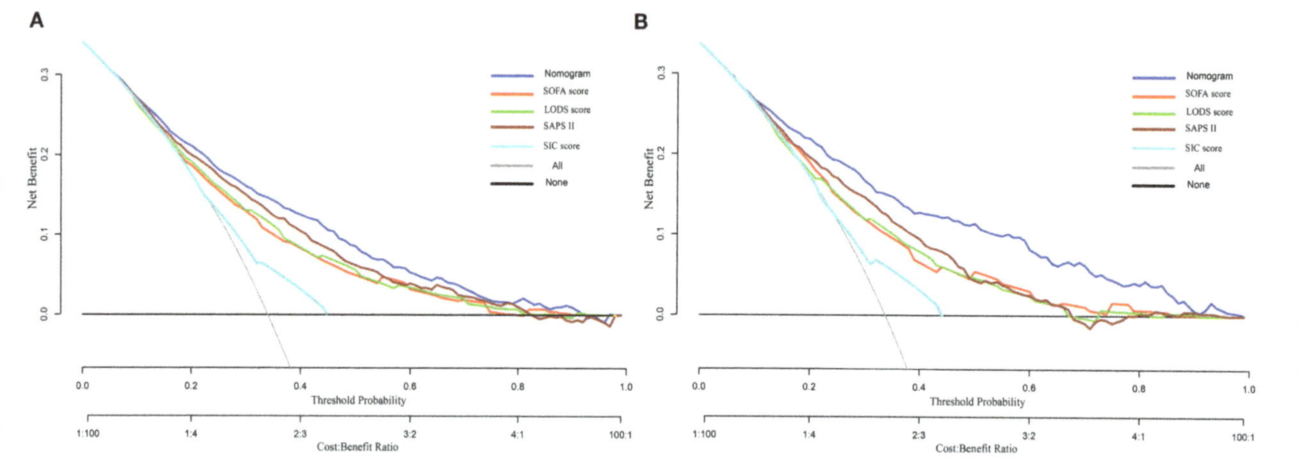


**FIGURE 4** | Decision curve analysis of the nomogram, SOFA, LODS, SAPS II and SIC. **(A)** Training set; **(B)** Validation set.

significantly higher than in patients without liver diseases (29). Vital signs were widely used to develop the prediction model of sepsis (30, 31) and were also included in the nomogram. Furthermore, SIC was normally characterized by reduced platelets and prolonged PT or INR. Notably, a decreased mortality rate of SIC patients was found in the present study when the PT values ranged from 16 to 18s. We supposed that a mildly prolonged PT might be more likely to gain the attention of the physician than a normal PT, which in turn would lead to earlier intervention. Alteration of the lactic levels reflects the situation of the microcirculatory perfusion. When lactic levels were >2.5 mmol/L, the probability of mortality increased with increasing lactic concentration, and this correlation was independent of vasopressor administration (32, 33).

Currently, no specialized prediction models for the assessment of the 28-day mortality risk in SIC patients are available. As defined in the Surviving Sepsis Campaign 2016 guideline, sepsis is induced by infections and eventually leads to systemic multiple organ dysfunction. Therefore, several scoring systems applied to evaluate organ functional status were useful in predicting the prognosis of sepsis patients. The SOFA and LODS were widely applied in the ICU, and may be more appropriate to reflect the acute changes in organ function of sepsis patients (34). However, the effectiveness of these scoring systems in predicting the 28-day mortality risk of SIC patients remained unknown. Therefore, we compared the predictive ability of the proposed nomogram with some common clinical rating scales, including the SOFA, LODS, SAPS II and SIC score, based on the AUROC. We found that the nomogram performed best. Furthermore, the DCA curve and IDI and NRI indices also supported this conclusion. Additionally, the nomogram could effectively discriminate the real positive patients with a high risk for 28-day mortality in both the training and validation sets. In the present study, we attempted to develop other machine-learning models, including RF and SVM, to improve the accuracy of the prediction. However, the AUROC of these models decreased dramatically in the process of validation, which indicated poor generalization ability. On the basis of predictive power and clinical interpretability, we chose multivariate logistic regression as the final model to construct the proposed nomogram. However, we are currently developing an XGBoost model using a new external database.

The nomogram developed here performed well in the discrimination of 28-day mortality risk, as reflected by a high C-index of 0.81 and an acceptable calibration. When obtaining a nomogram, physicians only need to calculate the scores corresponding to each indicator based on the first row, and then add up each point to obtain a final total points value. Finally, the 28-day mortality can be determined based on the final row. In the calculation process, vital signs and the laboratory test values of the SIC patients during the first 24 h since ICU admission are necessary.

The present study also had several limitations. First, according to the sepsis 3.0 criterion, infection and suspected infection diagnosing requires an exact time of the sampling culture and antibiotic use. These were difficult to obtain from the MIMIC III database. Therefore, we referred to the Angus criterion to extract the infectious patients (35). Second, in the PT were inherent defects reflecting the pro-coagulant and anti-coagulant processes (36, 37). Some new coagulation markers and examinations, including thrombin-antithrombin-III complex, plasmin-α2-antiplasmin complex and thromboelastography, are becoming useful tools in coagulopathy diagnosis (38, 39). Combining these parameters with the current optimization model may further optimize the capacity for 28-day mortality prediction in SIC patients; however, they were not recorded in the MIMIC III database. Third, nomogram as a visualization tool, could make the analyses more intuitive and convenient, but it has been used for years. In addition to nomogram, clinical scoring scale and web-based risk calculators were commonly used. For some models that are harder to explain, such as integrated tree model and neural network model, SHAP algorithm may be useful. In recent years, increasing efforts have been put into improving the interpretability of black-box artificial intelligence and designing more interpretable models for clinical prediction (40, 41). This will be our future direction.

In conclusion, on the basis of logistic regression analysis, a nomogram including 13 conventional clinical variables was conducted. This model provided an optimal prediction of the 28-day mortality risk in SIC patients and through the internal validation. Using this model, the 28-day mortality risk of an individual SIC patient can be determined, which can lead to an improved prognostic assessment. However, external validation is required for further generalizability improvement of this nomogram.

## ETHICS STATEMENT

Ethical review and approval was not required for the study on human participants in accordance with the local legislation and institutional requirements. Written informed consent for participation was not required for this study in accordance with the national legislation and the institutional requirements.

## AUTHOR CONTRIBUTIONS

MY and JZ: concept. ZL and JZ: methodology and writing of the manuscript and contributed equally. JH and JW: data processing. YL and WX: software. MY and TH: review and editing. All authors contributed to the article and approved the submitted version.

## ACKNOWLEDGMENTS

We thanks all participants in the Second Affiliated Hospital of Anhui Medical University and AnHui University. We also thank Robert Blakytny, DPhil, from Liwen Bianji, Edanz Editing China, for editing the English text of a draft of this manuscript.

## SUPPLEMENTARY MATERIAL

**Supplementary Figure 1 |** Flowchart of data extraction and study design.

**Supplementary Figure 2 |** K-M curves estimated the 7-day **(A)** and 28-day **(B)** survival probability of SIC and non-SIC patients. The log-rank results showed that the 7-day and 28-day survival of SIC patients was significantly lower than that of non-SIC patients.

**Supplementary Figure 3 |** After PSM processed, K-M curves estimated the 7-day **(A)** and 28-day **(B)** survival probability of SIC and non-SIC patients. The log-rank results showed that the 7-day and 28-day survival of SIC patients was significantly lower than that of non-SIC patients.

**Supplementary Figure 4 |** The clinical impact curve of the nomogram, in which red solid curve indicates the number of people who are classified as high risk by the nomogram at each threshold probability; the blue dashed curve showed the number of true positive patients under each risk threshold. **(A)** Training set; **(B)** Validation set.

**Supplementary Table 1 |** The characteristics of SIC patients in the training set and validation set.

**Supplementary Table 2 |** Accuracy of the nomogram for predicting the risk of 28-day mortality in SIC patients.

## REFERENCES

1. Levi M, van der Poll T. Coagulation and sepsis. *Thromb Res.* (2017) 149:38–44. doi: 10.1016/j.thromres.2016.11.007
2. Fleischmann-Struzek C, Mellhammar L, Rose N, Cassini A, Rudd KE, Schlattmann P, et al. Incidence and mortality of hospital- and ICU-treated sepsis: results from an updated and expanded systematic review and meta-analysis. *Intensive Care Med.* (2020) 46:1552–62. doi: 10.1007/s00134-020-06151-x
3. Simmons J, Pittet JF. The coagulopathy of acute sepsis. *Curr Opin Anaesthesiol* (2015) 28:227–36. doi: 10.1097/ACO.0000000000000163
4. Lipinska-Gediga M. Coagulopathy in sepsis - a new look at an old problem. *Anaesthesiol Intensive Ther.* (2016) 48:352–9. doi: 10.5603/AIT.a2016.0051

5. Vincent JL, Francois B, Zabolotskikh I, Daga MK, Lascarrou JB, Kirov MY, et al. Effect of a recombinant human soluble thrombomodulin on mortality in patients with sepsis-associated coagulopathy: the SCARLET randomized clinical trial. *JAMA.* (2019) 321:1993–2002. doi: 10.1001/jama.2019.5358
6. Saito S, Uchino S, Hayakawa M, Yamakawa K, Kudo D, Iizuka Y, et al. Epidemiology of disseminated intravascular coagulation in sepsis and validation of scoring systems. *J Crit Care.* (2019) 50:23–30. doi: 10.1016/j.jcrc.2018.11.009
7. Tiru B, DiNino EK, Orenstein A, Mailloux PT, Pesaturo A, Gupta A, et al. The economic and humanistic burden of severe sepsis. *Pharmacoeconomics.* (2015) 33:925–37. doi: 10.1007/s40273-015-0282-y
8. Jhang WK, Park SJ. Evaluation of sepsis-induced coagulopathy in critically ill pediatric patients with septic shock. *Thromb Haemost.* (2020). doi: 10.1055/s-0040-1718736. [Epub ahead of print].
9. Iba T, Nisio MD, Levy JH, Kitamura N, Thachil J. New criteria for sepsis-induced coagulopathy (SIC) following the revised sepsis definition: a retrospective analysis of a nationwide survey. *BMJ Open.* (2017) 7:e017046. doi: 10.1136/bmjopen-2017-017046
10. Iba T, Arakawa M, Di Nisio M, Gando S, Anan H, Sato K, et al. Newly proposed sepsis-induced coagulopathy precedes international society on thrombosis and haemostasis overt-disseminated intravascular coagulation and predicts high mortality. *J Intensive Care Med.* (2020) 35:643–9. doi: 10.1177/0885066618773679
11. Ding R, Wang Z, Lin Y, Liu B, Zhang Z, Ma X. Comparison of a new criteria for sepsis-induced coagulopathy and International Society on Thrombosis and Haemostasis disseminated intravascular coagulation score in critically ill patients with sepsis 3.0: a retrospective study. *Blood Coagul Fibrinolysis.* (2018) 29:551–8. doi: 10.1097/MBC.0000000000000755
12. Li X, Fan Y, Dong Y, Cheng Y, Zhou J, Wang Z, et al. Development and validation of nomograms predicting the overall and the cancer-specific survival in endometrial cancer patients. *Front Med.* (2020) 7:614629. doi: 10.21203/rs.3.rs-68463/v1
13. Xun Y, Chen M, Liang P, Tripathi P, Deng H, Zhou Z, et al. A novel clinical-radiomics model pre-operatively predicted the stone-free rate of flexible ureteroscopy strategy in kidney stone patients. *Front Med.* (2020) 7:576925. doi: 10.3389/fmed.2020.576925
14. Ge H, Jiang Y, Jin Q, Wan L, Qian X, Zhang Z. Nomogram for the prediction of postoperative hypoxemia in patients with acute aortic dissection. *BMC Anesthesiol.* (2018) 18:146. doi: 10.1186/s12871-018-0612-7
15. Johnson AE, Pollard TJ, Shen L, Lehman LW, Feng M, Ghassemi M, et al. MIMIC-III, a freely accessible critical care database. *Sci Data.* (2016) 3:160035. doi: 10.1038/sdata.2016.35
16. Collins GS, Reitsma JB, Altman DG, Moons KG. Transparent Reporting of a multivariable prediction model for Individual Prognosis Or Diagnosis (TRIPOD). *Ann Intern Med.* (2015) 162:735–6. doi: 10.7326/L15-5093-2
17. Singer M, Deutschman CS, Seymour CW, Shankar-Hari M, Annane D, Bauer M, et al. The third international consensus definitions for sepsis and septic shock (Sepsis-3). *JAMA.* (2016) 315:801–10. doi: 10.1001/jama.2016.0287
18. Lyons PG, Micek ST, Hampton N, Kollef MH. Sepsis-associated coagulopathy severity predicts hospital mortality. *Crit Care Med.* (2018) 46:736–42. doi: 10.1097/CCM.0000000000002997
19. Piriyakhuntorn P, Tantiworawit A, Rattanathammethee T, Chai-Adisaksopha C, Rattarittamrong E, Norasetthada L. The role of red cell distribution width in the differential diagnosis of iron deficiency anemia and non-transfusiondependent thalassemia patients. *Hematol Rep.* (2018) 10:7605. doi: 10.4081/hr.2018.7605
20. Huidong L, Bo X. Evaluation of the influence of red blood cell distribution width on the prognosis of patients with sepsis based on data mining. *J Clin Emerg.* (2019) 20:263–7. doi: 10.13201/j.issn.1009-5918.2019.04.002
21. Kim CH, Park JT, Kim EJ, Han JH, Han JS, Choi JY, et al. An increase in red blood cell distribution width from baseline predicts mortality in patients with severe sepsis or septic shock. *Crit Care.* (2013) 17:R282. doi: 10.1186/cc13145
22. Van Koeverden ID, den Ruijter HM, Scholtes VPW, G E H Lam M, Haitjema S, Buijsrogge MP, et al. A single preoperative blood test predicts postoperative sepsis and pneumonia after coronary bypass or open aneurysm surgery. *Eur J Clin Invest.* (2019) 49:e13055. doi: 10.1111/eci.13055
23. Straat M, van Bruggen R, de Korte D, Juffermans NP. Red blood cell clearance in inflammation. *Transfus Med Hemother.* (2012) 39:353–61. doi: 10.1159/000342229
24. Kolls JK. Oxidative stress in sepsis: a redox redux. *J Clin Invest.* (2006) 116:860–3. doi: 10.1172/JCI28111
25. Mahé I, Caulin C, Bergmann JF. Age, an independent risk factor for thrombosis. Epidemiologic data. *Presse Med.* (2005) 34:878–86. doi: 10.1016/S0755-4982(05)84068-0
26. Xie JF, Wang HL, Kang Y, Zhou LX, Liu ZM, Qin BY, et al. The epidemiology of sepsis in Chinese ICUs: a national cross-sectional survey. *Crit Care Med.* (2020) 48:e209–19. doi: 10.1097/CCM.0000000000004155
27. He XL, Liao XL, Xie ZC, Han L, Yang XL, Kang Y. Pulmonary infection is an independent risk factor for long-term mortality and quality of life for sepsis patients. *Biomed Res Int.* (2016) 2016:4213712. doi: 10.1155/2016/4213712
28. Brun-Buisson C, Meshaka P, Pinton P, Vallet B, EPISEPSIS Study Group. EPISEPSIS: a reappraisal of the epidemiology and outcome of severe sepsis in French intensive care units. *Intensive Care Med.* (2004) 30:580–8. doi: 10.1007/s00134-003-2121-4
29. Yan J, Li S, Li S. The role of the liver in sepsis. *Int Rev Immunol.* (2014) 33:498–510. doi: 10.3109/08830185.2014.889129
30. Faisal M, Scally A, Richardson D, Beatson K, Howes R, Speed K, et al. Development and external validation of an automated computer-aided risk score for predicting sepsis in emergency medical admissions using the patient's first electronically recorded vital signs and blood test results. *Crit Care Med.* (2018) 46:612–8. doi: 10.1097/CCM.0000000000002967
31. Churpek MM, Snyder A, Han X, Sokol S, Pettit N, Howell MD, et al. Quick sepsis-related organ failure assessment, systemic inflammatory response syndrome, and early warning scores for detecting clinical deterioration in infected patients outside the intensive care unit. *Am J Respir Crit Care Med.* (2017) 195:906–11. doi: 10.1164/rccm.201604-0854OC
32. Thomas-Rueddel DO, Poidinger B, Weiss M, Bach F, Dey K, Häberle H, et al. Hyperlactatemia is an independent predictor of mortality and denotes distinct subtypes of severe sepsis and septic shock. *J Crit Care.* (2015) 30:439.e1-439.e4396. doi: 10.1016/j.jcrc.2014.10.027
33. Meiring C, Dixit A, Harris S, MacCallum NS, Brealey DA, Watkinson PJ, et al. Optimal intensive care outcome prediction over time using machine learning. *PLoS ONE.* (2018) 13:e0206862. doi: 10.1371/journal.pone.0206862
34. Seymour CW, Liu VX, Iwashyna TJ, Brunkhorst FM, Rea TD, Scherag A, et al. Assessment of clinical criteria for sepsis: for the third international consensus definitions for sepsis and septic shock (Sepsis-3). *JAMA.* (2016) 315:762–74. doi: 10.1001/jama.2016.0288
35. Angus DC, Linde-Zwirble WT, Lidicker J, Clermont G, Carcillo J, Pinsky MR. Epidemiology of severe sepsis in the United States: analysis of incidence, outcome, and associated costs of care. *Crit Care Med.* (2001) 29:1303–10. doi: 10.1097/00003246-200107000-00002
36. Zeerleder S, Hack CE, Wuillemin WA. Disseminated intravascular coagulation in sepsis. *Chest.* (2005) 128:2864–75. doi: 10.1378/chest.128.4.2864
37. Scarlatescu E, Juffermans NP, Thachil J. The current status of viscoelastic testing in septic coagulopathy. *Thromb Res.* (2019) 183:146–52. doi: 10.1016/j.thromres.2019.09.029
38. Gall LS, Davenport RA. Fibrinolysis and antifibrinolytic treatment in the trauma patient. *Curr Opin Anaesthesiol.* (2018) 31:227–33. doi: 10.1097/ACO.0000000000000561
39. Müller MC, Meijers JC, Vroom MB, Juffermans NP. Utility of thromboelastography and/or thromboelastometry in adults with sepsis: a systematic review. *Crit Care.* (2014) 18:R30. doi: 10.1186/cc13721
40. Xie F, Chakraborty B, Ong MEH, Goldstein BA, Liu N. AutoScore: a machine learning-based automatic clinical score generator and its application to mortality prediction using electronic health records. *JMIR Med Inform.* (2020) 8:e21798. doi: 10.2196/21798
41. Zhang Z, Navarese EP, Zheng B, Meng Q, Liu N, Ge H, et al. Analytics with artificial intelligence to advance the treatment of acute respiratory distress syndrome. *J Evid Based Med.* (2020) 13:301–12. doi: 10.1111/jebm.12418

17

# Registered Trials on Artificial Intelligence Conducted in Emergency Department and Intensive Care Unit

*Guina Liu*[1,2†], *Nian Li*[3*†], *Lingmin Chen*[4], *Yi Yang*[5] *and Yonggang Zhang*[1,6,7*]

[1] Department of Periodical Press and National Clinical Research Center for Geriatrics, West China Hospital, Sichuan University, Chengdu, China, [2] West China School of Medicine, Sichuan University, Chengdu, China, [3] Department of Medical Administration, West China Hospital, Sichuan University, Chengdu, China, [4] Department of Anesthesiology and National Clinical Research Center for Geriatrics, West China Hospital, Sichuan University and The Research Units of West China (2018RU012), Chinese Academy of Medical Sciences, Chengdu, China, [5] Department of Clinical Medicine, Gansu University of Traditional Chinese Medicine, Lanzhou, China, [6] Chinese Evidence-based Medicine Center, West China Hospital, Sichuan University, Chengdu, China, [7] Nursing Key Laboratory of Sichuan Province, Chengdu, China

***Correspondence:**
Nian Li
linian@wchscu.cn
Yonggang Zhang
jebm_zhang@yahoo.com

† These authors have contributed equally to this work

**Objective:** Clinical trials contribute to the development of clinical practice. However, little is known about the current status of trials on artificial intelligence (AI) conducted in emergency department and intensive care unit. The objective of the study was to provide a comprehensive analysis of registered trials in such field based on ClinicalTrials.gov.

**Methods:** Registered trials on AI conducted in emergency department and intensive care unit were searched on ClinicalTrials.gov up to 12th January 2021. The characteristics were analyzed using SPSS21.0 software.

**Results:** A total of 146 registered trials were identified, including 61 in emergency department and 85 in intensive care unit. They were registered from 2004 to 2021. Regarding locations, 58 were conducted in Europe, 58 in America, 9 in Asia, 4 in Australia, and 17 did not report locations. The enrollment of participants was from 0 to 18,000,000, with a median of 233. Universities were the primary sponsors, which accounted for 43.15%, followed by hospitals (35.62%), and industries/companies (9.59%). Regarding study designs, 85 trials were interventional trials, while 61 were observational trials. Of the 85 interventional trials, 15.29% were for diagnosis and 38.82% for treatment; of the 84 observational trials, 42 were prospective, 14 were retrospective, 2 were cross-sectional, 2 did not report clear information and 1 was unknown. Regarding the trials' results, 69 trials had been completed, while only 10 had available results on ClinicalTrials.gov.

**Conclusions:** Our study suggest that more AI trials are needed in emergency department and intensive care unit and sponsors are encouraged to report the results.

**Keywords: artificial intelligence, emergency department, intensive care unit, ClinicalTrials.gov, cross-sectional, trial**

## INTRODUCTION

Artificial intelligence (AI), described as the science and engineering of making intelligent machines (1), is a broad term that implies the use of a computer to model intelligent behavior with minimal human intervention, generally at a speed and scale that exceed human capability (2–5). With the achievement of computer science, AI is involved in clinical practice, including tracking data (6, 7), diagnosis (8), and support of decision making (9, 10). AI has been widely used in clinical practices, such as in prediction, decision support, and the delivery of personalized health care (11–13), especially in diagnosis and treatment of acute events (14) to improve outcomes (15–17).

Emergency and critical care focus on resuscitating unstable patients and allowing time for recovery or the effect of specific therapies (18), and it can be provided in emergency department (ED) or intensive care unit (ICU) (18, 19). Emergency and critical care can be affected by levels of staffs, equipment and knowledge (18, 20). Adverse emergency and critical care will result in burdens and adverse outcomes, including weakness, dysfunction, contractures, pain, depression, anxiety, post-traumatic stress disorder, and even death (21–23). Early and fast diagnosis could save lives. Thus, using AI tools to fastly and accurately diagnostic will help a lot (10), especially to assist in uncertainty (24) or to further developing strategies (25). Will AI tools help physicians or patients in ED and ICU (26), there is still limited information and it should be assessed by well-deigned trials.

Well-designed trials can assist clinical practice (27, 28) and transparency is the key characteristic for well-designed trials. Pre-registered in public registries is the most important strategy to ensure transparency (29) and now been required for all trials by The International Committee of Medical Journal Editors (ICMJE). Thus, analyzing registered trials will know the progress in such field, and many studies have been published to analyze registered trials in Clinicaltrials.gov, such as acupuncture (30), ventilator-associated pneumonia (VAP) (31), old populations with infectious diseases (32), and cancer diagnosis (33). However, there is no such study for AI in ED and ICU. Thus, we conducted the current study to provide a comprehensive analysis of the development of AI for ED and ICU.

## MATERIALS AND METHODS

### Reporting Guideline

This is a cross-sectional study, and it was reported according to STROBE (34).

### Data Source

A cross-sectional study about registered trials for AI in ED and ICU on ClinicalTrials.gov was carried out, and the searched words were as follows: artificial intelligence, AI, computational intelligence, machine intelligence, machine learning, deep learning, algorithms, computer reasoning, computer vision system, knowledge acquisition (computer), knowledge representation (computer), natural language processing, neural networks of computer, robotics. All information was downloaded, and duplicates were removed by Excel (Office 365, Microsoft, Redmond, WA, USA) according to the trials' national clinical trial (NCT) number.

### Data Selection and Eligible Trials

We selected trials mainly according to their conditions or study descriptions. Inclusion criteria: Trials on AI and only conducted at ED and ICU. Exclusion criteria: trials not related to artificial intelligence; trials excluded conditions in the ED or ICU; trials conducted in general wards.

### Studied Variables

The studied variables included study type, start year, enrollment, participant age, participant gender, status, phase, study results, sponsor, main funding source, number of funding sources, location, number of centers, primary purpose, intervention, allocation, intervention model, masking, observational model, and time perspective.

### Statistical Analysis

The characteristics were analyzed by descriptive methods. The continuous variables were characterized as median and interquartile ranges (IQR), and the categorical variables were reported as frequencies and percentages. The study types included interventional trials and observational trials. The start year was when the trial was first posted on ClinicalTrial.gov, including 2004–2010, 2011–2016, and 2017–2021. Whether the results were available or unavailable was also analyzed. The sponsor included university, hospital, industry/company, or others, including individuals, institutions, or some organizations that cannot be included in other categories. The main funding resources included industry, the federal reserve of United States (U.S. fed), or other resources, such as universities, individuals, and organizations that cannot be divided into subtypes. Data analysis was performed using SPSS21.0 software.

## RESULTS

### Basic Characteristics

Up to 12th January 2021, 4990 trials were identified after the initial search. After reviewing all information, a total of 146 registered trials were included (**Figure 1**). The characteristics of the included trials are shown in **Table 1**. Among the 146 trials, 85 (58.22%) were interventional trials, and 61 (41.78%) were observational trials. Seventy-five (51.37%) trials registered after 2017, while 25 (17.12%) and 46 (31.51%) registered in 2004–2010 and 2011–2016, respectively. Sample sizes were from 0 to 18,000,000, with a median of 233. For genders, 143 (97.95%) trials recruited both male and female participants; however, three trials (2.05%) recruited females only. For age, 112 (76.71%) trials only recruited adults, 11 (7.53%) only recruited children, while 23 (15.75%) recruited both adults and children. For status, 23 (15.75%) trials were not yet recruiting, 30 (20.55%) were recruiting, 69 (47.26%) were completed, 1 was suspended, 10 were terminated or withdrawn and 13 were in unknown status. For results, only 10 (6.85%) trials reported results on ClinicalTrials.gov, while 136 (93.15%) did not report results. For sponsors, 63 (43.15%) were sponsored by

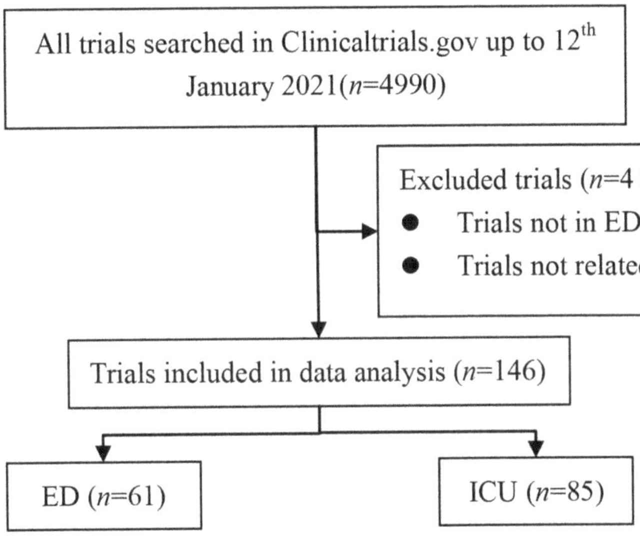


**FIGURE 1** | Flowchart of recruited trials registered in ClinicalTrials.gov up to 12th January 2021.

universities, 52 (35.62%) were sponsored by hospitals, 14 (9.59%) were sponsored by industries/companies, and 17 (11.64%) were sponsored by other institutions. For funding, 15 (10.27%) were funded by industries, and 131 (89.73%) did not report clear funding sources. For locations, 58 (39.73%) trials were conducted in America, 58 (39.73%) in Europe, 9 (6.16%) in Asia, 4 (2.74%) in Australia, and 17 (11.64%) did not report locations.

## Characteristics of Study Design

### Interventional Study

The characteristics of the 85 interventional studies are shown in **Table 2**. Thirteen (15.29%) trials were for diagnosis, 33 (38.82%) for treatment, 16 (18.82%) for prevention, 15 (17.65%) for supportive care, 6 (7.06%) for health services research and 2 (2.35%) did not report the clear purpose. Twety-one (24.71%) trials were for behavioral intervention, 28 (32.94%) for intervention device, 6 (7.06%) for diagnostic test, 7 (8.24%) for the procedure and 23 (27.06%) did not have clear information on intervention. For the types of assignments, 53 (62.35%) were parallel assignment, 24 (28.24%) were single group assignment, 1 (1.18%) was factorial assignment, 3(3.53%) were crossover assignment, 3(3.6%) were sequential assignment and 1(1.2%) was unknown, respectively. For allocation, 59 (69.41%) were randomized, 11 (12.94%) were nonrandomized, 14 (16.47%) were not applicable and 1 (1.18%) was unknown. For masking, 52 (61.18%) were open-labeled, 20 (23.53%) were single-masked, 8 (9.41%) were double-masked, 2(2.35%) were triple-masked, 2(2.35%) were quadruple-masked and 1 (1.18%) had no information. For sample size, 24 (28.23%) trials recruited more than 500 participants, while 39 (45.88%) recruited <100 participants and 22 (25.88%) recruited 100–500 participants. For gender, 1 (1.18%) trial included female only and 84 (98.82%) recruited both male and female. For age, 63 (74.12%) trials recruited adult only, while 8 (9.41%) trials recruited child only and 14 (16.47%) trials recruited both child and adult. One (1.18%) trial was in phase 2, 1 (1.18%) in phase 2/3, 3(3.53%) in phase 3, 1 (1.18%) in phase 4 and 79 had no clear information. For status, 46 (54.12%) trials were completed, 15 (17.65%) were recruiting, 9 (10.59%) were not recruiting, 7 (8.24%) were terminated or withdrawn, 1 (1.18%) was suspended and 7 (8.24%) had no information. Among all 85 interventional trials, only 10 trials reported results on Clinicaltrials.gov. For sponsors, 43 (50.59%) were sponsored by universities, 25 (29.41%) were sponsored by hospitals, 8 (9.41%) were sponsored by industries/companies, and 9 (10.59) were sponsored by other institutions. For funding, 8 (9.41%) trials were funded by industries and 77 (90.59%) did not report funding sources. For locations, 42 (49.41%) were from America, 28 (32.94%) were from Europe, 4 (4.71%) were from Asia, 4 (4.71%) were from Australia and 7 (8.24%) did not report location information.

### Observational Study

The characteristics of the 61 observational studies are shown in **Table 3**. Among them, 35 (57.38%) were cohort studies, 9 (14.75%) were case-only studies, 8 (13.11%) were case-control studies and one was case-crossover study, while 6 (9.84%) had no clear information and 2 (3.28%) did not provide information. Forty-two (68.85%) were prospective studies, 14 (22.95%) were retrospective studies, 2 (3.28%) were cross-sectional studies, 2 (3.28%) were other designed studies and one did not report related information. For sample size, 21 (34.43%) recruited more than 500 participants, while 14 (22.95%) recruited <100 participants and 25 (40.98%) recruited 100–500 participants. For gender, only 2 studies included female only and 59 (96.72%) recruited both male and female. For age, 49 (80.33%) recruited adult only, while 3 (4.92%) recruited child only and 9 (14.75%) recruited both child and adult. For status, 23 (37.70%) were

**TABLE 1** | The characteristics of the 146 trials registered on ClinicalTrial.gov.

| Characteristics | | Number | Percentage (%) |
|---|---|---|---|
| **Study type** | | | |
| | Interventional | 85 | 58.22 |
| | Observational | 61 | 41.78 |
| **Registered year** | | | |
| | 2004–2010 | 25 | 17.12 |
| | 2011–2016 | 46 | 31.51 |
| | 2017–2021 | 75 | 51.37 |
| **Enrollment** | | | |
| | 0–100 | 53 | 36.30 |
| | 100–500 | 47 | 32.19 |
| | >500 | 45 | 30.82 |
| | Unknown | 1 | 0.68 |
| **Gender** | | | |
| | Female only | 3 | 2.05 |
| | Both | 143 | 97.95 |
| **Participant age (year)** | | | |
| | <18 | 11 | 7.53 |
| | ≥18 | 112 | 76.71 |
| | Both | 23 | 15.75 |
| **Status** | | | |
| | Not recruiting | 23 | 15.75 |
| | Recruiting | 30 | 20.55 |
| | Completed | 69 | 47.26 |
| | Suspended | 1 | 0.68 |
| | Terminated/withdrawn | 10 | 6.85 |
| | Unknown | 13 | 8.91 |
| **Study results** | | | |
| | Has results | 10 | 6.85 |
| | No results available | 136 | 93.15 |
| **Sponsor** | | | |
| | University | 63 | 43.15 |
| | Hospital | 52 | 35.62 |
| | Industry/company | 14 | 9.59 |
| | Other | 17 | 11.64 |
| **Funding source** | | | |
| | Industry | 15 | 10.27 |
| | Other | 131 | 89.73 |
| **Location** | | | |
| | America | 58 | 39.73 |
| | Europe | 58 | 39.73 |
| | Asia | 9 | 6.16 |
| | Australia | 4 | 2.74 |
| | Unknown | 17 | 11.64 |

completed, 15 (24.59%) were recruiting, 14 (22.95%) were not recruiting, 3 (4.92%) were terminated or withdrawn and 6 (9.84%) had no information. Among all 61 observational studies, none of them reported results on Clinicaltrials.gov. For sponsors, 20 (32.79%) were sponsored by universities, 27 (44.26%) were sponsored by hospitals, 6 (9.84%) were sponsored by industries/companies, and 8 (13.11%) were sponsored by

**TABLE 2** | Designs of 85 interventional trials registered with ClinicalTrial.gov.

| Characteristics | | Number | Percentage (%) |
|---|---|---|---|
| **Primary purpose** | | | |
| | Diagnosis | 13 | 15.29 |
| | Treatment | 33 | 38.82 |
| | Prevention | 16 | 18.82 |
| | Supportive care | 15 | 17.65 |
| | Health services research | 6 | 7.06 |
| | Unknown | 2 | 2.35 |
| **Intervention** | | | |
| | Behavioral | 21 | 24.71 |
| | Device | 28 | 32.94 |
| | Diagnostic test | 6 | 7.06 |
| | Procedure | 7 | 8.24 |
| | Other | 23 | 27.06 |
| **Intervention model** | | | |
| | Parallel assignment | 53 | 62.35 |
| | Factorial assignment | 1 | 1.18 |
| | Crossover assignment | 3 | 3.53 |
| | Single group assignment | 24 | 28.24 |
| | Sequential assignment | 3 | 3.53 |
| | Unknown | 1 | 1.18 |
| **Allocation** | | | |
| | Randomized | 59 | 69.41 |
| | Nonrandomized | 11 | 12.94 |
| | N/A | 14 | 16.47 |
| | Unknown | 1 | 1.18 |
| **Masking** | | | |
| | Single | 20 | 23.53 |
| | Double | 8 | 9.41 |
| | Triple | 2 | 2.35 |
| | Quadruple | 2 | 2.35 |
| | None (open-label) | 52 | 61.18 |
| | Unknown | 1 | 1.18 |
| **Enrollment** | | | |
| | 0–100 | 39 | 45.88 |
| | 100–500 | 22 | 25.88 |
| | >500 | 24 | 28.23 |
| **Gender** | | | |
| | Both | 84 | 98.82 |
| | Female | 1 | 1.18 |
| **Participant age (year)** | | | |
| | <18 | 8 | 9.41 |
| | ≥18 | 63 | 74.12 |
| | Both | 14 | 16.47 |
| **Status** | | | |
| | Not recruiting | 9 | 10.59 |
| | Recruiting | 15 | 17.65 |
| | Completed | 46 | 54.12 |
| | Suspended | 1 | 1.18 |
| | Terminated/withdrawn | 7 | 8.24 |
| | Unknown | 7 | 8.24 |

*(Continued)*

**TABLE 2 |** Continued

| Characteristics | | Number | Percentage (%) |
|---|---|---|---|
| **Results** | | | |
| | Has results | 10 | 11.76 |
| | No results available | 75 | 88.24 |
| **Sponsor** | | | |
| | University | 43 | 50.59 |
| | Hospital | 25 | 29.41 |
| | Industry/company | 8 | 9.41 |
| | Other | 9 | 10.59 |
| **Funding source** | | | |
| | Industry | 8 | 9.41 |
| | Other | 77 | 90.59 |
| **Location** | | | |
| | America | 42 | 49.41 |
| | Europe | 28 | 32.94 |
| | Asia | 4 | 4.71 |
| | Australia | 4 | 4.71 |
| | Unknown | 7 | 8.24 |

other institutions. For funding, 7 (11.48%) were funded by industries, and 54 (88.52%) did not report clear funding sources. For locations, 30 (49.18%) were from Europe, 16 (26.23%) were from America, 5 (8.20%) were from Asia and 10 (16.39%) did not report locations.

## Characteristics of Trials at Emergency Department

**Table 4** shows the characteristics of trials conducted in ED. Among the 61 trials, 37 (60.66%) were interventional trials, and 24 (39.34%) were observational trials. Thirty-four (55.73%) trials registered after 2017, while 8 (13.11%) and 19 (31.15%) were registered in 2004–2010 and 2011–2016, respectively. For sample size, 27 (44.26%) trials recruited more than 500 participants, while 14 (22.95%) recruited <100 participants and 20 (32.79%) recruited 100 to 500 participants. For genders, 60 trials (98.36%) recruited both male and female participants; however, 1 (1.64%) recruited females only. For age, 39 trials (63.93%) only recruited adults, 6 (9.84%) only recruited children, while 16 (26.23%) recruited both adults and children. For status, 9 (14.75%) were not yet recruiting, 10 (16.39%) were recruiting, 30 (49.18%) were completed, six were terminated or withdrawn and six were in unknown status. For results, only three trials reported results on Clinicaltrials.gov, while 58 (95.08%) did not report results. For sponsors, 28 (45.90%) were sponsored by universities, 25 (40.98%) were sponsored by hospitals, 4 (6.56%) were sponsored by industries/companies, and 4 (6.56%) were sponsored by other institutions. For funding, 4 trials (6.56%) were funded by industries and 57 (93.44%) did not report clear funding sources. For locations, 28 (45.90%) were in America, 26 (42.62%) in Europe, 1 (1.64%) in Asia and 6 (9.84%) did not report locations.

**TABLE 3 |** Designs of 61 observational trials registered on ClinicalTrial.gov.

| Characteristics | | Number | Percentage (%) |
|---|---|---|---|
| **Observational model** | | | |
| | Case-control | 8 | 13.11 |
| | Case-only | 9 | 14.75 |
| | Case-crossover | 1 | 1.64 |
| | Cohort | 35 | 57.38 |
| | Other | 6 | 9.84 |
| | Unknown | 2 | 3.28 |
| **Time perspective** | | | |
| | Prospective | 42 | 68.85 |
| | Retrospective | 14 | 22.95 |
| | Cross-sectional | 2 | 3.28 |
| | Other | 2 | 3.28 |
| | Unknown | 1 | 1.64 |
| **Enrollment** | | | |
| | 0–100 | 14 | 22.95 |
| | 100–500 | 25 | 40.98 |
| | >500 | 21 | 34.43 |
| | Unknown | 1 | 1.64 |
| **Participant gender** | | | |
| | Female only | 2 | 3.28 |
| | Both | 59 | 96.72 |
| **Participant age (year)** | | | |
| | <18 | 3 | 4.92 |
| | ≥18 | 49 | 80.33 |
| | Both | 9 | 14.75 |
| **Status** | | | |
| | Not recruiting | 14 | 22.95 |
| | Recruiting | 15 | 24.59 |
| | Completed | 23 | 37.70 |
| | Terminated/withdrawn | 3 | 4.92 |
| | Unknown | 6 | 9.84 |
| **Results** | | | |
| | Has results | 0 | 0.00 |
| | No results available | 61 | 100.00 |
| **Sponsor** | | | |
| | University | 20 | 32.79 |
| | Hospital | 27 | 44.26 |
| | Industry/company | 6 | 9.84 |
| | Other | 8 | 13.11 |
| **Funding source** | | | |
| | Industry | 7 | 11.48 |
| | Other | 54 | 88.52 |
| **Location** | | | |
| | America | 16 | 26.23 |
| | Europe | 30 | 49.18 |
| | Asia | 5 | 8.20 |
| | Unknown | 10 | 16.39 |

## Characteristics of Trials at ICU

**Table 5** shows the characteristics of trials on AI conducted in emergency department. Among the 85 trials, 48 (56.47%) were interventional trials, and 37 (43.53%) were observational

**TABLE 4** | The characteristics of the 61 trials in ED registered on ClinicalTrial.gov.

| Characteristics | | Number | Percentage (%) |
|---|---|---|---|
| **Study type** | | | |
| | Interventional | 37 | 60.66 |
| | Observational | 24 | 39.34 |
| **Start year** | | | |
| | 2004–2010 | 8 | 13.11 |
| | 2011–2016 | 19 | 31.15 |
| | 2017–2021 | 34 | 55.73 |
| **Enrollment** | | | |
| | 0–100 | 14 | 22.95 |
| | 100–500 | 20 | 32.79 |
| | >500 | 27 | 44.26 |
| **Gender** | | | |
| | Female only | 1 | 1.64 |
| | Both | 60 | 98.36 |
| **Participant age (year)** | | | |
| | <18 | 6 | 9.84 |
| | ≥18 | 39 | 63.93 |
| | Both | 16 | 26.23 |
| **Status** | | | |
| | Not recruiting | 9 | 14.75 |
| | Recruiting | 10 | 16.39 |
| | Completed | 30 | 49.18 |
| | Terminated/withdrawn | 6 | 9.84 |
| | Unknown | 6 | 9.84 |
| **Study results** | | | |
| | Has results | 3 | 4.92 |
| | No results available | 58 | 95.08 |
| **Sponsor** | | | |
| | University | 28 | 45.90 |
| | Hospital | 25 | 40.98 |
| | Industry/company | 4 | 6.56 |
| | Other | 4 | 6.56 |
| **Funding source** | | | |
| | Industry | 4 | 6.56 |
| | Other | 57 | 93.44 |
| **Location** | | | |
| | America | 28 | 45.90 |
| | Europe | 26 | 42.62 |
| | Asia | 1 | 1.64 |
| | Unknown | 6 | 9.84 |

**TABLE 5** | The characteristics of the 85 trials in ICU registered on ClinicalTrial.gov.

| Characteristics | | Number | Percentage (%) |
|---|---|---|---|
| **Study type** | | | |
| | Interventional | 48 | 56.47 |
| | Observational | 37 | 43.53 |
| **Start year** | | | |
| | 2004–2010 | 17 | 20.00 |
| | 2011–2016 | 27 | 31.76 |
| | 2017–2021 | 41 | 48.24 |
| **Enrollment** | | | |
| | 0–100 | 39 | 45.88 |
| | 100–500 | 27 | 31.76 |
| | >500 | 18 | 21.18 |
| | Unknown | 1 | 1.18 |
| **Gender** | | | |
| | Female only | 2 | 2.35 |
| | Both | 83 | 97.65 |
| **Participant age (year)** | | | |
| | <18 | 5 | 5.88 |
| | ≥18 | 73 | 85.88 |
| | Both | 7 | 8.24 |
| **Status** | | | |
| | Not recruiting | 14 | 16.47 |
| | Recruiting | 20 | 23.53 |
| | Completed | 39 | 45.88 |
| | Suspended | 1 | 1.18 |
| | Terminated/withdrawn | 4 | 4.71 |
| | Unknown | 7 | 8.24 |
| **Study results** | | | |
| | Has results | 7 | 8.24 |
| | No results available | 78 | 91.76 |
| **Sponsor** | | | |
| | University | 35 | 41.18 |
| | Hospital | 27 | 31.76 |
| | Industry/company | 10 | 11.76 |
| | Other | 13 | 15.29 |
| **Funding source** | | | |
| | Industry | 11 | 12.94 |
| | Other | 74 | 87.06 |
| **Location** | | | |
| | America | 30 | 35.29 |
| | Europe | 32 | 37.65 |
| | Asia | 8 | 9.41 |
| | Australia | 4 | 4.71 |
| | Unknown | 11 | 12.94 |

trials. Forty-one (48.24%) trials registered after 2017, while 17 (20.00%) and 27 (31.76%) registered in 2004–2010 and 2011–2016, respectively. For sample size, 18 (21.18%) trials recruited more than 500 participants, 39 (45.88%) recruited <100 participants, 27 (31.76%) recruited 100–500 participants and 1 was unknown. For genders, 83 trials (97.65%) recruited both male and female participants; however, 2 (2.35%) trials recruited females only. For age, 73 trials (85.88%) only recruited adults, 5 (5.88%) trials only recruited children, while 7 (8.24%) recruited both adults and children. For status, 14 (16.47%) were not yet recruiting, 20 (23.53%) were recruiting, 39 (45.88%) were completed, while one was suspended, four were terminated or withdrawn and seven were in unknown status. For results, only seven trials reported results on Clinicaltrials.gov, while 78 (91.76%) did not report results. For sponsors, 35 (41.18%) trials were sponsored by universities, 27 (31.76%) were sponsored by hospitals, 10

(11.76%) were sponsored by industries/companies, and 13 (15.29%) were sponsored by other institutions. For funding, 11 trials (12.94%) were funded by industries and 74 (87.06%) did not report clear funding sources. For locations, 30 (35.29%) were in America, 32 (37.65%) were in Europe, 8 (9.41%) in Asia, 4 (4.71%) in Australia and 11 (12.94%) did not report locations.

## DISCUSSION

Clinical trials have played important roles in changing clinical practice (19, 35, 36). Analyzing registered trials could provide a comprehensive analysis of progress in a specific field; thus, numerous studies have been published to analyze registered trials on Clinicaltrials.gov. Considering AI is important tool and have been applied in ED and ICU, we performed the current study to analyze registered trials on AI conducted in ED and ICU.

A total of 146 registered trials were identified, including 61 trials in ED and 85 in ICU, which is similar with our previous study for cancer (33). Over half trials registered after 2017, and it was consistent with the development of industry 4.0, which depended on AI to empower medicine (37). Research in children was often challenging due to scientific, ethical, and practical factors, so only 23.29% trials enrolled children, and 17% enrolled children from 2007 to 2010 (38). More work is needed to ensure that children are equally involved in trials on AI in ED and ICU. In our study, most registered trials included relatively large samples, which would help to reduce the potential risk of statistical error (39). It is interesting to know that no trials were funded by NIH, which did not mean NIH did not fund trials in such field, because academic institutions/medical centers might have been funded by NIH to perform the trials, and they did not report it clearly in the website of Clinicaltrials.gov (30).

Reporting trials' results is very important. In our study, 47.26% trials had been completed, but only 6.85% reported results on ClinicalTrials.gov, suggesting a lack of transparency (40). Although the completion rate was higher than all trials from 2007 to 2010 (38), but reported results was significantly lower than other study (31). The possible explanation might be positive results were submitted more rapidly after completion, and studies sponsored by industries or companies were not likely to report negative results (41, 42). As a public registry platform, ClinicalTrials.gov is expected to make research more transparent and to reduce reporting bias, and sponsors are encouraged to publish their outcomes on ClinicalTrials.gov with no delay (31). Feasibility, lacking funding, unforeseen issues, poor recruitment and change project will also affect the progress of trials. In our study, 6.85% trials were suspended, terminated, or withdrawn, which was not high than previous study (38), suggesting supporting are good for such field.

In our study, a total of 37.64% trials were blinded, and 61.18% were open-labeled, the results were lower than all trials in Clinicaltrials.gov from 2007 to 2010 (38). Randomization is a hallmark of trials, and randomization with blinding can help reduce bias (43). Most trials were observational designs. Observational studies are subjected to a number of potential problems that might cause bias in the results; however, the main methodological issues can be avoided by using specific study designs (44). Therefore, more well-designed trials on AI in ED and ICU are needed to help the progress of prevention, diagnosis, and treatment of emergency and critical illness.

Trials increased a lot in the past several years. With the assistant of AI, the management of patients in ED and ICU will be greatly improved (45). In spite of advantages, we found some deficiencies of trials in this field, such as lack of results reporting, clear information losing and short of trials quantities. Thus, more efforts are needed to help registered trials in this field.

The limitations should be acknowledged. Firstly, ClinicalTrials.gov does not include all trials because some investigators and sponsors may register on other registry platforms. Secondly, our study provided only the characteristics of the registered trials. The actual strengths and weaknesses of the trials were not assessed, and some missing data may bring bias to this study. Thirdly, we did not check whether the registered trials have been published in journals. These results should be analyzed in future.

In conclusion, the current study is the first study to study registered AI trilas in ED and ICU, more trials are needed and sponsors are encouraged to report the results.

## AUTHOR CONTRIBUTIONS

YZ and NL visualized the presented idea and supervised the project, YZ and GL contributed to manuscript writing, GL and YZ contributed to trial searches and preparing the manuscript draft, NL, LC, and YY revised the manuscript. All authors contributed to the article and approved the submitted version.

## ACKNOWLEDGMENTS

The paper has been carefully revised by native English speakers and scientific editors of Enliven LLC to improve grammar and readability.

## REFERENCES

1. Hamet P, Tremblay J. Artificial intelligence in medicine. *Metab Clin Exp.* (2017) 69s:S36–s40. doi: 10.1016/j.metabol.2017.01.011
2. Maddox TM, Rumsfeld JS, Payne PRO. Questions for artificial intelligence in health care. *JAMA.* (2019) 321:31–2. doi: 10.1001/jama.2018.18932
3. Miller DD, Brown EW. Artificial intelligence in medical practice: the question to the answer? *Am J Med.* (2018) 131:129–33. doi: 10.1016/j.amjmed.2017.10.035
4. Goldhahn J, Rampton V, Spinas GA. Could artificial intelligence make doctors obsolete? *BMJ (Clinical research ed).* (2018) 363:k4563. doi: 10.1136/bmj.k4563
5. Rampton V. Artificial intelligence versus clinicians. *BMJ (Clinical research ed).* (2020) 369:m1326. doi: 10.1136/bmj.m1326

6. Vaishya R, Javaid M, Khan IH, Haleem A. Artificial Intelligence (AI) applications for COVID-19 pandemic. *Diabetes Metab Syndrome.* (2020) 14:337–9. doi: 10.1016/j.dsx.2020.04.012
7. Schwalbe N, Wahl B. Artificial intelligence and the future of global health. *Lancet.* (2020) 395:1579–86. doi: 10.1016/S0140-6736(20)30226-9
8. Bi WL, Hosny A, Schabath MB, Giger ML, Birkbak NJ, Mehrtash A, et al. Artificial intelligence in cancer imaging: clinical challenges and applications. *CA Cancer J Clin.* (2019) 69:127–57. doi: 10.3322/caac.21552
9. Stead WW. Clinical implications and challenges of artificial intelligence and deep learning. *JAMA.* (2018) 320:1107–8. doi: 10.1001/jama.2018.11029
10. Liang H, Tsui BY, Ni H, Valentim CCS, Baxter SL, Liu G, et al. Evaluation and accurate diagnoses of pediatric diseases using artificial intelligence. *Nat Med.* (2019) 25:433–8. doi: 10.1038/s41591-018-0335-9
11. Abbasi J. Artificial intelligence tools for sepsis and cancer. *JAMA.* (2018) 320:2303. doi: 10.1001/jama.2018.19383
12. Knaus WA, Marks RD. New phenotypes for sepsis: the promise and problem of applying machine learning and artificial intelligence in clinical research. *JAMA.* (2019) 321:1981–2. doi: 10.1001/jama.2019.5794
13. Matheny ME, Whicher D, Thadaney Israni S. artificial intelligence in health care: a report from the national academy of medicine. *JAMA.* (2020) 323:509–10. doi: 10.1001/jama.2019.21579
14. Zhang Z, Navarese EP, Zheng B, Meng Q, Liu N, Ge H, et al. Analytics with artificial intelligence to advance the treatment of acute respiratory distress syndrome. *J Evid Based Med.* (2020) 13:301–12. doi: 10.1111/jebm.12418
15. Lynch CJ, Liston C. New machine-learning technologies for computer-aided diagnosis. *Nat Med.* (2018) 24:1304–5. doi: 10.1038/s41591-018-0178-4
16. Goto S, Kimura M, Katsumata Y, Goto S, Kamatani T, Ichihara G, et al. Artificial intelligence to predict needs for urgent revascularization from 12-leads electrocardiography in emergency patients. *PLoS One.* (2019) 14:e0210103. doi: 10.1371/journal.pone.0210103
17. Mao Q, Jay M, Hoffman JL, Calvert J, Barton C, Shimabukuro D, et al. Multicentre validation of a sepsis prediction algorithm using only vital sign data in the emergency department, general ward and ICU. *BMJ open.* (2018) 8:e017833. doi: 10.1136/bmjopen-2017-017833
18. Schell CO, Gerdin Wärnberg M, Hvarfner A, Höög A, Baker U, Castegren M, et al. The global need for essential emergency and critical care. *Crit Care (London, England).* (2018) 22:284. doi: 10.1186/s13054-018-2219-2
19. Vincent JL. Critical care–where have we been and where are we going? *Critical Care (London, England).* (2013) 17(Suppl 1):S2. doi: 10.1186/cc11500
20. Singer M, Deutschman CS, Seymour CW, Shankar-Hari M, Annane D, Bauer M, et al. The Third International Consensus Definitions for Sepsis and Septic Shock (Sepsis-3). *JAMA.* (2016) 315:801–10. doi: 10.1001/jama.2016.0287
21. Adhikari NK, Fowler RA, Bhagwanjee S, Rubenfeld GD. Critical care and the global burden of critical illness in adults. *Lancet.* (2010) 376:1339–46. doi: 10.1016/S0140-6736(10)60446-1
22. Hensley MK, Prescott HC. Bad brains, bad outcomes: acute neurologic dysfunction and late death after sepsis. *Crit Care Med.* (2018) 46:1001–2. doi: 10.1097/CCM.0000000000003097
23. Vincent JL, Marshall JC, Namendys-Silva SA, François B, Martin-Loeches I, Lipman J, et al. Assessment of the worldwide burden of critical illness: the intensive care over nations (ICON) audit. *Lancet Respir Med.* (2014) 2:380–6. doi: 10.1016/S2213-2600(14)70061-X
24. Patel VL, Shortliffe EH, Stefanelli M, Szolovits P, Berthold MR, Bellazzi R, et al. The coming of age of artificial intelligence in medicine. *Artif Intell Med.* (2009) 46:5–17. doi: 10.1016/j.artmed.2008.07.017
25. Loftus TJ, Tighe PJ, Filiberto AC, Efron PA, Brakenridge SC, Mohr AM, et al. Artificial intelligence and surgical decision-making. *JAMA Surg.* (2020) 155:148–58. doi: 10.1001/jamasurg.2019.4917
26. Sanchez-Pinto LN, Luo Y, Churpek MM. Big data and data science in critical care. *Chest.* (2018) 154:1239–48. doi: 10.1016/j.chest.2018.04.037
27. Faraoni D, Schaefer ST. Randomized controlled trials vs. observational studies: why not just live together? *BMC Anesthesiol.* (2016) 16:102. doi: 10.1186/s12871-016-0265-3
28. Feizabadi M, Fahimnia F, Mosavi Jarrahi A, Naghshineh N, Tofighi S. Iranian clinical trials: an analysis of registered trials in International Clinical Trial Registry Platform (ICTRP). *J Evid Based Med.* (2017) 10:91–6. doi: 10.1111/jebm.12248
29. DeAngelis CD, Drazen JM, Frizelle FA, Haug C, Hoey J, Horton R, et al. Clinical trial registration: a statement from the International Committee of Medical Journal Editors. *Arch Otolaryngol Head Neck Surg.* (2005) 131:479–80. doi: 10.1001/archotol.131.6.479
30. Chen J, Huang J, Li JV, Lv Y, He Y, Zheng Q. The Characteristics of TCM Clinical Trials: a systematic review of ClinicalTrials.gov. *Evid Based Complem Altern Med.* (2017) 2017:9461415. doi: 10.1155/2017/9461415
31. Chen L, Su Y, Quan L, Zhang Y, Du L. Clinical trials focusing on drug control and prevention of ventilator-associated pneumonia: a comprehensive analysis of trials registered on ClinicalTrials.gov. *Front Pharmacol.* (2018) 9:1574. doi: 10.3389/fphar.2018.01574
32. Chen L, Wang M, Yang Y, Shen J, Zhang Y. Registered interventional clinical trials for old populations with infectious diseases on ClinicalTrials.gov: a cross-sectional study. *Front Pharmacol.* (2020) 11:942. doi: 10.3389/fphar.2020.00942
33. Dong J, Geng Y, Lu D, Li B, Tian L, Lin D, et al. Clinical trials for artificial intelligence in cancer diagnosis: a cross-sectional study of registered trials in ClinicalTrials.gov. *Front Oncol.* (2020) 10:1629. doi: 10.3389/fonc.2020.01629
34. Yao X, Florez ID, Zhang P, Zhang C, Zhang Y, Wang C, et al. Clinical research methods for treatment, diagnosis, prognosis, etiology, screening, and prevention: a narrative review. *J Evid Based Med.* (2020) 13:130–6. doi: 10.1111/jebm.12384
35. Tiguman GMB. Characteristics of Brazilian clinical studies registered in ClinicalTrials.gov between 2010 and 2020. *J Evid Based Med.* (2020) 13:261–4. doi: 10.1111/jebm.12415
36. Heredia P, Alarcon-Ruiz CA, Roque-Roque JS, De La Cruz-Vargas JA, Quispe AM. Publication and associated factors of clinical trials registered in Peru. *J Evid Based Med.* (2020) 13:284–91. doi: 10.1111/jebm.12413
37. Jha S, Topol EJ. Adapting to artificial intelligence: radiologists and pathologists as information specialists. *JAMA.* (2016) 316:2353–4. doi: 10.1001/jama.2016.17438
38. Califf RM, Zarin DA, Kramer JM, Sherman RE, Aberle LH, Tasneem A. Characteristics of clinical trials registered in ClinicalTrials.gov, 2007-2010. *Jama.* (2012) 307:1838–47. doi: 10.1001/jama.2012.3424
39. Inrig JK, Califf RM, Tasneem A, Vegunta RK, Molina C, Stanifer JW, et al. The landscape of clinical trials in nephrology: a systematic review of Clinicaltrials.gov. *Am J Kidney Dis.* (2014) 63:771–80. doi: 10.1053/j.ajkd.2013.10.043
40. Roberto A, Radrezza S, Mosconi P. Transparency in ovarian cancer clinical trial results: ClinicalTrials.gov versus PubMed, Embase and Google scholar. *J Ovarian Res.* (2018) 11:28. doi: 10.1186/s13048-018-0404-1
41. Ioannidis JP. Effect of the statistical significance of results on the time to completion and publication of randomized efficacy trials. *JAMA.* (1998) 279:281–6. doi: 10.1001/jama.279.4.281
42. Lundh A, Lexchin J, Mintzes B, Schroll JB, Bero L. Industry sponsorship and research outcome. *Cochrane Database Syst Rev.* (2017) 2:Mr000033. doi: 10.1002/14651858.MR000033.pub3
43. Berger VW, Alperson SY. A general framework for the evaluation of clinical trial quality. *Rev Recent Clin Trials.* (2009) 4:79–88. doi: 10.2174/157488709788186021
44. Hammer GP, du Prel JB, Blettner M. Avoiding bias in observational studies: part 8 in a series of articles on evaluation of scientific publications. *Dtsch Arztebl Int.* (2009) 106:664–8. doi: 10.3238/arztebl.2009.0664
45. Fleuren LM, Klausch TLT, Zwager CL, Schoonmade LJ, Guo T, Roggeveen LF, et al. Machine learning for the prediction of sepsis: a systematic review and meta-analysis of diagnostic test accuracy. *Intens Care Med.* (2020) 46:383–400. doi: 10.1007/s00134-019-05872-y

# 18

# Development and Validation of a Machine-Learning Model for Prediction of Extubation Failure in Intensive Care Units

*Qin-Yu Zhao[1†], Huan Wang[2†], Jing-Chao Luo[2†], Ming-Hao Luo[3], Le-Ping Liu[4], Shen-Ji Yu[2], Kai Liu[2], Yi-Jie Zhang[2], Peng Sun[5], Guo-Wei Tu[2*] and Zhe Luo[2,6*]*

*[1] College of Engineering and Computer Science, Australian National University, Canberra, ACT, Australia, [2] Department of Critical Care Medicine, Zhongshan Hospital, Fudan University, Shanghai, China, [3] Shanghai Medical College, Fudan University, Shanghai, China, [4] Department of Blood Transfusion, The Third Xiangya Hospital of Central South University, Changsha, China, [5] Artificial Intelligence Institute, Shanghai Jiao Tong University, Shanghai, China, [6] Department of Critical Care Medicine, Xiamen Branch, Zhongshan Hospital, Fudan University, Xiamen, China*

***Correspondence:**
*Guo-Wei Tu*
*tu.guowei@zs-hospital.sh.cn*
*Zhe Luo*
*luo.zhe@zs-hospital.sh.cn*

*[†] These authors have contributed equally to this work and share first authorship*

**Background:** Extubation failure (EF) can lead to an increased chance of ventilator-associated pneumonia, longer hospital stays, and a higher mortality rate. This study aimed to develop and validate an accurate machine-learning model to predict EF in intensive care units (ICUs).

**Methods:** Patients who underwent extubation in the Medical Information Mart for Intensive Care (MIMIC)-IV database were included. EF was defined as the need for ventilatory support (non-invasive ventilation or reintubation) or death within 48 h following extubation. A machine-learning model called Categorical Boosting (CatBoost) was developed based on 89 clinical and laboratory variables. SHapley Additive exPlanations (SHAP) values were calculated to evaluate feature importance and the recursive feature elimination (RFE) algorithm was used to select key features. Hyperparameter optimization was conducted using an automated machine-learning toolkit (Neural Network Intelligence). The final model was trained based on key features and compared with 10 other models. The model was then prospectively validated in patients enrolled in the Cardiac Surgical ICU of Zhongshan Hospital, Fudan University. In addition, a web-based tool was developed to help clinicians use our model.

**Results:** Of 16,189 patients included in the MIMIC-IV cohort, 2,756 (17.0%) had EF. Nineteen key features were selected using the RFE algorithm, including age, body mass index, stroke, heart rate, respiratory rate, mean arterial pressure, peripheral oxygen saturation, temperature, pH, central venous pressure, tidal volume, positive end-expiratory pressure, mean airway pressure, pressure support ventilation (PSV) level, mechanical ventilation (MV) durations, spontaneous breathing trial success times, urine output, crystalloid amount, and antibiotic types. After hyperparameter optimization, our model had the greatest area under the receiver operating characteristic (AUROC: 0.835) in internal validation. Significant differences in mortality, reintubation rates, and NIV rates were shown between patients with a high predicted risk and those with a low predicted risk. In the prospective validation, the superiority of our model was also observed (AUROC: 0.803). According to the SHAP values, MV duration and PSV level were the most important features for prediction.

**Conclusions:** In conclusion, this study developed and prospectively validated a CatBoost model, which better predicted EF in ICUs than other models.

**Keywords: extubation failure, recursive feature elimination, hyperparameter optimization, categorical boosting, prospective validation**

# INTRODUCTION

Extubation, the process of removing an artificial airway to liberate a patient from mechanical ventilation (MV), leads to non-negligible risks due to significant respiratory and circulatory changes. Although MV is an advanced respiratory support widely used in intensive care units (ICUs) (1), prolonged ventilation is associated with poorer prognosis and should be avoided (2, 3). However, premature extubation in unprepared patients will cause extubation failure (EF), leading to a higher risk of ventilator-associated pneumonia, extended hospital stays, and higher mortality (25–50%) (4, 5). Therefore, it is significant to accurately predict the EF risk and optimize the timing of MV weaning.

Many factors have been assessed by prior studies for EF prediction, including Rapid Shallow Breathing Index (RSBI, f/Vt) (6), prolonged MV (7, 8), and cough strength (9, 10). Unfortunately, it was shown that these factors as well as physicians' judgments were not as accurate as expected (11, 12). As a result, the current weaning criteria based on these factors are still unsatisfactory. 10–29% of patients who have met these criteria still experience reintubation (1, 3).

With the rapid development of precision medicine, machine-learning approaches, respected as a deep analysis "vehicle," have derived predictive tools in a vast range of clinical applications (13–15). Some previous studies have explored the ability of machine-learning models to accurately predict EF in recent years (11, 16, 17). Despite remarkable accuracy, these studies had a limited sample size, including only hundreds of observations. Although data resampling methods were applied, the models might overfit specific populations and therefore, lack generalization ability. Other studies developed models based on larger datasets, but they failed to validate their model on an external dataset (12, 18). Furthermore, score variables such as Acute Physiology Age Chronic Health Evaluation (APACHE)-II and Therapeutic Intervention Scoring System (TISS) are included in all these models, probably making the models inconvenient for use in clinical settings.

In this study, we aimed to develop and validate a machine-learning model with good accuracy for a general population. To this end, we explored a large-scale public database to develop a prediction model, using features selected according to their importance and clinical availability. In addition, our model was further validated in a university teaching hospital prospectively.

# MATERIALS AND METHODS

## Source of Data

The model was developed and internally validated based on a sizeable critical care database called the Medical Information Mart for Intensive Care (MIMIC)-IV (19), which consists of comprehensive and high-quality data of patients admitted to ICUs at the Beth Israel Deaconess Medical Center between 2008 and 2019. One author (QZ) obtained access to the database and was responsible for data extraction. For external validation, a prospective cohort was developed in the Cardiac Surgical ICU (CSICU) of Zhongshan Hospital, Fudan University (ZS cohort). This cohort was approved by its institutional ethics committee (Approval No. B2019-075R). The study was reported according to the recommendations of the Transparent Reporting of a multivariable prediction model for Individual Prognosis Or Diagnosis (TRIPOD) statement (20).

## Selection of Participants

In the MIMIC-IV cohort, patients who underwent extubation during ICU stays were included. The exclusion criteria were as follows: (i) age < 18 years, (ii) unplanned extubation, (iii) not the first extubation during the hospital stay, or (iv) no MV records before extubation. In the ZS cohort, all eligible patients that did not meet the exclusion criteria described above from December 2020 to January 2021, were prospectively enrolled. Written consent was obtained from patients' legally authorized representatives upon admission to the ICU.

## Data Collection and Outcome Definition

In the MIMIC-IV cohort, clinical and laboratory variables were extracted within 4 h before extubation (**Supplementary Table 1**), including patient characteristics (age, gender, and ethnicity), laboratory data (arterial blood gas, full blood count, liver function, and renal function), vital signs (respiratory rate, blood pressure, heart rate, peripheral oxygen saturation ($SpO_2$), and temperature). For some variables with multiple measurements, average values were assessed. The average amount per hour of transfusion (red blood cells, platelets, and fresh frozen plasma) and fluid balance (urine output, crystalloid bolus, and colloid bolus) were calculated within 24 h before extubation, and were then normalized by patient weight. Comorbidities were also assessed based on the recorded International Classification of Diseases (ICD)-9 and ICD-10 codes (21), and the Charlson Comorbidity Index was calculated (22). In addition, data on medications such as heparin, antibiotics and vasopressors, as well as continuous renal replacement therapy (CRRT) were extracted. Finally, the 28-day mortality, reintubation, and initiation of non-invasive ventilation (NIV) after extubation were also assessed. In the ZS cohort, due to limited manpower, we did not collect all the variables; instead, key candidate variables were recorded when

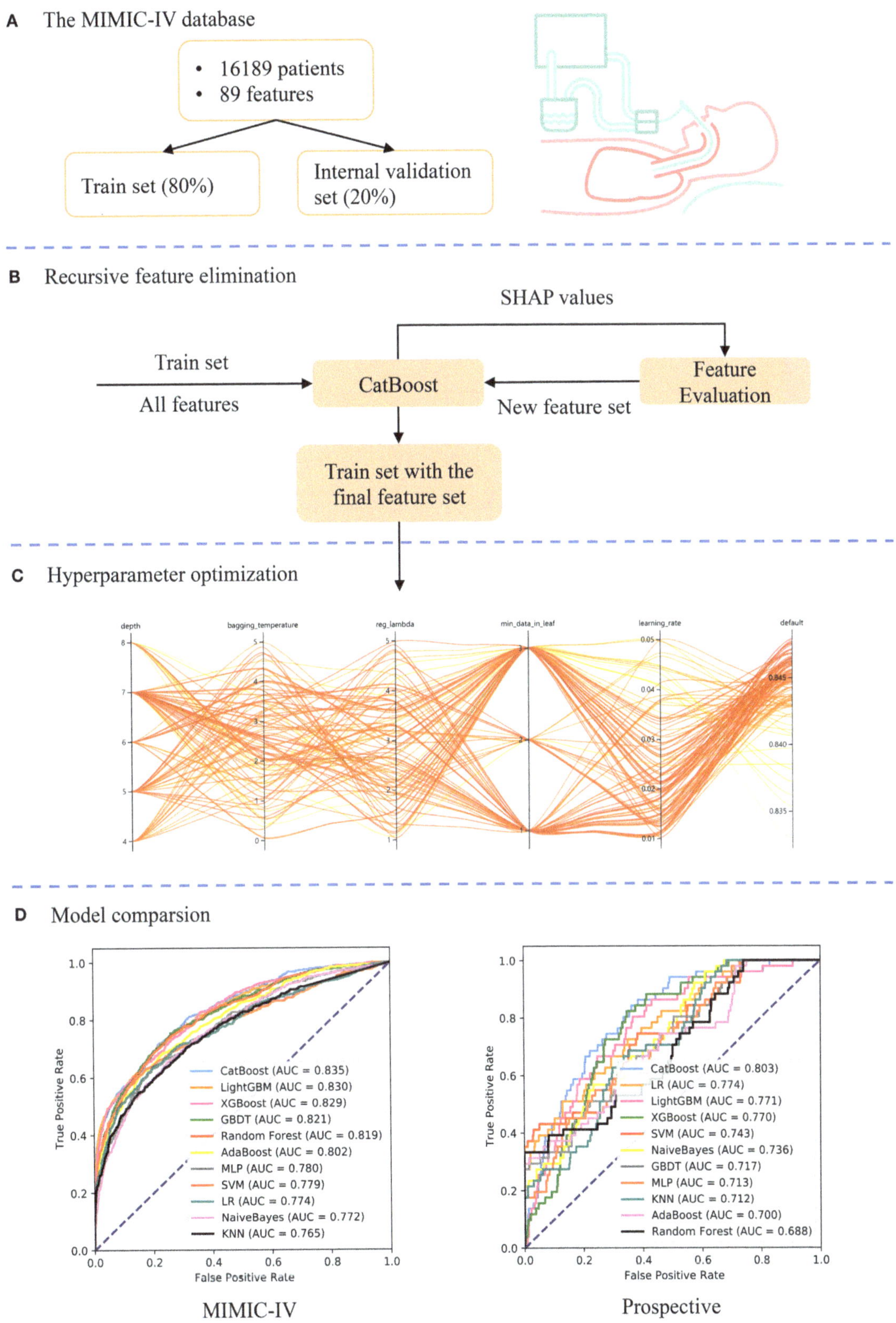


**FIGURE 1** | Schematic illustration of the study design. **(A)** Patients who underwent extubation in the Medical Information Mart for Intensive Care (MIMIC)-IV database were included in the study and 89 variables were extracted. The dataset was divided into train set (80%) and internal validation set (20%). **(B)** The recursive feature elimination algorithm was performed based on the train set, and key features were selected. **(C)** Hyperparameters was optimized using an automated machine learning toolkit on the train set. **(D)** The developed CatBoost model outperformed other models both in the internal validation and prospective validation sets.

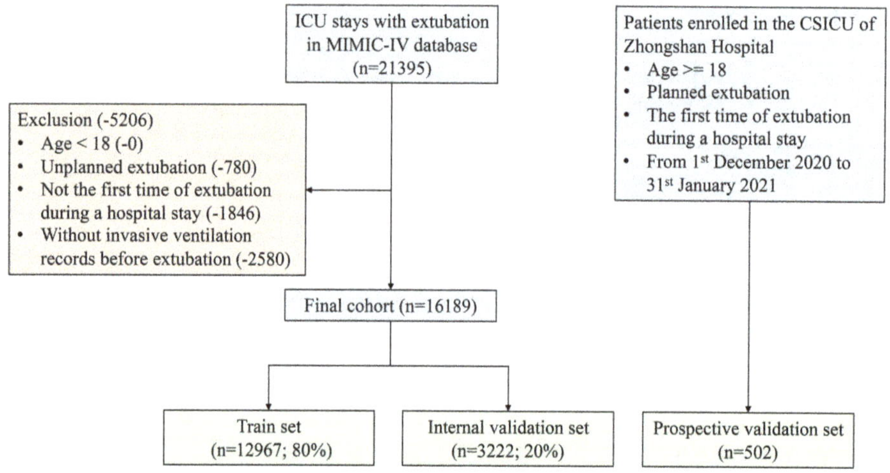


**FIGURE 2** | Flow chart of patient selection. MIMIC-IV, Medical Information Mart for Intensive Care-IV; ICU, intensive care unit.

patients underwent extubation. Patients were followed up until discharge or death.

The primary outcome of the present study was EF, which was defined as the need for ventilatory support (NIV or reintubation) or death within 48 h following planned extubation (5, 23).

## Statistical Analysis

Baseline characteristics were compared between the successful extubation group and the EF group in the MIMIC-IV and ZS cohorts. For continuous variables, values are presented as the means (standard deviations) (if normal) or medians [interquartile ranges] (if non-normal), and comparisons were made using Student's *t*-test or the rank-sum test, as appropriate. For categorical variables, values are presented as total numbers [percentages] and the Chi-square test or Fisher's exact test were used, as appropriate, to examine differences between the two groups.

An advanced machine-learning model called CatBoost was developed using the Catboost Python package (version 0.24). As shown in **Figure 1**, the MIMIC-IV dataset was first randomly split into the train set (80%) and internal validation set (20%). Categorical variables or missing values were not processed, as the CatBoost algorithm could handle them automatically. Second, the recursive feature elimination (RFE) algorithm based on SHapley Additive exPlanations values was performed to screen out key features, as shown in **Figure 1B**. Thus, a full CatBoost model was developed based on the train set with all available variables to predict EF. Second-order variables were calculated based on other variables, such as RSBI, Sequential Organ Failure Assessment (SOFA) and Simplified Acute Physiology Score (SAPS)-II, were manually excluded. The effects of remaining features on prediction scores were then measured using the functions of the SHAP Python package (version 0.32.1), which assessed the importance of each feature using a game-theoretic approach (24). The feature with the smallest effect on the prediction was eliminated in each loop, and a new CatBoost model was recursively fitted based on smaller feature sets until a significant decrease in model performance was observed (25). Finally, key features were selected that had the greatest importance and were easy to collect in clinical settings.

To further improve the model performance, hyperparameter tuning was conducted using an automated machine learning toolkit called Neural Network Intelligence (NNI) designed by Microsoft Research. We chose the Tree-structured Parzen Estimator (TPE), one of the sequential model-based optimization algorithms, as the tuning algorithm. TPE sequentially constructed models to approximate the performance of hyperparameters based on historical measurements, and then subsequently chose new hyperparameters to test based on this model (26). The hyperparameter search domain is summarized in **Supplementary Table 2**. One hundred trials were carried out and the parameters with the greatest area under the receiver operating characteristic (AUROC) were saved. A compact CatBoost model using the saved parameters was then trained based on the selected features, and then validated in the validation sets.

AUROCs were also calculated to compare our model and other predictive factors commonly used in the ICU, such as RSBI, SOFA, SAPS-II, and ROX (the ratio of pulse oximetry/fraction of inspired oxygen to respiratory rate). Additionally, 10 different models were derived in the train set and compared with our CatBoost model, including K-Nearest Neighbor (KNN), AdaBoost, Multi-Layer Perceptron (MLP), Support Vector Machine (SVM), Logistic Regression (LR), NaiveBayes, Gradient Boosting Decision Tree (GBDT), random forest, eXtremely Gradient Boosting (XGBoost) and LightGBM (15). Note that most of these models could not analyze data with missing values, and therefore, datasets were imputed by multiple imputation (27). In addition, categorical variables were converted to one-hot encoding and data were centered to zero and scaled before training the KNN, MLP, SVM, LR, and NaiveBayes models. These models and our CatBoost model were compared both in the internal and prospective validation sets.

**TABLE 1** | Baseline characteristics of the MIMIC-IV and ZS cohorts.

| | MIMIC-IV cohort | | | Zhongshan hospital cohort | | |
|---|---|---|---|---|---|---|
| | Success ($n$ = 13,433) | Failure ($n$ = 2,756) | $P$-value | Success ($n$ = 451) | Failure ($n$ = 51) | $P$-value |
| Age | 64 (16) | 68 (15) | <0.001 | 60 (13) | 63 (12) | 0.073 |
| BMI | 30 (7) | 30 (9) | <0.001 | 24 (12) | 26 (4) | 0.135 |
| Strokes, $n$ (%) | 968 (7) | 543 (20) | <0.001 | 23 (5) | 7 (14) | 0.024 |
| Heart rate (/min) | 83 (15) | 88 (18) | <0.001 | 85 (14) | 95 (20) | 0.002 |
| Respiratory rate (/min) | 18 (4) | 20 (5) | <0.001 | 20 (8) | 23 (6) | <0.001 |
| MAP (mmHg) | 79 (12) | 76 (15) | <0.001 | 81 (10) | 80 (15) | 0.508 |
| $SpO_2$ (%), median [Q1,Q3] | 99 [97,100] | 98 [96,99] | <0.001 | 99 [98,100] | 99 [97,100] | 0.433 |
| Temperature (°C) | 37.0 (0.6) | 37.1 (0.9) | <0.001 | 36.8 (0.6) | 36.9 (0.7) | 0.183 |
| pH | 7.39 (0.05) | 7.36 (0.11) | <0.001 | 7.41 (0.04) | 7.44 (0.03) | 0.197 |
| CVP (mmHg) | 10 (4) | 12 (5) | <0.001 | 11 (2) | 12 (3) | 0.125 |
| Tidal volume (mL/kg), median [Q1,Q3] | 5.8 [4.7,7.1] | 5.6 [4.4,6.9] | <0.001 | 7.2 [6.3,8.5] | 6.9 [5.5,8.2] | 0.557 |
| PEEP ($cmH_2O$) | 4.6 (1.7) | 6.0 (3.0) | <0.001 | 5 (0.0) | 5 (0.0) | 1.000 |
| Mean airway pressure ($cmH_2O$) | 7.3 (2.2) | 9.3 (4.1) | <0.001 | 7.1 (0.7) | 7.4 (0.8) | 0.017 |
| PSV Level ($cmH_2O$), median [Q1,Q3] | 5.0 [5.0,5.0] | 5.0 [5.0,7.5] | <0.001 | 5 [5.0, 5.0] | 5 [5.0, 5.0] | 1.000 |
| MV durations (h), median [Q1,Q3] | 15.9 [7.2,37.0] | 36.9 [15.0,89.6] | <0.001 | 16.0 [13.0,20.0] | 36.0 [16.8,61.0] | <0.001 |
| SBT success times, $n$ (%) | | | | | | |
| 0 | 7,803 (58) | 1,677 (61) | <0.001 | 0 (0.00) | 0 (0.00) | <0.001 |
| 1 | 3,645 (27) | 531 (19) | | 449 (100) | 45 (88) | |
| 2 | 1,025 (8) | 230 (8) | | 2 (0) | 4 (8) | |
| ≥3 | 960 (7) | 318 (12) | | 0 (0.00) | 2 (4) | |
| Urine output (mL/kg/h), median [Q1,Q3] | 0.9 [0.6,1.5] | 0.7 [0.3,1.2] | <0.001 | 1.5 [1.2,1.9] | 1.4 [1.1,1.6] | 0.024 |
| Antibiotic types, $n$ (%) | | | | | | |
| 0 | 10,288 (77) | 1,764 (64) | <0.001 | 0 (0.00) | 0 (0.00) | 1.000 |
| 1 | 2,192 (16) | 428 (16) | | 451 (100) | 51 (100) | |
| 2 | 752 (6) | 334 (12) | | 0 (0.00) | 0 (0.00) | |
| 3 | 169 (1) | 169 (6) | | 0 (0.00) | 0 (0.00) | |
| ≥4 | 32 (0) | 61 (2) | | 0 (0.00) | 0 (0.00) | |
| Failure type, $n$ (%) | | | | | | |
| Death | / | 1,504 (55) | | / | 4 (8) | |
| NIV | / | 411 (15) | | / | 43 (84) | |
| Reintubation | / | 902 (33) | | / | 14 (27) | |

*Values are presented as mean (SD) if not otherwise specified. MIMIC-IV, Medical Information Mart for Intensive Care-IV; ZS, Zhongshan; BMI, body mass index; MAP, mean arterial pressure; $SpO_2$, peripheral oxygen saturation; CVP, central venous pressure; PEEP, positive end-expiratory pressure; PSV, pressure support ventilation; MV, mechanical ventilation; SBT, spontaneous breathing trial; NIV, non-invasive ventilation.*

All statistical analyses in the present study were performed using Python (version 3.7.6); $p < 0.05$ was considered statistically significant.

## RESULTS

### Baseline Characteristics

As shown in **Figure 2**, a total of 16,189 and 502 patients who underwent extubation were ultimately included in the MIMIC-IV and ZS cohorts, respectively. The MIMIC-IV dataset was then divided into the train set ($n = 12,967$) and the internal validation set ($n = 3,222$).

A comparison of baseline characteristics between the successful extubation and EF groups in the MIMIC-IV and ZS cohorts is summarized in **Table 1**. In both cohorts, patients in the failure group had a higher rate of stroke, higher heart rate and respiratory rate, and mean airway pressure ($p < 0.05$). Significant prolonged MV duration and lower urine output were also observed in the failure group in both cohorts. No significant difference in pressure support ventilation (PSV) between the successful extubation and EF group was observed in the ZS cohort as a PSV level of 5 was routinely set at the beginning (28), and the level was elevated when the target tidal volume could not be reached, but not if the patients were unable to tolerate that.

### Development of CatBoost Model

The RFE algorithm was performed, and 19 key features were finally selected, including age, body mass index (BMI), stroke, heart rate, respiratory rate, mean arterial pressure (MAP), $SpO_2$, temperature, pH, central venous pressure

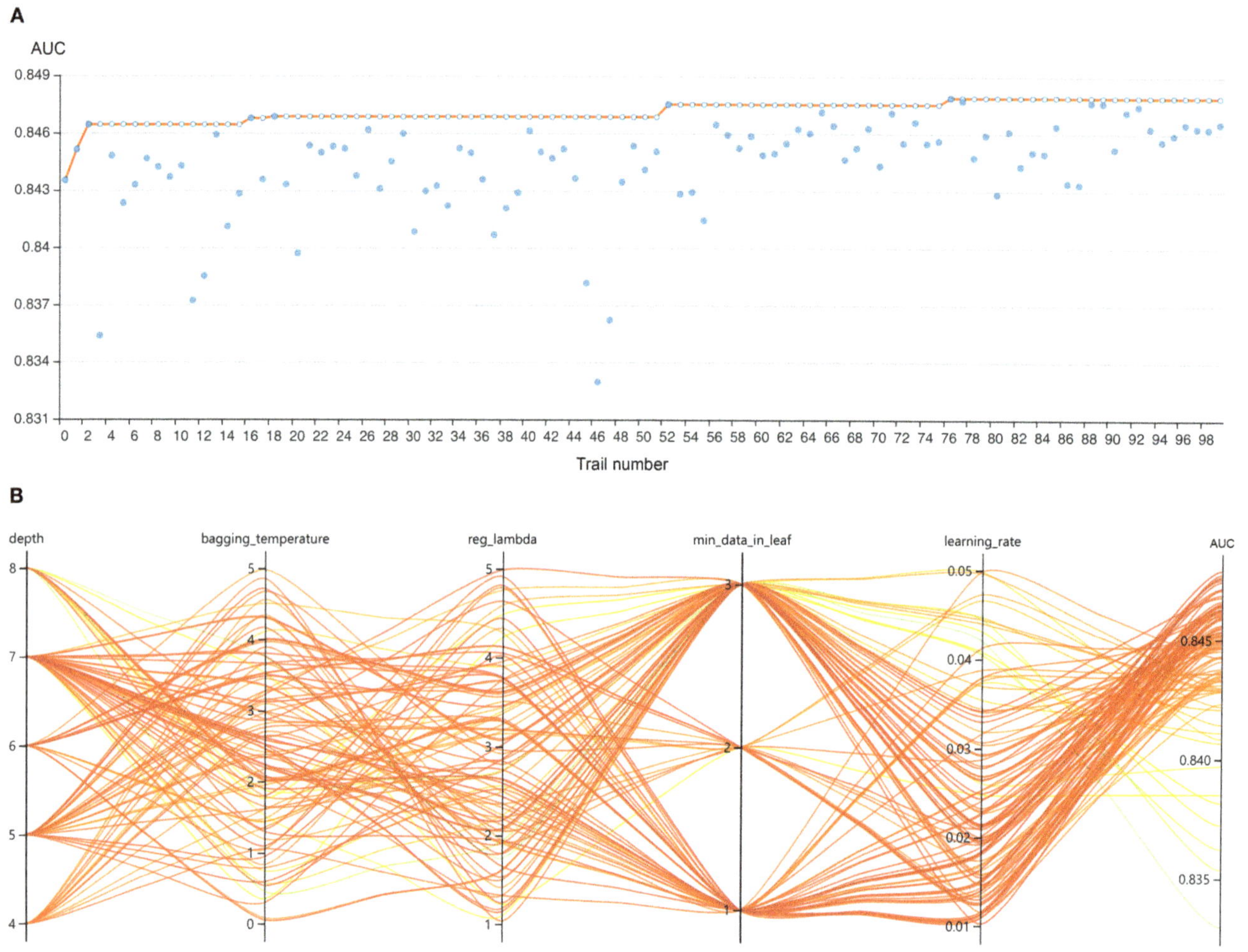


**FIGURE 3 |** Hyperparameter optimization using an automated machine learning toolkit. **(A)** Each blue point represents the result of a trial, and the dark orange line represents the best area under the receiver operating characteristic curve (AUROC). **(B)** Each line represents a trial, and the green to red color represents its AUROC.

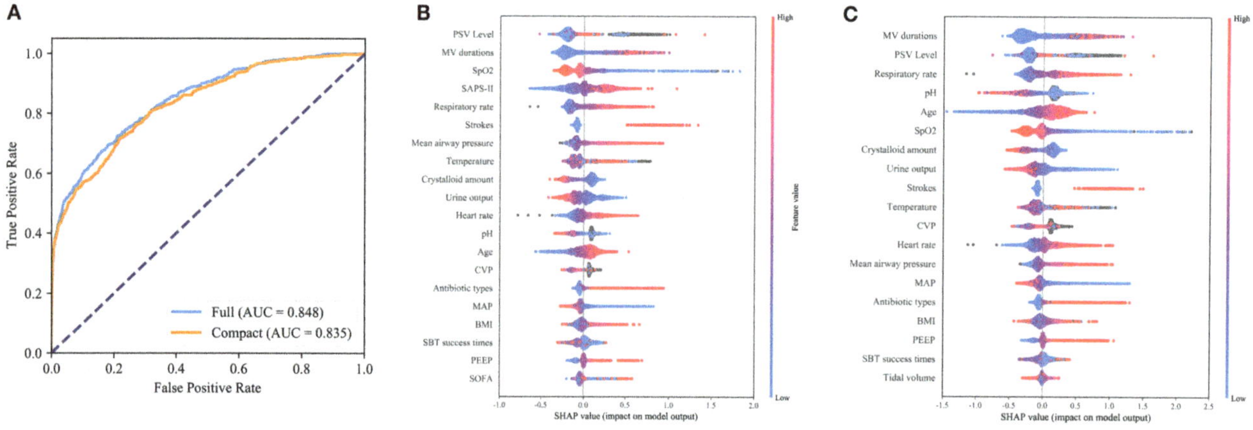


**FIGURE 4 |** Comparison of the full and the compact CatBoost models. The full model was developed based on all available features while the compact was derived based on key features selected by the recursive feature elimination algorithm. Both models had optimized hyperparameters. **(A)** Receiver operating characteristic curves (ROCs) of the full and the compact models. Distribution of the impacts each feature had on the output of the full model **(B)** or compact model **(C)** estimated using the SHapley Additive exPlanations (SHAP) values. The plot sorts features by the sum of SHAP value magnitude over all samples. The blue to red color represents the feature value (red high, blue low). The x-axis measures the impacts on the model output (right positive, left negative).

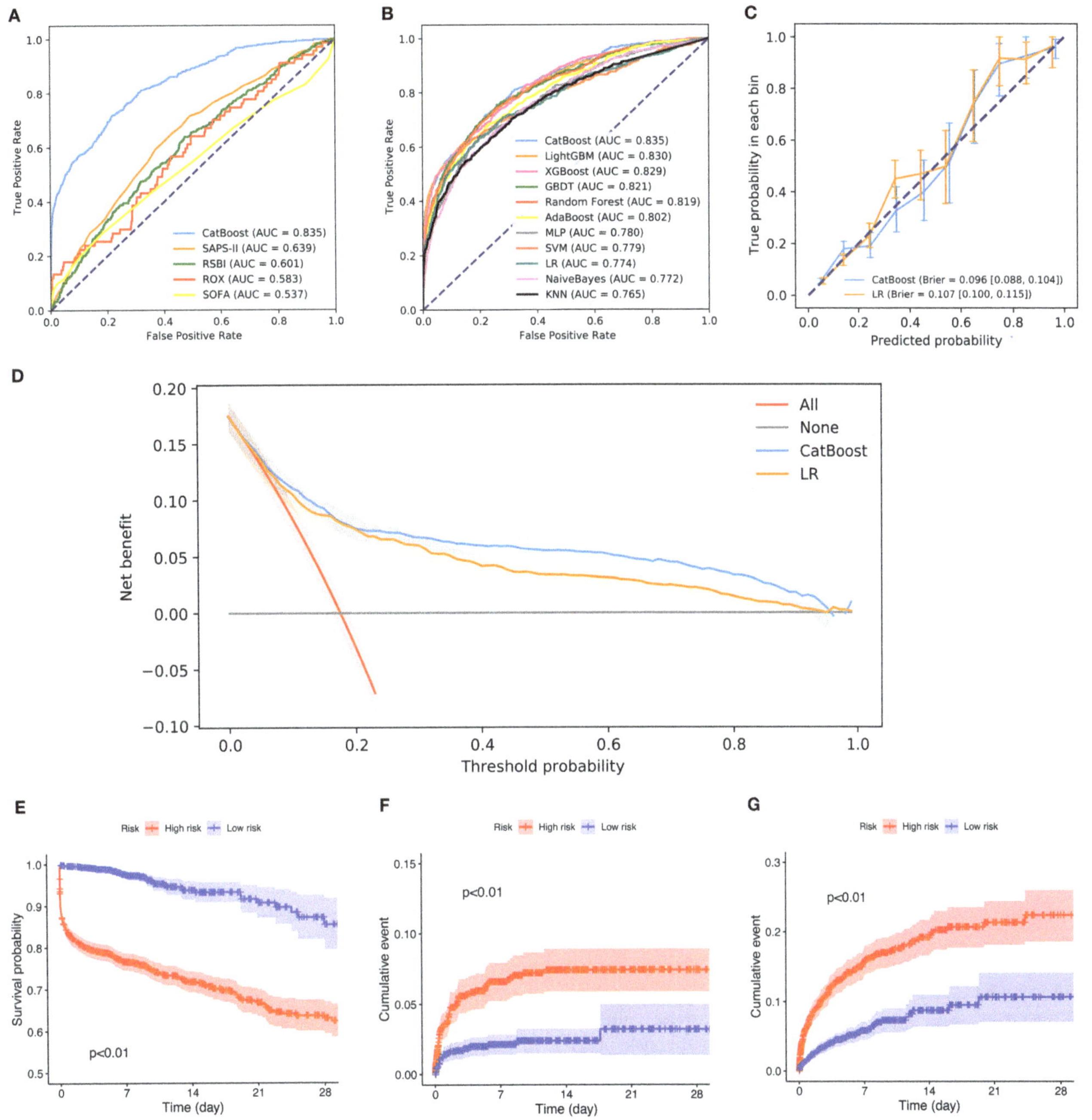


**FIGURE 5 |** Comparison of model performance in the internal validation set. **(A)** Receiver operating characteristic curves (ROCs) of CatBoost and other predictive factors. **(B)** Receiver operating characteristic curves (ROCs) of different models. **(C)** Calibration plot of CatBoost model and Logistic Regression (LR). **(D)** Decision curve analysis of CatBoost and LR. **(E)** Kaplan Meier analysis of 28-day survival in the high- and low-risk groups; **(F)** Cumulative NIV events in the high- and low-risk groups; **(G)** Cumulative reintubation events in the high- and low-risk groups. AUC, area under the curve; RSBI, Rapid Shallow Breathing Index; SOFA, Sequential Organ Failure Assessment; SAPS-II, Simplified Acute Physiology Score-II; ROX, the ratio of pulse oximetry/fraction of inspired oxygen to respiratory rate; XGBOOST, eXtremely Gradient Boosting; GBDT, Gradient Boosting Decision Tree; KNN, K-Nearest Neighbor; SVM, Support Vector Machine; MLP, Multi-Layer Perceptron; LR, Logistic Regression; PPV, Positive Predictive Value; NPV, Negative Predictive Value.

(CVP), tidal volume, positive end-expiratory pressure (PEEP), mean airway pressure, PSV level, MV duration, spontaneous breathing trial (SBT) success time, urine output, crystalloid amount, and antibiotic types. Hyperparameter optimization was then conducted (shown in **Figure 3**). After 100 trials, a CatBoost model with the greatest AUROC was obtained. The final settings of the hyperparameter search are listed in **Supplementary Table 2**.

**TABLE 2** | Model performance in the internal and prospective validation sets.

| Model | AUROC | Best cutoff | Gray zone | Values in gray zone | Youden index (%) | Sensitivity (%) | Specificity (%) | PPV (%) | NPV (%) |
|---|---|---|---|---|---|---|---|---|---|
| **Internal validation** | | | | | | | | | |
| CatBoost | **0.84 (0.82–0.85)** | 0.148 | 0.07–0.24 | 1,276 (39.60%) | **50** | 72 (68–76) | 78 (76–79) | 41 (38–44) | **93 (92–94)** |
| LightGBM | 0.83 (0.81–0.85) | 0.147 | 0.06–0.24 | 1,269 (39.39%) | 49 | 70 (66–74) | 79 (77–80) | 41 (38–44) | 93 (92–94) |
| XGBoost | 0.83 (0.81–0.85) | 0.156 | 0.04–0.23 | 1182 (36.69%) | 47 | 64 (60–68) | 84 (82–85) | 45 (42–49) | 92 (91–93) |
| GBDT | 0.82 (0.80–0.84) | 0.144 | 0.08–0.25 | 1380 (42.62%) | 50 | **76 (72–79)** | 74 (73–76) | 38 (36–41) | 93 (92–95) |
| Random forest | 0.82 (0.80–0.84) | 0.183 | 0.08–0.29 | 1472 (45.46%) | 49 | 73 (70–77) | 75 (74–77) | 39 (36–42) | 93 (92–94) |
| AdaBoost | 0.80 (0.78–0.82) | 0.493 | 0.49–0.50 | 1046 (32.30%) | 45 | 61 (57–65) | 84 (83–86) | 45 (41–49) | 91 (90–92) |
| MLP | 0.78 (0.76–0.80) | 0.173 | 0.02–0.35 | 1737 (53.64%) | 43 | 63 (59–67) | 80 (79–82) | 40 (37–43) | 91 (90–92) |
| SVM | 0.78 (0.76–0.80) | 0.142 | 0.09–0.16 | 2004 (61.89%) | 46 | 60 (56–64) | **86 (85–87)** | **47 (44–51)** | 91 (90–92) |
| LR | 0.77 (0.75–0.80) | 0.179 | 0.06–0.25 | 1840 (56.83%) | 44 | 64 (60–68) | 80 (79–81) | 40 (37–43) | 91 (90–92) |
| NaiveBayes | 0.77 (0.75–0.79) | 0.058 | 0.00–0.49 | 2711 (83.72%) | 41 | 65 (62–70) | 75 (74–77) | 36 (33–39) | 91 (90–92) |
| KNN | 0.77 (0.74–0.79) | 0.188 | 0.05–0.21 | 1428 (44.10%) | 40 | 55 (51–59) | 85 (84–86) | 44 (40–47) | 90 (89–91) |
| **Prospective validation** | | | | | | | | | |
| CatBoost | **0.80 (0.74–0.86)** | 0.049 | 0.04–0.09 | 198 (39.36%) | **48** | 85 (74–93) | 64 (59–68) | 21 (15–26) | 97 (95–99) |
| LR | 0.77 (0.70–0.84) | 0.834 | 0.37–0.88 | 246 (48.91%) | 38 | 51 (37–65) | 87 (84–90) | 31 (21–42) | 94 (92–96) |
| LightGBM | 0.77 (0.70–0.84) | 0.053 | 0.04–0.10 | 260 (51.69%) | 44 | 81 (69–91) | 63 (59–68) | 20 (15–26) | 97 (95–99) |
| XGBoost | 0.77 (0.71–0.82) | 0.045 | 0.03–0.13 | 217 (43.14%) | 48 | 83 (71–93) | 65 (61–70) | 21 (15–27) | 97 (95–99) |
| SVM | 0.74 (0.67–0.82) | 0.956 | 0.33–0.85 | 254 (50.50%) | 38 | 41 (28–55) | 97 (95–98) | 60 (43–77) | 94 (91–96) |
| NaiveBayes | 0.74 (0.66–0.80) | 0.377 | 0.42–0.87 | 230 (45.73%) | 35 | **96 (90–100)** | 39 (34–43) | 15 (12–19) | **99 (97–100)** |
| GBDT | 0.72 (0.64–0.79) | 0.495 | 0.34–0.85 | 261 (51.89%) | 30 | 81 (68–91) | 49 (44–54) | 15 (11–19) | 96 (93–98) |
| MLP | 0.71 (0.64–0.78) | 0.781 | 0.37–0.90 | 275 (54.67%) | 31 | 55 (42–69) | 76 (72–80) | 20 (14–27) | 94 (91–96) |
| KNN | 0.71 (0.65–0.78) | 0.63 | 0.42–0.88 | 239 (47.51%) | 33 | 69 (55–81) | 65 (60–69) | 18 (13–24) | 95 (92–97) |
| AdaBoost | 0.70 (0.62–0.78) | 0.992 | 0.34–0.88 | 271 (53.88%) | 30 | 31 (19–44) | **98 (97–100)** | **70 (50–88)** | 93 (90–95) |
| Random forest | 0.69 (0.62–0.77) | 0.64 | 0.32–0.85 | 278 (55.27%) | 33 | 48 (31–58) | 85 (74–92) | 60 (49–72) | 93 (91–95) |

*Models are ordered according to their areas under receiver operating characteristic curves. Youden index was defined as sensitivity + specificity − 1. The bold values indicate the best performance of the 10 models in the internal or prospective validation. XGBOOST, eXtremely Gradient Boosting; GBDT, Gradient Boosting Decision Tree; KNN, K-Nearest Neighbor; SVM, Support Vector Machine; MLP, Multi-Layer Perceptron; LR, Logistic Regression; PPV, Positive Predictive Value; NPV, Negative Predictive Value.*

As shown in **Figure 4A**, the CatBoost model with all available variables had a remarkable AUROC of 0.848, while the compact model with 19 selected variables had a slightly lower AUROC of 0.835. SHAP values for the two models were assessed in the internal validation set, and are shown in **Figures 4B,C**, respectively. Feature values were indicated by a spectrum with blue representing the lowest value. A positive SHAP value represents an increase in the risk of EF and vice versa. Features were ranked according to the sum of absolute SHAP values over all samples. As shown, MV duration is the most important feature for prediction of EF in the final model, and a longer duration indicates a higher EF risk.

**Figures 5A,B** depicts the comparison between the CatBoost model and other predictive factors or models. As shown, our CatBoost model significantly outperformed other predictive factors or models and had the greatest AUROC. To further elucidate the performance of our model, a calibration plot (**Figure 5C**) and decision curve analysis (**Figure 5D**) were performed (29). For simplicity, only the results of CatBoost and LR are demonstrated. The sensitivity and specificity analysis of these predictive methods in the internal validation set is summarized in **Table 2**. Although the CatBoost model was not the best on all measures, it had the greatest Youden Index (0.499) which is considered a more comprehensive evaluation approach.

Additionally, patients in the internal validation set were divided into high- and low-risk groups, according to whether their failure risks predicted by CatBoost were greater than the median risk in the set. **Figures 5E–G** shows the survival curves, cumulative NIV curves, and cumulative reintubation curves of the two groups, respectively. Log rank $p$-values are lower than 0.01 in **Figures 5E–G**, indicating significant differences between the high- and low-risk groups.

## Prospective Validation and a Web-Based Tool

The results of prospective validation are shown in **Figure 6A**. It can be seen that our model also had a better generalization ability (AUROC: 0.803 [95%CI: 0.74–0.86]) than the other models. The sensitivity and specificity analyses are summarized in **Table 2**.

In addition, a web-based tool was established for clinicians to use the compact model, http://www.aimedicallab.com/tool/aiml-extfailure.html. An example of using our tool is depicted in **Figure 6B**. A user needs to enter the variable values when weaning, leaving missing values blank and clicking the "predict" button. The risk of EF assessed by the CatBoost model, and the

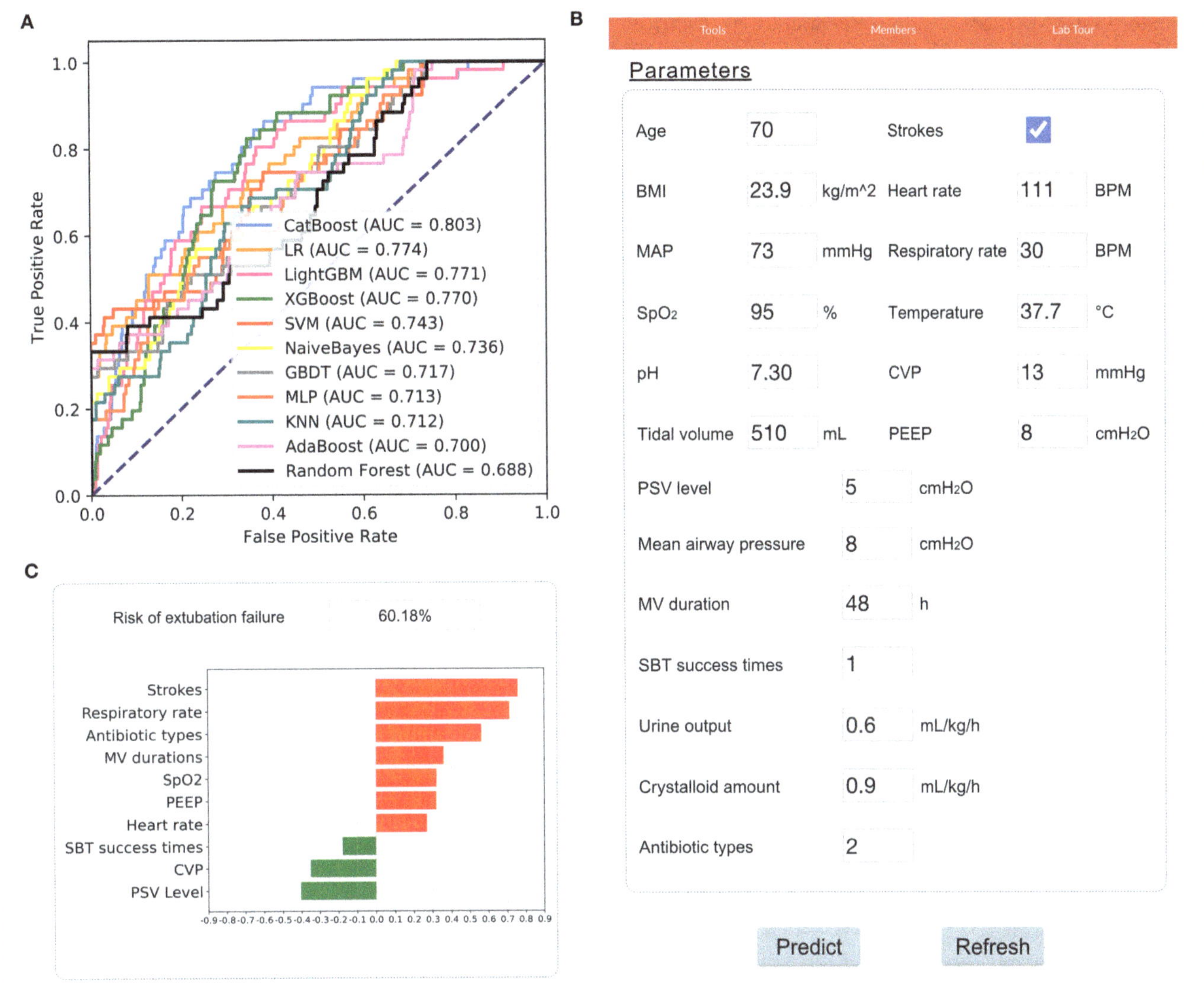


**FIGURE 6 |** Application of the CatBoost model. **(A)** Receiver operating characteristic curves of different models in the prospective validation set. **(B)** An example of the web-based tool. **(C)** The prediction results of the CatBoost model and the top 10 important features were summarized. A green bar indicates a protective factor while a red bar represents a risk factor. The bar length corresponds to the magnitude of protection or risk.

top 10 important features will be shown to the user, as shown in **Figure 6C**.

## DISCUSSION

In this study, we developed and validated an accurate machine-learning model for predicting EF in ventilated critically ill patients. To our knowledge, this is the first model constructed on a large-scale public database and then further validated in a university teaching hospital prospectively. Moreover, different to previously published models, we provide an open and accessible data interface for the public to use and validate our model.

Eighty-nine variables were evaluated, and key features were screened out, improving model usability compared with previous studies. We eventually selected 19 key features that could be more easily obtained, including age, BMI, stroke, heart rate, respiratory rate, MAP, $SpO_2$, temperature, pH, CVP, tidal volume, PEEP, mean airway pressure, PSV level, MV duration, SBT success time, urine output, crystalloid amount, and antibiotic types. As expected, the slight decrease in the AUROC of the compact model based on selected features (shown in **Figure 4A**), demonstrated that other variables could be excluded without a marked negative effect on the model performance.

Previous studies indicated that age and BMI are two important factors associated with an increased risk of EF (6, 30–32). Elderly or overweight patients have a higher prevalence of comorbidities, a decline in cardiac and lung functions, and a higher risk of respiratory failure, leading to a worse outcome following extubation. Increasing evidence supports that stroke patients suffer a higher risk of EF, and airway management remains a clinical challenge in this population (33, 34).

In addition, abnormal vital signs, such as heart rate, respiratory rate, MAP, $SpO_2$, and temperature were related to a higher EF risk (35, 36). These basic factors are commonly used in ICUs, representing the vital status of a patient, and were included in many prediction models. Arterial pH was another key feature in our study, which monitors the body's acid-base balance. A lower-than-normal pH indicates hypoventilation or severe pulmonary disease, and was a remarkable predictive factor for EF according to its SHAP values.

Our study also showed that CVP contributed to EF prediction. As shown in **Figure 4C**, gray points of CVP representing missing values, had positive SHAP values as shown, which suggested that patients without CVP measures had a higher failure rate. Prior research has explored the benefit of CVP measurement in septic patients (37). In our study, it was shown that CVP monitoring might also be associated with improved outcomes following extubation. More studies are needed to confirm this.

As expected, SBT success time and parameters of MV such as tidal volume, PEEP and mean airway pressure, helped to accurately predict EF in our study. By assessing SHAP values, we found that MV duration and PSV level were the most important features for prediction, which is consistent with previous studies (7, 38–41). Additionally, fluid balance (only urine output, crystalloid amount in our study) and antibiotic types were included in the final model. Evidence suggests that fluid balance was associated with failed extubation and was consistent with our findings (32, 42). The number of antibiotics administered to a patient reflected his or her infectious status. As shown in **Figure 4C**, a greater number of antibiotics administered was related to a higher EF risk.

Although SAPS-II, APACHE-II, and other risk scores showed great importance for prediction in previous studies (16, 17) as well as in our study, we excluded these features for two main reasons. Firstly, the extracted features covered most components of these scores, leading to negligible benefits of including these scores. Previous research has shown that excluding these scores did not impede the development of an accurate model (43). Secondly, including these scores such as APACHE-II and SOFA, would make our model inconvenient to use in clinical settings.

Based on these key features, a CatBoost model was derived with optimized hyperparameters and outperformed other predictive factors and 10 models in the MIMIC-IV dataset. CatBoost, a member of the gradient boosting algorithm family, has not been widely adopted in critical care research, despite the fact that CatBoost significantly outperformed other machine-learning models in various tasks in some previous studies (44). Its main advantage is that it can successfully handle categorical features and missing values automatically, and takes advantage of dealing with them during training instead of preprocessing time (45). Therefore, categorical features no longer need to be encoded, and missing values do not need to be imputed. Another advantage of the algorithm is that it uses a new schema to calculate leaf values when selecting the tree structure. The schema helps to reduce overfitting, the major problem that constrains the generalization ability of machine-learning models (45).

Apart from internal validation, we enrolled more than 500 patients in the CSICU of Zhongshan Hospital, Fudan University to prospectively validate our model. As shown in **Figure 6**, our model had a greater AUROC than others, indicating a remarkable generalization ability and clinical value. To help clinicians use the model, a web-based tool was developed, which provides a user-friendly interface. After entering the variables, the risk of EF, as well as the top 10 important features were shown. These results will help clinical decision-makers to understand the patient's status and prepare an appropriate treatment strategy.

More importantly, our model is a promising tool for improving the prognosis of patients who undergo extubation and can have a positive impact both medically and financially. As shown in previous studies, either EF or reintubation is independently associated with higher mortality (3, 46). Reintubation is also accompanied by the occurrence of complications such as acute respiratory distress syndrome, sepsis, ventilator-associated pneumonia, prolonged ICU stay, and increased medical cost (4, 5). By adopting this model, if a patient is predicted to have a high risk of EF, weaning from MV can be delayed, and more intensive monitoring will be granted, which may avoid injuries caused by EF and reduce mortality. In addition, extra medical costs due to further medical investigations and treatments could be prevented as low-risk patients would be less likely to develop severe complications. The clinical value of this model will be further assessed and reported in future prospective studies.

Several limitations of this study should be considered. Firstly, there is still disagreement on the definition of EF. The definition adopted in the present study included the need for NIV, reintubation and death within 48 h following extubation. High-flow oxygen therapy, with the potential to prevent reintubation, was excluded. Further studies should be carried to include the use of a high-flow nasal cannula as EF. A different time interval (e.g., 72 h following extubation) could also be studied. Secondly, the majority of routine ventilation methods following surgery were included in our study, which have a minimal risk of EF. This could have led to biased results. Our future study is to fine-tune our model or develop new models for patients who undergo difficult or prolonged weaning. These patients have a significantly higher risk of EF in ICUs. Thirdly, novel parameters or techniques proposed in recent studies were not included in the present study, such as central venous-to-arterial $P_{CO2}$ difference (36), the cuff leak test (47), thenar oxygen saturation (48), and diaphragm dysfunction (49). We argue that these parameters or techniques need multiple measurements or complex calculations, leading to difficult application in clinical settings. The variables selected in our study are rapidly available and directly measured, improving model practicality. Fourthly, the sensitivity and specificity of our model were 72 and 78%, respectively, indicating that the false negative rate could be relatively high. A number of patients with EF may be missed, which is important as they have a non-negligible mortality. Lastly, patients enrolled in the prospective validation set were all from one CSICU; thus, this dataset can only validate the efficacy of our model in a limited patient population. More large-scale prospective studies are needed to validate our model.

## CONCLUSIONS

In conclusion, the present study screened out 19 key features associated with EF and developed a CatBoost model which can better predict EF than other predictive methods in ICUs.

## ETHICS STATEMENT

The establishment of the MIMIC-IV database was approved by the Massachusetts Institute of Technology (Cambridge, MA) and Beth Israel Deaconess Medical Center (Boston, MA), and consent was obtained for the original data collection. Therefore, the ethical approval statement and the need for informed consent were waived for the studies on this database. Besides, the prospective study involving human participants was reviewed and approved by Ethics Committee of Zhongshan Hospital, Fudan University. The patients/participants provided their written informed consent to participate in this study.

## AUTHOR CONTRIBUTIONS

Q-YZ, HW, and J-CL: conception, design, data analysis, and interpretation. G-WT and ZL: administrative support. Q-YZ and HW: collection and collation of data. All authors: manuscript writing and final approval of manuscript.

## REFERENCES


1. Penuelas O, Frutos-Vivar F, Fernandez C, Anzueto A, Epstein SK, Apezteguia C, et al. Characteristics and outcomes of ventilated patients according to time to liberation from mechanical ventilation. *Am J Respir Crit Care Med.* (2011) 184:430–7. doi: 10.1164/rccm.201011-1887OC
2. Fernandez-Zamora MD, Gordillo-Brenes A, Banderas-Bravo E, Arboleda-Sanchez JA, Hinojosa-Perez R, Aguilar-Alonso E, et al. Prolonged mechanical ventilation as a predictor of mortality after cardiac surgery. *Respir Care.* (2018) 63:550–7. doi: 10.4187/respcare.04915
3. Frutos-Vivar F, Esteban A, Apezteguia C, Gonzalez M, Arabi Y, Restrepo MI, et al. Outcome of reintubated patients after scheduled extubation. *J Crit Care.* (2011) 26:502–9. doi: 10.1016/j.jcrc.2010.12.015
4. Thille AW, Harrois A, Schortgen F, Brun-Buisson C, Brochard L. Outcomes of extubation failure in medical intensive care unit patients. *Crit Care Med.* (2011) 39:2612–8. doi: 10.1097/CCM.0b013e3182282a5a
5. Perren A, Previsdomini M, Llamas M, Cerutti B, Gyorik S, Merlani G, et al. Patients' prediction of extubation success. *Intensive Care Med.* (2010) 36:2045–52. doi: 10.1007/s00134-010-1984-4
6. Frutos-Vivar F, Ferguson ND, Esteban A, Epstein SK, Arabi Y, Apezteguia C, et al. Risk factors for extubation failure in patients following a successful spontaneous breathing trial. *Chest.* (2006) 130:1664–71. doi: 10.1378/chest.130.6.1664
7. Silva-Cruz AL, Velarde-Jacay K, Carreazo NY, Escalante-Kanashiro R. Risk factors for extubation failure in the intensive care unit. *Rev Bras Ter Intensiva.* (2018) 30:294–300. doi: 10.5935/0103-507X.20180046
8. Thille AW, Boissier F, Ben Ghezala H, Razazi K, Mekontso-Dessap A, Brun-Buisson C. Risk factors for and prediction by caregivers of extubation failure in ICU patients: a prospective study. *Crit Care Med.* (2015) 43:613–20. doi: 10.1097/CCM.0000000000000748
9. Su WL, Chen YH, Chen CW, Yang SH, Su CL, Perng WC, et al. Involuntary cough strength and extubation outcomes for patients in an ICU. *Chest.* (2010) 137:777–82. doi: 10.1378/chest.07-2808
10. Khamiees M, Raju P, DeGirolamo A, Amoateng-Adjepong Y, Manthous CA. Predictors of extubation outcome in patients who have successfully completed a spontaneous breathing trial. *Chest.* (2001) 120:1262–70. doi: 10.1378/chest.120.4.1262
11. Mueller M, Almeida JS, Stanislaus R, Wagner CL. Can machine learning methods predict extubation outcome in premature infants as well as clinicians? *J Neonatal Biol.* (2013) 2:1000118. doi: 10.1109/IJCNN.2013.6707058
12. Hsieh MH, Hsieh MJ, Chen CM, Hsieh CC, Chao CM, Lai CC. An artificial neural network model for predicting successful extubation in intensive care units. *J Clin Med.* (2018) 7:240. doi: 10.3390/jcm7090240
13. Zhang Z, Ho KM, Hong Y. Machine learning for the prediction of volume responsiveness in patients with oliguric acute kidney injury in critical care. *Crit Care.* (2019) 23:112. doi: 10.1186/s13054-019-2411-z
14. Zhang Z, Zhao Y, Canes A, Steinberg D, Lyashevska O, written on behalf of AMEB-DCTCG. Predictive analytics with gradient boosting in clinical medicine. *Ann Transl Med.* (2019) 7:152. doi: 10.21037/atm.2019.03.29
15. Luo JC, Zhao QY, Tu GW. Clinical prediction models in the precision medicine era: old and new algorithms. *Ann Transl Med.* (2020) 8:274. doi: 10.21037/atm.2020.02.63
16. Tsai TL, Huang MH, Lee CY, Lai WW. Data science for extubation prediction and value of information in surgical intensive care unit. *J Clin Med.* (2019) 8:1709. doi: 10.3390/jcm8101709
17. Fabregat A, Magret M, Ferre JA, Vernet A, Guasch N, Rodriguez A, et al. A Machine Learning decision-making tool for extubation in Intensive Care Unit patients. *Comput Methods Programs Biomed* (2020) 200:105869. doi: 10.1016/j.cmpb.2020.105869
18. Chen T, Xu J, Ying H, Chen X, Feng R, Fang X, et al. Prediction of extubation failure for intensive care unit patients using light gradient boosting machine. *IEEE Access.* (2019) 7:150960–8. doi: 10.1109/ACCESS.2019.2946980
19. Goldberger AL, Amaral LA, Glass L, Hausdorff JM, Ivanov PC, Mark RG, et al. PhysioBank, PhysioToolkit, and PhysioNet: components of a new research resource for complex physiologic signals. *Circulation.* (2000) 101:E215–20. doi: 10.1161/01.CIR.101.23.e215
20. Collins GS, Reitsma JB, Altman DG, Moons KG. Transparent reporting of a multivariable prediction model for individual prognosis or diagnosis (TRIPOD): the TRIPOD Statement. *BMC Med.* (2015) 13:1. doi: 10.1186/s12916-014-0241-z
21. Quan H, Sundararajan V, Halfon P, Fong A, Burnand B, Luthi JC, et al. Coding algorithms for defining comorbidities in ICD-9-CM and ICD-10 administrative data. *Med Care.* (2005) 43:1130–9. doi: 10.1097/01.mlr.0000182534.19832.83
22. Charlson ME, Pompei P, Ales KL, MacKenzie CR. A new method of classifying prognostic comorbidity in longitudinal studies: development and validation. *J Chronic Dis.* (1987) 40:373–83. doi: 10.1016/0021-9681(87)90171-8
23. Boles JM, Bion J, Connors A, Herridge M, Marsh B, Melot C, et al. Weaning from mechanical ventilation. *Eur Respir J.* (2007) 29:1033–56. doi: 10.1183/09031936.00010206
24. Lundberg SM, Erion G, Chen H, DeGrave A, Prutkin JM, Nair B, et al. From local explanations to global understanding with explainable AI for trees. *Nat Mach Intell.* (2020) 2:56–67. doi: 10.1038/s42256-019-0138-9
25. Zhang Z. Variable selection with stepwise and best subset approaches. *Ann Transl Med.* (2016) 4:136. doi: 10.21037/atm.2016.03.35
26. Bergstra J, Bardenet R, Bengio Y, Kégl B. Algorithms for hyper-parameter optimization. *Proceedings of the 24th International Conference on Neural Information Processing Systems.* Granada, Spain: Curran Associates Inc. (2011). p. 2546–54. doi: 10.5555/2986459.2986743
27. Zhang Z. Multiple imputation with multivariate imputation by chained equation (MICE) package. *Ann Transl Med.* (2016) 4:30. doi: 10.3978/j.issn.2305-5839.2015.12.63
28. Schmidt GA, Girard TD, Kress JP, Morris PE, Ouellette DR, Alhazzani W, et al. Official executive summary of an American thoracic society/American college of chest physicians clinical practice guideline: liberation from mechanical

ventilation in critically ill adults. *Am J Respir Crit Care Med.* (2017) 195:115–9. doi: 10.1164/rccm.201610-2076ST
29. Zhang Z, Rousson V, Lee WC, Ferdynus C, Chen M, Qian X, et al. Decision curve analysis: a technical note. *Ann Transl Med.* (2018) 6:308. doi: 10.21037/atm.2018.07.02
30. El Solh AA, Bhat A, Gunen H, Berbary E. Extubation failure in the elderly. *Respir Med.* (2004) 98:661–8. doi: 10.1016/j.rmed.2003.12.010
31. De Jong A, Wrigge H, Hedenstierna G, Gattinoni L, Chiumello D, Frat JP, et al. How to ventilate obese patients in the ICU. *Intensive Care Med.* (2020) 46:2423–35. doi: 10.1007/s00134-020-06286-x
32. Maezawa S, Kudo D, Miyagawa N, Yamanouchi S, Kushimoto S. Association of body weight change and fluid balance with extubation failure in intensive care unit patients: a single-center observational study. *J Intensive Care Med.* (2021) 36:175–81. doi: 10.1177/0885066619887694
33. Castro AA, Cortopassi F, Sabbag R, Torre-Bouscoulet L, Kumpel C, Ferreira Porto E. Respiratory muscle assessment in predicting extubation outcome in patients with stroke. *Arch Bronconeumol.* (2012) 48:274–9. doi: 10.1016/j.arbr.2012.06.007
34. Suntrup-Krueger S, Schmidt S, Warnecke T, Steidl C, Muhle P, Schroeder JB, et al. Extubation readiness in critically ill stroke patients. *Stroke.* (2019) 50:1981–8. doi: 10.1161/STROKEAHA.118.024643
35. Xie J, Cheng G, Zheng Z, Luo H, Ooi OC. To extubate or not to extubate: risk factors for extubation failure and deterioration with further mechanical ventilation. *J Card Surg.* (2019) 34:1004–11. doi: 10.1111/jocs.14189
36. Mallat J, Baghdadi FA, Mohammad U, Lemyze M, Temime J, Tronchon L, et al. Central venous-to-arterial PCO2 difference and central venous oxygen saturation in the detection of extubation failure in critically ill patients. *Crit Care Med.* (2020) 48:1454–61. doi: 10.1097/CCM.0000000000004446
37. Chen H, Zhu Z, Zhao C, Guo Y, Chen D, Wei Y, et al. Central venous pressure measurement is associated with improved outcomes in septic patients: an analysis of the MIMIC-III database. *Crit Care.* (2020) 24:433. doi: 10.1186/s13054-020-03109-9
38. Vidotto MC, Sogame LC, Gazzotti MR, Prandini MN, Jardim JR. Analysis of risk factors for extubation failure in subjects submitted to non-emergency elective intracranial surgery. *Respir Care.* (2012) 57:2059–66. doi: 10.4187/respcare.01039
39. Vidotto MC, Sogame LC, Calciolari CC, Nascimento OA, Jardim JR. The prediction of extubation success of postoperative neurosurgical patients using frequency-tidal volume ratios. *Neurocrit Care.* (2008) 9:83–9. doi: 10.1007/s12028-008-9059-x
40. Brochard L, Rauss A, Benito S, Conti G, Mancebo J, Rekik N, et al. Comparison of three methods of gradual withdrawal from ventilatory support during weaning from mechanical ventilation. *Am J Respir Crit Care Med.* (1994) 150:896–903. doi: 10.1164/ajrccm.150.4.7921460
41. Farhadi R, Lotfi HR, Alipour A, Nakhshab M, Ghaffari V, Hashemi SA. Comparison of two levels of pressure support ventilation on success of extubation in preterm neonates: a randomized clinical trial. *Glob J Health Sci.* (2015) 8:240–7. doi: 10.5539/gjhs.v8n2p240
42. Upadya A, Tilluckdharry L, Muralidharan V, Amoateng-Adjepong Y, Manthous CA. Fluid balance and weaning outcomes. *Intensive Care Med.* (2005) 31:1643–7. doi: 10.1007/s00134-005-2801-3
43. Liu L, Xie J, Wu W, Chen H, Li S, He H, et al. A simple nomogram for predicting failure of non-invasive respiratory strategies in adults with COVID-19: a retrospective multicentre study. *Lancet Digit Health* (2021) 3:e166–74. doi: 10.1016/S2589-7500(20)30316-2
44. Zhao QY, Liu LP, Luo JC, Luo YW, Wang H, Zhang YJ, et al. A machine-learning approach for dynamic prediction of sepsis-induced coagulopathy in critically ill patients with sepsis. *Front Med.* (2020) 7:637434. doi: 10.3389/fmed.2020.637434
45. Prokhorenkova L, Gusev G, Vorobev A, Dorogush AV, Gulin A. CatBoost: unbiased boosting with categorical features. In: *Proceedings of the 32nd International Conference on Neural Information Processing Systems.* Montréal, QC: Curran Associates Inc. (2018). p. 6639–49.
46. Fot EV, Izotova NN, Yudina AS, Smetkin AA, Kuzkov VV, Kirov MY. Automated weaning from mechanical ventilation after off-pump coronary artery bypass grafting. *Front Med.* (2017) 4:31. doi: 10.3389/fmed.2017.00031
47. Kuriyama A, Jackson JL, Kamei J. Performance of the cuff leak test in adults in predicting post-extubation airway complications: a systematic review and meta-analysis. *Crit Care.* (2020) 24:640. doi: 10.1186/s13054-020-03358-8
48. Mesquida J, Gruartmoner G, Espinal C, Masip J, Sabatier C, Villagra A, et al. Thenar oxygen saturation (StO2) alterations during a spontaneous breathing trial predict extubation failure. *Ann Intensive Care.* (2020) 10:54. doi: 10.1186/s13613-020-00670-y
49. Dres M, Goligher EC, Dube BP, Morawiec E, Dangers L, Reuter D, et al. Diaphragm function and weaning from mechanical ventilation: an ultrasound and phrenic nerve stimulation clinical study. *Ann Intensive Care.* (2018) 8:53. doi: 10.1186/s13613-018-0401-y

# 19

# Risk Factors for Patient–Ventilator Asynchrony and its Impact on Clinical Outcomes: Analytics Based on Deep Learning Algorithm

*Huiqing Ge*[1,2], *Kailiang Duan*[1], *Jimei Wang*[1], *Liuqing Jiang*[1], *Lingwei Zhang*[3], *Yuhan Zhou*[3], *Luping Fang*[3], *Leo M. A. Heunks*[4], *Qing Pan*[3*] *and Zhongheng Zhang*[5*]

[1] *Department of Respiratory Care, Sir Run Run Shaw Hospital, Zhejiang University School of Medicine, Hangzhou, China,* [2] *Regional Medical Center for National Institute of Respiratory Diseases, Bethesda, MD, United States,* [3] *College of Information Engineering, Zhejiang University of Technology, Hangzhou, China,* [4] *Department of Intensive Care Medicine, Amsterdam UMC, Amsterdam, Netherlands,* [5] *Department of Emergency Medicine, Sir Run Run Shaw Hospital, Zhejiang University School of Medicine, Hangzhou, China*

***Correspondence:**
*Zhongheng Zhang*
*zh_zhang1984@zju.edu.cn*
*Qing Pan*
*pqpq@zjut.edu.cn*

**Background and objectives:** Patient–ventilator asynchronies (PVAs) are common in mechanically ventilated patients. However, the epidemiology of PVAs and its impact on clinical outcome remains controversial. The current study aims to evaluate the epidemiology and risk factors of PVAs and their impact on clinical outcomes using big data analytics.

**Methods:** The study was conducted in a tertiary care hospital; all patients with mechanical ventilation from June to December 2019 were included for analysis. Negative binomial regression and distributed lag non-linear models (DLNM) were used to explore risk factors for PVAs. PVAs were included as a time-varying covariate into Cox regression models to investigate its influence on the hazard of mortality and ventilator-associated events (VAEs).

**Results:** A total of 146 patients involving 50,124 h and 51,451,138 respiratory cycles were analyzed. The overall mortality rate was 15.6%. Double triggering was less likely to occur during day hours (RR: 0.88; 95% CI: 0.85–0.90; $p < 0.001$) and occurred most frequently in pressure control ventilation (PCV) mode (median: 3; IQR: 1–9 per hour). Ineffective effort was more likely to occur during day time (RR: 1.09; 95% CI: 1.05–1.13; $p < 0.001$), and occurred most frequently in PSV mode (median: 8; IQR: 2–29 per hour). The effect of sedatives and analgesics showed temporal patterns in DLNM. PVAs were not associated mortality and VAE in Cox regression models with time-varying covariates.

**Conclusions:** Our study showed that counts of PVAs were significantly influenced by time of the day, ventilation mode, ventilation settings (e.g., tidal volume and plateau pressure), and sedatives and analgesics. However, PVAs were not associated with the hazard of VAE or mortality after adjusting for protective ventilation strategies such as tidal volume, plateau pressure, and positive end expiratory pressure (PEEP).

**Keywords: patient ventilator asynchrony, mortality, deep learning, mechanical ventilalion, critical care**

# INTRODUCTION

Patient–ventilator asynchrony (PVA) is common in intensive care unit (ICU) patients (1, 2). PVA can be defined as a mismatch between patient respiratory effort and ventilator support. Most prevalent types of asynchrony include ineffective efforts, double triggering (DT), and early/late cycling off (3). Well-known risk factors for PVA include inappropriate level of inspiratory assist, ventilator mode, and the level of sedation (3). Several techniques have been used clinically to evaluate patient–ventilator interaction, including esophageal pressure, diaphragm electrical activity (4), and software algorithms analyzing ventilator flow and pressure curves (2). There is evidence showing that PVA is associated with adverse clinical outcomes, including mortality (5). However, previous epidemiological studies have important limitations. First, most techniques for the detection of PVA requires the physical presence of an expert physician at the bedside and is thus only feasible during short periods (3, 6–8). Second, risk factors were explored in a simplified time-fixed manner (9, 10). In reality, both well-known risk factors and PVAs are time varying; in addition, some risk factors may take time (lag) to take effect. In this situation, both the magnitude and time lag between exposure and PVA should be accounted for. Third, the association of PVA and mortality risk was mainly explored in small studies (5, 11), and the association was explored by dividing patients into groups with different degrees of PVA severity as represented by the asynchrony index (AI) (2). Since PVA is a time-varying covariate, it is important to appropriately account for the time-varying property of the PVA, while avoiding the immortal time bias (12).

The current study employed high-granularity data from multiparameter monitors and ventilators to explore the risk factors of PVA, the association with ventilator-associated events (VAEs), and mortality. We hypothesized that time of day, ventilation mode, ventilator settings, and sedatives could affect the PVA. In a multivariable regression model, we adjusted the sedatives and analgesics to see whether time of day was still independently associated with PVA. Secondly, we hypothesize that PVA has a negative impact on clinically important outcomes such as VAE and mortality.

# METHODS

## Study Design and Setting

The study was conducted in an academic medical center from June 2019 to December 2019. The last follow-up date was on December 31, 2019, when the last patient was discharged home. Patients' electronic medical records (EMRs) were retrospectively reviewed. The study was approved by the ethics committee of the Sir Run Run Shaw Hospital (20190916-16). Informed consent was waived by the institutional review board due to the retrospective nature of the study. The study was conducted in accordance with the Helsinki declaration. The study was reported in accordance to the REporting of OBservational studies Conducted using Observational Routinely-collected Data (RECORD) checklist (13).

## Participants

Patients receiving invasive mechanical ventilation (IMV) at ICU admission were potentially eligible for the study. Patients were excluded if they (1) were younger than 15 years; (2) signed a do-not-resuscitate order; (3) were transferred from other ICUs for long-term care; (4) were terminally ill with an expected length of ICU stay of <48 h; (5) had no mechanical ventilation (MV) waveforms available. Since volume-controlled ventilation was seldom used in our institution (<5% ventilation hours), effective identification of PVA was impossible by our deep learning algorithms. Thus, patients with volume-controlled ventilation was excluded.

## Variables

Variables were extracted from EMR including demographics, reasons for MV, sequential organ failure assessment (SOFA) score, source of ICU admission, and vital status on hospital discharge. Time-varying covariates were recorded during MV, including VAE, ventilation mode, ventilator setting, sedatives, and analgesics. VAE was defined as either two or more baseline days of stable or decreasing daily minimum positive end expiratory pressure (PEEP) values followed by at least 2 days of daily minimum PEEP values 3 cm $H_2O$ above each of the two baseline days' values or two or more baseline days of stable or decreasing daily minimum $FiO_2$ values followed by at least 2 days of daily minimum $FiO_2$ values 0.20 above each of the 2 baseline days' values (14). VAE was used as a study end-point because (1) VAE can be included as a time-varying covariate in our longitudinal dataset; (2) it can be more objectively defined than ventilator-associated pneumonia; and (3) the impact of PVA on mortality might be mediated via VAE. Missing values were handled with single imputation.

## Identification of Four Types of Asynchrony

A one-dimensional interpretable convolutional neural network (1D-CNN) model was developed to detect DT, ineffective inspiratory effort during expiration (IEE), prolonged cycling (PC), and short cycling (SC). The model follows the classical AlexNet structure, which has excellent performance for image processing (15). The features in the ventilator waveforms were extracted by the convolutional layers, concatenated, and processed by a global averaging pooling (GAP) layer and a softmax layer for the final binary classification. The GAP layer allows us to highlight which segments contribute to the classification results mostly, thus providing a visual interpretation of the PVA classification. Individual deep learning models were developed under all ventilation modes. Under each ventilation mode, four models were established for detecting DT, IEE, PC, and SC. Each model uses the raw ventilator waveforms (airway pressure and flow) as input for a binary classification (PVA or non-PVA). Datasets were annotated by a group of clinical professionals for training and validating the models following the same approach proposed in our previous study (16). Fivefold cross-validation shows that the PVA recognition accuracy reached above 95% for all types of PVA in all the ventilation modes. Details of the data annotation, algorithm development, and validation are described in the ESM.

## Statistical Methods

Descriptive statistics were reported and compared by convention. Continuous data were expressed as mean and standard deviation (SD) or median and interquartile range (IQR) as appropriate. They were compared between survivors and non-survivors by using $t$-test or rank sum test. Categorical data were expressed as the number and percentage and were compared between different outcome groups by chi-square test or Fisher's exact test (17).

Potential risk factors associated with PVA such as ventilator mode, time of day, and ventilator settings were explored using the negative binomial regression because it is suitable for the description of the probabilities of the occurrence of whole numbers $\geq 0$. Unlike Poisson regression, it does not require for the variance and the mean of the outcome count to be equivalent (18).

The association of sedatives/analgesics with PVA was explored using the distributed lag non-linear model (DLNM), which allows for lagged effect of these drugs (19). Drug exposure was considered in two dimensions of drug dose and time lag after the exposure. All other factors such as ventilator type, clock hours, and ventilator setting were adjusted in the model as a unidimensional variable.

The potential impact of PVA on clinical outcomes (VAE and mortality) was explored with the Cox regression model with time-varying covariates (20, 21). That is, the PVA counts were entered into the model for every hour before the occurrence of the outcome. Other time-varying covariates included ventilator parameters such as plateau pressure, PEEP, tidal volume, and work of breathing (WOB). Time-fixed variables included age, BMI, gender, admission type, reasons for MV, and SOFA score.

# RESULTS

## Participants and Descriptive Data

A total of 160 patients were screened during the study period. After the exclusion of 14 patients due to missing waveform data, ventilation of <24 h, presence of volume-controlled ventilation, and presence of a do-not-resuscitate order, we finally included 146 patients for analysis. A total of 50,124 h involving 51,451,138 respiratory cycles was analyzed (e.g., an average of 51,451,138/50,124/60 = 17 cycles per minute). The overall mortality rate was 15.6%. Non-survivors showed greater SOFA [9.5 (7, 13) vs. 6.5 (5, 9); $p = 0.009$] and NUTRIC score (6.62 ± 2.2 vs. 4.94 ± 2.06; $p = 0.077$, **Table 1**), but there was no difference in mortality rate between VAE and non-VAE groups

**TABLE 1** | Comparisons between survivors and non-survivors.

| Variables | Total ($n$ = 146) | Survivors ($n$ = 123) | Non-survivors ($n$ = 23) | $p$ |
|---|---|---|---|---|
| Age (years), median (IQR) | 69 (56, 77) | 67 (56.5, 75.5) | 72 (54, 84.5) | 0.289 |
| BMI (kg/m$^2$), median (IQR) | 61.5 (33.25, 91.75) | 64 (34.5, 93) | 42 (31.5, 79) | 0.267 |
| Reasons for MV, $n$ (%) | | | | 0.545 |
| Cardiac disease | 16 (11) | 13 (11) | 3 (13) | |
| Neuromuscular disease# | 48 (33) | 44 (36) | 4 (17) | |
| Post-operation | 17 (12) | 13 (11) | 4 (17) | |
| COPD | 12 (8) | 9 (7) | 3 (13) | |
| Sepsis | 30 (21) | 25 (20) | 5 (22) | |
| Systemic disease* | 13 (9) | 10 (8) | 3 (13) | |
| Trauma | 9 (6) | 8 (7) | 1 (4) | |
| SOFA, median (IQR) | 7 (5, 10) | 6.5 (5, 9) | 9.5 (7, 13.25) | 0.009 |
| APACHE II, mean ± SD | 22.42 ± 8.34 | 22.06 ± 8 | 24.22 ± 9.91 | 0.334 |
| VAE, $n$ (%) | 26 (18) | 19 (15) | 7 (30) | 0.132 |
| ICU LOS (days), median (IQR) | 12.91 (7.72, 22.12) | 12.91 (7.95, 22.66) | 12.48 (5.92, 19.38) | 0.271 |
| NUTRIC score, mean ± SD | 5.27 ± 2.17 | 4.94 ± 2.06 | 6.62 ± 2.2 | 0.077 |

*MV, mechanical ventilation; IQR, interquartile range; SD, standard deviation; SOFA, sequential organ failure assessment; COPD, chronic obstructive pulmonary disease; APACHE, Acute Physiology and Chronic Health Evaluation; LOS, length of stay; ICU, intensive care unit; NUTRIC, nutrition Risk in the Critically ill.*

*#Neuromuscular disease included disorders such as respiratory failure caused by neuromuscular disorder like stroke and Guillain–Barre syndrome. *Systemic disease included autoimmune diseases such as SLE.*

**TABLE 2** | Clinical outcomes between VAE and non-VAE groups.

| Variables | Total ($n$ = 147) | Non-VAE ($n$ = 121) | VAE ($n$ = 26) | $p$ |
|---|---|---|---|---|
| ICU LOS (days), median (IQR) | 12.91 (7.72, 22.12) | 12.24 (7.18, 18.99) | 21.82 (17.01, 29.82) | <0.001 |
| MV days, median (IQR) | 9.93 (6.05, 15.9) | 8.46 (5.93, 12.6) | 18.18 (13.83, 25.94) | <0.001 |
| Mortality, $n$ (%) | 23 (16) | 16 (13) | 7 (27) | 0.132 |

*IQR, interquartile range; MV, mechanical ventilation; LOS, length of stay; ICU, intensive care unit; VAE, ventilator associated events.*

**TABLE 3** | The performance of the PVA detection models under different ventilation modes.

| | Modes | ACC | SEN | SPE |
|---|---|---|---|---|
| IEE | PCV | 0.972 ± 0.001 | 0.975 ± 0.003 | 0.969 ± 0.003 |
| | PSV | 0.993 ± 0.003 | 0.994 ± 0.002 | 0.991 ± 0.005 |
| DT | PCV | 0.986 ± 0.001 | 0.992 ± 0.004 | 0.979 ± 0.006 |
| | PSV | 0.985 ± 0.002 | 0.986 ± 0.008 | 0.984 ± 0.006 |
| Prolonged cycling | PCV | 0.979 ± 0.002 | 0.977 ± 0.007 | 0.982 ± 0.005 |
| | PSV | 0.973 ± 0.004 | 0.973 ± 0.004 | 0.973 ± 0.008 |
| Short cycling | PCV | 0.970 ± 0.005 | 0.975 ± 0.008 | 0.966 ± 0.004 |
| | PSV | 0.985 ± 0.003 | 0.987 ± 0.003 | 0.984 ± 0.005 |

*ACC, accuracy; SPE, specificity; SEN, sensitivity; PCV, pressure control ventilation; PSV, pressure support ventilation; DT, double triggering; IEE, ineffective effort.*

(**Table 2**). The VAE group showed longer ICU length of stay [21.82 (17.01, 29.82) vs. 12.24 (7.18, 18.99) days; $p < 0.001$] and MV duration [18.18 (13.83, 25.94) vs. 8.46 (5.93, 12.6) days; $p < 0.001$] than did the non-VAE group (**Table 2**).

## The Performance of the PVA Detection Models Under Different Ventilation Modes

Eight independent binary classifiers were developed for different types of PVA under different ventilation modes, i.e., $H_{PCV-IEE}$, $H_{PCV-DT}$, $H_{PCV-Prol}$, $H_{PCV-Short}$, $H_{PSV-IEE}$, $H_{PSV-DT}$, $H_{PSV-Prol}$, and $H_{PSV-Short}$. The performance of the models was evaluated by a fivefold cross-validation. The average accuracy, sensitivity, and specificity are given in **Table 3**. We intended to interpret the PVA recognition using a class activation map (CAM) technique (22). The technique replaced the FC layer in the CNN model with a GAP layer to allow visualization of the sections that the CNN model focuses on. In other words, the sections that contribute mostly to the classification results will be highlighted. In this way, we may understand why the CNN model decides a certain breath manifests PVA. The interpretation of the classification under the three involved ventilation modes is illustrated in **Figure 1**.

## Risk Factors of PVA

With the ML model used to detect PVA, the occurrence of PVA varied depending on the time of day (**Figure 2**). DT, PC, and SC were less likely to occur during 0–3 o'clock (**Figure 2**). To examine whether the difference in the effect of day vs. night was attributable to the difference of the use of sedatives and analgesics, we adjusted for the use of analgesics and sedatives in the negative binomial regression model (**Figure 2**). DT was less likely to occur during day hours (RR: 0.88; 95% CI: 0.85–0.90; $p < 0.001$). IEE (RR: 1.09; 95% CI: 1.05–1.13; $p < 0.001$), PC (RR: 2.23; 95% CI: 2.14–2.32; $p < 0.001$), and SC (RR: 1.27; 95% CI: 1.21–1.32; $p < 0.001$) were more likely to occur during daytime. Ventilator mode (PSV vs. PCV) was also significantly associated with the incidence of PVA (**Figure 3**). DT was more likely to occur in PCV than in PSV (median [IQR]: 3 [1–9] vs. 2 [1–6] per hour), whereas IEE occurred more frequently in PSV than in PCV (8 [2–29] vs. 3 [0–17] per hour). In the DLNM model, each drug was considered in two dimensions of dosage and time after exposure (time lag after instantaneous exposure to a certain dose of the drug). Propofol was able to reduce the incidence of DT 30–60 min after exposure (i.e., the drug was discontinued after infusion at a dose of 1–3 mg/kg/h); however, the count of DT increased after 2–4 h following discontinuation after infusion at a dose of 1–4 mg/kg/h (**Figure 4**). The effects of midazolam and sufentanil are shown in SEM (**Supplementary Figures 1, 2**). Finally, all risk factors were entered into negative binomial regression models with each asynchrony type as the response variable (**Table 4**). The result showed that day hour, ventilator mode, tidal volume, PEEP, and WOB were all associated with PVAs.

## Impact of PVA on Clinical Outcomes

PVA was entered into a Cox regression model as a time-varying covariate. After adjusting for baseline characteristics and other

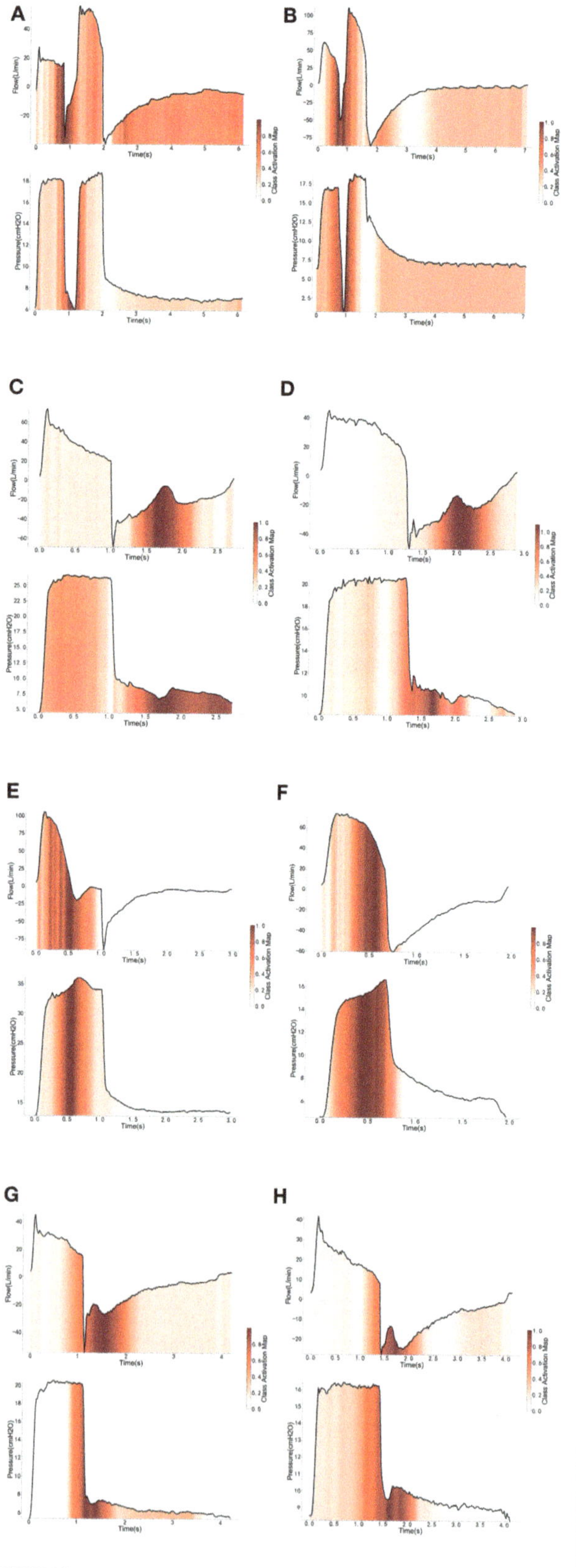


**FIGURE 1** | Interpretation of the cycles classified as PVA under PCV mode **(A,C,E,G)** and PSV mode **(B,D,F,H)**.

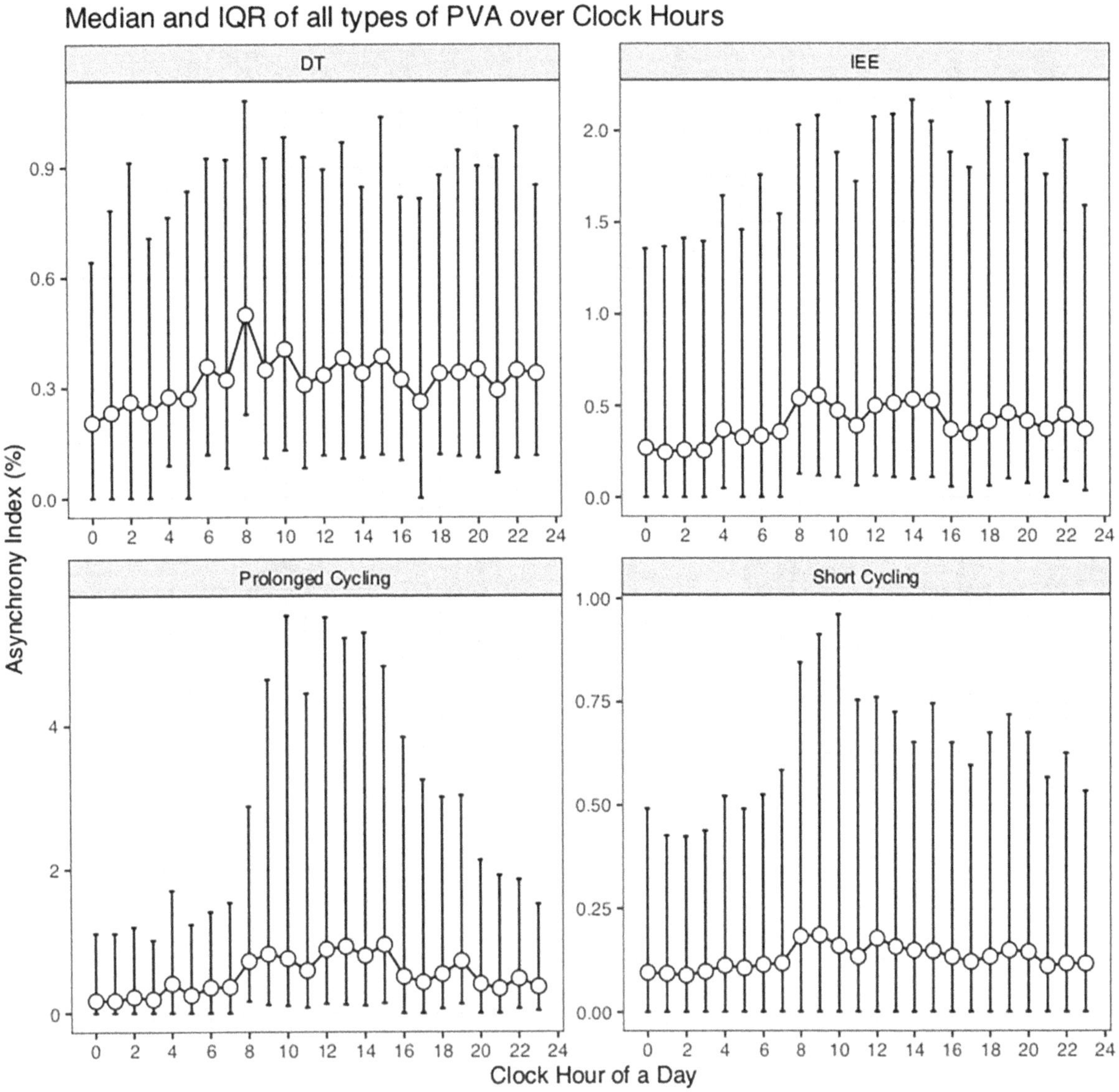


| | RR for DT [95% CI] | p value | RR for IEE [95% CI] | p value |
|---|---|---|---|---|
| Day vs. Night | 0.88 [0.85, 0.90] | <0.001 | 1.09 [1.05, 1.13] | <0.001 |
| Propofol | 1.45 [1.40, 1.51] | <0.001 | 0.58 [0.55, 0.61] | <0.001 |
| Sufentanil | 1.40 [1.35, 1.45] | <0.001 | 1.00 [0.95, 1.05] | 0.937 |
| Midazolam | 0.97 [0.90, 1.05] | 0.423 | 0.54 [0.49, 0.59] | <0.001 |

| | RR for PC [95% CI] | p value | RR for SC [95% CI] | p value |
|---|---|---|---|---|
| Day vs. Night | 2.23 [2.14, 2.32] | <0.001 | 1.27 [1.21, 1.32] | <0.001 |
| Propofol | 1.21 [1.15, 1.28] | <0.001 | 1.26 [1.20, 1.32] | <0.001 |
| Sufentanil | 1.03 [0.97, 1.09] | 0.260 | 1.45 [1.37, 1.53] | <0.001 |
| Midazolam | 0.96 [0.87, 1.07] | 0.435 | 1.13 [1.01, 1.26] | 0.034 |

**FIGURE 2** | Impact of day hours on four types of asynchrony. AI was defined as the percentage of respiratory cycles with the presence of relevant types of PVA. A negative binomial regression model was built to adjust for the confounding effect of analgesics and sedatives. IEE, ineffective effort; DT, double triggering; SC, short cycling, PC, prolonged cycling.

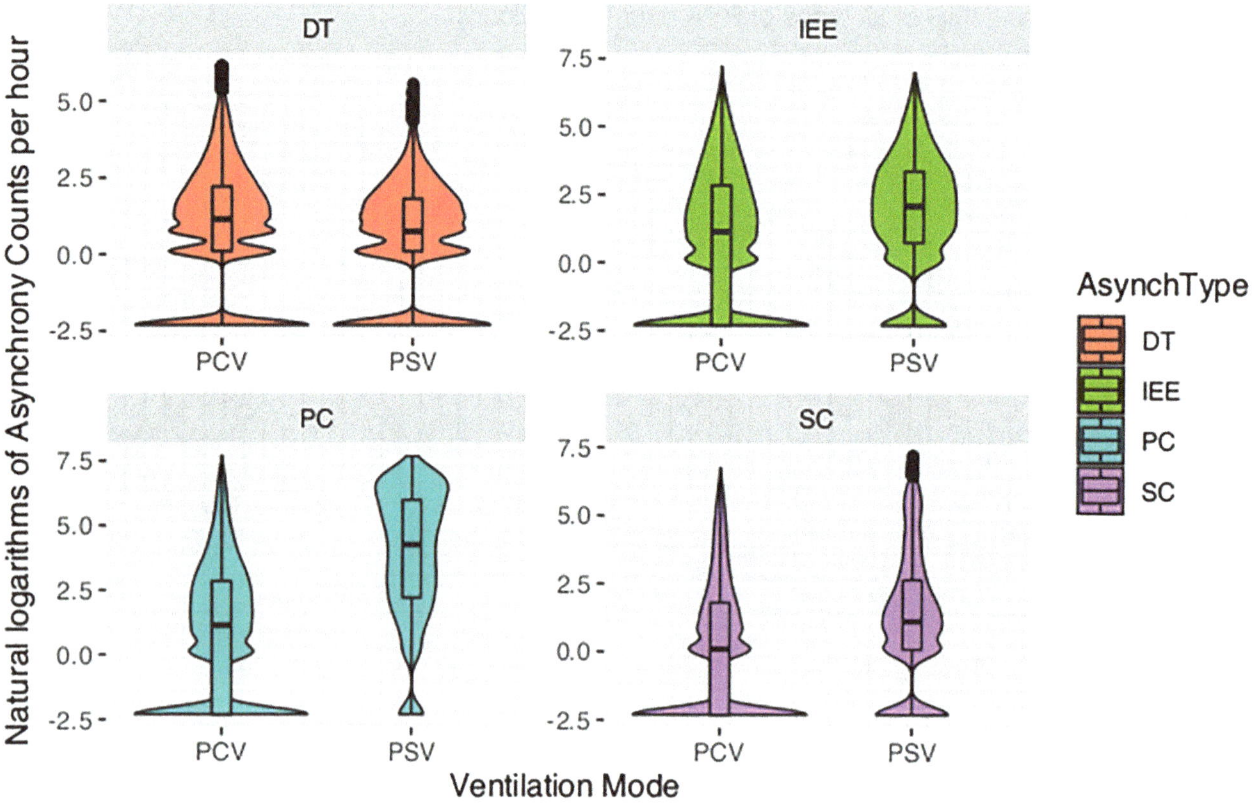


| Variables | PCV (n = 43857) | PSV (n = 6267) | p |
|---|---|---|---|
| IEE, Median (IQR) | 3 (0, 17) | 8 (2, 29) | < 0.001 |
| DT, Median (IQR) | 3 (1, 9) | 2 (1, 6) | < 0.001 |
| SC, Median (IQR) | 1 (0, 6) | 3 (1, 14) | < 0.001 |
| PC, Median (IQR) | 3 (0, 17) | 70 (9, 392.5) | < 0.001 |

**FIGURE 3 |** Violin plot showing the impact of ventilation mode on four types of asynchrony. Violin-and-box plots are used to visualize the distribution of the asynchrony counts (transformed by natural logarithms) and their probability density. The table at the bottom shows the number of asynchrony counts per hour. IEE, ineffective effort; DT, double triggering; SC, short cycling; PC, prolonged cycling; PCV, pressure control ventilation; PSV, pressure support ventilation.

time-varying covariates, PVA was not associated with increased risk of mortality or VAE (**Table 5**). Interestingly, high plateau pressure (>30 cm $H_2O$) was a significant risk factor for both mortality (HR: 26.95; 95% CI: 1.95–372.59; $p = 0.014$) and VAE (HR: 9.30; 95% CI: 1.34–64.38; $p = 0.024$). Large tidal volume (>10 ml/kg) was associated with increased risk of fatality (HR: 11.22; 95% CI: 1.27–99.28; $p = 0.03$). Other significant risk/protective factors for VAE were admission from emergency department (HR: 0.23; 95% CI: 0.07–0.83; $p = 0.024$), SOFA (HR: 1.21; 95% CI: 1.03–1.43; $p = 0.019$), and MV due to systematic disorders such as systematic lupus erythematosus (HR: 0.04; 95% CI: 0.00–0.44; $p = 0.008$).

## DISCUSSION

This is the most comprehensive study to investigate the epidemiology and clinical consequences of PVA in ICU patients. The main findings can be summarized as follows: First, our study shows that day hours, ventilation mode, ventilator parameters, sedatives, and analgesics were important risk factors for all types of asynchrony. The effect of sedatives and analgesics showed time-dependent patterns. Second, PVAs were not associated with either VAE or mortality after adjusting for covariates. Third, ventilator parameters such as tidal volume and plateau pressure were significantly associated with VAE and mortality in

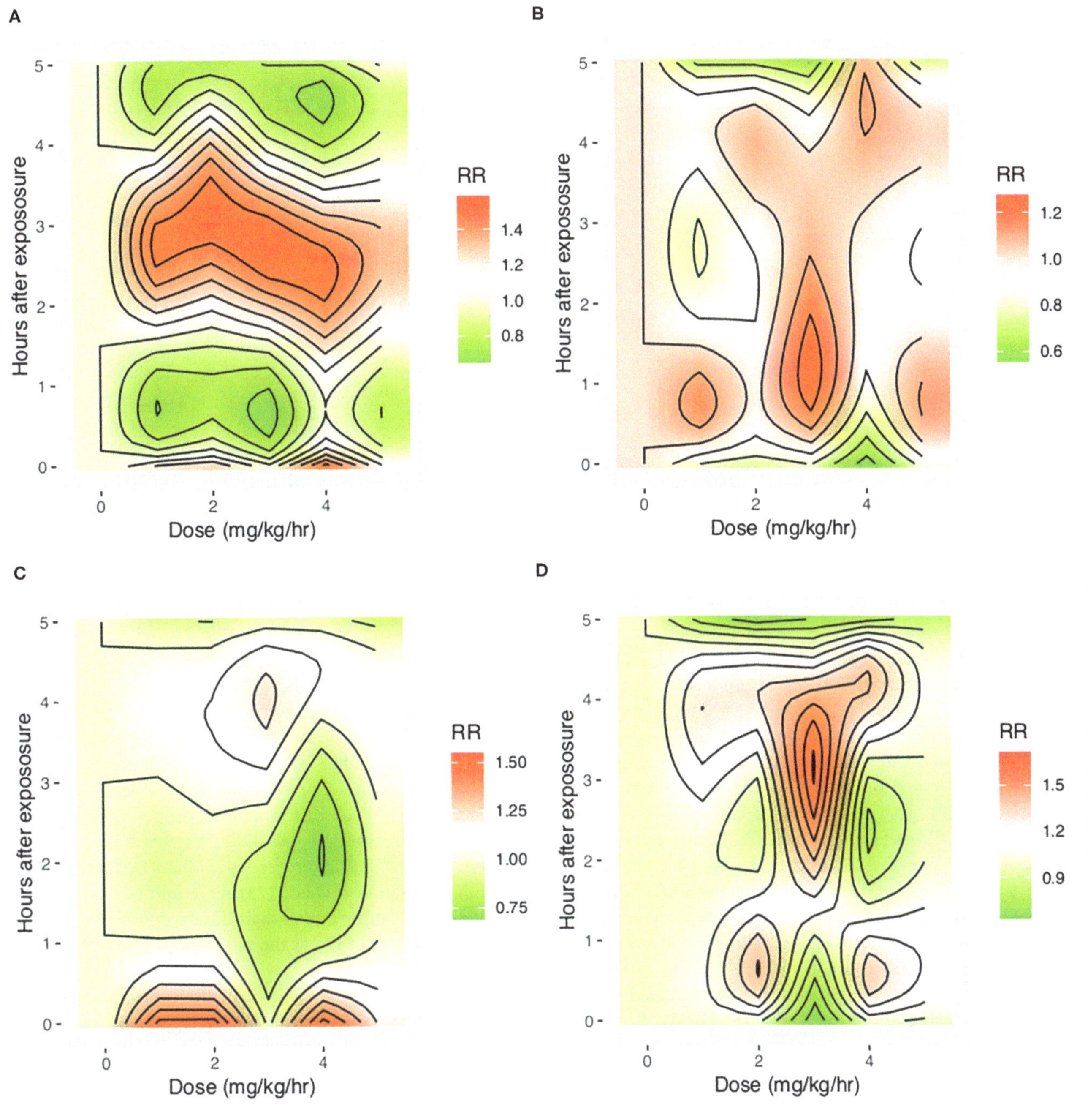


**FIGURE 4 |** Impact of propofol on four types of asynchrony. Propofol was entered into the distributed lag non-linear model with two dimensions: dose and time lag. The y-axis shows the time after instantaneous exposure of propofol, so the drug was assumed to be discontinued after a certain dose exposure. Other covariates including tidal volume, WOB, PEEP, plateau pressure, mode of ventilation, and day hours were adjusted. The red color shows increased risk of asynchrony, and the green color shows reduced risk of asynchrony. **(A)** Impact on DT, **(B)** Impact on IEE, **(C)** Impact on PC, and **(D)** Impact on SC. IEE, ineffective effort; DT, double triggering; SC, short cycling; PC, prolonged cycling.

a Cox regression model with time-varying covariates. Our study indicates that although protective ventilation strategies such as low tidal volume and low plateau pressure were associated with increased PVA, it is unwise to increase the TV and plateau pressure in order to reduce PVA, because increasing TV and plateau pressure would increase the hazard of VAE and mortality. Our deep learning algorithm can be used in a standard ICU for real-time monitoring of PVAs. High frequency or intensity of PVAs can trigger warnings from the machine, and measures can be taken to modify some risk factors as identified in our study.

One strength of our study was that different types of PVAs were identified by using deep learning algorithms and

**TABLE 4** | Negative binomial regression model exploring the risk factors for the four types of asynchronies.

| Variables | RR for IEE (95% CI) | $p$ | RR for DT (95% CI) | $p$ | RR for SC (95% CI) | $p$ | RR for PC (95% CI) | $p$ |
|---|---|---|---|---|---|---|---|---|
| Day hours (night as reference)* | 1.063 (1.026, 1.101) | <0.001 | 0.994 (0.964, 1.024) | 0.666 | 0.963 (0.923, 1.006) | 0.084 | 1.243 (1.196, 1.293) | <0.001 |
| Ventilation mode (PCV as reference) | 1.186 (1.111, 1.267) | <0.001 | 0.402 (0.381, 0.424) | <0.001 | 1.388 (1.285, 1.499) | <0.001 | 4.398 (4.103, 4.715) | <0.001 |
| **TV (<6 ml/kg as reference)** | | | | | | | | |
| 6–8 ml/kg | 0.654 (0.612, 0.699) | <0.001 | 0.718 (0.684, 0.753) | <0.001 | 1.139 (1.06, 1.223) | <0.001 | 1.43 (1.339, 1.526) | <0.001 |
| 8–10 ml/kg | 0.425 (0.392, 0.46) | <0.001 | 0.541 (0.511, 0.573) | <0.001 | 1.47 (1.349, 1.6) | <0.001 | 1.87 (1.725, 2.026) | <0.001 |
| >10 ml/kg | 0.239 (0.215, 0.267) | <0.001 | 0.419 (0.387, 0.454) | <0.001 | 1.519 (1.346, 1.715) | <0.001 | 5.159 (4.575, 5.818) | <0.001 |
| **WOB (<10 J/ml/kg as reference)** | | | | | | | | |
| 10–15 J/ml/kg | 1.26 (1.182, 1.343) | <0.001 | 0.948 (0.904, 0.995) | 0.04 | 0.473 (0.442, 0.506) | <0.001 | 0.415 (0.388, 0.444) | <0.001 |
| 15–20 J/ml/kg | 1.167 (1.068, 1.275) | <0.001 | 1.239 (1.162, 1.322) | <0.001 | 0.556 (0.507, 0.61) | <0.001 | 0.216 (0.197, 0.237) | <0.001 |
| >20 J/ml/kg | 0.867 (0.776, 0.969) | 0.008 | 2.114 (1.949, 2.292) | <0.001 | 1.206 (1.067, 1.364) | 0.003 | 0.154 (0.136, 0.174) | <0.001 |
| **PEEP (≤5 cm $H_2O$ as reference)** | | | | | | | | |
| 5–10 cm $H_2O$ | 0.638 (0.61, 0.668) | <0.001 | 1.236 (1.191, 1.282) | <0.001 | 1.218 (1.155, 1.286) | <0.001 | 1.443 (1.369, 1.521) | <0.001 |
| >10 cm $H_2O$ | 1.063 (0.94, 1.205) | 0.313 | 2.018 (1.823, 2.238) | <0.001 | 6.702 (5.722, 7.869) | <0.001 | 4.446 (3.875, 5.116) | <0.001 |
| **Plateau pressure (<20 cm $H_2O$ as reference)** | | | | | | | | |
| 20–30 cm $H_2O$ | 1.39 (1.317, 1.467) | <0.001 | 0.64 (0.613, 0.668) | <0.001 | 0.538 (0.506, 0.571) | <0.001 | 1.354 (1.271, 1.441) | <0.001 |
| >30 cm $H_2O$ | 0.768 (0.703, 0.838) | <0.001 | 0.318 (0.296, 0.341) | <0.001 | 0.079 (0.071, 0.088) | <0.001 | 0.96 (0.87, 1.06) | 0.401 |

*RR, relative risk; CI, confidence interval; DT, double triggering; IEE, ineffective effort; SC, short cycling; PC, prolonged cycling; PEEP, positive end expiratory pressure; WOB, work of breathing; VCV, volume control ventilation; PCV, pressure control ventilation; VC+, volume control plus; APRV, airway pressure release ventilation; PSV, pressure support ventilation; CPAP, continuous positive airway pressure; TV, tidal volume. Four negative binomial regression models were built by using each type of asynchrony as the dependent variable. All variables in the table were entered into the models to adjust for confounding effects. *Day hours were categorized by visually inspecting the asynchrony–day hour trend curve.*

were analyzed separately (16). We believe that different PVAs have different underlying mechanisms, and risk factors and its consequences can be different (3). Previous studies have analyzed PVAs as a composite outcome that all types of PVAs were aggregated as a single index called AI (2, 10). Our study found that risk factors for different PVAs were different. For example, while IEE, PC, and SC were more likely to occur during daytime, DT was less likely to occur during daytime after adjustment for the use of sedatives and analgesics (**Figure 1**). Pathophysiologically, DT is the result of high inspiratory demand and excessive inspiratory effort (23). Inspiratory demand can be high during daytime because of the diurnal variation pattern (24). Furthermore, patients are more likely to be awake and influenced by medical procedures during day hours. Propofol also showed differing effects on IEE and DT. At 30-60 min after propofol discontinuation, the risk of DT decreased, but the risk of IEE increased (**Figure 3**). Propofol could reduce patient inspiratory efforts and thus DT. Recall that DT could be the result of excessive inspiratory efforts (25). However, when there is too much sedative, some normal inspiratory efforts are reduced such that they fail to trigger a respiratory cycle, leading to increased IEE. Such differing effects on different types of PVAs were also noted in another randomized controlled trial (26).

A novel finding in our study was that the effect of sedatives and analgesics on PVA followed distinct temporal patterns. Although previous studies have shown that sedatives were associated with reduced IEE (9), data from 1 day were binned in their studies, making it difficult to explore the causal/temporal relationship of sedatives and PVA. For example, the attending physician may give more sedative for a patient with increased PVAs, and sedatives may also change the risk of PVAs. The sedatives and PVAs construct a cyclic causal diagram. Our study employed DLNM to explore the temporal effect of sedatives on different types of PVA. It was interesting to find that the risk of DT first decreased at 30–60 min after propofol infusion and then increased at 3–4 h after propofol discontinuation, which was probably due to the short half-life of the drug (30–60 min) and increased risk of delirium after propofol infusion (27). In a controlled experimental study, Vaschetto and colleagues showed that deep propofol sedation increased asynchronies, while light sedation did not (25). Our finding was consistent with Vaschetto's study in that high-dose propofol was associated with increased risk of DT at the same hour of propofol infusion (**Figure 3**).

Our study was the first to systematically explore the association of protective ventilation strategy on PVAs. We found that protective ventilation strategies such as low tidal volume, low plateau pressure, and high PEEP were all significantly associated with the risk of PVAs, after adjusting for other risk factors in negative binomial regression models. Other studies also observed some patients with strong inspiratory effort and patient–ventilator mismatch when the tidal volume was given below 6.5 ml/kg (28). The protective ventilation strategy usually cannot meet patient requirements, and thus PVAs are common; thus, more sedatives and neuromuscular blocking agents are usually required to deliver protective ventilation strategies (29). In Cox regression models with PVAs and ventilation parameters as time-varying covariates, we did not find independent associations between PVAs and the hazard of mortality and VAE, which was consistent with other studies (10, 11, 30). However, this finding does not mean that we shall no longer pay attention to the PVA phenomenon. The reasons for our study not finding

**TABLE 5 |** Cox regression model with time-varying covariates.

| Variables | HR for VAE (95% CI) | *p* | HR for mortality (95% CI) | *p* |
|---|---|---|---|---|
| Age (for every 1-year increase) | 0.97 (0.92, 1.02) | 0.246 | 1.01 (0.97, 1.05) | 0.509 |
| BMI (for every 1-point increase) | 0.98 (0.96, 1.00) | 0.010 | 1.00 (0.99, 1.01) | 0.674 |
| Gender (female as reference) | 0.83 (0.25, 2.74) | 0.765 | 1.96 (0.46, 8.38) | 0.364 |
| **Admission type (from ward as reference)** | | | | |
| Emergency room | 0.23 (0.07, 0.83) | 0.024 | 2.41 (1.05, 5.52) | 0.038 |
| Others | 0.84 (0.13, 5.49) | 0.859 | 1.67 (0.30, 9.20) | 0.558 |
| SOFA (for every 1-point increase) | 1.21 (1.03, 1.43) | 0.019 | 1.23 (0.99, 1.53) | 0.065 |
| **Reasons for MV (cardiac disease as reference)** | | | | |
| Neuromuscular disease | 0.35 (0.04, 3.13) | 0.347 | 0.64 (0.10, 4.18) | 0.644 |
| Post-operation | 0.25 (0.04, 1.75) | 0.162 | 0.78 (0.11, 5.41) | 0.804 |
| COPD | 0.39 (0.06, 2.64) | 0.331 | 1.87 (0.34, 10.42) | 0.474 |
| Sepsis | 0.31 (0.07, 1.33) | 0.114 | 1.75 (0.35, 8.63) | 0.494 |
| Systemic disease | 0.04 (0.00, 0.44) | 0.008 | 1.19 (0.26, 5.46) | 0.821 |
| Trauma | 2.98 (0.38, 23.19) | 0.297 | 1.24 (0.12, 12.95) | 0.857 |
| IEE (for every increase per hour) | 1.00 (1.00, 1.01) | 0.250 | 1.00 (0.99, 1.00) | 0.139 |
| DT (for every increase per hour) | 1.00 (0.99, 1.01) | 0.687 | 1.00 (0.98, 1.01) | 0.677 |
| SC (for every increase per hour) | 1.02 (0.99, 1.04) | 0.183 | 0.83 (0.61, 1.13) | 0.239 |
| PC (for every increase per hour) | 0.69 (0.40, 1.21) | 0.197 | 0.70 (0.39, 1.27) | 0.242 |
| **WOB (<10 J/ml/kg as reference)** | | | | |
| 10–15 J/ml/kg | 0.27 (0.03, 2.12) | 0.215 | 0.27 (0.02, 3.04) | 0.289 |
| 15–20 J/ml/kg | 0.88 (0.12, 6.54) | 0.899 | 0.14 (0.01, 2.43) | 0.179 |
| >20 J/ml/kg | 0.98 (0.09, 10.63) | 0.988 | 0.06 (0.00, 1.91) | 0.111 |
| **TV (<6 ml/kg as reference)** | | | | |
| 6–8 ml/kg | 2.43 (0.13, 46.21) | 0.554 | 3.07 (0.77, 12.30) | 0.113 |
| 8–10 ml/kg | 2.86 (0.14, 60.39) | 0.499 | 2.26 (0.38, 13.34) | 0.370 |
| >10 ml/kg | 5.31 (0.19, 145.37) | 0.323 | 11.22 (1.27, 99.28) | 0.030 |
| **Plateau pressure (<20 cm $H_2O$ as reference)** | | | | |
| 20–30 cm $H_2O$ | 4.03 (1.20, 13.58) | 0.025 | 5.63 (0.64, 49.22) | 0.118 |
| >30 cm $H_2O$ | 9.30 (1.34, 64.38) | 0.024 | 26.95 (1.95, 372.59) | 0.014 |

*HR, hazard ratio; CI, confidence interval; WOB, work of breathing; TV, tidal volume; IEE, ineffective effort; DT, double triggering; SC, short cycling; PC, prolonged cycling; SOFA, sequential organ failure assessment; COPD, chronic obstructive pulmonary disease; BMI, body mass index.*

statistically significant results might be that there are numerous factors that can influence mortality and that the effect size of a single variable is very small. The sample size or statistical power must be very large to reach the statistical significance level. PVA can cause patient discomfort and may be a sign of inappropriate ventilation setting. However, the use of protective ventilation strategy was associated with mortality and VAE. These results indicate that we should not increase tidal volume or plateau pressure in order to reduce PVAs. If VAE is the primary concern, we could use sedatives and neuromuscular blocking agents to safely deliver the protective ventilation strategy while avoiding PVAs (31).

Several limitations must be acknowledged in the study. First, reverse triggering was not distinguished from DT, because we did not have data on esophageal pressure monitoring. There has been evidence that reverse triggering is different from other types of PVAs from a pathophysiological view (3, 32). Ideally, it should be analyzed independently. Clinical findings of the present study are based on the accuracy of the method for detecting PVA coming from a machine learning model, and the results are limited by its accuracy. Second, the study included heterogeneous MV patients including those with ARDS and COPD. Although we have adjusted our results by disease type, the sample sizes in some disease groups were limited. Third, the study was carried out in a single center, and it is unknown whether the results are generalizable to other hospitals. The limited sample size and small number of mortality event make our model preliminary, especially the results related to the mortality outcome. The model should be verified in studies with a larger sample size. Finally, the models trained in our study were not externally validated. Thus, further studies are required to validate current findings.

In conclusion, with the ML model used to detect PVA, our study showed that counts of PVAs were significantly influenced by day hours, ventilation mode, ventilation parameters, and the use of sedatives and analgesics. However, PVAs were not associated with the hazard of VAE and mortality after adjusting for protective ventilation strategies such as tidal volume, plateau pressure, and PEEP.

## TAKE HOME MESSAGE

- Our study showed that counts of PVAs were significantly influenced by time of day, ventilation mode, ventilation settings (e.g., tidal volume and plateau pressure), and sedatives and analgesics.
- PVAs were not associated with the hazard of VAE or mortality after adjusting for protective ventilation strategies such as tidal volume, plateau pressure, and PEEP.

## ETHICS STATEMENT

The study was approved by the ethics committee of Sir Run Run Shaw hospital (20190916-16). Written informed consent for participation was not required for this study in accordance with the national legislation and the institutional requirements.

## AUTHOR CONTRIBUTIONS

ZZ and HG conceived the idea, performed the analysis, and drafted the manuscript. KD, JW, and LJ collected the data. LZ, YZ, LF, and QP analyzed respiratory mechanics using deep learning methods. LH interpreted the results and helped revise the manuscript. All authors contributed to the article and approved the submitted version.

## REFERENCES


1. Bein T, Weber-Carstens S. The BREATHE-appeal: harmonize interaction between patient and ventilator! *J. Thorac. Dis.* (2016) 8:E1647–50. doi: 10.21037/jtd.2016.12.35
2. Blanch L, Villagra A, Sales B, Montanyà J, Lucangelo U, Luján M, et al. Asynchronies during mechanical ventilation are associated with mortality. *Intensive Care Med.* (2015) 41:633–41. doi: 10.1007/s00134-015-3692-6
3. De Haro C, Ochagavia A, López-Aguilar J, Fernandez-Gonzalo S, Navarra-Ventura G, Magrans R, et al. Patient-ventilator asynchronies during mechanical ventilation: current knowledge and research priorities. *Intensive Care Med. Exp.* (2019) 7:43–14. doi: 10.1186/s40635-019-0234-5
4. Doorduin J, van Hees HWH, van der Hoeven JG, Heunks LMA. Monitoring of the respiratory muscles in the critically ill. *Am. J. Respir. Crit. Care Med.* (2013) 187:20–7. doi: 10.1164/rccm.201206-1117CP
5. Subirà C, De Haro C, Magrans R, Fernández R, Blanch L. Minimizing asynchronies in mechanical ventilation: current and future trends. *Respir. Care.* (2018) 63:464–78. doi: 10.4187/respcare.05949
6. Conti G, Ranieri VM, Costa R, Garratt C, Wighton A, Spinazzola G, et al. Effects of dexmedetomidine and propofol on patient-ventilator interaction in difficult-to-wean, mechanically ventilated patients: a prospective, open-label, randomised, multicentre study. *Crit. Care.* (2016) 20:206–8. doi: 10.1186/s13054-016-1386-2
7. Ramírez II, Adasme RS, Arellano DH, Rocha ARM, Andrade FMD, Núñez-Silveira J, et al. Identifying and managing patient-ventilator asynchrony: an international survey. *Med. Intensiva.* (2019). doi: 10.1016/j.medin.2019.09.004. [Epub ahead of print].
8. See KC, Sahagun J, Taculod J. Defining patient-ventilator asynchrony severity according to recurrence. *Intensive Care Med.* (2020) 32:1515. doi: 10.1007/s00134-020-05974-y
9. De Haro C, Magrans R, López-Aguilar J, Montanyà J, Lena E, Subirà C, et al. Effects of sedatives and opioids on trigger and cycling asynchronies throughout mechanical ventilation: an observational study in a large dataset from critically ill patients. *Crit. Care.* (2019) 23:245. doi: 10.1186/s13054-019-2531-5
10. de Araújo Sousa ML, Magrans R, Hayashi FK, Blanch L, Kacmarek RM, Ferreira JC. Predictors of asynchronies during assisted ventilation and its impact on clinical outcomes: the EPISYNC cohort study. *J. Crit. Care.* (2020) 57:30–5. doi: 10.1016/j.jcrc.2020.01.023
11. Vaporidi K, Babalis D, Chytas A, Lilitsis E, Kondili E, Amargianitakis V, et al. Clusters of ineffective efforts during mechanical ventilation: impact on outcome. *Intensive Care. Med.* (2017) 43:184–91. doi: 10.1007/s00134-016-4593-z
12. Lévesque LE, Hanley JA, Kezouh A, Suissa S. Problem of immortal time bias in cohort studies: example using statins for preventing progression of diabetes. *BMJ.* (2010) 340:b5087. doi: 10.1136/bmj.b5087
13. Benchimol EI, Smeeth L, Guttmann A, Harron K, Moher D, Petersen I, et al. The REporting of studies conducted using observational routinely-collected health data (RECORD) statement. *PLoS Med.* (2015) 12:e1001885. doi: 10.1371/journal.pmed.1001885
14. Magill SS, Klompas M, Balk R, Burns SM, Deutschman CS, Diekema D, et al. Developing a new, national approach to surveillance for ventilator-associated events. *Crit. Care Med.* (2013) 41:2467–75. doi: 10.1097/CCM.0b013e3182a262db
15. Krizhevsky A, Sutskever I, Hinton GE. *ImageNet Classification with Deep Convolutional Neural Networks.* Red Hook, NY: Curran Associates Inc. (2012). p. 1097–105.
16. Zhang L, Mao K, Duan K, Fang S, Lu Y, Gong Q, et al. Detection of patient-ventilator asynchrony from mechanical ventilation waveforms using a two-layer long short-term memory neural network. *Comput. Biol. Med.* (2020) 120:103721. doi: 10.1016/j.compbiomed.2020.103721
17. Zhang Z, Gayle AA, Wang J, Zhang H, Cardinal-Fernández P. Comparing baseline characteristics between groups: an introduction to the CBCgrps package. *Ann. Transl. Med.* (2017) 5:484. doi: 10.21037/atm.2017.09.39
18. Donoghoe MW, Marschner IC. Estimation of adjusted rate differences using additive negative binomial regression. *Stat. Med.* (2016) 35:3166–78. doi: 10.1002/sim.6960
19. Gasparrini A, Armstrong B, Kenward MG. Distributed lag non-linear models. *Stat. Med.* (2010) 29:2224–34. doi: 10.1002/sim.3940
20. Fisher LD, Lin DY. Time-dependent covariates in the cox proportional-hazards regression model. *Ann. Rev. Public Health.* (1999) 20:145–57. doi: 10.1146/annurev.publhealth.20.1.145
21. Zhang Z, Reinikainen J, Adeleke KA, Pieterse ME, Groothuis-Oudshoorn CGM. Time-varying covariates and coefficients in cox regression models. *Ann. Transl. Med.* (2018) 6:121. doi: 10.21037/atm.2018.02.12
22. Zhou B, Khosla A, Lapedriza A, Oliva A, Torralba A. Learning deep features for discriminative localization. In: *2016 IEEE Conference on Computer Vision and Pattern Recognition (CVPR).* Las Vegas, NV (2015). doi: 10.1109/CVPR.2016.319
23. Sheehy RD, Duce B, Edwards TP, Churton JA, Sharma R, Hukins CA. Double-triggering during noninvasive ventilation in a simulated lung model. *Respir. Care.* (2020) 65:1333–38. doi: 10.4187/respcare.07280
24. Carroll MS, Ramirez J-M, Weese-Mayer DE. Diurnal variation in autonomic regulation among patients with genotyped Rett syndrome. *J. Med. Genet.* (2020) 57:786–93. doi: 10.1136/jmedgenet-2019-106601
25. Vaschetto R, Cammarota G, Colombo D, Longhini F, Grossi F, Giovanniello A, et al. Effects of propofol on patient-ventilator synchrony and interaction during pressure support ventilation and neurally adjusted ventilatory assist. *Crit. Care Med.* (2014) 42:74–82. doi: 10.1097/CCM.0b013e318 29e53dc
26. Bassuoni AS, Elgebaly AS, Eldabaa AA, Elhafz AAA. Patient-ventilator asynchrony during daily interruption of sedation versus no sedation protocol. *Anesth. Essays Res.* (2012) 6:151–6. doi: 10.4103/0259-1162. 108296
27. Brown KE, Mirrakhimov AE, Yeddula K, Kwatra MM. Propofol and the risk of delirium: exploring the anticholinergic properties of propofol. *Med. Hypotheses.* (2013) 81:536–9. doi: 10.1016/j.mehy.2013.06.027
28. Diniz-Silva F, Moriya HT, Alencar AM, Amato MBP, Carvalho CRR, Ferreira JC. Neurally adjusted ventilatory assist vs. pressure support to deliver protective mechanical ventilation in patients with acute respiratory distress syndrome: a randomized crossover trial. *Ann. Intensive Care.* (2020) 10:18–10. doi: 10.1186/s13613-020-0638-0
29. Chang W, Sun Q, Peng F, Xie J, Qiu H, Yang Y. Validation of neuromuscular blocking agent use in acute respiratory distress syndrome: a meta-analysis of randomized trials. *Crit. Care.* (2020) 24:54–8. doi: 10.1186/s13054-02 0-2765-2
30. Rue M, Andrinopoulou E-R, Alvares D, Armero C, Forte A, Blanch L. Bayesian joint modeling of bivariate longitudinal and competing risks data: an application to study patient-ventilator asynchronies in critical care patients. *Biom. J.* (2017) 59:1184–203. doi: 10.1002/bimj.2016 00221
31. Beitler JR, Sands SA, Loring SH, Owens RL, Malhotra A, Spragg RG, et al. Quantifying unintended exposure to high tidal volumes from breath stacking dyssynchrony in ARDS: the BREATHE criteria. *Intensive Care Med.* (2016) 42:1427–36. doi: 10.1007/s00134-016-4423-3
32. Rodriguez PO, Tiribelli N, Gogniat E, Plotnikow GA, Fredes S, Fernandez Ceballos I, et al. Automatic detection of reverse-triggering related asynchronies during mechanical ventilation in ARDS patients using flow and pressure signals. *J. Clin. Monit. Comput.* (2019) 307:2526. doi: 10.1007/s10877-019-00444-3

20

# Deep Learning-Based Pain Classifier Based on the Facial Expression in Critically Ill Patients


*Chieh-Liang Wu*[1,2,3,4†], *Shu-Fang Liu*[5†], *Tian-Li Yu*[6], *Sou-Jen Shih*[5], *Chih-Hung Chang*[6], *Shih-Fang Yang Mao*[7], *Yueh-Se Li*[7], *Hui-Jiun Chen*[5], *Chia-Chen Chen*[7*] and *Wen-Cheng Chao*[1,4,8,9*]

*[1] Department of Critical Care Medicine, Taichung Veterans General Hospital, Taichung, Taiwan, [2] Department of Industrial Engineering and Enterprise Information, Tunghai University, Taichung, Taiwan, [3] Artificial Intelligence Studio, Taichung Veterans General Hospital, Taichung, Taiwan, [4] Colledge of Medicine, National Chung Hsing University, Taichung, Taiwan, [5] Department of Nursing, Taichung Veterans General Hospital, Taichung, Taiwan, [6] Department of Electrical Engineering, National Taiwan University, Taipei, Taiwan, [7] Electronic and Optoelectronic System Research Laboratories, Industrial Technology Research Institute, Hsinchu, Taiwan, [8] Department of Automatic Control Engineering, Feng Chia University, Taichung, Taiwan, [9] Big Data Center, National Chung Hsing University, Taichung, Taiwan*

***Correspondence:**
*Chia-Chen Chen*
*ChiaChen@itri.org.tw*
*Wen-Cheng Chao*
*cwc081@hotmail.com*

*† These authors have contributed equally to this work*



**Objective:** Pain assessment based on facial expressions is an essential issue in critically ill patients, but an automated assessment tool is still lacking. We conducted this prospective study to establish the deep learning-based pain classifier based on facial expressions.

**Methods:** We enrolled critically ill patients during 2020–2021 at a tertiary hospital in central Taiwan and recorded video clips with labeled pain scores based on facial expressions, such as relaxed (0), tense (1), and grimacing (2). We established both image- and video-based pain classifiers through using convolutional neural network (CNN) models, such as Resnet34, VGG16, and InceptionV1 and bidirectional long short-term memory networks (BiLSTM). The performance of classifiers in the test dataset was determined by accuracy, sensitivity, and F1-score.

**Results:** A total of 63 participants with 746 video clips were eligible for analysis. The accuracy of using Resnet34 in the polychromous image-based classifier for pain scores 0, 1, 2 was merely 0.5589, and the accuracy of dichotomous pain classifiers between 0 vs. 1/2 and 0 vs. 2 were 0.7668 and 0.8593, respectively. Similar accuracy of image-based pain classifier was found using VGG16 and InceptionV1. The accuracy of the video-based pain classifier to classify 0 vs. 1/2 and 0 vs. 2 was approximately 0.81 and 0.88, respectively. We further tested the performance of established classifiers without reference, mimicking clinical scenarios with a new patient, and found the performance remained high.

**Conclusions:** The present study demonstrates the practical application of deep learning-based automated pain assessment in critically ill patients, and more studies are warranted to validate our findings.



**Keywords: pain, critically ill patients, facial expression, artificial intelligence, classifier**

## BACKGROUND

Pain is an essential medical issue but somehow difficult to assess in critically ill patients who cannot report their pain (1). Therefore, the Critical-Care Pain Observation Tool (CPOT) has been developed to grade the pain through assessing behavior alternations, such as facial expressions, among critically ill patients in the past two decades (2). The facial expression is the fundamental behavior alternation in CPOT and consists of relaxed, tense, and grimacing (pain score 0, 1, and 2) (3). Currently, facial expression-based pain assessment is graded by the nurse, and there is an unmet need to develop an automated pain assessment tool based on facial expression to relieve the medical staff from the aforementioned workload (4).

A number of automated recognition of facial expressions of pain and emotion has been developed through using distinct approaches (5–9). Pedersen et al. used Support Vector Machine (SVM) as a facial expression-based pain classifier in UNBC-McMaster Shoulder Pain Expression Archive Database, consisting of 200 video sequences obtained from 25 patients with shoulder pain, and reported that the accuracy of the leave-one-subject-out 25-fold cross was 0.861 (7). Given that video sequences contain temporal information with respect to pain, two studies were used Recurrent Neural Network (RNN) and hybrid network to extract the time-frame feature among images and reported an improved performance (8, 9). Furthermore, recent studies have employed fusion network architectures and further improved the F1 score to ~0.94 (10, 11). Therefore, the recent advancements in deep learning might enable us to establish a facial expressed-based pain assessment tool in critically ill patients.

Notably, the application of the aforementioned methods in critically ill patients might not be straightforward due to real-world difficulties to obtain standardized and whole unmasked facial images of patients admitted to the intensive care unit (ICU) (12). Unlike the high-quality whole facial image in the UNBC-McMaster Shoulder Pain Expression Archive Database, critically ill patients may have masks on the face due to needed medical devices, such as endotracheal tube, nasoesophageal tube, and oxygen mask. Furthermore, pain-associated facial muscle movements might hence be subtle due to sedation and tissue oedema in critically ill patients. Therefore, there is a substantial need for using facial images obtained in sub-optimal real-world conditions at ICUs to establish an automated facial expression-based assessment tool for pain in critically ill patients. In the present prospective study, we recorded facial video clips in critically ill patients at the ICUs of Taichung Veterans General Hospital (TCVGH) and employed an ensemble of three Convolutional Neural Network (CNN) models as well as RNN to establish the pain classifier based on facial expressions.

## MATERIALS AND METHODS

### Ethical Approval

This study was approved by the Institutional Review Board approval of the Taichung Veterans General Hospital (CE20325A). Informed consent was obtained from all of the participants prior to the enrollment in the study and collection of data.

### Study Population

We conducted this prospective study by enrolling patients who were admitted to medical and surgical ICUs at TCVGH, a referral hospital with 1,560 beds in central Taiwan, between 2020-Nov and 2021-Nov. The CPOT is a standard of care in the study hospital, and grading of the facial expression-based pain score is in accordance with the guideline (3). In detail, a score of 0 is given if there is no observed muscle tension in the face, and the score of 1 is composed of a tensed muscle contraction, such as the presence of frowning, brow lowering, orbit tightening as well as levator muscle contraction. The score of 2 consists of grimacing, which is a contraction of facial muscles, particularly muscles nearby the eyebrow area, plus eyelid tightly closed.

### Video Sequences With Labeled Pain Grade Based on Facial Expression

**Figure 1** depicts the protocol of video record, labeling, and image preprocessing of the present study (**Figure 1**). Video record and labeling were performed by three experienced nurses after training for inter-rater concordance, and the labeling was further validated by two senior registered nurses. To mitigate information bias and synchronize the recording and labeling, we designed a user interface that enables the study nurse to observe the patient for 10 s, to record a video for 20 s, and then label the pain score at the end of the video. To further reduce the potential sampling errors, we recorded three labeled videos in each observation; therefore, each 90-s video sequence has three 20-s clips (**Figure 1A**). Given the nature of observation of this study, we conducted the recording per day during the ICU admission of participants, particularly before and after suction, dressing change as well as invasive procedures, to obtain the videos with distinct pain grades in individual critically ill patients. With regards to the hardware, the frame per second of the applied camera was 30, and the total frames of a 20-s video clip were nearly 400–600 frames per clip. To standardize the video clips, we used 50 frames in each 20-s clip; therefore, there were 2.5 representative frames per second for the following experiments. To avoid any interference with critical care, we designed a portable camera rack that enables us to take high-quality video ~1–2 m from the patient.

### Image Preprocessing

We used a facial landmark tracker to locate the facial area (13). Due to the face that was masked by the aforementioned medical devices might not be detected by the facial landmark tracker, we further used multi-task CNN to locate the facial area if the face was not located by the facial landmark tracker (14). Given that the area nearby the eyebrow is the key area to interpret pain score, we hence cropped the face between hairline and nose not only to focus on the eyebrow area, but also to avoid the confounding of the aforementioned medical devices. We further cropped the central part of the eyebrow area with a fixed ratio of height/width (3/4) for the following experiments. Given that facial images with extreme angles may lead to the facial landmark misalignment

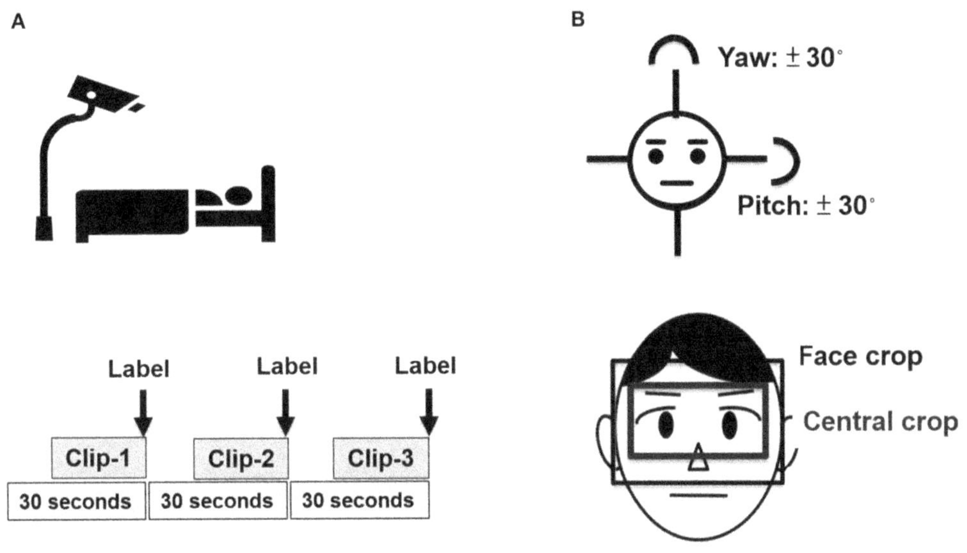


**FIGURE 1** | Schematic diagram of image acquisition and preprocessing. **(A)** Recording of video clips with labeling and **(B)** Preprocessing of video sequences.

and affect the following experiments, we hence excluded the faces with yaw or pitch angle over 30 degrees (**Figure 1B**).

## Image-Based Pain Classifiers

**Figure 2** illustrates the deep learning-based Siamese network architectures for image- and video-based pain classifiers in this study (15) (**Figure 2**). To reduce the need for an extremely high number of labeled but unrelated images for learning, we employed a relation network architecture for the image-based pain classifier (16). In brief, the aforementioned relation network is designed for learning to compare the differences among labeled images of each individual patient; therefore, the essential need is the images with distinct grades among individual patients, instead of a high number of unrelated images from patients with high heterogeneity. Therefore, we used the data of the 63 participants who had images of all of 0, 1, 2 labeled images. In detail, by feeding grade-0 facial expression image and grade 1/2 images into CNN encoder, two vectors were obtained to represent the subtle difference between the image of grade-0 and grade-1/2, instead of calculating the complex distance metric of two images in high dimensions. Indeed, the application of relation network should be in line with clinical grading of pain by the nurse, who had to recognize the baseline facial appearance of an individual patient prior to grade pain-score based on the facial expression. In this study, we used three CNN models that have fewer vanishing gradient issues, such as Resnet34, VGG16, and inceptionV1, as well as two types of the fully connected layer set up with one and two layers (17–19). Therefore, there were a total of six combinations for the image-based pain classifier, and we applied the voting to optimize the classifier performance through averaging outputs of different models. With regards to the main hyperparameters, we used the cross-entropy loss as the loss function in the image-based pain classifier, and the learning rate, optimizer, and trained epochs were 1e-4, Adam, and 60 epochs, respectively.

## Video-Based Pain Classifiers

With regard to the video-based pain classifier, we employed a many-to-one sequence model given that the output of this study is a one pain grade. Similar to the image-based pain classifier, we used a Siamese network architecture as feature extractors. Given that multiple CNN encoders were used in the present study, we hence processed the image through three CNN encoders to get three vectors and concatenate these vectors to a relatively low-dimensional space. The concatenated output vectors of each frame were then fed into the bidirectional long short-term memory networks (BiLSTM) for the classification of pain (20). Given that the CNN encoder had been trained in the image-based pain classifier, we hence reduced the learning rate to 1e-5 on the video-based pain classifier and froze the weights of the CNN encoder in the first 10 epochs, and this approach may facilitate to focus on training BiLSTM in the first 10 epochs. The other parameters, such as loss function, optimizer, and trained epochs, were in line with those used in the image-based pain classifier.

## Statistical Analyses

Data were expressed in frequency of occurrence (percentages) for categorical variables and as means ± *SD* for continuous variables. Differences between the survivor and non-survivor groups were analyzed using Student's *t*-test for continuous variables and Fisher's exact test for categorical variables. The proportion of train, validation, and test datasets were 60, 20, and 20%, respectively. The performance of the pain classifier in the test dataset was determined by accuracy, sensitivity, and F1-score. Python version 3.8, PyTorch 1.9.1, and CUDA 11.1 were used in this study.

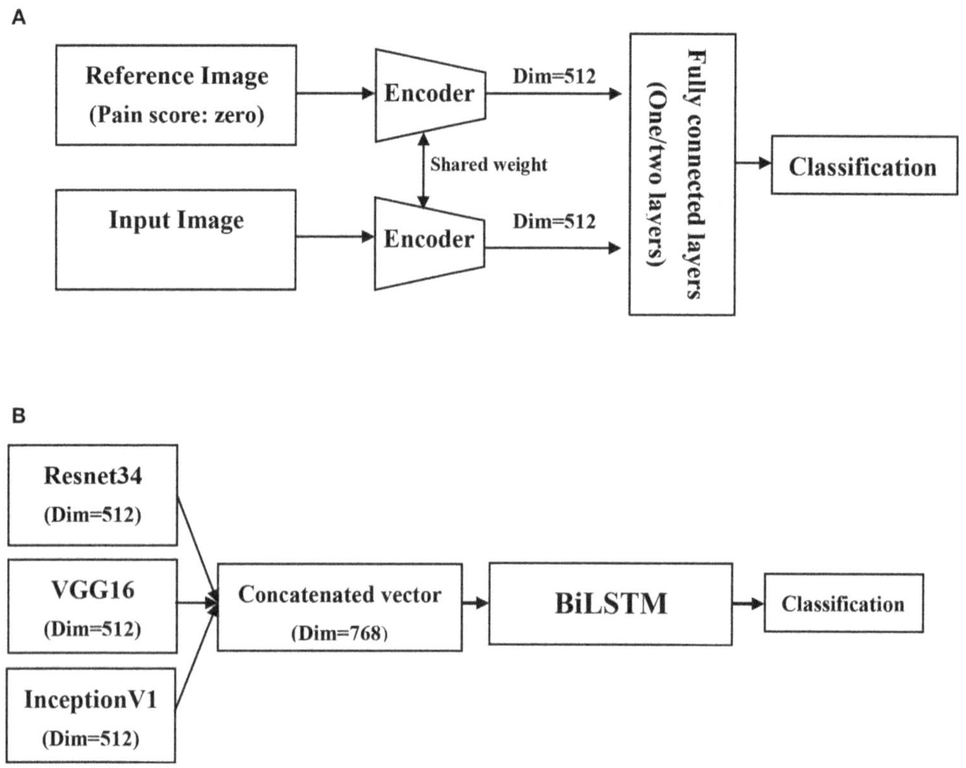


**FIGURE 2** | Schematic diagram of network architectures in the present study. **(A)** Image-based pain classifiers using relation and siamese network architecture, **(B)** Video-base pain classifier using bidirectional long short-term memory networks (BiLSTM).

# RESULTS

## Patients' Characteristics

A total of 341 participants were enrolled, and there were 7,813 qualified videos, of which the number of scores 0, 1, and 2 were 5,717, 1,714, and 382, respectively. Given that we employed relation network architecture in this study, we hence used images among 63 participants who had all of the pain-score 0, 1, and 2 labeled video clips, and the number of videos with 0, 1, and 2 were 351, 253, and 142, respectively. The mean age of included patients for analyses was 69.3 ± 14.6 years, and 55.6 (35/63) of them was male (**Table 1**). The majority (81.0%, 51/63) of enrolled participants were critically ill patients who were admitted to medical ICUs. The ICU severity scores of acute physiology and chronic health evaluation II (APACHE II), sequential organ failure assessment (SOFA) day-1, SOFA day-3, and SOFA day-7 were 25.3 ± 5.7, 9.0 ± 3.7, 8.5 ± 4.1, and 8.2 ± 3.8, respectively.

## Performance of Image-Based Pain Classifiers

In image-based pain classifiers, we attempted to classify with three pain categories (0, 1, and 2) and dichotomous pain classifiers (0 vs. 1/2 and 0 vs. 2) given pain score = 2 reflects a clinical warning signaling requiring immediate clinical evaluation and management (**Table 2**). In Resnet34 with one fully connected layer (1024, 3), the performance of the polychromous classifier for 0, 1, and 2 appeared to be suboptimal, with the accuracy, sensitivity, and F1 score were merely 0.5589, 0.5589, and 0.5495, respectively. The performance of the two dichotomous image-based pain classifiers was much higher than that in polychromous pain classifier. The accuracy, sensitivity, and F1 score were 0.7668, 0.8422, and 0.8593 to classify 0 vs. 1/2 and were 0.8593, 0.8925, and 0.8638 to classify 0 vs. 2. We further tested the performance of using VGG16, InceptionV1, and two fully connected layers. The performances of Resnet34 and VGG16 were slightly higher than that of InceptionV1. For example, the accuracy of dichotomous pain classifier between 0 vs. 1/2 in Resnet34, VGG16, and Inception were 0.7668, 0.7578, and 0.7055, respectively. With regard to the efficacy of using two fully connected layers ([1024, 256] followed by [256, 3]), the performance tended to improve in a few models, such as dichotomous pain classifier between 0 vs. 1/2 in InceptionV1 (accuracy increased from 0.7055 to 0.7587).

## Performance of Video-Based Pain Classifiers and the Pain Classifier Without Reference

We then examined the performance of a video-based pain classifier through concatenating vectors of the aforementioned three CNN encoders and BiLSTM with distinct hidden layers (**Table 3**). We found that the performance of video-based

**TABLE 1 |** Characteristics of the enrolled 63 participants who had videos with all of three pain-score categories.

| Basic data | |
|---|---|
| Age, years | 69.3 ± 14.6 |
| Sex (male) | 35 (55.6%) |
| Height (cm) | 160.1 ± 8.0 |
| Body weight (kgs) | 57.3 ± 10.0 |
| **ICU types** | |
| Medical ICUs | 51 (81.0%) |
| Surgical ICUs | 12 (19.0%) |
| **Laboratory data (Day-1)** | |
| White blood cell counts (/ml) | 13,670.7 ± 11,259.5 |
| Hematocrit (%) | 28.8 ± 8.4 |
| Creatinine (mg/dl) | 1.9 ± 1.4 |
| Sodium (mg/dl) | 140.3 ± 5.5 |
| Potassium (mg/dl) | 4.0 ± 0.7 |
| **Severity scores** | |
| APACHE II score | 25.3 ± 5.7 |
| SOFA score, day-1 | 9.0 ± 3.7 |
| SOFA score, day-3 | 8.5 ± 4.1 |
| SOFA score, day-7 | 8.2 ± 3.8 |

*Data were presented as mean ± standard deviation and number (percentage). ICU, intensive care unit; APACHE II, acute physiology and chronic health evaluation II; SOFA, sequential organ failure assessment.*

**TABLE 2 |** Performance image-based pain classifiers with pain score zero as the reference in different settings.

| | CNN model | Fully connected layers | Pain score 0 vs. 1 vs. 2 | Pain score 0 vs. 1/2 | Pain score 0 vs. 2 |
|---|---|---|---|---|---|
| Accuracy | Resnet34 | 1 layer | 0.5589 | 0.7668 | 0.8593 |
| Sensitivity | | (1024, 3) | 0.5589 | 0.8422 | 0.8925 |
| F1-score | | | 0.5495 | 0.7832 | 0.8638 |
| Accuracy | | 2 layers | 0.6032 | 0.7711 | 0.8568 |
| Sensitivity | | (1,024, 256) | 0.6032 | 0.8380 | 0.8514 |
| F1-score | | (256, 3) | 0.5969 | 0.7855 | 0.8561 |
| Accuracy | VGG16 | 1 layer | 0.5914 | 0.7578 | 0.8557 |
| Sensitivity | | (1024, 3) | 0.5914 | 0.6665 | 0.8499 |
| F1-score | | | 0.5867 | 0.7141 | 0.8548 |
| Accuracy | | 2 layers | 0.5871 | 0.7578 | 0.8276 |
| Sensitivity | | (1,024, 256) | 0.5871 | 0.6908 | 0.8064 |
| F1-score | | (256, 3) | 0.5811 | 0.7405 | 0.8239 |
| Accuracy | InceptionV1 | 1 layer | 0.5872 | 0.7055 | 0.8302 |
| Sensitivity | | (1024, 3) | 0.5872 | 0.8216 | 0.8782 |
| F1-score | | | 0.5788 | 0.7362 | 0.8380 |
| Accuracy | | 2 layers | 0.5567 | 0.7587 | 0.8035 |
| Sensitivity | | (1,024, 256) | 0.5567 | 0.8159 | 0.8338 |
| F1-score | | (256, 3) | 0.5556 | 0.7718 | 0.8093 |

*CNN, convolutional neural network.*

**TABLE 3 |** Performance of video-based pain classifiers with different numbers of hidden layers in bidirectional long short-term memory (BiLSTM) networks.

| | Hidden layers | Pain score 0 vs. 1 vs. 2 | Pain score 0 vs. 1/2 | Pain score 0 vs. 2 |
|---|---|---|---|---|
| Accuracy | 64 | 0.6144 | 0.8145 | 0.8810 |
| Sensitivity | | 0.6144 | 0.7947 | 0.8755 |
| F1-score | | 0.6123 | 0.8107 | 0.8803 |
| Accuracy | 128 | 0.5941 | 0.8054 | 0.8461 |
| Sensitivity | | 0.5942 | 0.7858 | 0.7589 |
| F1-score | | 0.5902 | 0.8015 | 0.8314 |
| Accuracy | 256 | 0.6006 | 0.8268 | 0.8367 |
| Sensitivity | | 0.6006 | 0.8244 | 0.7500 |
| F1-score | | 0.5948 | 0.8264 | 0.8212 |

*BiLSTM, bidirectional long short-term memory.*

pain classifiers among the polychromous classifier and two dichotomous classifiers was higher than those in the image-based pain classifier. The accuracy in classifying 0 vs. 1/2 was nearly 0.8 and reached ~0.88 to classify 0 vs. 2. Additionally, we further tested the performance of the established classifier without reference, mimicking the clinical scenario in a new patient without an image score of 0 as the reference (**Table 4**). We found that the performance of both image- and video-based classifiers slightly decreased in classifiers without reference. Notably, the performance of a video-based classifier without reference to differentiate 2 from 0 was up to 0.8906, indicating the established classifier had learned the difference between 0 and 2. Collectively, we established the image and video facial expression-based pain classifier in critically ill patients, with the accuracy to classify 0 vs. 1/2 and 0 vs. 2 were ~0.8 and 0.9, respectively.

## DISCUSSION

In this prospective study, we developed a protocol to obtain video clips of facial expressions in critically ill patients and employed the deep learning-based approach to establish the facial expression-based pain classifier. We focused on the area nearby eyebrow that is less likely to be masked by medical devices and employed an ensemble of three CNN models, such as Resnet34, VGG16, and InceptionV1, to learn pain-associated facial features and BiLSTM for temporal relation between video frames. The accuracy of the dichotomous classifier to differentiate tense/grimacing (1/2) from relaxed (0) facial expression was ~80%, and the accuracy to detect grimacing (2) was nearly 90%. The present study demonstrates the practical application of deep learning-based automated pain assessment in ICU, and the findings shed light on the application of medical artificial intelligence (AI) not only to improve patient care, but also to relieve healthcare workers from the routine workload.

Pain is the fifth vital sign in hospitalized patients but is somehow difficult to assess in critically ill patients who cannot self-report the pain (21, 22). Facial expressions of pain consist of coordinated pain-indicative muscle movements, particularly the contraction of muscles surrounding the eyes, i.e., orbicularis oculi muscle (23). Notably, facial pain responses appear to be

**TABLE 4** | Accuracy of proposed image- and video-based pain classifiers with and without reference.

| | Reference | Pain score 0 vs. 1 vs. 2 | Pain score 0 vs. 1/2 | Pain score 0 vs. 2 |
|---|---|---|---|---|
| **Image-based pain classifiers** | | | | |
| Accuracy | Pain score 0 | 0.6347 | 0.8000 | 0.8937 |
| Sensitivity | | 0.6347 | 0.8022 | 0.8826 |
| F1-score | | 0.6321 | 0.8004 | 0.8953 |
| Accuracy | No reference | 0.6421 | 0.7954 | 0.8771 |
| Sensitivity | | 0.6421 | 0.7974 | 0.9074 |
| F1-score | | 0.6371 | 0.7947 | 0.8724 |
| **Video-based pain classifiers** | | | | |
| Accuracy | Pain score 0 | 0.6144 | 0.8268 | 0.8810 |
| Sensitivity | | 0.6144 | 0.8244 | 0.8755 |
| F1-score | | 0.6123 | 0.8264 | 0.8803 |
| Accuracy | No reference | 0.6130 | 0.7858 | 0.8906 |
| Sensitivity | | 0.6130 | 0.8016 | 0.8344 |
| F1-score | | 0.6102 | 0.7892 | 0.8841 |

consistent across distinct types of pain stimulation, such as pressure, temperature, electrical current, and ischemia (23, 24). A number of studies have explored the physiological basis of how pain signaling leads to pain-indicative muscle movement. Kuramoto et al. recently used facial myogenic potential topography in 18 healthy adult participants to investigate the facial myogenic potential and subsequent facial expressions (25). Furthermore, Kunz used functional MRI (fMRI) to address the association between brain responses in areas that processed the sensory dimension of pain and activation of the orbicularis oculi muscle (26). Although promising, monitoring of facial myogenic potential might be infeasible in critically ill patients given that contact device-associated issues regarding infection control and the potential interference with critical care (27). The possibility of application of fMRI in ICU appears to be low; therefore, using a portable camera to take high-quality video ~1–2 m from the patient as well as AI-based image analyses focusing on eyebrow area as we have shown in the present study has high applicative value in critically ill patients.

It is estimated that more than 50% of patients in ICU experienced experience moderate to severe pain at rest, and 80% of critically ill patients experience pain during procedures (28, 29). Therefore, CPOT, as well as Behavioral Pain Scale (BPS), has been introduced for pain assessment in patients at ICUs in the past two decades, and facial expression is the fundamental domain in both BPS and CPOT given that muscle tension in facial areas, particularly facial area nearby eyebrow, can be directly observed by the caring staff without contact (3, 30). Notably, contactless monitoring in ICU is of increasing importance in the post-coronavirus disease (COVID) era (27). A number of AI-based tools, such as the dynamic relationship of facial landmarks or CNN-learned facial features, have been developed to assess pain in non-ICU patients (7, 23, 31). Nevertheless, the subtle pain-associated movement of facial muscles/landmarks in the non-ICU patient is largely distinct from those in critically ill patients under sedation. Given that patients in ICU often received mechanical ventilation, experienced fear were deprived of normal sleep, felt isolation; therefore, appropriate sedation, at least light sedation, is recommended as a standard of care in critically ill patients and hence leads to difficulties to identify pain based on facial expressions (32). In addition to the impact of sedation on pain assessment, subtle facial muscle movements might also be confounded by facial oedema resulting from fluid overload, which is highly prevalent in critically ill patients who underwent fluid resuscitation, as we have shown in our previous studies (33, 34). Collectively, automated pain assessment based on facial expressions in critically ill patients is currently an unmet need in the research field of medical AI due to the aforementioned difficulties.

Intriguingly, we found a suboptimal performance in the polychromous classifier, whereas the performance in dichotomous classifiers was high. We postulated that the relatively little difference between pain grades 1 and 2 may lead to the reduced performance to differentiate between 1 and 2, and the performance of dichotomous classifiers was high due to the apparent difference between 0 and 1/2. We found a higher performance in video classifiers than those in image classifiers, and this finding indicates that the temporal relation among image frames is crucial to classify pain by facial expressions. A similar finding has been found in pain classifiers using the UNBC-McMaster shoulder pain database (7–9). The accuracy of the leave-one-subject-out 25-fold cross in facial expression-based pain classifier by machine learning approach was ~0.861 using the UNBC-McMaster database (7). Similar to our approach, Rodriguez et al. used VGG to learn basic facial features as well as LSTM to exploit the temporal relation between video frames and reported a further increased accuracy (0.933) in the aforementioned UNBC-McMaster database (8). Similarly, Huang *et al.* proposed an end-to-end hybrid network to extract multidimensional features including time-frame features from images of the UNBC-McMaster database and also found an improved performance (9). Recently, Semwal and Londhe further used distinct fusion network architectures, including CNN-based fusion network to learn both the spatial appearance and shape-based descriptors, as well as decision-level fusion network to learn the domain-specific spatial appearance and complementary features, to improve the performance of pain intensity assessment, with the F1 score, was ~0.94 (10, 11). This evidence highlights the potential application of automated pain assessment based on facial expressions in hospital.

The inevitable medical devices and high heterogeneity in critically ill patients have led to technical difficulties as we have shown in this study. We choose to crop the facial area nearby the eyebrow area, and this approach not only keeps the essential area to detect painful facial expressions but also is essential to extend the established model to clinical scenarios with distinct facial masks, such as the increasing prevalence of wearing a facial mask in the post-COVID era. Moreover, we used a pain score of 0 to train the pain classifiers in this study and further tested the performance of established classifiers without reference (**Table 4**). Notably, the performance of dichotomous classifiers, particularly the 0 vs. 2 classifier, remains high without reference, indicating that the established model has learned the pain-associated facial expression in critically ill patients.

Timely detection of severe pain, such as pain score 2, is crucial in critical care. Frequent pain assessment is substantial for the identification of the existence of pain and the adjustment dosage of pharmacological analgesic agents or the intensity of non-pharmacological management (1). The previous studies have shown that regular pain assessment is associated with a better outcome, such as ventilator-day, in critically ill patients (35, 36). Severe pain may reflect not only inadequate pain control, but also the potential deterioration of critical illness. For example, increasing pain has been implicated with anxiety, delirium, and poor both short-term and long-term outcomes in critically ill patients (37). Therefore, the automated AI-based pain assessment, particularly timely identification of severe pain/pain score 2, should serve as an actionable AI target, i.e., the detection of pain score 2 indicates the need for immediate evaluation and management by the healthcare worker. Additionally, we have established the user interface to guide the user with regard to quality of the image and the real-time classification of pain based on facial expressions, and the application of the established model should hence reach level 5 of technology readiness level (TRL) (**Supplementary Demonstration Video 1**) (38, 39).

There are limitations in this study. First, this study is a single center study. However, the pain relevant management in the study hospital is in accordance with the guideline; therefore, the generalization issue should be at least partly mitigated. Second, we recorded the video for 90 s in each record, and a longer duration could further improve the accuracy. Third, we focused on the facial expression in the present study, and more sensors for the other domains of CPOT/BPS are warranted in the future.

## CONCLUSION

Autonomous facial expression-based pain assessment is an essential issue in critical care but is somehow difficult in critically ill patients due to inevitable masked areas by medical devices and relatively subtle muscle movement resulting from sedation/oedema. In the present prospective study, we established the deep learning-based pain classifier based on facial expression focusing on the area nearby eyebrow, with the accuracy to detect tense/grimacing and grimacing were ~80 and 90%, respectively. These findings indicate a real-world application of AI-based pain assessment based on the facial expression in ICU, and more studies are warranted to validate the performance of the automated pain assessment tool.

## ETHICS STATEMENT

The study was approved by the Institutional Review Board of Taichung Veterans General Hospital (TCVGH: CE20325A). The patients/participants provided their written informed consent to participate in this study.

## AUTHOR CONTRIBUTIONS

C-LW, S-JS, S-FY, C-CC, and W-CC: study concept and design. S-FL, S-JS, and H-JC: acquisition of data. T-LY, C-HC, S-FY, Y-SL, C-CC, and W-CC: analysis and interpretation of data. C-LW and W-CC: drafting the manuscript.

## REFERENCES


1. Devlin JW, Skrobik Y, Gelinas C, Needham DM, Slooter AJC, Pandharipande PP, et al. Clinical practice guidelines for the prevention and management of pain, agitation/sedation, delirium, immobility, and sleep disruption in adult patients in the ICU. *Crit Care Med.* (2018) 46:e825–e73. doi: 10.1097/CCM.0000000000003259
2. Payen JF, Bru O, Bosson JL, Lagrasta A, Novel E, Deschaux I, et al. Assessing pain in critically ill sedated patients by using a behavioral pain scale. *Crit Care Med.* (2001) 29:2258–63. doi: 10.1097/00003246-200112000-00004
3. Gelinas C, Fillion L, Puntillo KA, Viens C, Fortier M. Validation of the critical-care pain observation tool in adult patients. *Am J Crit Care.* (2006) 15:420–7. doi: 10.4037/ajcc2006.15.4.420
4. Buchanan C, Howitt ML, Wilson R, Booth RG, Risling T, Bamford M. Predicted influences of artificial intelligence on the domains of nursing: scoping review. *JMIR Nurs.* (2020) 3:e23939. doi: 10.2196/23939
5. Bartlett MS, Littlewort GC, Frank MG, Lee K. Automatic decoding of facial movements reveals deceptive pain expressions. *Curr Biol.* (2014) 24:738–43. doi: 10.1016/j.cub.2014.02.009
6. Sikka K, Ahmed AA, Diaz D, Goodwin MS, Craig KD, Bartlett MS, et al. Automated assessment of children's postoperative pain using computer vision. *Pediatrics.* (2015) 136:e124–31. doi: 10.1542/peds.2015-0029
7. Pedersen H. Learning appearance features for pain detection using the Unbc-mcmaster shoulder pain expression archive database. *Computer Vision Syst.* (2015) 15:12. doi: 10.1007/978-3-319-20904-3_12
8. Rodriguez P, Cucurull G, Gonalez J, Gonfaus JM, Nasrollahi K, Moeslund TB, et al. Deep pain: exploiting long short-term memory networks for facial expression classification. *IEEE Trans Cybern.* (2017) 17:2199. doi: 10.1109/TCYB.2017.2662199
9. Huang Y, Qing L, Xu S, Wang L, Peng Y. HybNet: a hybrid network structure for pain intensity estimation. *Visual Comput.* (2021) 21:56. doi: 10.1007/s00371-021-02056-y
10. Semwal A, Londhe ND. Computer aided pain detection and intensity estimation using compact CNN based fusion network. *Appl Soft Comput.* (2021) 112:107780. doi: 10.1016/j.asoc.2021.107780
11. Semwal A, Londhe ND. MVFNet: A multi-view fusion network for pain intensity assessment in unconstrained environment. *Biomed Signal Process Control.* (2021) 67:102537. doi: 10.1016/j.bspc.2021.102537
12. Davoudi A, Malhotra KR, Shickel B, Siegel S, Williams S, Ruppert M, et al. Intelligent ICU for autonomous patient monitoring using pervasive sensing and deep learning. *Sci Rep.* (2019) 9:8020. doi: 10.1038/s41598-019-44004-w
13. Sanchez-Lozano E, Tzimiropoulos G, Martinez B, Torre F, Valstar M. A functional regression approach to facial landmark tracking. *IEEE Trans Pattern Anal Mach Intell.* (2018) 40:2037–50. doi: 10.1109/TPAMI.2017.2745568
14. Ge H, Dai Y, Zhu Z, Wang B. Robust face recognition based on multi-task convolutional neural network. *Math Biosci Eng.* (2021) 18:6638–51. doi: 10.3934/mbe.2021329
15. Chicco D. Siamese neural networks: an overview. *Methods Mol Biol.* (2021) 2190:73–94. doi: 10.1007/978-1-0716-0826-5_3
16. Sung F, Yang Y, Zhang L, Xiang T, Torr PHS, Hospedales TM. "Learning to

compare: relation network for few-shot learning," in *IEEE/CVF Conference on Computer Vision and Pattern Recognition.* (2018), p. 1199–208.
17. Kaiming He, Xiangyu Zhang, Shaoqing Ren, Sun. J. "Deep residual learning for image recognition," in *Proceedings of the IEEE Conference on Computer Vision and Pattern Recognition.* (2016), p. 770-8.
18. Karen S, Zisserman A. "Very deep convolutional networks for large-scale image recognition," in *Proceedings of the IEEE Conference on Computer Vision and Pattern Recognition* (2014).
19. Szegedy C, Wei L, Yangqing J, Sermanet P, Reed S, Anguelov D, et al. "Going deeper with convolutions," in *2015 IEEE Conference on Computer Vision and Pattern Recognition (CVPR).* (2015), pp. 7–12.
20. Sharfuddin AA, Tihami MN, Islam MS, "A deep recurrent neural network with BiLSTM model for sentiment classification," in *2018 International Conference on Bangla Speech and Language Processing (ICBSLP).* (2018), p. 21–22.
21. Quality improvement guidelines for the treatment of acute pain and cancer pain. American Pain Society Quality of Care Committee. *JAMA.* (1995) 274:1874–80. doi: 10.1001/jama.274.23.1874
22. Arif-Rahu M, Grap MJ. Facial expression and pain in the critically ill non-communicative patient: state of science review. *Intensive Crit Care Nurs.* (2010) 26:343–52. doi: 10.1016/j.iccn.2010.08.007
23. Kunz M, Meixner D, Lautenbacher S. Facial muscle movements encoding pain-a systematic review. *Pain.* (2019) 160:535–49. doi: 10.1097/j.pain.0000000000001424
24. Prkachin KM. The consistency of facial expressions of pain: a comparison across modalities. *Pain.* (1992) 51:297–306. doi: 10.1016/0304-3959(92)90213-U
25. Kuramoto E, Yoshinaga S, Nakao H, Nemoto S, Ishida Y. Characteristics of facial muscle activity during voluntary facial expressions: Imaging analysis of facial expressions based on myogenic potential data. *Neuropsychopharmacol Rep.* (2019) 39:183–93. doi: 10.1002/npr2.12059
26. Kunz M, Chen JI, Rainville P. Keeping an eye on pain expression in primary somatosensory cortex. *Neuroimage.* (2020) 217:116885. doi: 10.1016/j.neuroimage.2020.116885
27. Lyra S, Mayer L, Ou L, Chen D, Timms P, Tay A, et al. A deep learning-based camera approach for vital sign monitoring using thermography images for ICU patients. *Sensors (Basel).* (2021) 21:1495. doi: 10.3390/s21041495
28. Chanques G, Sebbane M, Barbotte E, Viel E, Eledjam JJ, Jaber S. A prospective study of pain at rest: incidence and characteristics of an unrecognised symptom in surgical and trauma versus medical intensive care unit patients. *Anesthesiology.* (2007) 107:858–60. doi: 10.1097/01.anes.0000287211.98642.51
29. Puntillo KA, Max A, Timsit JF, Vignoud L, Chanques G, Robleda G, et al. Determinants of procedural pain intensity in the intensive care unit. *The Europain(R) study. Am J Respir Crit Care Med.* (2014) 189:39–47. doi: 10.1164/rccm.201306-1174OC
30. Chanques G, Payen JF, Mercier G, de Lattre S, Viel E, Jung B, et al. Assessing pain in non-intubated critically ill patients unable to self report: an adaptation of the Behavioral Pain Scale. *Intensive Care Med.* (2009) 35:2060–7. doi: 10.1007/s00134-009-1590-5
31. Neshov N, Manolova A. "Pain detection from facial characteristics using supervised descent method," in *IEEE 8th International Conference on Intelligent Data Acquisition and Advanced Computing Systems: Technology and Applications (IDAACS).* (2015), p. 251–6.
32. Chanques G, Constantin JM, Devlin JW, Ely EW, Fraser GL, Gelinas C, et al. Analgesia and sedation in patients with ARDS. *Intensive Care Med.* (2020) 46:2342–56. doi: 10.1007/s00134-020-06307-9
33. Chen YC, Zheng ZR, Wang CY, Chao WC. Impact of early fluid balance on 1-year mortality in critically ill patients with cancer: a retrospective study in Central Taiwan. *Cancer Control.* (2020) 27:1073274820920733. doi: 10.1177/1073274820920733
34. Wu CL, Pai KC, Wong LT, Wang MS, Chao WC. Impact of early fluid balance on long-term mortality in critically ill surgical patients: a retrospective cohort study in Central Taiwan. *J Clin Med.* (2021) 10:73. doi: 10.3390/jcm10214873
35. Payen JF, Bosson JL, Chanques G, Mantz J, Labarere J, Investigators D. Pain assessment is associated with decreased duration of mechanical ventilation in the intensive care unit: a post Hoc analysis of the DOLOREA study. *Anesthesiology.* (2009) 111:1308–16. doi: 10.1097/ALN.0b013e3181c0d4f0
36. Georgiou E, Hadjibalassi M, Lambrinou E, Andreou P, Papathanassoglou ED. The impact of pain assessment on critically ill patients' outcomes: a systematic review. *Biomed Res Int.* (2015) 2015:503830. doi: 10.1155/2015/503830
37. Reade MC, Finfer S. Sedation and delirium in the intensive care unit. *N Engl J Med.* (2014) 370:444–54. doi: 10.1056/NEJMra1208705
38. Martínez-Plumed F, Gómez E, Hernández-Orallo J. Futures of artificial intelligence through technology readiness levels. *Telematics and Informatics.* (2021) 58:101525. doi: 10.1016/j.tele.2020.101525
39. Komorowski M. Artificial intelligence in intensive care: are we there yet? *Intensive Care Med.* (2019) 45:1298–300. doi: 10.1007/s00134-019-05662-6

21

# Machine Learning Prediction Model for Acute Renal Failure After Acute Aortic Syndrome Surgery

*Jinzhang Li*[1,2,3]*, Ming Gong*[2,3*]*, Yashutosh Joshi*[4]*, Lizhong Sun*[2]*, Lianjun Huang*[5]*, Ruixin Fan*[6]*, Tianxiang Gu*[7]*, Zonggang Zhang*[8]*, Chengwei Zou*[9]*, Guowei Zhang*[10]*, Ximing Qian*[11]*, Chenhui Qiao*[12]*, Yu Chen*[13]*, Wenjian Jiang*[2,3,4*] *and Hongjia Zhang*[1,2,3*]

[1] Department of Physiology and Pathophysiology, School of Basic Medical Sciences, Capital Medical University, Beijing, China, [2] Department of Cardiac Surgery, Beijing Anzhen Hospital, Capital Medical University, Beijing, China, [3] Beijing Lab for Cardiovascular Precision Medicine, Beijing, China, [4] Department of Cardiothoracic Surgery, St Vincent's Hospital, Sydney, NSW, Australia, [5] Department of Interference Diagnosis and Treatment, Beijing Anzhen Hospital, Capital Medical University, Beijing, China, [6] Department of Cardiovascular Surgery, Guangdong Provincial People's Hospital, Guangzhou, China, [7] Department of Cardiac Surgery, First Affiliated Hospital, China Medical University, Shenyang, China, [8] Department of Cardiac Surgery, People's Hospital of Xinjiang Uygur Autonomous Region, Urumqi, China, [9] Department of Cardiovascular Surgery, Shandong Provincial Hospital Affiliated With Shandong First Medical University, Jinan, China, [10] Department of Cardiovascular Surgery, The First Affiliated Hospital of Harbin Medical University, Harbin, China, [11] Department of Cardiac Surgery, School of Medicine, Sir Run Run Shaw Hospital, Zhejiang University, Hangzhou, China, [12] Department of Cardiovascular Surgery, The First Affiliated Hospital of Zhengzhou University, Zhengzhou, China, [13] Department of Cardiac Surgery, Peking University People's Hospital, Beijing, China

***Correspondence:**
*Hongjia Zhang*
*zhanghongjia722@ccmu.edu.cn*
*Wenjian Jiang*
*jiangwenjian@ccmu.edu.cn*
*Ming Gong*
*gongmaster@126.com*

**Background:** Acute renal failure (ARF) is the most common major complication following cardiac surgery for acute aortic syndrome (AAS) and worsens the postoperative prognosis. Our aim was to establish a machine learning prediction model for ARF occurrence in AAS patients.

**Methods:** We included AAS patient data from nine medical centers ($n$ = 1,637) and analyzed the incidence of ARF and the risk factors for postoperative ARF. We used data from six medical centers to compare the performance of four machine learning models and performed internal validation to identify AAS patients who developed postoperative ARF. The area under the curve (AUC) of the receiver operating characteristic (ROC) curve was used to compare the performance of the predictive models. We compared the performance of the optimal machine learning prediction model with that of traditional prediction models. Data from three medical centers were used for external validation.

**Results:** The eXtreme Gradient Boosting (XGBoost) algorithm performed best in the internal validation process (AUC = 0.82), which was better than both the logistic regression (LR) prediction model (AUC = 0.77, $p < 0.001$) and the traditional scoring systems. Upon external validation, the XGBoost prediction model (AUC =0.81) also performed better than both the LR prediction model (AUC = 0.75, $p = 0.03$) and the traditional scoring systems. We created an online application based on the XGBoost prediction model.

**Conclusions:** We have developed a machine learning model that has better predictive performance than traditional LR prediction models as well as other existing risk scoring systems for postoperative ARF. This model can be utilized to provide early warnings when high-risk patients are found, enabling clinicians to take prompt measures.

**Keywords: machine learning, acute renal failure, acute aortic syndrome, prediction model, eXtreme Gradient Boosting**

## INTRODUCTION

Acute aortic syndrome (AAS) is a serious and life-threatening disease process involving the ascending aorta and aortic arch. Traditionally, surgical intervention is the best way to treat AAS (1). Acute renal failure (ARF) is an important complication affecting the prognosis of AAS patients after surgery. This complication indicates that the patient has a poor prognosis, and it can increase postoperative mortality and morbidity (2). While renal replacement therapy (RRT) is a feasible treatment modality, it is arguably more important to identify the risk factors for postoperative ARF and identify potential patients with a higher likelihood of developing ARF in the postoperative setting. Some scoring systems already exist for predicting ARF after cardiac surgery (3–6), but they are usually employed for coronary artery bypass graft or heart valve surgery. Whether these scoring systems can be used in AAS-related surgery is unclear.

In recent years, machine learning has become increasingly widely used in medicine; it can help us process large amounts of data and find potential data relationships. Multiple excellent algorithms have been developed in the field of machine learning so that we can use them to build predictive models.

The main purpose of this study was to establish a predictive model for the occurrence of ARF in AAS patients after surgery through machine learning, thereby helping to identify potential patients who may develop ARF, and compare it with a traditional logistic regression (LR) prediction model and other scoring systems. This study followed the recommendations of the *Transparent Reporting of a Multivariable Prediction Model for Individual Prognosis or Diagnosis* statement (7).

## MATERIALS AND METHODS

### Participants

A total of 1,637 AAS patients undergoing surgery and treatment at nine medical centers in China from January 1, 2015, to December 31, 2019 were recruited for this study. The ethics committee of Beijing Anzhen Hospital approved this retrospective cohort study (No. 2018015; Date: 2018-10-18). Patients' written informed consent was waived due to the retrospective nature of the study. We collected demographic, surgical, and clinical data with a potential relationship to the renal function of patients from admission through discharge. Patients who had renal failure before surgery, incomplete surgical data, or surgery involving the abdominal aorta and below were excluded. All patients were diagnosed with Stanford type-A AAS through aortic computed tomography angiography (CTA) by experienced imaging specialists and cardiovascular surgeons. The diagnosis of ARF was established according to the Kidney Disease: Improving Global Outcomes guidelines (8). Postoperative ARF was defined as an increase of >3 times or an increase of >4.0 mg/dL (353.6 μmol/L) in postoperative serum creatinine (Scr) or the initiation of RRT compared to baseline. The estimated glomerular filtration rate (eGFR) was calculated using the Chronic Kidney Disease Epidemiology Collaboration formula (CKD-EPI) (9). Surgery was performed by the surgical team of the medical center at the time of the patient's admission.

### Surgical Details

Anesthesia was maintained by either total intravenous anesthetics (propofol and sufentanil) or an inhalational agent (sevoflurane) with vecuronium bromide. Tranexamic acid was used for coagulation support. Cardiopulmonary bypass (CPB) was routinely instituted at 2.2 to 2.5 L/min/m$^2$. When the lesion involved the aortic arch, arterial cannulation was performed in the right axillary and/or femoral artery and/or ascending aorta; venous cannulations were bicaval. Cold blood cardioplegia for myocardial protection was perfused through the left and right coronary arteries. If the distal aorta or aortic arch needed reconstruction, this process was performed under deep or moderate hypothermia and circulatory arrest. Once the distal reconstruction was complete, the aortic graft was clamped proximally. Selective anterograde perfusion was most often instituted through the innominate arteries. During core cooling, accompanying cardiac procedures, including aortic valve repair or replacement, sinus reconstruction, and root replacement, were performed if necessary. If the lesion involved only the ascending aorta, arterial cannulation was performed in the ascending aorta; venous cannulations were bicaval. Subsequently, reconstruction of the ascending aorta was performed.

### Data Pre-processing

For missing data, we used the k-nearest neighbors approach to fill in missing values (10). By calculating the Euclidean distance between each case, the missing value was imputed using the mean value from the five nearest neighbors. When the data were in the range of 0 to 1, most machine learning algorithms had excellent performance. To improve the performance of machine learning, we used the method provided by the MinMaxScaler function to scale the data during data pre-processing.

### Statistical Analysis

The description of the data and basic statistical analysis were performed using IBM SPSS Statistics for Windows Version 25.0. Continuous variables are expressed as the median (along with the first and third quartile values). Categorical variables are expressed as frequencies (n) with percentages (%). Statistical analysis of continuous variables was performed using the Mann–Whitney U test, while categorical variables were analyzed using the chi-squared test and Fisher's exact test. The area under the curve (AUC) of the receiver operating characteristic (ROC) curve was compared with the machine learning prediction model. DeLong's test (11) was used to calculate the P value. A $P <$ 0.05 was considered statistically significant, and all statistical tests were two-sided.

## Establishment of Prediction Model

We used Python for programming and used the scikit-learn 0.22.1 package to build machine learning classifiers (12). The concise process of establishing and evaluating the prediction model is shown in **Supplementary Figure 1**.

The machine learning prediction model used data from 1,637 patients from nine medical centers in China. Among them, 1,318 patient data points from six medical centers in Beijing, Zhejiang, Shandong, Liaoning and Henan provinces were used for machine learning training and internal validation. Training and validation data were divided by ten-fold cross-validation, each time 90% of the data was used as training data, and 10% of the data was used as validation data. And 319 patient data points from three medical centers in Heilongjiang and Guangdong provinces and Xinjiang Uygur Autonomous Region were used for external validation of the prediction model. The division of internal validation and external validation data was determined by the geographic location of the medical centers. The six medical centers used for machine learning training and internal validation were located in central China, and the three medical centers used for external validation were located in northern, southern and western China. This division method was suitable for evaluating the generalization ability of predictive models.

For the selection of machine learning algorithms, we chose the support vector machine classifier (SVC) linear kernel and Nu-SVC with the radial basis function kernel in the SVC algorithm. These are two classic algorithms that use the classifier with the largest interval in the feature space for classification, and can perform data classification after linear-range or high-dimensional mapping. It is still valid when the feature has a high-dimensional relationship. Among them, SVC uses a linear algorithm, while Nu-SVC uses a radial basis function. At the same time, we chose the AdaBoost algorithm (13) and the eXtreme Gradient Boosting (XGBoost) algorithm (14) in the ensemble methods, which are popular algorithms in machine learning classifiers and can combine the predictions of several base estimators so that they have excellent performance. AdaBoost integrates multiple basic decision trees, uses misclassified data points to identify problems, and improves the model by adjusting the weights of misclassified data points. XGBoost uses negative gradients to identify problems, and calculates negative gradients to improve the model. In addition, we also tested the combination of two algorithms. This combination uses two independent algorithms to build prediction models separately, and uses the results of the two prediction models as features to retrain the new prediction model, which is also called a stacking algorithm. We tested the combination of XGBoost + random forest algorithm and XGBoost + decision tree algorithm.

## Feature Selection

To make the prediction model more accurate, we selected all demographic characteristics and preoperative clinical data as the features for machine learning. At the beginning of model training, all 134 features were used (**Supplementary Table 3**), and Shapley additive explanations (SHAP) was used to judge the importance of each feature. In the machine learning prediction model, SHAP can analyse the impact of each feature of each patient on the prediction result (15). Finally, the features that were considered important in all prediction models were used as the final features of the machine learning model.

## Ten-Fold Cross-Validation

Ten-fold cross-validation is considered a reliable method for model evaluation and performance improvement (16), and it was used for parameter adjustment and algorithm comparison. Since machine learning algorithms usually cannot use training data as test data, 10-fold cross-validation is generally used to evaluate machine learning algorithms. Ten-fold cross-validation can divide the data into 10 parts. The classifier used nine of them for training, and the remaining part was used for testing. Ten repetitions constituted a 10-fold cross-validation (**Supplementary Figure 2**). The average of 10 test results was used to evaluate the predictive ability of machine learning algorithms and parameters.

Each classifier algorithm had many parameter settings, and the choice of parameters had a great impact on the results of the classifier. We used the grid-search algorithm and internal validation data to determine the best parameters for each classifier algorithm.

The grid-search algorithm used 10-fold cross-validation to select the parameters of the machine learning algorithm. We told the grid search algorithm the potential optimal parameter range of the classifier, and the grid search algorithm used 10-fold cross validation to calculate the predictive ability of each set of parameters. After the grid-search algorithm calculated each set of parameter combinations, it told us the optimal parameter combination. After constantly changing the parameter range used by the grid search algorithm, the optimal parameter combination of this machine learning algorithm was finally obtained.

Similarly, 10-fold cross-validation was used to compare classifier algorithms. The ROC curve and AUC were calculated at each validation, and the mean and standard deviation of each AUC were compared to obtain the optimal classifier algorithm.

## Evaluation of Predictive Models

To compare the machine learning prediction model with the traditional prediction model, we used multivariable LR analysis to establish an LR prediction model with ARF as the end point. In addition, the Cleveland scoring system (3), the simplified renal index (SRI) scoring system (5) and the Leicester scoring system (6) were selected as representatives of the traditional prediction model. The endpoints of these three classic scoring systems were renal failure and RRT, and they were also scored for complex surgery. To evaluate the prediction model, we compared the machine learning prediction model with the four traditional prediction models. The ROC curve and AUC of the prediction model were calculated using internal validation data. The machine learning prediction model used 10-fold cross-validation to calculate the mean ROC curve and the AUC. In the external validation, the machine learning predictive model was trained using internal validation data. Then, we used the parametric approach based on Platt's logistic model to calibrate the probability of the machine learning model (17) and evaluated the discrimination and calibration of the model by calculating the Brier score. The trained machine learning prediction model was compared with the traditional prediction models using external validation data to evaluate the generalization ability of the prediction model.

## RESULTS

### Patient Characteristics

A total of 1,637 patients were enrolled in the study, with 1,318 of these cases being used for machine learning training and internal validation. The main characteristics of patients in the internal validation group are presented in **Table 1**. The median age of the patients was 50.0 (42.0–57.0) years; 301 (22.8%) patients were female.

### Incidence and Prognosis of Postoperative ARF

The incidence of ARF after aortic surgery was 11.5% (151 in 1,318). The prognostic characteristics of the patients are presented in **Supplementary Table 1**. Patients with postoperative ARF had a poor prognosis and had longer ICU stays (204.0 (104.5–308.2) h vs. 43.0 (20.0–112.5) h, $P < 0.001$) as well as longer ventilator use times (114.0 (62.0–179.0) h vs. 20.0 (15.0–48.0) h, $P < 0.001$). Postoperative ARF may be related to the use of more blood products and drug infusions. Furthermore, patients with postoperative ARF had more postoperative complications (74.8 vs. 34.5%, $P < 0.001$). Most importantly, there were significant differences in mortality between patients with and without ARF (12.6 vs. 0.8%, respectively, $P < 0.001$).

### Risk Factors for Postoperative ARF

As a comparison with machine learning models, we used traditional statistical methods to analyse all preoperative and intraoperative factors that either had significant differences or were clinically believed to be related to ARF and calculated the risk factors for postoperative ARF. A multivariable binary LR with the "Forward: LR" method was conducted to determine the risk factors for postoperative ARF (**Table 2**). The results showed that, among the preoperative factors, older age, a higher pulse rate, emergency surgery, and an increased absolute value of leukocytes in the preoperative setting were all risk factors. It was also noted that an increased estimated glomerular filtration rate (eGFR) and platelet count were protective factors against postoperative ARF. In the combined analysis of preoperative and intraoperative factors, in addition to the aforementioned preoperative factors, longer cardiopulmonary bypass time, lower rectal temperature when circulatory arrest, and surgery with circulatory arrest were risk factors for postoperative ARF. We used preoperative factors to establish an LR prediction model for the predictive model to have the ability to predict postoperative ARF of patients before surgery (**Table 2**).

## Machine Learning Prediction Model

### Feature Selection

In the initial stage, we built machine learning models using all the preoperative features and unoptimized parameters. We analyzed the feature importance of these machine learning models through SHAP (15) and finally selected 15 features for building machine learning prediction models (**Table 3**).

Among the 15 features used to establish these models, we collected complete demographic and renal function data. However, as AAS patients may require emergency surgery, occasionally, the blood test results were partially missing. We used the k-nearest neighbors approach to fill in missing values. **Supplementary Table 2** shows the details of missing values.

### Internal Validation

Machine learning models were trained using internal validation data, and the performance of the machine learning models was evaluated using 10-fold cross-validation. The results showed the mean ROC curve and AUC of each machine learning model after 10-fold cross-validation (**Figure 1**). We found that among the prediction models established by a single algorithm, the XGBoost machine learning model performed best (AUC = 0.82, 95% confidence interval (CI): 0.79–0.85), and the combination of XGBoost and other algorithms did not improve performance (**Supplementary Figure 3**); thus, we chose the XGBoost model as the final machine learning model to evaluate its performance. This model had 750 gradient boosted trees, the maximum tree depth was eight, the learning rate was 0.01, the subsample ratio of columns when constructing each tree was 0.75, and the subsample ratio of the training instance was 0.68.

Subsequently, the importance of each feature of the XGBoost model was analyzed by the SHAP method. **Figure 2** shows the results of the feature importance analysis, with more important features distributed on the top and relatively unimportant features on the bottom. Most of the characteristics, either positively or negatively, correlated with the prediction results; however, activated partial thromboplastin time (APTT), fasting blood glucose, body mass index (BMI), international normalized ratio (INR), and alanine aminotransferase (ALT) that were either too high or too low increased the risk of ARF. At the same time, we also analyzed the feature importance based on the fitted trees of the XGBoost model (**Supplementary Figure 4**), and the result is similar to the result of SHAP.

We used internal validation data to calculate the ROC curve and the AUC of the four traditional prediction models (**Figure 3**) and found that the XGBoost model (AUC = 0.82, 95% CI: 0.79–0.85) performed better than the LR prediction model (AUC = 0.77, 95% CI: 0.73–0.81, P<0.001), the Cleveland scoring system (AUC = 0.73, 95% CI: 0.69–0.77, P<0.001), the SRI scoring system (AUC = 0.72, 95% CI: 0.68–0.76, P<0.001), and the

**TABLE 1** | Main characteristics of patients in the internal validation groups.

| | Overall | Without ARF | Combined ARF | *P* value |
|---|---|---|---|---|
| Number of patients (cases) | 1,318 | 1,167 | 151 | |
| Gender, female (cases) | 301 (22.8%) | 269 (23.1%) | 32 (21.2%) | 0.61 |
| Age (years) | 50.0 (42.0–57.0) | 49.0 (41.0–57.0) | 53.0 (46.0–60.0) | < 0.001 |
| **Information on admission** | | | | |
| Pulse (beats/min) | 80.0 (75.0–85.0) | 80.0 (75.0–85.0) | 80.0 (77.0–88.0) | 0.003 |
| Height (cm) | 170.0 (166.0–175.0) | 170.0 (166.0–175.0) | 170.0 (165.0–175.0) | 0.06 |
| Weight (kg) | 75.0 (65.0–82.4) | 75.0 (65.0–83.0) | 73.2 (65.0–80.0) | 0.62 |
| Body mass index (kg/m$^2$) | 25.4 (22.9–27.8) | 25.4 (22.9–27.8) | 25.4 (23.4–28.0) | 0.35 |
| Systolic pressure (mmHg) | 130.0 (120.0–142.0) | 130.0 (120.0–143.0) | 129.0 (110.0–140.0) | 0.009 |
| Diastolic pressure (mmHg) | 78.0 (70.0–84.1) | 78.0 (70.0–85.0) | 78.0 (70.0–82.0) | 0.10 |
| **Medical history** | | | | |
| Smoking history (cases) | 507 (38.5%) | 449 (38.5%) | 58 (38.4%) | 0.99 |
| History of previous cardiac surgery (cases) | 107 (8.1%) | 98 (8.4%) | 9 (6.0%) | 0.30 |
| Peripheral vascular disease history (cases) | 9 (0.7%) | 9 (0.8%) | 0 (0.0%) | 0.61 |
| **Echocardiographic results** | | | | |
| Left ventricular ejection fraction (%) | 63.0 (60.0–66.0) | 63.0 (60.0–66.0) | 62.0 (58.0–65.0) | 0.21 |
| **Preoperative laboratory examination results** | | | | |
| Absolute value of leukocytes (10$^9$/L) | 9.69 (7.00–13.18) | 9.30 (6.80–12.90) | 12.33 (10.29–15.33) | < 0.001 |
| Platelets (10$^9$/L) | 185.0 (147.0–228.3) | 189.0 (150.0–231.0) | 158.0 (126.0–201.0) | < 0.001 |
| Hemoglobin (g/L) | 137.0 (122.0–148.0) | 137.0 (123.0–148.0) | 136.0 (121.0–144.0) | 0.12 |
| CK–MB (ng/mL) | 1.88 (0.90–9.30) | 1.70 (0.80–8.20) | 7.10 (1.60–15.00) | < 0.001 |
| Lactate dehydrogenase (U/L) | 221.5 (179.0–288.3) | 214.0 (176.0–279.0) | 277.0 (225.0–332.2) | < 0.001 |
| D–dimer (ng/mL) | 1,100.0 (270.8–3,269.3) | 940.0 (231.0–2,887.0) | 3,328.0 (1,120.0–14,485.0) | < 0.001 |
| INR | 31.9 (28.9–36.5) | 31.9 (28.8–36.3) | 32.2 (29.5–37.8) | 0.02 |
| APTT (s) | 48.8 (39.6–60.1) | 48.6 (39.5–60.0) | 51.4 (40.5–65.1) | 0.03 |
| Blood amylase (U/dL) | 21.0 (15.0–34.0) | 21.0 (15.0–33.0) | 27.0 (16.0–45.0) | 0.07 |
| ALT (U/mL) | 22.0 (18.0–32.0) | 22.0 (17.0–30.0) | 29.0 (21.0–46.0) | 0.005 |
| AST (U/mL) | 39.1 (35.6–42.1) | 39.2 (35.6–42.2) | 38.9 (35.2–40.7) | < 0.001 |
| Albumin (g/mL) | 78.3 (64.6–99.6) | 76.7 (63.9–95.8) | 99.7 (78.0–138.6) | 0.08 |
| Creatinine (μmol/L) | 6.30 (4.99–8.10) | 6.10 (4.90–7.78) | 8.20 (6.01–10.30) | < 0.001 |
| BUN (mmol/mL) | 95.0 (73.1–107.1) | 97.1 (77.0–108.4) | 69.1 (49.0–93.4) | < 0.001 |
| eGFR (ml/min/1.73 m$^2$) | 6.49 (5.39–7.77) | 6.38 (5.30–7.67) | 7.26 (6.28–8.48) | < 0.001 |
| Fasting blood glucose (mmol/L) | 9.69 (7.00–13.18) | 9.30 (6.80–12.90) | 12.33 (10.29–15.33) | < 0.001 |
| **Diagnosis** | | | | |
| Coronary artery disease (cases) | 35 (2.7%) | 33 (2.8%) | 2 (1.3%) | 0.42 |
| Congestive heart failure (cases) | 26 (2.0%) | 23 (2.0%) | 3 (2.0%) | 1.00 |
| Chronic respiratory disease (cases) | 31 (2.4%) | 28 (2.4%) | 3 (2.0%) | 1.00 |
| Hypertension (cases) | 905 (68.7%) | 786 (67.4%) | 119 (78.8%) | 0.004 |
| Diabetes (cases) | 62 (4.7%) | 54 (4.6%) | 8 (5.3%) | 0.71 |
| **Surgery** | | | | |
| Operative duration (min) | 405.0 (340.0–479.0) | 396.0 (330.0–465.0) | 454.6 (390.0–520.0) | < 0.001 |
| Emergency surgery (cases) | 650 (49.3%) | 536 (45.9%) | 114 (75.5%) | < 0.001 |
| Cardiopulmonary bypass time (min) | 186.0 (144.0–224.0) | 181.0 (140.0–218.0) | 224.0 (188.0–266.0) | < 0.001 |
| Aortic cross–clamp time (min) | 104.0 (82.6–131.0) | 102.0 (80.0–127.0) | 125.0 (103.0–149.0) | < 0.001 |
| With circulatory arrest (cases) | 997 (75.6%) | 855 (73.3%) | 142 (94.0%) | < 0.001 |
| Circulatory arrest time (min) | 21.0 (17.4–27.0) | 21.0 (17.6–26.6) | 21.0 (17.0–27.0) | 0.88 |
| Nasopharyngeal temperature when circulatory arrest (°C) | 24.1 (23.1–24.9) | 24.1 (23.2–24.9) | 23.5 (22.5–24.5) | < 0.001 |
| Rectal temperature when circulatory arrest (°C) | 25.6 (24.8–26.7) | 25.8 (24.9–26.8) | 25.0 (24.0–26.0) | < 0.001 |
| RBC transfusion volume (U) | 4.00 (0.00–6.00) | 3.50 (0.00–6.00) | 5.50 (4.00–8.00) | < 0.001 |

*INR, international normalized ratio; APTT, activated partial thromboplastin time; ALT, alanine aminotransferase; AST, aspartate transaminase; BUN, blood urea nitrogen; eGFR, estimated glomerular filtration rate.*

**TABLE 2** | Multivariable binary logistic regression results.

| Characteristics | B | Standard error | *P* value | OR value | OR 95%CI |
|---|---|---|---|---|---|
| **Preoperative factors only** | | | | | |
| Age (years) | 0.028 | 0.010 | 0.003 | 1.029 | 1.010–1.048 |
| Absolute value of leukocyte | 0.076 | 0.022 | 0.001 | 1.079 | 1.033–1.127 |
| Pulse (beats/min) | 0.021 | 0.008 | 0.006 | 1.021 | 1.006–1.037 |
| eGFR (ml/min/1.73m$^2$) | −0.019 | 0.004 | < 0.001 | 0.982 | 0.974–0.989 |
| Platelet ($10^9$/L) | −0.005 | 0.002 | 0.003 | 0.995 | 0.992–0.998 |
| Emergency surgery | 0.779 | 0.216 | < 0.001 | 2.179 | 1.426–3.331 |
| Constant | −4.207 | 1.057 | < 0.001 | 0.015 | |
| **Preoperative and intraoperative factors** | | | | | |
| Age (years) | 0.032 | 0.010 | 0.001 | 1.032 | 1.012–1.052 |
| Absolute value of leukocyte | 0.062 | 0.023 | 0.008 | 1.064 | 1.017–1.114 |
| Pulse (beats/min) | 0.023 | 0.008 | 0.004 | 1.023 | 1.007–1.039 |
| eGFR (ml/min/1.73m$^2$) | −0.017 | 0.004 | < 0.001 | 0.983 | 0.976–0.991 |
| Platelet ($10^9$/L) | −0.004 | 0.002 | 0.011 | 0.996 | 0.993–0.999 |
| Emergency surgery | 0.587 | 0.222 | 0.008 | 1.799 | 1.164–2.781 |
| Cardiopulmonary bypass time (min) | 0.006 | 0.002 | < 0.001 | 1.006 | 1.003–1.010 |
| Surgery with circulatory arrest | 0.875 | 0.379 | 0.021 | 2.400 | 1.142–5.042 |
| Rectal temperature when circulatory arrest (°C) | −0.129 | 0.054 | 0.017 | 0.879 | 0.792–0.977 |
| Constant | −3.315 | 1.842 | 0.072 | 0.036 | |

*eGFR, Estimated Glomerular Filtration Rate.*

**TABLE 3** | Features used to build machine learning prediction model.

| |
|---|
| **Information on admission** |
| Age (years) |
| Pulse (beats/min) |
| BMI (kg/m$^2$) |
| Diastolic pressure (mmHg) |
| **Echocardiographic results** |
| Left ventricular ejection fraction (%) |
| **Preoperative laboratory examination results** |
| Absolute value of leukocytes ($10^9$/L) |
| Platelets ($10^9$/L) |
| D-dimer (ng/mL) |
| INR |
| APTT (s) |
| ALT (U/mL) |
| Albumin (g/mL) |
| eGFR (ml/min/1.73 m$^2$) |
| Fasting blood glucose (mmol/L) |
| **Surgery** |
| Emergency surgery |

*BMI, body mass index; INR, international normalized ratio; APTT, activated partial thromboplastin time; ALT, alanine aminotransferase; eGFR, estimated glomerular filtration rate.*

Leicester scoring system (AUC = 0.72, 95% CI: 0.68–0.77, $P <$ 0.001) (**Table 4**).

### External Validation

The external validation group included 319 patients. The comparison of the internal and external validation group characteristics is presented in **Table 5**. The median of the average age of patients in the external validation group was 50.0 (16.0) years. The incidence of ARF after aortic surgery was similar to that in the internal validation group (11.0 vs. 11.5%, $P = 0.807$).

After probability calibration, the Brier score of the machine learning prediction model using the external validation data was 0.087, which showed that the prediction model had good discrimination and calibration. Using external validation data for evaluation, we found that the XGBoost model after probability calibration (AUC = 0.81, 95% CI: 0.75–0.88) performed better than the LR prediction model (AUC = 0.75, 95% CI: 0.67–0.83, $P = 0.03$), the Cleveland scoring system (AUC = 0.71, 95% CI: 0.63–0.80, $P = 0.04$), the SRI scoring system (AUC = 0.70, 95% CI: 0.61–0.79, $P = 0.02$), and the Leicester scoring system (AUC = 0.67, 95% CI: 0.59–0.75, $P = 0.002$) (**Table 4**).

Finally, to make the XGBoost prediction model easy to use, we developed an application (https://ljzyal.github.io/ARF/) for clinical use. The application used a probability-calibrated XGBoost prediction model, which had the same performance as the prediction model in external validation. We set the cut-off value based on the results of external validation. The prediction model had a sensitivity of 82.9% and a specificity of 67.6%. The risk calculated by the application increased with the possibility of postoperative ARF.

# DISCUSSION

## Factors Influencing Postoperative ARF and the Role of a Prediction Model

ARF is the end stage of acute kidney injury, and it is the most common major complication following cardiac surgery (18).

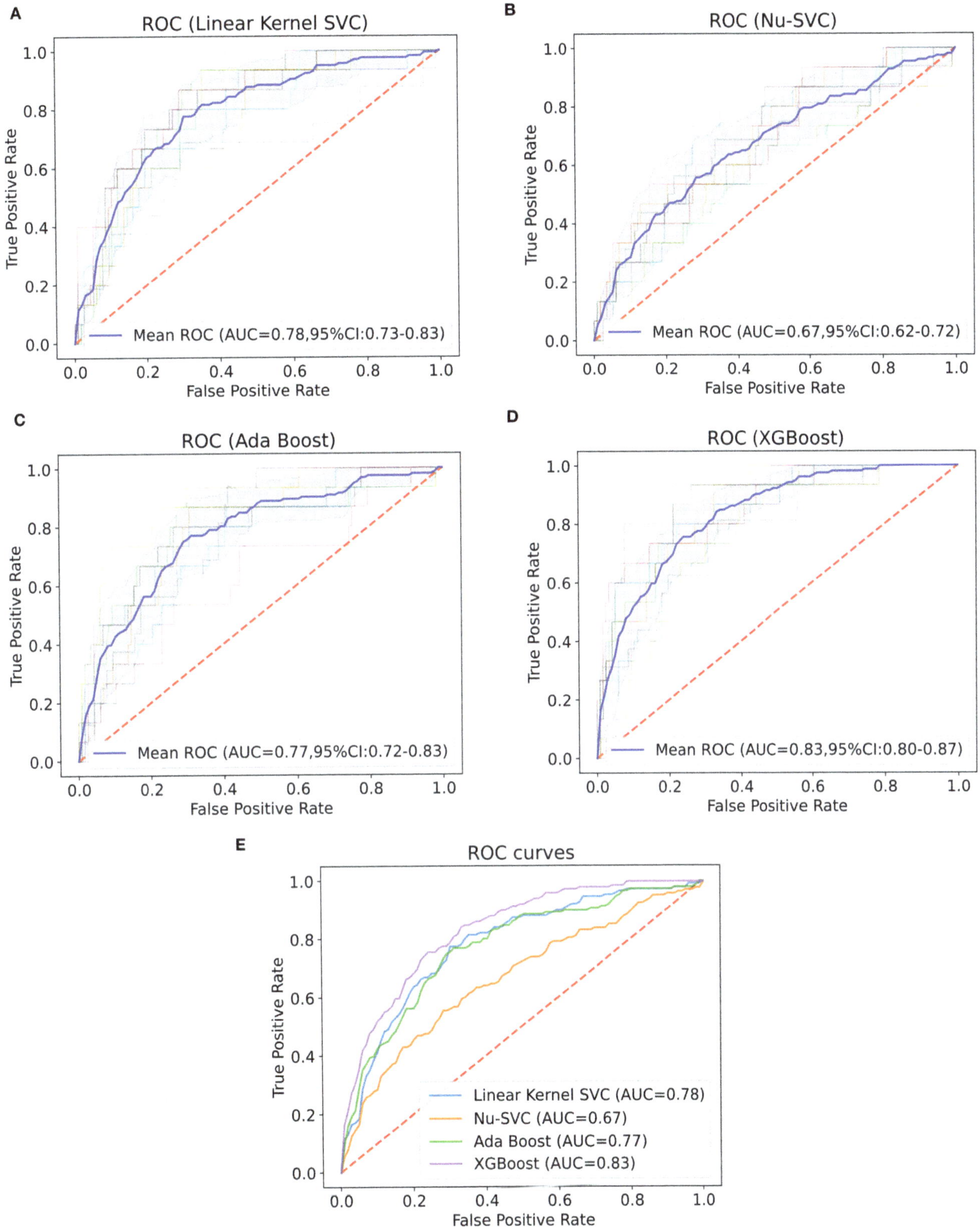


**FIGURE 1** | Mean ROC curve and AUC of machine learning models. This figure depicts the mean ROC curve and AUC of the linear kernel SVC **(A)**, Nu-SVC **(B)**, AdaBoost **(C)** and XGBoost **(D)** using internal validation data (*n* = 1,318). The blue line represents the mean of each ROC curve after 10-fold cross-validation. The shaded area is the 95% confidence interval of the mean ROC curve. The other translucent lines are ROC curves for each cross-validation. **(E)** Comparison of the mean ROC curves for each algorithm.

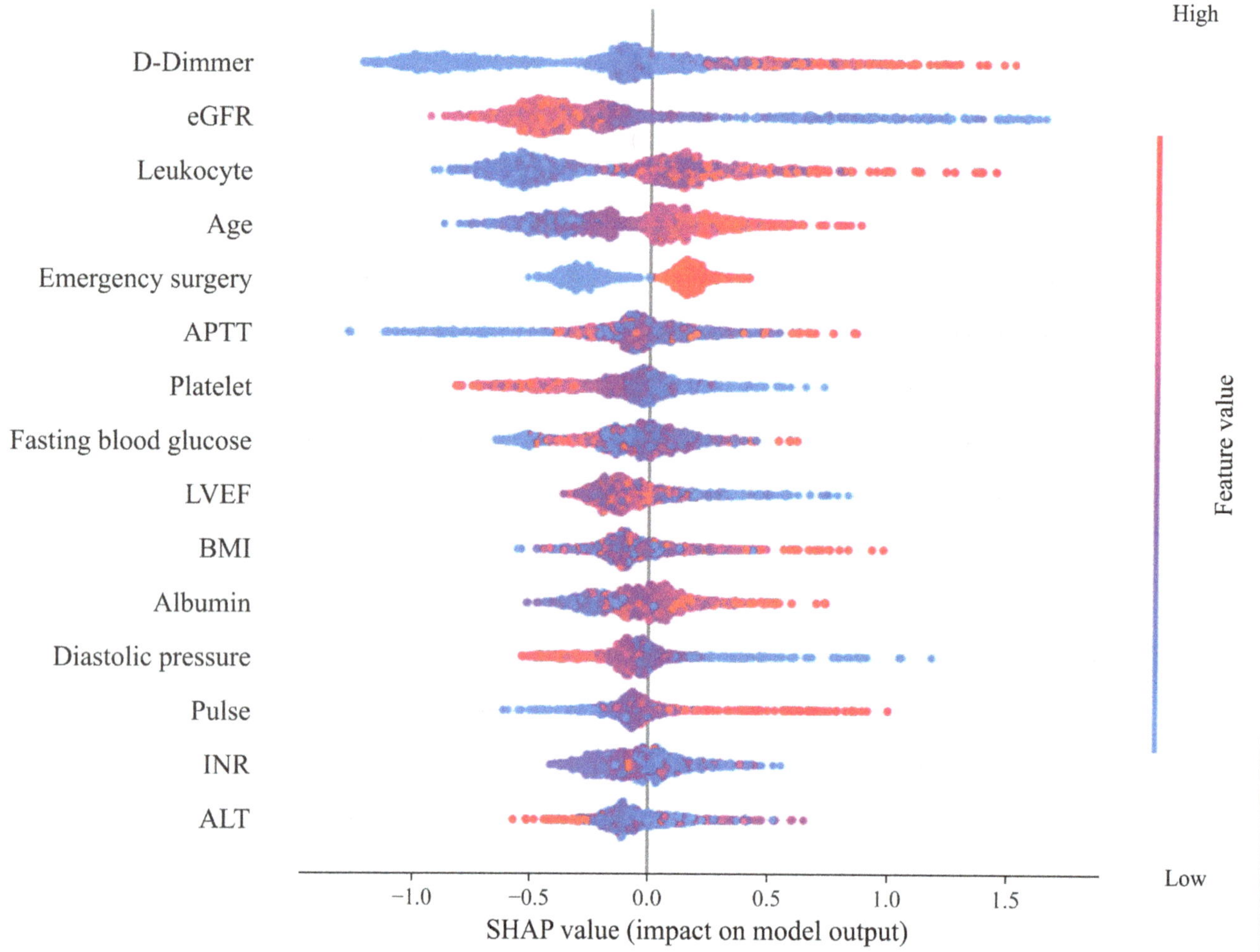


**FIGURE 2 |** Feature importance analysis. This figure shows the results of the analysis on the importance of the features in the XGBoost model through the SHAP method. Each feature value of each patient is marked as a dot on the graph. The color of the dot represents the degree of deviation of the feature value from the overall value according to the ordinate, and purple represents that the feature of the patient is close to the mean of the feature of the overall patient value. The SHAP value of the dot indicates the influence of the feature on the prediction result. A negative SHAP value indicates that the patient's risk of ARF is reduced, while a positive SHAP value indicates that the patient's risk of ARF is increased.

ARF can lead to poor patient prognosis and is independently associated with increased morbidity and mortality after cardiac surgery (19). In this study, the incidence of postoperative ARF in AAS patients reached 11.5%, and patients with ARF had a longer ICU length of stay, longer ventilator use time and a worse prognosis.

The mechanism of ARF after cardiac surgery remains to be elucidated, and its pathogenesis is currently thought to be related to renal hypoperfusion, tissue ischaemia-reperfusion injury and the inflammatory response (20). Previous studies have shown that risk factors for ARF include female sex, advanced age, previous heart surgery, chronic obstructive pulmonary disease, diabetes, complex heart surgery, prolonged cardiopulmonary bypass, rapid heart rate, emergency surgery, and intraoperative infusion of 2 or more packed red blood cell (RBC) units (21–23). In this study, we found that patients with AAS have more complex risk factors for postoperative ARF. In addition to the above factors, we found that postoperative ARF was also related to preoperative leukocyte and platelet counts, which may be because the occurrence of ARF is related to the inflammatory response (20). The higher preoperative leukocyte count may indicate that the inflammatory response caused by AAS is more serious. This effect may continue to play a role after surgery, making postoperative ARF more likely to occur. Furthermore, abnormal blood coagulation is another potential mechanism of ARF (24). Lower preoperative platelets may be a manifestation of a hypercoagulable state and intravascular coagulation, which makes AAS patients with higher preoperative platelet counts less prone to postoperative ARF.

Early identification of patients with a higher ARF risk can help clinicians strengthen patient monitoring and take measures to prevent ARF. Many studies have used risk factors or novel

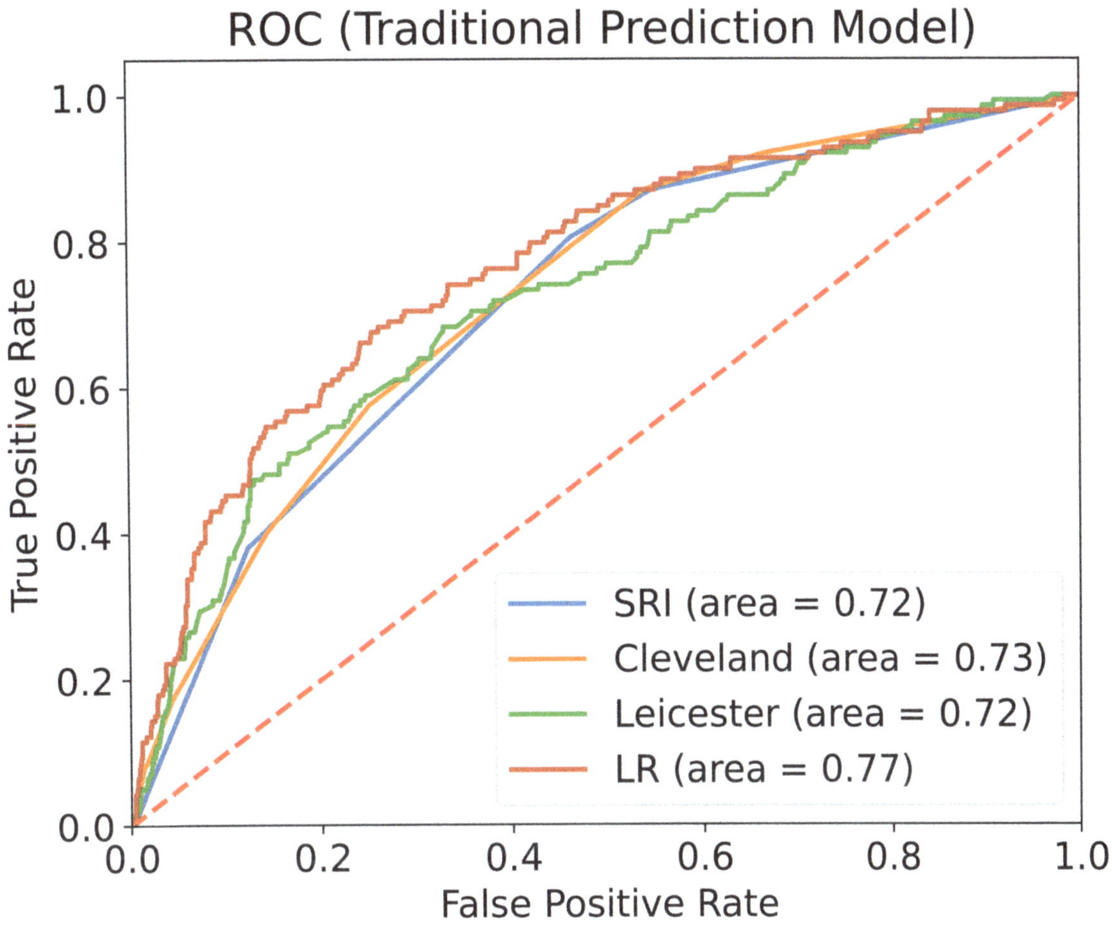


**FIGURE 3 |** ROC curve and AUC of the traditional prediction models with internal validation data. This figure describes the ROC curve and the AUC of the Cleveland scoring system, the SRI scoring system, the Leicester scoring system and the LR prediction model with internal validation data ($n = 1{,}318$).

biomarkers to build prediction models for ARF (3–6, 25). Novel biomarker-related prediction methods, however, are usually cumbersome, and no new biomarker has been widely accepted (25). Currently, the best-performing large-sample model is poor at predicting ARF after complex surgery (6). Aortic surgery usually results in a higher incidence of postoperative ARF; therefore, postoperative ARF prediction methods for complex heart and aortic surgeries are necessary.

## Clinical Applications and Strategies

According to the results of this study, we recommend the following measures to reduce the occurrence of ARF. Once the model is used to predict the postoperative risk of ARF, for those with a low predicted risk, it is recommended to perform surgery in a timely fashion once the patient is surgically prepared.

For patients with a higher predicted risk of ARF, it is recommended to attempt to ameliorate the modifiable risk factors that are included in the prediction model. This could be achieved by improving preoperative preparations, such as administering antimicrobials, considering platelet transfusion, controlling blood glucose levels, maintaining adequate diastolic blood pressure, and controlling heart rate. In addition, during the operation, it is recommended to pay more attention to renal function and to maintain renal perfusion by taking measures to maintain circulatory stability. In addition to the aforementioned modifications, intraoperative innovations in surgical methods should be adopted, which can help reduce the operative and CPB time.

Additionally, for patients noted to be at a higher risk of ARF, it is also recommended to use stricter monitoring and more favorable preventive and treatment measures in perioperative management, which could include minimizing the use of nephrotoxic drugs and administering treatment for renal injury as soon as possible to prevent patients from progressing to ARF.

## Features of Machine Learning Prediction Models

Risk prediction plays an important role in cardiovascular disease research. As the most commonly used traditional predictive model, LR sometimes cannot handle complex clinical data

**TABLE 4 |** Performance of machine learning prediction model and scoring system.

| | Prediction methods | AUC | 95% CI of AUC | *P value* |
|---|---|---|---|---|
| Internal validation | | | | |
| | Machine learning prediction model (XGBoost) | 0.82 | 0.79–0.85 | |
| | LR prediction model | 0.77 | 0.73–0.81 | < 0.001 |
| | Cleveland scoring system | 0.73 | 0.69–0.77 | < 0.001 |
| | SRI scoring system | 0.72 | 0.68–0.76 | < 0.001 |
| | Leicester scoring system | 0.72 | 0.68–0.77 | < 0.001 |
| External validation | | | | |
| | Machine learning prediction model (XGBoost) | 0.81 | 0.75–0.88 | |
| | LR prediction model | 0.75 | 0.67–0.83 | 0.03 |
| | Cleveland scoring system | 0.71 | 0.63–0.80 | 0.04 |
| | SRI scoring system | 0.70 | 0.61–0.79 | 0.02 |
| | Leicester scoring system | 0.67 | 0.59–0.75 | 0.002 |

*AUC, area under the receiver operating characteristic (ROC) curve; XGBoost, eXtreme Gradient Boosting; LR, logistic regression; SRI, simplified renal index.*
*The AUC of the ROC curve was compared with a machine learning prediction model (XGBoost), and DeLong's test was used to calculate the P value.*

and thus cannot obtain an ideal predictive model. Conversely, machine learning can handle complex clinical data and thus potentially has more advantages (26). In this study, by selecting AAS as a disease process for focused research, we found that the performance of machine learning predictive models is better than that of traditional predictive models. This suggests that machine learning algorithms are more suitable for building clinical prediction models and have a higher performance than LR.

In this study, we found that the XGBoost algorithm has the best prediction performance and still has excellent performance in external validation. XGBoost is a machine learning algorithm that uses classification and regression trees as weak classifiers (14). Compared with other algorithms, the XGBoost algorithm allows easy adjustment of parameters and can deal with nonlinear features. It usually has higher sensitivity and specificity when overfitting is avoided. In most cases, XGBoost has higher prediction performance than other algorithms (27, 28).

Machine learning algorithms are also suitable for the construction of other predictive models, which have excellent performance and can be continuously trained with new data to have greater potential. After the prediction model is established, the newly collected data can be used to continue training, thereby enhancing the generalization ability of the prediction model.

Machine learning algorithms have been considered a black box in the past, which is the main disadvantage compared to LR. However, the SHAP method can explain the machine learning prediction model. We used the SHAP method to analyse the importance of particular features in the prediction model. This method can analyse the impact of each variable on each patient so the prediction model is interpretable. We found that the SHAP method is effective in determining the importance of particular individual features.

To compare with LR, all features included in an LR are also considered important features in machine learning prediction models. Concurrently, however, the SHAP method also judges other features, those that are not considered statistically significant in the LR, as important features. This possibly results in LR not including certain relevant features, whereas the SHAP method does not exclude such features. According to the results of the feature importance analysis, we can also judge the impact of each variable on the results to determine the patient's treatment direction to prevent postoperative ARF.

## Limitations

First, all data for this study were sourced from China. Due to ethnic differences, the performance of our predictive model in other countries may decrease. However, our research method is innovative, and it is feasible to establish such a model in other countries through this investigational method. Second, machine learning algorithms are more complex than LR, and model representation is also very complicated (29). Our predictive model cannot be similar to LR, and it does not provide a scoring system for clinicians. We have therefore developed an online application for convenience. Third, our machine learning prediction model needs more extensive data for verification. Finally, although the performance of our prediction model was better than that of LR, some data were not involved in the initial data collection, such as detailed laboratory test results, detailed medical history and detailed documentation of the use of nephrotoxic drugs. Supervised machine learning can improve the model after supplementing these data, and consequently, our predictive model has the potential to improve.

In summary, our findings suggest that machine learning prediction models can provide better prediction performance than traditional LR prediction models and other existing risk scoring systems for AAS and complex cardiac and aortic surgeries. This predictive model is helpful for the early detection of patients with high ARF risk, thus enabling clinicians to take early measures to prevent and treat ARF.

**TABLE 5 |** Comparison of characteristics in the internal and external validation groups.

| | Internal validation group | External validation group | *P* value |
|---|---|---|---|
| Number of patients (cases) | 1,318 | 319 | |
| Incidence of postoperative ARF | 151 (11.5%) | 35 (11.0%) | 0.81 |
| Need CRRT treatment (cases) | 137 (90.7%) | 30 (85.7%) | 0.36 |
| **Information on admission** | | | |
| Gender, female (cases) | 301 (22.8%) | 65 (20.4%) | 0.34 |
| Age (years) | 50.0 (42.0–57.0) | 50.0 (43.0–59.0) | 0.10 |
| Pulse (beats/min) | 80.0 (75.0–85.0) | 80.0 (74.0–85.0) | 0.62 |
| Height (cm) | 170.0 (166.0–175.0) | 170.0 (165.0–175.0) | 0.59 |
| Weight (kg) | 75.0 (65.0–82.4) | 74.0 (65.0–83.0) | 0.42 |
| Body mass index (kg/m$^2$) | 25.4 (22.9–27.8) | 25.4 (23.1–27.8) | 0.71 |
| Systolic pressure (mmHg) | 130.0 (120.0–142.0) | 135.0 (120.0–160.0) | < 0.001 |
| Diastolic pressure (mmHg) | 78.0 (70.0–84.1) | 80.0 (70.0–95.0) | < 0.001 |
| **Medical history** | | | |
| Smoking history (cases) | 507 (38.5%) | 96 (30.1%) | 0.005 |
| History of previous cardiac surgery (cases) | 107 (8.1%) | 20 (6.3%) | 0.27 |
| Peripheral vascular disease history (cases) | 9 (0.7%) | 3 (0.9%) | 0.71 |
| **Echocardiographic results** | | | |
| Left ventricular ejection fraction (%) | 63.0 (60.0–66.0) | 61.0 (57.0–66.0) | 0.02 |
| **Preoperative laboratory examination results** | | | |
| Absolute value of leukocytes (10$^9$/L) | 9.69 (7.00–13.18) | 11.08 (7.78–14.29) | < 0.001 |
| Platelets (10$^9$/L) | 185.0 (147.0–228.3) | 184.0 (143.0–236.0) | 0.93 |
| Hemoglobin (g/L) | 137.0 (122.0–148.0) | 134.0 (122.0–147.0) | 0.19 |
| CK-MB (ng/mL) | 1.88 (0.90–9.30) | 3.30 (1.00–11.60) | < 0.001 |
| Lactate dehydrogenase (U/L) | 221.5 (179.0–288.3) | 224.0 (189.0–277.4) | 0.32 |
| D-dimer (ng/mL) | 1,100.0 (270.8–3,269.3) | 715.9 (18.4–4,230.0) | < 0.001 |
| INR | 31.9 (28.9–36.5) | 34.0 (29.1–39.7) | 0.39 |
| APTT (s) | 48.8 (39.6–60.1) | 50.4 (43.0–58.4) | < 0.001 |
| Blood amylase (U/dL) | 21.0 (15.0–34.0) | 23.0 (15.0–36.0) | 0.14 |
| ALT (U/mL) | 22.0 (18.0–32.0) | 22.0 (18.0–33.0) | 0.14 |
| AST (U/mL) | 39.1 (35.6–42.1) | 38.5 (35.0–42.0) | 0.56 |
| Albumin (g/mL) | 78.3 (64.6–99.6) | 80.4 (66.8–101.6) | 0.12 |
| Creatinine (μmol/L) | 6.30 (4.99–8.10) | 6.40 (5.10–8.70) | 0.48 |
| BUN (mmol/mL) | 95.0 (73.1–107.1) | 92.3 (70.4–107.3) | 0.05 |
| eGFR (ml/min/1.73 m$^2$) | 6.49 (5.39–7.77) | 6.63 (5.40–7.65) | 0.22 |
| Fasting blood glucose (mmol/L) | 9.69 (7.00–13.18) | 11.08 (7.78–14.29) | 0.94 |
| **Diagnosis** | | | |
| Coronary artery disease (cases) | 35 (2.7%) | 6 (1.9%) | 0.43 |
| Congestive heart failure (cases) | 26 (2.0%) | 1 (0.3%) | 0.04 |
| Chronic respiratory disease (cases) | 31 (2.4%) | 15 (4.7%) | 0.02 |
| Hypertension (cases) | 905 (68.7%) | 216 (67.7%) | 0.74 |
| Diabetes (cases) | 62 (4.7%) | 13 (4.1%) | 0.63 |
| **Surgery** | | | |
| Operative duration (min) | 405.0 (340.0–479.0) | 390.0 (321.2–480.0) | 0.21 |
| Emergency surgery (cases) | 650 (49.3%) | 164 (51.4%) | 0.50 |
| Cardiopulmonary bypass time (min) | 186.0 (144.0–224.0) | 184.0 (135.2–236.0) | 0.70 |
| Aortic cross-clamp time (min) | 104.0 (82.6–131.0) | 108.0 (82.0–140.0) | 0.13 |
| With circulatory arrest (cases) | 997 (75.6%) | 223 (69.9%) | 0.04 |
| Circulatory arrest time (min) | 21.0 (17.4–27.0) | 21.2 (17.0–28.0) | 0.63 |
| Nasopharyngeal temperature when circulatory arrest (°C) | 24.1 (23.1–24.9) | 24.2 (23.0–25.0) | 0.32 |
| Rectal temperature when circulatory arrest (°C) | 25.6 (24.8–26.7) | 25.8 (24.5–27.0) | 0.84 |
| RBC transfusion volume (U) | 4.00 (0.00–6.00) | 4.00 (2.00–6.00) | 0.006 |

*CRRT, continuous renal replacement therapy; INR, international normalized ratio; APTT, activated partial thromboplastin time; ALT, alanine aminotransferase; AST, aspartate transaminase; BUN, blood urea nitrogen; eGFR, estimated glomerular filtration rate.*

## ETHICS STATEMENT

The studies involving human participants were reviewed and approved by the Ethics Committee of Beijing Anzhen Hospital. Written informed consent for participation was not required for this study in accordance with the national legislation and the institutional requirements.

## AUTHOR CONTRIBUTIONS

HZ and WJ designed the research. JL and MG analyzed the data and wrote the paper. YJ analyzed the data and revised the manuscript. LS, LH, RF, TG, ZZ, CZ, GZ, XQ, CQ, and YC were responsible for the data collection. All authors read and approved the final manuscript.

## REFERENCES


1. Erbel R, Aboyans V, Boileau C, Bossone E, Bartolomeo RD, Eggebrecht H, et al. 2014 ESC Guidelines on the diagnosis and treatment of aortic diseases: Document covering acute and chronic aortic diseases of the thoracic and abdominal aorta of the adult. The Task Force for the Diagnosis and Treatment of Aortic Diseases of the European Society of Cardiology (ESC). *Eur Heart J.* (2014) 35:2873–926. doi: 10.1093/eurheartj/ehu281
2. Englberger L, Suri RM, Greason KL, Burkhart HM, Sundt TM. 3rd, Daly RC, et al. Deep hypothermic circulatory arrest is not a risk factor for acute kidney injury in thoracic aortic surgery. *J Thorac Cardiovasc Surg.* (2011) 141:552–8. doi: 10.1016/j.jtcvs.2010.02.045
3. Thakar CV, Arrigain S, Worley S, Yared JP, Paganini EP, A. clinical score to predict acute renal failure after cardiac surgery. *J Am Soc Nephrol.* (2005) 16:162–8. doi: 10.1681/ASN.2004040331
4. Mehta RH, Grab JD, O'Brien SM, Bridges CR, Gammie JS, Haan CK, et al. Bedside tool for predicting the risk of postoperative dialysis in patients undergoing cardiac surgery. *Circulation.* (2006) 114:2208–16. doi: 10.1161/CIRCULATIONAHA.106.635573
5. Wijeysundera DN, Karkouti K, Dupuis JY, Rao V, Chan CT, Granton JT, et al. Derivation and validation of a simplified predictive index for renal replacement therapy after cardiac surgery. *JAMA.* (2007) 297:1801–9. doi: 10.1001/jama.297.16.1801
6. Birnie K, Verheyden V, Pagano D, Bhabra M, Tilling K, Sterne JA, et al. Predictive models for kidney disease: improving global outcomes (KDIGO) defined acute kidney injury in UK cardiac surgery. *Crit Care.* (2014) 18:606. doi: 10.1186/s13054-014-0606-x
7. Collins GS, Reitsma JB, Altman DG, Moons KG, Group T. Transparent reporting of a multivariable prediction model for individual prognosis or diagnosis (TRIPOD): the TRIPOD statement. The TRIPOD group. *Circulation.* (2015) 131:211–9. doi: 10.1161/CIRCULATIONAHA.114.014508
8. Kellum JA, Lameire N, Group KAGW. Diagnosis, evaluation, and management of acute kidney injury: a KDIGO summary (Part 1). *Crit Care.* (2013) 17:204. doi: 10.1186/cc11454
9. Levey AS, Stevens LA, Schmid CH, Zhang YL, Castro AF. 3rd, Feldman HI, et al. A new equation to estimate glomerular filtration rate. *Ann Intern Med.* (2009) 150:604–12. doi: 10.7326/0003-4819-150-9-200905050-00006
10. Troyanskaya O, Cantor M, Sherlock G, Brown P, Hastie T, Tibshirani R, et al. Missing value estimation methods for DNA microarrays. *Bioinformatics.* (2001) 17:520–5. doi: 10.1093/bioinformatics/17.6.520
11. DeLong ER, DeLong DM, Clarke-Pearson DL. Comparing the areas under two or more correlated receiver operating characteristic curves: a nonparametric approach. *Biometrics.* (1988) 44:837–45. doi: 10.2307/2531595
12. Pedregosa F, Varoquaux G, Gramfort A, Michel V, Thirion B, Grisel O, et al. Scikit-learn: machine learning in Python. *J Mach Learn Res.* (2011) 12:2825–30.
13. Freund Y, Schapire RE, editors. A desicion-theoretic generalization of on-line learning and an application to boosting. *European conference on computational learning theory.* Springer. (1995) doi: 10.1007/3-540-59119-2_166
14. Chen T, Guestrin C. XGBoost: A Scalable Tree Boosting System. *Proceedings of the 22nd ACM SIGKDD International Conference on Knowledge Discovery and Data Mining.* San Francisco, California, USA: Association for Computing Machinery (2016). p. 785–94. doi: 10.1145/2939672.2939785
15. Lundberg SM, Lee S-I, A. Unified Approach to Interpreting Model Predictions. *Adv Neural Inf Process Syst.* (2017) 30:4765–74.
16. Motwani M, Dey D, Berman DS, Germano G, Achenbach S, Al-Mallah MH, et al. Machine learning for prediction of all-cause mortality in patients with suspected coronary artery disease: a 5-year multicentre prospective registry analysis. *Eur Heart J.* (2017) 38:500–7. doi: 10.1093/eurheartj/ehw188
17. Platt JC. *Probabilistic Outputs for Support Vector Machines and Comparisons to Regularized Likelihood Methods.* Advances in Large Margin Classifiers. (1999).
18. Bove T, Monaco F, Covello RD, Zangrillo A. Acute renal failure and cardiac surgery. *HSR Proc Intensive Care Cardiovasc Anesth.* (2009) 1:13–21.
19. Ortega-Loubon C, Fernandez-Molina M, Carrascal-Hinojal Y, Fulquet-Carreras E. Cardiac surgery-associated acute kidney injury. *Ann Card Anaesth.* (2016) 19:687–98. doi: 10.4103/0971-9784.191578
20. Chew STH, Hwang NC. Acute Kidney Injury After Cardiac Surgery: A Narrative Review of the Literature. *J Cardiothorac Vasc Anesth.* (2019) 33:1122–38. doi: 10.1053/j.jvca.2018.08.003
21. Pacini D, Pantaleo A, Di Marco L, Leone A, Barberio G, Parolari A, et al. Risk factors for acute kidney injury after surgery of the thoracic aorta using antegrade selective cerebral perfusion and moderate hypothermia. *J Thorac Cardiovasc Surg.* (2015) 150:127–33 e1. doi: 10.1016/j.jtcvs.2015.04.008
22. Khan UA, Coca SG, Hong K, Koyner JL, Garg AX, Passik CS, et al. Blood transfusions are associated with urinary biomarkers of kidney injury in cardiac surgery. *J Thorac Cardiovasc Surg.* (2014) 148:726–32. doi: 10.1016/j.jtcvs.2013.09.080
23. Shiao CC, Huang YT, Lai TS, Huang TM, Wang JJ, Huang CT, et al. Perioperative body weight change is associated with in-hospital mortality in cardiac surgical patients with postoperative acute kidney injury. *PLoS ONE.* (2017) 12:e0187280. doi: 10.1371/journal.pone.0187280
24. Nguyen TC, Cruz MA, Carcillo JA. Thrombocytopenia-associated multiple organ failure and acute kidney injury. *Crit Care Clin.* (2015) 31:661–74. doi: 10.1016/j.ccc.2015.06.004
25. Wang Y, Bellomo R. Cardiac surgery-associated acute kidney injury: risk factors, pathophysiology and treatment. *Nat Rev Nephrol.* (2017) 13:697–711. doi: 10.1038/nrneph.2017.119
26. Hamet P, Tremblay J. Artificial intelligence in medicine. *Metabolism.* (2017) 69S:S36–S40. doi: 10.1016/j.metabol.2017.01.011
27. Ruan Y, Bellot A, Moysova Z, Tan GD, Lumb A, Davies J, et al. Predicting the risk of inpatient hypoglycemia with machine learning using electronic health records. *Diabetes Care.* (2020) 43:1504–11. doi: 10.2337/dc19-1743
28. Leung WK, Cheung KS Li B, Law SYK, Lui TKL. Applications of machine learning models in the prediction of gastric cancer risk in patients after Helicobacter pylori eradication. *Aliment Pharmacol Ther.* (2021) 53:864–72. doi: 10.1111/apt.16272
29. Goldstein BA, Navar AM, Carter RE. Moving beyond regression techniques in cardiovascular risk prediction: applying machine learning to address analytic challenges. *Eur Heart J.* (2017) 38:1805–14. doi: 10.1093/eurheartj/ehw302

# 22

# Prediction Models for Sepsis-Associated Thrombocytopenia Risk in Intensive Care Units Based on a Machine Learning Algorithm

*Xuandong Jiang, Yun Wang, Yuting Pan and Weimin Zhang**

*Intensive Care Unit, Dongyang Hospital of Wenzhou Medical University, Jinhua, China*

***Correspondence:**
*Weimin Zhang*
*jalzhan@163.com*

Sepsis-associated thrombocytopenia (SAT) is a common complication in the intensive care unit (ICU), which significantly increases the mortality rate and leads to poor prognosis of diseases. Machine learning (ML) is widely used in disease prediction in critically ill patients. Here, we aimed to establish prediction models for platelet decrease and severe platelet decrease in ICU patients with sepsis based on four common ML algorithms and identify the best prediction model. The research subjects were 1,455 ICU sepsis patients admitted to Dongyang People's Hospital affiliated with Wenzhou Medical University from January 1, 2015, to October 31, 2019. Basic clinical demographic information, biochemical indicators, and clinical outcomes were recorded. The prediction models were based on four ML algorithms: random forest, neural network, gradient boosting machine, and Bayesian algorithms. Thrombocytopenia was found to occur in 732 patients (49.7%). The mechanical ventilation time and length of ICU stay were longer, and the mortality rate was higher for the thrombocytopenia group than for the non-thrombocytopenia group. The models were validated on an online international database (Medical Information Mart for Intensive Care III). The areas under the receiver operating characteristic curves (AUCs) of the four models for the prediction of thrombocytopenia were between 0.54 and 0.72. The AUCs of the models for the prediction of severe thrombocytopenia were between 0.70 and 0.77. The neural network and gradient boosting machine models effectively predicted the occurrence of SAT, and the Bayesian models had the best performance in predicting severe thrombocytopenia. Therefore, these models can be used to identify such high-risk patients at an early stage and guide individualized clinical treatment, to improve the prognosis of diseases.

**Keywords: sepsis-associated thrombocytopenia, intensive care unit, machine learning, artificial intelligence, prediction**

## INTRODUCTION

Artificial intelligence (AI) has enabled many cutting-edge scientific research achievements in the field of medical care, especially for acute and severe diseases. In fields such as disease risk assessment, early warning of disease deterioration, and early warning of death, AI can alert officials regarding potential risks earlier and more accurately. Machine learning (ML) is a branch of AI, and it has been used for predicting disease outcomes. Using the Medical Information Mart for Intensive Care (MIMIC) database, Garcia Gallo et al. (1) established a model to predict the mortality of patients with severe sepsis based on the ML algorithm, which achieved better evaluation results than traditional scoring systems such as Sequential (sepsis-related) Organ Failure Assessment (SOFA) Score and Simplified Acute Physiology Score II. Thorsen-Meyer et al. (2) applied the ML algorithm and further employed intensive care unit (ICU) time series data analysis to predict the 90-day mortality in real-time, thus improving the prognosis of diseases in ICU patients.

Sepsis-related thrombocytopenia (SAT) is a common complication in the ICU; in particular, the incidence of thrombocytopenia in patients with septic shock can be as high as 55% (3). SAT involves many mechanisms (4), which might include inflammation-mediated platelet production changes, endothelial dysfunction, abnormal blood coagulation function, and hemodilution. Thrombocytopenia can significantly increase the incidence of complications and mortality in patients with sepsis (5). A study by Azkárate et al. (6) showed that thrombocytopenia was associated with a 1.7-fold increased risk of mortality in severe sepsis patients. Thrombocytopenia may cause severe hemorrhage; a multicenter observational study (7) in UK ICU found that a total of 169 patients (9% of the study population) received platelet transfusion, and the prevalence of severe thrombocytopenia ($<50 \times 10(9)$ /L) was 12.4, and 35.4% of the patients finally died in the ICU. In actual clinical work, when a decrease in platelet count is observed for a patient, especially a severe decrease, platelets should be infused in time to reduce the risk of bleeding because platelets cannot be stored for a long time. However, patients may have to wait for 2–3 days from the beginning of platelet reservation to the actual infusion of platelets. In this process, the patients are at a high risk of bleeding and may even experience hemorrhagic shock, which is life-threatening. Early detection of platelet decrease is crucial for critically ill patients.

Presently, there are many related models for predicting sepsis using artificial intelligence (8, 9), which can enhance doctors' medical decision-making ability for patients with sepsis. However, research on predicting SAT and severe thrombocytopenia in the ICU is lacking, and effective models for predicting SAT using ML algorithms have not yet been established. Therefore, we used a large amount of real-time data from the ICU to establish prediction models for thrombocytopenia in ICU sepsis patients for the early identification of patients with a high risk of thrombocytopenia, which would help reduce the occurrence of bleeding events and improve the prognosis of diseases in patients.

## MATERIALS AND METHODS

### Study Design and Research Subjects

Our study was reported according to the guidelines of the TRIPOD (10) statement (Checklist in **Additional File 1**). A retrospective study was conducted with 1,455 sepsis patients who were admitted to the ICU of Dongyang People's Hospital between January 1, 2015, and October 31, 2019. External validation was performed using the MIMIC III dataset (11), a freely accessible online critical care database. The inclusion criteria were age $\geq 18$ years and admission to the ICU with sepsis. The exclusion criteria were patients who had hematological malignancy, cirrhosis patients who had underlying thrombocytopenia before ICU admission, and patients who had undergone splenectomy.

This study was approved by the Ethics Committee of Dongyang People's Hospital (DRY-2021-YX-178). The need for informed consent was waived because of the retrospective, observational study design. The data were anonymously analyzed after the removal of personal information from the data. One author (XJ) obtained permission for accessing the MIMIC database after the completion of "Protecting Human Research Participants," an online training course launched by the National Institutes of Health (certification number: 7632299).

### Data Collection and Grouping

#### Data Collection

Data were collected using the medical record information mining software provided by Shanghai Le9 Healthcare Technology Co., Ltd. The collected information included the following: (1) basic clinicodemographic information [age, sex, disease severity (Acute Physiology and Chronic Health Evaluation, APACHE II score, SOFA score), smoking history, alcohol abuse history, and complications]; (2) blood gas, blood routine, biochemistry, and liver function indicators on the first day of ICU admission; and (3) clinical outcomes (mortality, time on ventilator, length of ICU stay, length of hospital stay, and hospitalization cost).

#### Diagnostic Criteria

Definition of SAT: Sepsis patients with thrombocytopenia.

Thrombocytopenia (12, 13):Platelet count $<100 \times 109$/L or a 30% relative decrease of the baseline platelet count during ICU stay; the baseline platelet count was defined as the highest value over the past seven days before ICU admission. We used the initial platelet count in ICU admission as baseline platelet count for patients without platelet count measurement before ICU admission.

Severe thrombocytopenia (14, 15): Platelet count $<50 \times 109$/L during ICU stay.

Sepsis 3.0 (16): Organ dysfunction triggered by an infection that endangers the patient's life and rapid increase in the SOFA score, with a total score of two points.

Sepsis shock (16): The patient with sepsis requiring vasopressors to maintain mean blood pressure at 65 mmHg or higher and having a serum lactate level higher than 2 mmol/L (18 mg/dL) after fluid resuscitation.

### Data Processing

#### Selection of Independent Variables

Sixty-five potentially related variables were preliminarily screened. After excluding three variables with more than 15% of missing values, the remaining 62 variables were subjected to data preprocessing using CARET in R language. Thirteen variables showing a strong correlation (correlation coefficient $>0.9$) with other independent variables were eliminated. The remaining 57 variables were then subjected to feature

**TABLE 1** | Comparison of the additional evaluation metrics of four machine learning models in external validation.

| | Models for predicting thrombocytopenia | | | |
|---|---|---|---|---|
| | **RF** | **Bayesian** | **NNET** | **GBM** |
| Accuracy | 0.61 | 0.55 | 0.68 | 0.67 |
| Precision | 0.61 | 0.59 | 0.71 | 0.67 |
| Recall | 0.72 | 0.40 | 0.65 | 0.74 |
| Specificity | 0.50 | 0.70 | 0.71 | 0.61 |
| | **Models for predicting severe thrombocytopenia** | | | |
| | **RF** | **Bayesian** | **NNET** | **GBM** |
| Accuracy | 0.71 | 0.68 | 0.72 | 0.72 |
| Precision | 0.47 | 0.45 | 0.48 | 0.48 |
| Recall | 0.55 | 0.84 | 0.59 | 0.49 |
| Specificity | 0.77 | 0.62 | 0.77 | 0.81 |

*RF, random forest; NNET, neural network; GBM, gradient boosting machine.*

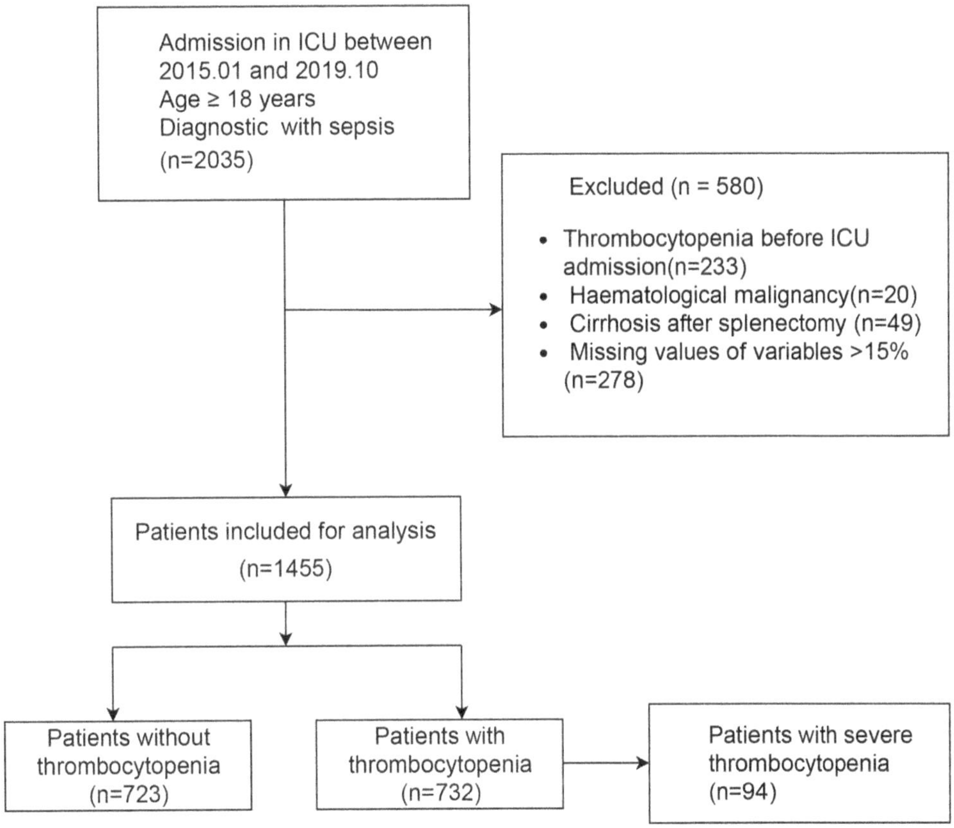


**FIGURE 1** | Flow chart of the study. ICU, Intensive Care Unit.

selection using the backward selection method, random forest (RF) sampling, and 10% cross-checking. Then, the efficiency (precision, recall, accuracy, and specificity, the cutoff point was 0.5) was calculated, and the variables were ranked according to their importance. The 10 most important variables were retained.

## Handling of Missing Values

Variables with >15% missing values were deleted. If the incidence of missing values was <2%, the mean value of the variable was used to replace the missing values. The missing values of variables with loss rates of >2 and <15% were replaced using multiple imputations.

**TABLE 2** | Comparisons of baseline characteristics between with thrombocytopenia and without thrombocytopenia.

| | No-SAT ($n$ = 723) | SAT ($n$ = 732) | Total ($n$ = 1,455) | $P$ |
|---|---|---|---|---|
| Age (years) | 65.6 ± 16.1 | 65.6 ± 17.1 | 65.6 ± 16.6 | 0.97 |
| Male [$n$ (%)] | 455 (62.9) | 471 (64.3) | 926 (63.6) | 0.613 |
| Alcohol drinking [$n$ (%)] | 277 (38.3) | 262 (35.8) | 539 (37) | 0.347 |
| Smoking [$n$ (%)] | 275 (38) | 289 (39.5) | 564 (38.8) | 0.609 |
| CKD [$n$ (%)] | 17 (2.4) | 19 (2.6) | 36 (2.5) | 0.896 |
| Cancer [$n$ (%)] | 84 (11.6) | 82 (11.2) | 166 (11.4) | 0.867 |
| Diabetes [$n$ (%)] | 122 (16.9) | 108 (14.8) | 230 (15.8) | 0.3 |
| Hypertension [$n$ (%)] | 366 (50.6) | 311 (42.5) | 677 (46.5) | 0.002 |
| APACHE-II | 17.1 ± 6.1 | 19.7 ± 7 | 18.4 ± 6.7 | < 0.001 |
| SOFA | 6 ± 2.7 | 7.8 ± 3.3 | 6.9 ± 3.2 | < 0.001 |
| Sepsis_shock [$n$ (%)] | 44 (6.1) | 145 (19.8) | 189 (13) | < 0.001 |
| Antiplatelet drug used [$n$ (%)] | 185 (25.6) | 101 (13.8) | 286 (19.7) | < 0.001 |
| **Biochemical indexes on ICU admission** | | | | |
| Red blood cell (x$10^9$/L) | 3.8 ± 0.7 | 3.7 ± 0.8 | 3.8 ± 0.7 | 0.038 |
| Hematokrit (L/L) | 0.3 ± 0.1 | 0.3 ± 0.1 | 0.3 ± 0.1 | 0.045 |
| White blood cell (x$10^9$/L) | 11.3 (8.3, 14.77) | 12.03 (8.04, 16.71) | 11.54 (8.13, 15.39) | 0.052 |
| Neutrophil count (x$10^9$/L) | 9.82 (6.88, 13.19) | 10.47 (6.92, 14.93) | 10.06 (6.89, 13.93) | 0.013 |
| Lymphocyte count (x$10^9$/L) | 0.83 (0.5, 1.22) | 0.69 (0.43, 1.06) | 0.75 (0.47, 1.14) | < 0.001 |
| Platelet count (x$10^9$/L) | 193 (153, 243.5) | 211 (154, 274) | 201 (153, 256) | 0.002 |
| Platelet distribution width (%) | 16 (15.5, 16.4) | 16.2 (15.8, 16.5) | 16.1 (15.7, 16.5) | < 0.001 |
| Mean platelet volume (fl) | 9.8 ± 1.3 | 9.9 ± 1.3 | 9.8 ± 1.3 | 0.031 |
| pH | 7.42 (7.37, 7.47) | 7.38 (7.3, 7.43) | 7.4 (7.34, 7.45) | < 0.001 |
| Serum sodium (mmol/L) | 140.2 (137.5, 142.8) | 141.4 (138.6, 144.1) | 140.9 (138, 143.5) | < 0.001 |
| Serum calcium (mmol/L) | 2.1 ± 0.2 | 2 ± 0.2 | 2 ± 0.2 | < 0.001 |
| Serum lactic acid (mmol/L) | 1.7 (1.2, 2.6) | 3.1 (1.8, 5.2) | 2.2 (1.4, 3.85) | < 0.001 |
| Serum bicarbonate (mmol/L) | 96 ± 7.3 | 94.7 ± 8.7 | 95.4 ± 8 | 0.002 |
| Prothrombin time(s) | 14.4 (13.6, 15.3) | 15.4 (14.2, 17.03) | 14.8 (13.9, 16.1) | < 0.001 |
| Activated partial thromboplastin time(s) | 39.1 (35.4, 44.35) | 40.55 (36.07, 47.73) | 39.8 (35.7, 46) | < 0.001 |
| International normalized ratio | 1.12 (1.05, 1.23) | 1.23 (1.12, 1.41) | 1.17 (1.08, 1.3) | < 0.001 |
| D-dimer (μg/L) | 2.61 (1.28, 5.43) | 4.88 (2.21, 12.03) | 3.5 (1.58, 8.09) | < 0.001 |
| Alanine aminotransferase (U/L) | 20 (13, 37) | 24 (15, 55.25) | 23 (13, 44) | < 0.001 |
| Aspartate aminotransferase (U/L) | 29 (22, 54.5) | 45 (26, 99) | 36 (23, 70) | < 0.001 |
| Serum albumin (g/L) | 32.2 ± 5.1 | 30.5 ± 5.6 | 31.3 ± 5.4 | < 0.001 |
| C-reactive protein (mg/L) | 40 (9.95, 99.85) | 62.1 (21.27, 144.92) | 55.87 (14.61, 125.15) | < 0.001 |
| Serum urea (mmol/L) | 6.92 (5.08, 9.49) | 8.08 (5.74, 12.09) | 7.53 (5.43, 10.76) | < 0.001 |
| Serum creatinine (mmol/L) | 68 (53, 89) | 82 (59, 123.25) | 74 (56, 105.5) | < 0.001 |
| Procalcitonin (ug/L) | 0.41 (0.12, 1.5) | 1.04 (0.3, 5.74) | 0.67 (0.17, 2.92) | < 0.001 |

*Continuous variables are described by means and quarterbacks. Categories variables are analyzed by $\chi^2$ test and continuous variables are analyzed by Wilcoxon rank sum test. SAT, sepsis-associated thrombocytopenia; APACHE, acute physiology and chronic health evaluation; ICU, Intensive Care Unit; CKD, Chronic kidney disease; SOFA, Sepsis-related Organ Failure Assessment.*

## Handling of Outliers

Outliers were detected using the interquartile range (IQR), i.e., the difference between the upper and lower quartiles of the boxplot. We used 1.5 times of IQR as the standard, and points exceeding this criterion (the upper quartile + 1.5 times of IQR, or the lower quartile - 1.5 times of IQR) were defined as outliers. The excluded outliers were handled as missing values.

## Model Establishment

The following R packages for the ML method were used: caret, ipred, ranger, arm, nnet, and gbm. Samples were randomly divided into training set and test set in a 7:3 ratio. All ML models were evaluated using 10× cross-validation.

The hyperparameters were adjusted by grid search as follows. For the RF model, the number of trees and mtry parameters were adjusted. For the neural network (NNET) model, size and decay

**TABLE 3** | Comparison of infection site and clinical outcomes between groups.

| | No-SAT ($n$ = 723) | SAT ($n$ = 732) | Total ($n$ = 1,455) | $P$ |
|---|---|---|---|---|
| Ventilation duration (days) | 0.96 (0.28, 5) | 3.91 (0.8, 8.8) | 2.12 (0.47, 7.38) | <0.001 |
| ICU length of stay (days) | 3.88 (1.88, 8.47) | 6.97 (3.62, 12.02) | 5.22 (2.6, 10.65) | <0.001 |
| Hosp. LOS (days) | 19 (13, 29) | 18 (11, 28) | 19 (12, 28) | 0.022 |
| Hospital mortality [$n$ (%)] | 94 (13) | 221 (30.2) | 315 (21.6) | <0.001 |
| Cost (x10$^3$, yuan) | 51.2 (33.5, 79.0) | 55.54 (36.3, 87.6) | 53.6 (34.5, 82.7) | 0.002 |
| **Infection site [$n$ (%)]** | | | | |
| Pulmonary | 510 (70.5) | 509 (69.5) | 1019 (70) | 0.718 |
| Urinary | 54 (7.5) | 78 (10.7) | 132 (9.1) | 0.043 |
| Blood stream | 67 (9.3) | 150 (20.5) | 217 (14.9) | < 0.001 |

*Continuous variables are described by means and quarterbacks. Categories variables are analyzed by $\chi^2$ test and continuous variables are analyzed by Wilcoxon rank sum test. SAT, sepsis-associated thrombocytopenia; ICU, Intensive Care Unit; Hosp. LOS, length of hospital stay.*

parameters were adjusted. For the gradient boosting machine (GBM) model, n.trees, interaction.depth, and shrinkage were adjusted. Finally, the importance of variables was sorted using the function "varImpPlot" within the "caret" package in *R*.

### *Model Validation and Evaluation*

The area under the receiver operating characteristic curve (AUC), sensitivity, specificity, and 95% CI of each model were calculated. The confusion matrix was evaluated using accuracy, precision, and recall as parameters presented in **Table 1**. Local Interpretable Model-Agnostic Explanations (LIME) provides another method for model interpretation (17).

### Statistical Analysis

Descriptive statistics were analyzed conventionally using the CBCgrps package in R (18). Normally distributed measurement data were expressed as x ± s and compared between groups using the two-independent-samples $t$-test. Meanwhile, non-normally distributed data were expressed as M (P25, P75) and compared using the Mann–Whitney $U$ test. Enumeration data were expressed in terms of the rate and percentage and compared between the groups using the $\chi^2$ test. All statistical analyses were performed using R (software version 3.6.3). A $P$-value of 0.05 was considered significant.

# RESULTS

## Comparison of Basic Information and Clinical Outcomes

A total of 1,455 patients with sepsis were included in this study. The flow chart of the study is shown in **Figure 1**, including 732 SAT patients (49.7%). Regarding the sources of infection, pulmonary infection accounted for the highest proportion, with 1,019 cases (70%), followed by blood-borne infection, with 217 cases (14.9%), and urinary tract infection, with 132 cases (9.1%). There were 189 patients with septic shock, and 76.7% of them had SAT.

**Table 2** shows a comparison of general clinical information and clinical outcomes between the thrombocytopenia and non-thrombocytopenia groups. There was no significant difference in age and gender between the two groups, with an average age of 65.6 ± 16.6 years and 63.6% of subjects being male. The disease conditions in the thrombocytopenia group were more serious, and the APACHE and SOFA scores were significantly higher than those in the non-thrombocytopenia group, with statistically significant differences ($P$ < 0.001). There were significant differences in terms of mechanical ventilation time, length of ICU stays, length of hospital stays, and mortality between the two groups ($P$ < 0.001), and the clinical outcome of the thrombocytopenia group was worse. **Table 3** shows a comparison of infection site and clinical outcomes between the groups. We compared the baseline characteristics and clinical outcomes of the external validation set, shown in **Supplementary Table S1**. The comparison of feature distribution between the training, internal validation, and external validation is shown in in **Supplementary Table S2**. The incidence rate of SAT in the three groups of patients was similar, and there was no significant difference in age, SOFA score, and initial platelet count in ICU admission.

## Evaluation of Machine Learning Algorithm Models

**Figure 2** shows the ROC comparison of four ML models for thrombocytopenia prediction, with internal validation showing AUCs between 0.74 and 0.79 and external validation showing AUCs between 0.54 and 0.72. **Table 3** shows the pairwise comparison in external validation. Results of external validation show that NNET and GBM had the best prediction, with no significant difference between the two models, while the prediction accuracy of RF and Bayesian models was slightly worse. Additional evaluation metrics for the four machine learning models in external validation are presented in **Table 4**. We established the model for predicting severe thrombocytopenia using the same method. **Figure 3** shows the ROC comparison of ML models for the prediction of severe thrombocytopenia, with internal validation showing AUCs between 0.84 and 0.89 and external validation showing AUCs between 0.70 and 0.77. The prediction was better than for thrombocytopenia, with the Bayesian model showing the best results. The calibration curve analysis of models is

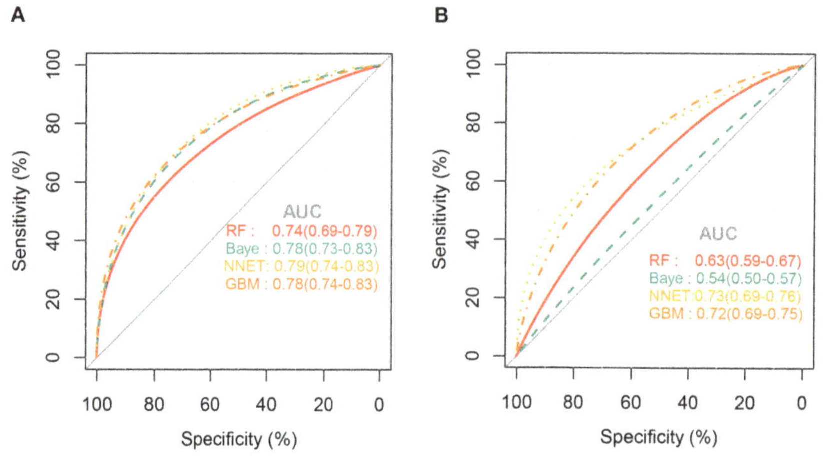


**FIGURE 2 |** ROC curves of the four machine learning models for predicting thrombocytopenia. **(A)**, Internal validation; **(B)**, external validation; RF, random forest; NNET, neural network; GBM, gradient boosting machine; Baye, bayesian.

**TABLE 4 |** Comparison of the area under the roc curve of four machine learning models in external validation.

| | | **Models for predicting thrombocytopenia** | | |
|---|---|---|---|---|
| | **RF** | **Bayesian** | **NNET** | **GBM** |
| RF | / | 0.001 | 0.001 | 0.001 |
| Bayesian | 0.001 | / | 0.001 | 0.001 |
| NNET | 0.001 | | / | 0.94 |
| GBM | 0.001 | 0.001 | 0.94 | / |
| | | **Models for predicting severe thrombocytopenia** | | |
| | **RF** | **Bayesian** | **NNET** | **GBM** |
| RF | / | 0.001 | 0.913 | 0.127 |
| Bayesian | 0.001 | / | 0.001 | 0.001 |
| NNET | 0.913 | 0.001 | / | 0.662 |
| GBM | 0.127 | 0.001 | 0.662 | / |

*ROC, Receiver operating characteristic; RF, random forest; NNET, neural network; GBM, gradient boosting machine.*

shown in **Supplementary Figure S1**. **Figures 4, 5** showed the top 10 variables of the four models ordered by importance. LIME provides explanations for any individual patient, and the contribution of a given variable may change depending on other features of the patient in **Supplementary Figures S2, S3** shows contributions by the variables for two patients (#2, #3). The red (blue) color indicates that the variable contradicts (supports) a given class.

## DISCUSSION

Our study found that SAT had high morbidity and mortality, as well as poor clinical outcomes in ICU, and RF, Bayesian, NNET, and GBM prediction models achieved good predictions.

Thrombocytopenia is very common in ICU patients, with sepsis being its main cause (12). Previous studies on SAT have shown that the incidence rate in critically ill patients (3, 19) was approximately 50%—similar to our findings. Platelets play crucial roles in inflammatory response (20), such as promoting immune response and blood coagulation activation. Presently, many published articles have shown that thrombocytopenia is significantly related to the poor prognosis of patients and is closely related to the degree of thrombocytopenia (21).

Thrombocytopenia is a common reason of platelet transfusion in the ICU. When the platelet count is $<50 \times 10^9$/ L, clinicians often transfuse platelets (22, 23) to reduce bleeding events. A British prospective multicenter observation study (7) showed that, in ICU patients with severe thrombocytopenia, the mortality rate was as high as 35.4%. Therefore, we also predicted severe thrombocytopenia in patients with sepsis. The models had higher accuracy and better prediction effect. For such patients, early discontinuation of antiplatelet drugs, use of platelet-increasing drugs, and early reservation of platelets might help prevent bleeding events and improve the prognosis of patients.

In this study, among the four ML models, the top variables in terms of importance scores were SOFA score, serum lactic acid, serum sodium bicarbonate, and dimer, which suggested that these factors had a significant correlation with SAT.

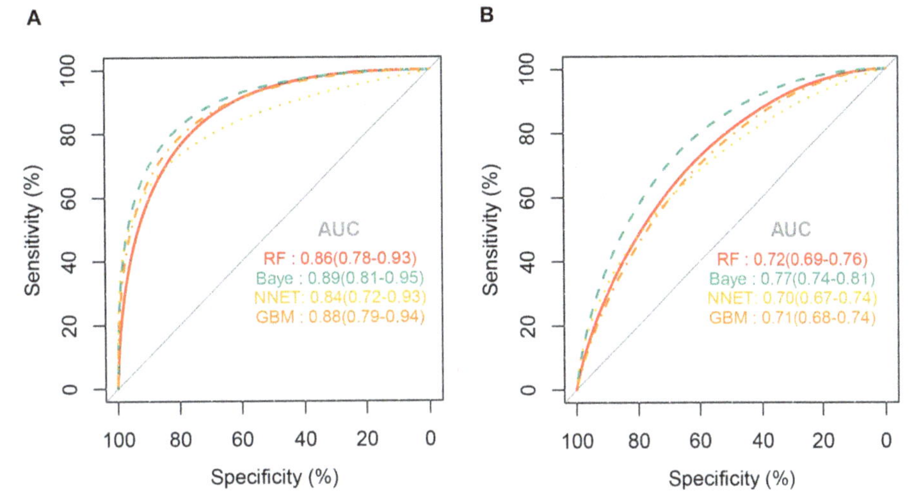


**FIGURE 3 |** ROC curves of the four machine learning models for predicting severe thrombocytopenia. **(A)**, Internal validation; **(B)**, external validation; RF, random forest; NNET, neural network; GBM, gradient boosting machine; Baye, bayesian.

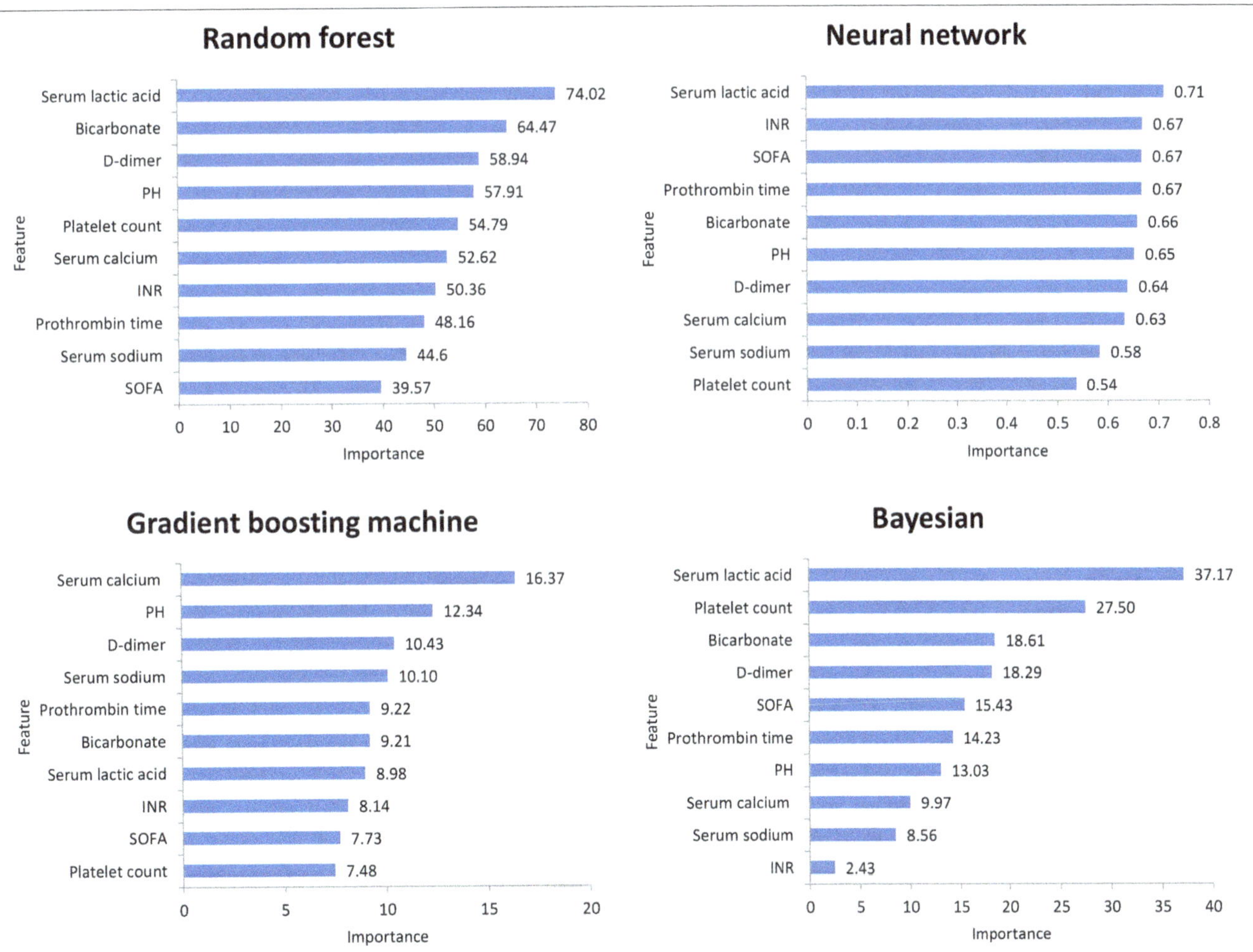


**FIGURE 4 |** Top 10 variables of the four machine learning models for predicting thrombocytopenia ordered by importance. SOFA, Sepsis-related Organ Failure Assessment; INR, International normalized ratio.

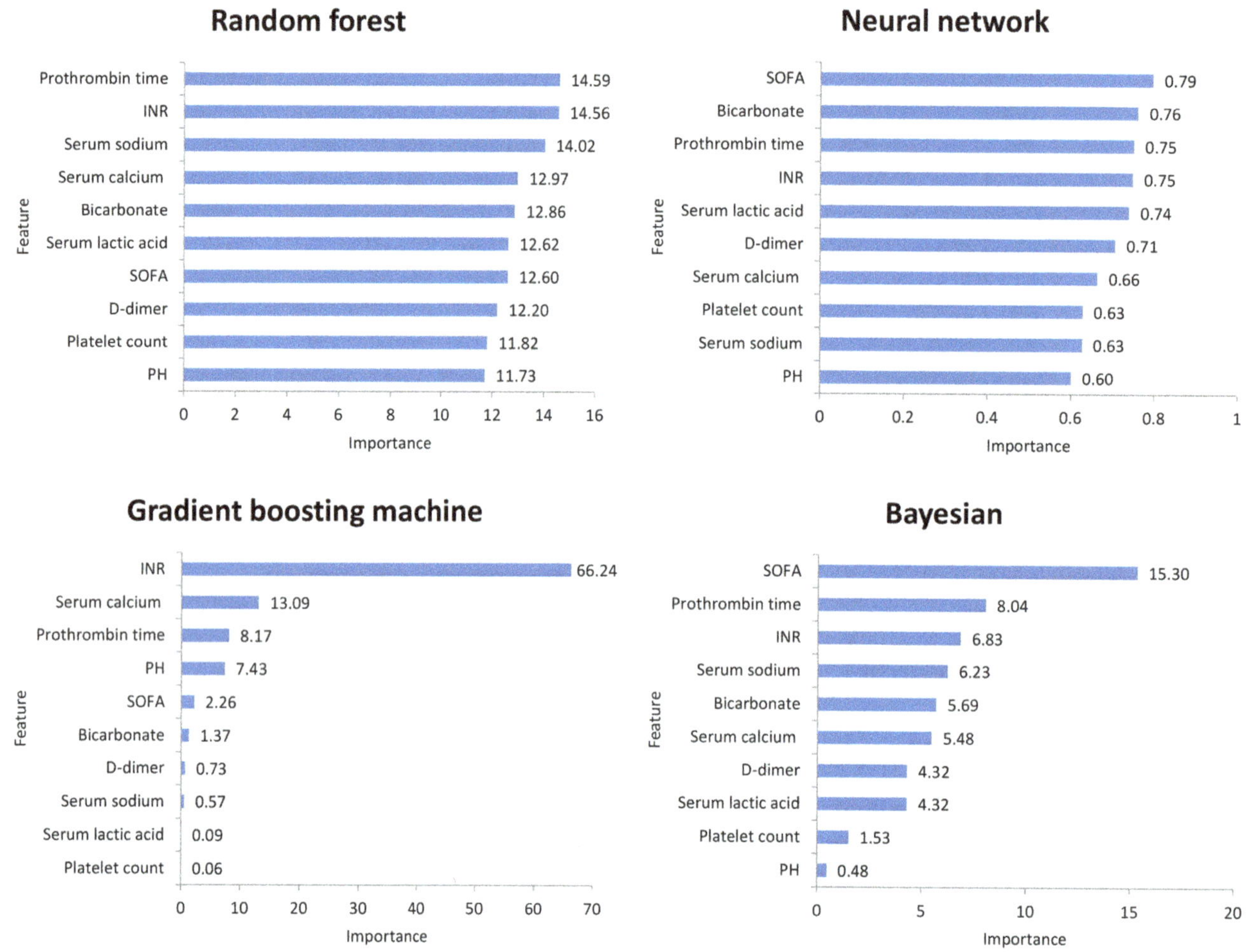


**FIGURE 5 |** Top 10 variables of the four machine learning models for predicting severe thrombocytopenia ordered by importance. SOFA, Sepsis-related Organ Failure Assessment; INR, International normalized ratio.

A retrospective study including 267 patients with abdominal infection showed that a high SOFA score was an important risk factor for hospital-acquired thrombocytopenia. A systematic evaluation (24) found that disease severity was an influencing factor of thrombocytopenia, while serum lactic acid and serum sodium bicarbonate were classic indicators reflecting the severity of the patient's disease. Plasma D-dimer is an important marker of thrombosis activity. In sepsis patients, fibrinolysis activation and D-dimer level have been independently correlated with mortality (25). Therefore, monitoring the SOFA score, serum lactic acid, serum sodium bicarbonate, and dimer levels is helpful for the early detection of thrombocytopenia patients.

This study has some limitations. First, this was a single-center, retrospective study, and some data were missing. We supplemented the data through multiple imputation functions of statistical software to reduce the bias of research results. Second, there are many reasons for thrombocytopenia. For example, some patients with sepsis were treated with hemodialysis, and heparin-induced thrombocytopenia was reported after using heparin. These patients were not excluded, which influenced the results. Third, due to the algorithm characteristics of ML, the models could not clarify the specific relationship between variables and thrombocytopenia, and they were not suitable for all people, which limited the performance of the models. Therefore, based on the algorithms, we showed the measurement of variable importance in the four models and LIME feature plot explained the relationship between variables in the models and thrombocytopenia to a certain extent. Finally, our ML models to predict SAT between ICU stays, the models to predict SAT each day of the ICU stays will be more clinically meaningful. In the future, we will develop software and join the electronic information system to predict SAT each day of the ICU stays.

## CONCLUSION

We established four ML models to predict SAT and severe thrombocytopenia. The models were validated in MIMIC III and can be used to identify such high-risk patients at an early stage and guide individualized clinical treatment. In the future, we will conduct a prospective cohort study and apply these models to clinical practice.

## ETHICS STATEMENT

The studies involving human participants were reviewed and approved by the Ethics Committee of Dongyang People's Hospital. Written informed consent for participation was not required for this study in accordance with the national legislation and the institutional requirements.

## AUTHOR CONTRIBUTIONS

YW and YP carried out the design and contributed to manuscript revision. XJ participated in data analysis and drafted the manuscript. WZ provided overall supervision and undertook the responsibility of submitting the manuscript for publication. All authors contributed to the article and approved the submitted version.

## ACKNOWLEDGMENTS

We would like to thank Editage (www.editage.cn) for English language editing.

## SUPPLEMENTARY MATERIAL

**Supplementary Figure S1 |** Calibration of four machine learning models. **(A)**: Models for predicting thrombocytopenia in Internal validation set; **(B)**: Models for predicting thrombocytopenia in external validation set. **(C)**: Models for predicting severe thrombocytopenia in Internal validation set; **(D)**: Models for predicting severe thrombocytopenia in external validation set; RF, random forest; NNET, neural network; GBM, gradient boosting machine; Baye, bayesian.

**Supplementary Figure S2 |** Heatmap plot showing the contribution of each variable to the classification of sample patients. The relative contribution of each variable was calculated using the LIME algorithm. Patients #2, #3 are shown as examples. Red (blue) color indicates that the relevant variable contradicts (supports) a given label. SOFA, Sepsis-related Organ Failure Assessment; INR, International normalized ratio; LIME, Local Interpretable Model-Agnostic Explanations.

**Supplementary Figure S3 |** LIME feature plot shows the contribution of each variable to the classification of sample patients. Red (blue) color indicates that the relevant variable contradicts (supports) a given label. SOFA, Sepsis-related Organ Failure Assessment; INR, International normalized ratio; LIME, Local Interpretable Model-Agnostic Explanations.

**Supplementary Table S1 |** Baseline characteristics and clinical outcomes between SAT and No-SAT groups in the MIMIC III cohort. Continuous variables are described by means and quarterbacks. Categories variables are analyzed by test and continuous variables are analyzed by Wilcoxon rank sum test. SAT, sepsis-associated thrombocytopenia; SOFA, Sepsis-related Organ Failure Assessment; DM, diabetes mellitus; COPD, Chronic Obstructive Pulmonary Disease; AST, aspartate aminotransferase; INR, International normalized ratio; PT, prothrombin time; Hosp. hospital, LOS length of stay; ICU LOS, ICU length of stay.

**Supplementary Table S2 |** Comparison of feature distribution between the training, internal validation, and external validation. Continuous variables are described by means and quarterbacks. Categories variables are analyzed by $\chi^2$ test and continuous variables are analyzed by Wilcoxon rank sum test. SAT, $\chi^2$ sepsis-associated thrombocytopenia; ICU, Intensive Care Unit; SOFA, Sepsis-related Organ Failure Assessment; Hosp. LOS, length of hospital stay.

## REFERENCES


1. García-Gallo JE, Fonseca-Ruiz NJ, Celi LA, Duitama-Muñoz JF. A machine learning-based model for 1-year mortality prediction in patients admitted to an Intensive Care Unit with a diagnosis of sepsis. *Med intensiva.* (2020) 44:160–70. doi: 10.1016/j.medin.2018.07.016
2. Thorsen-Meyer HC, Nielsen AB, Nielsen AP, Kaas-Hansen BS, Toft P, Schierbeck J, et al. Dynamic and explainable machine learning prediction of mortality in patients in the intensive care unit: a retrospective study of high-frequency data in electronic patient records. *Lancet Digit Health.* (2020) 2:e179–91. doi: 10.1016/S2589-7500(20)30018-2
3. Sharma B, Sharma M, Majumder M, Steier W, Sangal A, Kalawar M, et al. Thrombocytopenia in septic shock patients - a prospective observational study of incidence, risk factors and correlation with clinical outcome. *Anaesth Intensive Care.* (2007) 35:874–80. doi: 10.1177/0310057X0703500604
4. Bedet A, Razazi K, Boissier F, Surenaud M, Hue S, Giraudier S. Mechanisms of thrombocytopenia during septic shock: a multiplex cluster analysis of endogenous sepsis mediators. *Shock.* (2018) 49:641–8. doi: 10.1097/SHK.0000000000001015
5. Xie Y, Tian R, Xie H, Jin W, Du J, Huang P. The clinical significance of thrombocytopenia complicating sepsis: a meta-analysis. *J Infect.* (2019) 78:323–37. doi: 10.1016/j.jinf.2018.12.002
6. Azkárate I, Choperena G, Salas E, Sebastián R, Lara G, Elósegui I, et al. Epidemiology and prognostic factors in severe sepsis/septic shock. Evolution over six years. *Med Intensiva.* (2016) 40:18–25. doi: 10.1016/j.medine.2015.01.002
7. Stanworth SJ, Walsh TS, Prescott RJ, Lee RJ, Watson DM, Wyncoll DL, et al. Thrombocytopenia and platelet transfusion in UK critical care: a multicenter observational study. *Transfusion.* (2013) 53:1050-8. doi: 10.1111/j.1537-2995.2012.03866.x
8. Giannini HM, Ginestra JC, Chivers C, Draugelis M, Hanish A, Schweickert WD, et al. A machine learning algorithm to predict severe sepsis and septic shock: development, implementation, and impact on clinical practice. *Crit Care Med.* (2019) 47:1485–92. doi: 10.1097/CCM.0000000000003891
9. Giacobbe DR, Signori A, Del Puente F, Mora S, Carmisciano L, Briano F, et al. Early detection of sepsis with machine learning techniques: a brief clinical perspective. *Front Med.* (2021) 8:617486. doi: 10.3389/fmed.2021.617486
10. Collins, GS, Reitsma JB, Altman DG, Moons KG. Transparent reporting of a multivariable prediction model for individual prognosis or diagnosis (TRIPOD): the TRIPOD statement. *BMJ.* (2015) 350:g7594. doi: 10.1161/CIRCULATIONAHA.114.014508
11. Johnson A, Pollard T, Shen L, Lehman L, Feng M, Ghassemi M, et al. MIMIC-III, a freely accessible critical care database. *Sci Data.* (2016) 3:160035. doi: 10.1038/sdata.2016.35
12. Thiolliere F, Serre-Sapin AF, Reignier J, Benedit M, Constantin JM, Lebert C, et al. Epidemiology and outcome of thrombocytopenic patients in the intensive care unit: results of a prospective multicenter study. *Intensive Care Med.* (2013) 39:1460–8. doi: 10.1007/s00134-013-2963-3
13. Ben HC, Lauzet JY, Rézaiguia DS, Duvoux C, Cherqui D, Duvaldestin P, et al. Effect of severe thrombocytopenia on patient outcome after liver transplantation. *Intensive Care Med.* (2003) 29:756–62. doi: 10.1007/s00134-003-1727-x
14. Hui P, Cook DJ, Lim W, Fraser GA, Arnold DM. The frequency and clinical significance of thrombocytopenia complicating critical illness: a systematic review. *Chest.* (2011) 139:271–8. doi: 10.1378/chest.10-2243
15. Greinacher A, Selleng K. Thrombocytopenia in the intensive care unit patient. *Hematology Am Soc Hematol Educ Program.* (2010) 2010:135–43. doi: 10.1182/asheducation-2010.1.135
16. Singer M, Deutschman CS, Seymour CW, Shankar-Hari M, Annane D, Bauer M, et al. The third international consensus definitions for sepsis and septic shock (Sepsis-3). *JAMA.* (2016) 315:801–10. doi: 10.1001/jama.2016.0287

17. Zhang Zh, Chen L, Xu P, Hong YC. Predictive analytics with ensemble modeling in laparoscopic surgery: A technical note. *Laparosc Endosc Robot Surg.* (2022). doi: 10.1016/j.lers.2021.12.003
18. Zhang Z, Gayle AA, Wang J, Zhang H, Cardinal FP. Comparing baseline characteristics between groups: an introduction to the CBCgrps package. *Ann Transl Med.* (2017) 5:484. doi: 10.21037/atm.2017.09.39
19. Venkata C, Kashyap R, Farmer JC, Afessa B. Thrombocytopenia in adult patients with sepsis: incidence, risk factors, and its association with clinical outcome. *J Intensive Care.* (2013) 1:9. doi: 10.1186/2052-0492-1-9
20. Vardon BF, Ruiz S, Gratacap MP, Garcia C, Payrastre B, Minville V. Platelets are critical key players in sepsis. *Int J Mol Sci.* (2019) 20:3494. doi: 10.3390/ijms20143494
21. Vandijck DM, Blot SI, De WJ, Hoste EA, Vandewoude KH, Decruyenaere JM. Thrombocytopenia and outcome in critically ill patients with bloodstream infection. *Heart Lung.* (2010) 39:21–6. doi: 10.1016/j.hrtlng.2009.07.005
22. Ning S, Barty R, Liu Y, Heddle NM, Rochwerg B, Arnold DM. Platelet transfusion practices in the ICU: data from a large transfusion registry. *Chest.* (2016) 150:516–23. doi: 10.1016/j.chest.2016.04.004
23. Arnold DM, Crowther MA, Cook RJ, Sigouin C, Heddle NM, Molnar L, et al. Utilization of platelet transfusions in the intensive care unit: indications, transfusion triggers, and platelet count responses. *Transfusion.* (2006) 46:1286–91. doi: 10.1111/j.1537-2995.2006.00892.x
24. Jonsson AB, Rygård SL, Hildebrandt T, Perner A, Møller MH, Russell L. Thrombocytopenia in intensive care unit patients: a scoping review. *Acta Anaesthesiol Scand.* (2021) 65:2–14. doi: 10.1111/aas.13699
25. Semeraro F, Colucci M, Caironi P, Masson S, Ammollo CT, Teli R, et al. Platelet drop and fibrinolytic shutdown in patients with sepsis. *Crit Care Med.* (2018) 46:e221–8. doi: 10.1097/CCM.0000000000002919

23

# Efficacy and Safety of Anticoagulation Treatment in COVID-19 Patient Subgroups Identified by Clinical-Based Stratification and Unsupervised Machine Learning

*Yi Bian [1,2†], Yue Le [1,2†], Han Du [3], Junfang Chen [4], Ping Zhang [5], Zhigang He [1,2], Ye Wang [1,2], Shanshan Yu [1,2], Yu Fang [1,2], Gang Yu [1,2], Jianmin Ling [1,2], Yikuan Feng [1,2], Sheng Wei [6], Jiao Huang [7], Liuniu Xiao [1,2], Yingfang Zheng [1,2], Zhen Yu [8] and Shusheng Li [1,2*]*

*Department of Emergency Medicine, Tongji Medical College, Tongji Hospital, Huazhong University of Science and Technology, Wuhan, China, [2] Department of Critical Care Medicine, Tongji Medical College, Tongji Hospital, Huazhong University of Science and Technology, Wuhan, China, [3] Germany Research Center for Artificial Intelligence, Saarland Informatics Campus, Saarbrücken, Germany, [4] Intelligent Medicine Research Center, Greater Bay Area Institute of Precision Medicine (Guangzhou), Fudan University, Guangzhou, China, [5] Department of Neurology, Tongji Medical College, Tongji Hospital, Huazhong University of Science and Technology, Wuhan, China, [6] Ministry of Education Key Laboratory of Environment and Health, Department of Epidemiology and Biostatistics, School of Public Health, Tongji Medical College, Huazhong University of Science and Technology, Wuhan, China, [7] Center for Evidence-Based and Translational Medicine, Zhongnan Hospital of Wuhan, Wuhan, China, [8] Department of Critical Care Medicine, Renmin Hospital of Wuhan University, Wuhan, China*

***Correspondence:**
*Shusheng Li*
*lishusheng@hust.edu.cn*

*† These authors have contributed equally to this work and share first authorship*

**Objective:** To explore the efficacy of anticoagulation in improving outcomes and safety of Coronavirus disease 2019 (COVID-19) patients in subgroups identified by clinical-based stratification and unsupervised machine learning.

**Methods:** This single-center retrospective cohort study unselectively reviewed 2,272 patients with COVID-19 admitted to the Tongji Hospital between Jan 25 and Mar 23, 2020. The association between AC treatment and outcomes was investigated in the propensity score (PS) matched cohort and the full cohort by inverse probability of treatment weighting (IPTW) analysis. Subgroup analysis, identified by clinical-based stratification or unsupervised machine learning, was used to identify sub-phenotypes with meaningful clinical features and the target patients benefiting most from AC.

**Results:** AC treatment was associated with lower in-hospital death risk either in the PS matched cohort or by IPTW analysis in the full cohort. A higher incidence of clinically relevant non-major bleeding (CRNMB) was observed in the AC group, but not major bleeding. Clinical subgroup analysis showed that, at admission, severe cases of COVID-19 clinical classification, mild acute respiratory distress syndrome (ARDS) cases, and patients with a D-dimer level $\geq 0.5$ μg/mL, may benefit from AC. During the hospital stay, critical cases and severe ARDS cases may benefit from AC. Unsupervised machine learning analysis established a four-class clustering model. Clusters 1 and

2 were non-critical cases and might not benefit from AC, while clusters 3 and 4 were critical patients. Patients in cluster 3 might benefit from AC with no increase in bleeding events. While patients in cluster 4, who were characterized by multiple organ dysfunction (neurologic, circulation, coagulation, kidney and liver dysfunction) and elevated inflammation biomarkers, did not benefit from AC.

**Conclusions:** AC treatment was associated with lower in-hospital death risk, especially in critically ill COVID-19 patients. Unsupervised learning analysis revealed that the most critically ill patients with multiple organ dysfunction and excessive inflammation might not benefit from AC. More attention should be paid to bleeding events (especially CRNMB) when using AC.

**Keywords: COVID-19, anticoagulation, outcomes, mortality, bleeding events, unsupervised machine learning**

## INTRODUCTION

Coronavirus disease 2019 (COVID-19), caused by severe acute respiratory syndrome coronavirus 2 (SARS-CoV-2), has developed into a pandemic disease and affected nearly every country in the world. There is no comprehensive and strong clinical evidence to support the efficacy of any drugs that specifically target the SARS-CoV-2 (1). Previous research has found that coagulopathy is very common in COVID-19 patients, and includes thrombosis and coagulation abnormalities and dysfunction such as an elevated D-dimer level and prolonged prothrombin time (PT), respectively (2). Autopsy histopathologic analysis has identified widespread thrombosis and microangiopathy in small vessels and capillaries of the lung (3–5), which are different from the pathologies observed in respiratory failure caused by other diseases (3, 6–8). Some scholars have therefore proposed anticoagulation (AC) treatment as an integral part of systemic therapy in the early stage of COVID-19 (9). Generally, retrospective studies have suggested that AC may decrease mortality in COVID-19 patients (9, 10), However, these conclusions are not completely reliable nor applicable to all COVID-19 patients due to limitations in methodology such as no prospective control or matching cohort (9–11), large heterogeneity in anticoagulant therapy (9–12), and a lack of subgroup analysis (10, 11, 13). A recently completed randomized controlled trial (RCT) found that, compared with usual-care thromboprophylaxis, an initial strategy of therapeutic-dose anticoagulation did not result in a higher probability of survival in critically ill COVID-19 patients (14). The conclusion of this RCT may be inconsistent with that of previous retrospective studies. At present, the recommendations for empiric systemic AC treatment currently differ between COVID-19 management guidelines (15–17), with some recommending using anticoagulant drugs preventively for patients who have no contraindications to AC and a significantly increased D-dimer level, while others recommend that all hospitalized adults with COVID-19 should receive pharmacologic thromboprophylaxis with low molecular weight heparin (LMWH) rather than unfractionated heparin (UFH).

We conducted a retrospective cohort study using a comprehensive database of COVID-19 patients to investigate whether AC treatment was protective and safe for COVID-19 patients. Innovative analyses using propensity score matching (PSM) and inverse probability of treatment weighting (IPTW) were performed to balance baseline covariates, variates related to AC treatment assignment and variates related to the outcome between patients with or without AC treatment. Further sensitivity analyses were carried out to explore the association between outcome and duration, dosage and type of AC treatment. The second aim of the study was to identify the patients who benefited most from AC treatment using subgroup analysis that involved stratifying the data according to the severity of the acute respiratory distress syndrome (ARDS) (18), COVID-19 clinical classification (17), and D-dimer levels. Taking into account the heterogeneity of the patients, clinically relevant patient subpopulations were identified by unsupervised machine learning algorithms. The effectiveness of AC treatment was verified further in identified clusters.

## MATERIALS AND METHODS

### Ethics and Registration

This retrospective cohort study was approved by the ethics committee of Tongji Medical College, Huazhong University of Science and Technology (No. 2020-S220). The clinical trial was registered and verified by the Chinese Clinical Trial Registry (ChiCTR2000039855).

### Patient Population

This single-center retrospective cohort study was conducted in two designated branches for COVID-19 patients in Tongji Hospital, an academic hospital affiliated to Tongji Medical College, Huazhong University of Science and Technology in Wuhan, China. All patients with confirmed COVID-19 admitted consecutively to these two institutions between Jan 25 to Mar 23, 2020, were enrolled retrospectively in the study. Approval was obtained from the ethics committee at our institution that the patients did not need to provide informed consent for inclusion in the study. Patients were assigned to three groups, including one group of patients with systemic AC treatment for at least 7 days, one group of patients with systemic AC treatment for <7 days and one group of patients without AC treatment. The medications administered and clinical outcomes were followed up to June 4, 2020, when these two branches for exclusive COVID-19 treatment were closed. All COVID-19 patients were diagnosed according to the World Health Organization interim guidelines (19) and the Diagnosis and Treatment Protocol for COVID-19 Patients (Trial Version 8) (17). The exclusion criteria for the study were younger than 18 years, pregnant, length of stay <24 h, insufficient medical information, a history of severe comorbidities requiring surgical operation including, but not limited to, multiple trauma, a severe infection that required debridement, amputation or laparotomy, and patients who were classified again as COVID positive after RNA for SARS-CoV-2 was detected following their discharge from hospital.

## Anticoagulation Exposure

AC treatment was defined as receiving either UFH, LMWH, Fondaparinux sodium, Argatroban, or direct-acting oral anticoagulants (DOACs) (mainly Rivaroxaban). The initiation of AC treatment was decided by the bedside physicians. Possible reasons for AC treatment were extracted from electronic case files. Immortal time is a gap period between exposure and initiation of follow-up (20). We carried out a Cox proportional hazards model with a time-dependent manner for the drug exposure in this study.

## Outcomes, Definitions, and Data Collection

The primary outcome of this study was in-hospital mortality. The safety endpoints included bleeding events and thrombocytopenia. Major bleeding was defined according to the International Society on Thrombosis and Haemostasis (ISTH) statement (21) as those that resulted in death, were life-threatening, caused chronic sequelae, or consumed major healthcare resources. Hemorrhage that did not fit the criteria for the ISTH definition of major bleeding but required medical intervention was classified as clinically relevant non-major bleeding (CRNMB) (22). Other bleeding events which did not meet the criteria of either major bleeding or CRNMB, including bloody sputum, positive fecal occult blood test/gastric occult blood test and microscopic hematuria, were reported separately. Thrombocytopenia was defined as a platelet count $<100 \times 10^9$/L (23).

The CURB-65 score (21, 24), ARDS (18, 25, 26), and quick sequential organ failure assessment (qSOFA) (27) were defined according to the literature, while the COVID-19 clinical classification was made according to the Diagnosis and Treatment Protocol for COVID-19 Patients (Trial Version 8) (17). The detailed definition of ARDS and COVID-19 clinical classification is shown in **Supplementary Table 1**.

All the characteristics and clinical information of the patients were obtained from electronic medical and nursing record systems. This data included age, gender, current smoking history, comorbidities, laboratory results at admission, CURB-65 score and qSOFA score at admission, ARDS classification (18) and COVID-19 clinical classification at admission and during the hospital stay, antiviral therapies and other treatments during hospitalization, the level of oxygen therapy at admission, and the most intense level of oxygen therapy during hospitalization. Variables with missing data >20% were excluded from this analysis. Multiple imputations were conducted to address the presence of missing values.

## Unsupervised Clustering

For this work, we used the K-Medoids clustering algorithm to partition our data into subclasses in an unsupervised manner. The K-Medoids algorithm randomly selects K samples in the training data as the medoids. The remaining samples are assigned to each subclass based on the pairwise dissimilarities. The sample, which is more similar to the medoid, is assigned to the corresponding subclass. Next, the medoids are updated based on the new results of subgrouping. These two steps are iterated multiple times until there is no change in the assignments. In particular, we used the Partitioning Around Medoids (PAM), which is the most common implementation of K-Medoids. For the dissimilarity measure, we adopted the Manhattan distance because it has better performance than the Euclidean distance for the data containing both binary and category variables (28).

A total of 25 variables representing the patients' clinical characteristics were used as input features in the unsupervised learning method, which included demographic features, comorbidities, vital signs, biomarkers, and oxygen therapy types at admission and during the hospital stay. Each patient in our database was presented as a vector with 25 dimensions. To prepare each patient's case as a vector for modeling training, we converted the binary variable as (0, 1), with the category variable represented by the corresponding categorical index. Normalization of the numerical variables was performed. After the normalization, we made sure that each numerical variable had a normal distribution.

Two prominent probabilistic model selection methods: Bayesian information criterion (BIC) and Akaike information criterion (AIC) were used to determine the optimal number of clusters in this work. In general, the measurement of AIC and BIC scores are similar. BIC penalizes the complexity of the model more than AIC (29).

## Statistical Analysis

To minimize bias caused by the non-random allocation of potentially confounding covariates between the AC and non-AC groups, we adopted PSM methods (30). Propensity score (PS) was calculated using a logistic regression model, adjusted for the following covariates: level of oxygen therapy, clinical classification, high-sensitivity C reactive protein (hs-CRP), D-dimer levels, platelets count, CURB-65 score for the severity of pneumonia (31) at hospital admission, and the highest level of oxygen therapy during hospitalization. The match ratio was set at 1 to 3 and the maximum allowable distance (caliper) at 0.1 (32). To detect the selective bias potentially caused by this PSM, inverse probability of treatment weighting analysis (IPTW) was carried out based on the same variates used in PSM modeling (33).

Continuous variables were expressed as medians and interquartile ranges (IQR) and compared using the Mann-Whitney U test or Kruskal-Wallis H test. Categorical variables were compared using the Pearson $\chi 2$ test, continuity correction, or Fisher's exact test, as appropriate. Differences between clusters identified by unsupervised machine learning were judged by two-tailed Bonferroni correction *post hoc* tests, with a *P*-value < (0.05/6) considered statistically significant. A Kaplan-Meier curve was used to analyze survival during hospitalization, with the data stratified according to AC treatment and PAM clustering subphenotypes.

Univariate and multivariate Cox proportional hazards regression was used to determine the risk factors for in-hospital mortality in the PS matched cohort. Residual imbalanced variates were included in the multivariate Cox proportional hazards regression for the PSM cohort. Cox regression analysis with IPTW adjusted covariates of important demographic characteristics as well as variates associated with outcomes either reported previously (34–36) or by general clinic consensus, which included age, gender, platelets count, PT, D-dimer, total bilirubin, lactate dehydrogenase, urea and hs-CRP. Competing risk model analyses were carried out using Fine-Gray tests, which considered death as a competing event for the safety endpoints, including bleeding events and thrombocytopenia. Sensitivity analyses were carried out according to the AC exposure duration, type and dosage in the full cohort. In subgroups analysis among PS matched cohort, univariate and multivariate logistic regression analysis was used to explore the association of outcomes and AC treatment. Residual imbalanced variates were included in the multivariate logistic regression here. The interaction effect between AC treatment and subgroups was also analyzed by logistic regression.

SPSS version 26.0 software (IBM Corp., Armonk, New York, USA) and SAS version 9.4 (SAS Institute Inc. Cary, NC, USA) were used for the statistical analyses and PS matching. The Kaplan-Meier survival plot and forest plot were constructed using GraphPad Prism version 4.0 software (GraphPad Software Inc., La Jolla, CA, USA). All tests were two-tailed, with a $P < 0.05$ considered statistically significant.

# RESULTS

## Clinical Characteristics of the Patients at Presentation

Two thousand four hundred and sixty nine confirmed COVID-19 patients admitted to Tongji Hospital between Jan 25 and Mar 23, 2020, were consecutively and unselectively reviewed. After excluding 197 patients who did meet study exclusion criteria, a total of 2,272 patients were identified for IPTW analysis and sensitivity analyses. In PSM modeling, 78 patients who received AC treatment for <7 days were not included for matching. Finally, PS matching yielded 165 patients in the AC group (patients who received AC for 7 days or longer) and 393 in the non-AC group (patients who did not receive AC) (**Figure 1**). Detailed AC treatment type, dosage, duration, time of initiation from admission and possible reasons for AC treatment were shown in **Supplementary Figure 1**. In the PS matched cohort, compared to the non-AC group, patients in the AC group were older (69 years, interquartile range [IQR] 60–78 vs. 65 years, IQR 53–71 years, $P < 0.001$) and had more comorbidities at admission (75.2% vs. 58.5%, $P < 0.001$, **Table 1**).

## Primary and Secondary Outcomes

In the PS matched cohort, univariate Cox proportional hazard regression analysis showed a significantly lower probability of in-hospital death in the AC treatment group compared to that in the non-AC treatment group (hazard ratio [HR] = 0.450; 95% confidence interval [CI], 0.278 to 0.727; $P < 0.001$). Since there were still residual imbalances between AC and non-AC groups, multivariate Cox proportional hazard regression was carried out by adjusting imbalance covariates, including age, smoking, comorbidities, white blood cells, lactate dehydrogenase, urea, D-dimer, antiviral therapy, intravenous immunoglobulin, and oxygen therapy during hospitalization. Multivariate Cox analysis showed that AC treatment was associated with a lower probability of in-hospital mortality (adjusted HR = 0.249, 95% CI 0.143 to 0.436, $P < 0.001$, **Table 2**). To explore the immortal time bias, a further Cox proportional hazards model with a time-dependent manner for AC exposure was carried out in this study. This showed that the AC treatment was still associated with a lower probability of in-hospital death risk in the PS matched cohort (adjusted HR = 0.531, 95% CI 0.301 to 0.935, $P = 0.028$, **Figure 2**).

To detect the selective bias caused by PSM, IPTW analysis was performed in the full cohort including 2,272 patients. Multivariate Cox analysis again showed that AC treatment was associated with a lower probability of in-hospital mortality by comparing patients without AC treatment and patients with AC treatment for 7 days or longer (adjusted HR = 0.164; 95% CI: 0.104 to 0.260, $P < 0.001$). Sensitivity analyses were carried out according to the AC exposure duration, type and dosage in the full cohort. Duration of AC therapy <7 days was not associated with lower in-hospital mortality (adjusted HR = 1.018; 95% CI: 0.742 to 1.399, $P = 0.910$). In addition, AC treatment in all various dosages and types remained consistently associated with lower mortality (**Table 3**).

Secondary outcomes included bleeding events and thrombocytopenia. By adjusting baseline covariates and time-dependent AC exposure, it was revealed that AC treatment was associated with higher risk of total bleeding events (adjusted HR = 3.187, 95% CI, 1.846 to 5.504, $P < 0.001$), CRNMB (adjusted HR = 3.713 95% CI, 1.446 to 9.532, $P = 0.006$) and microscopic hematuria (adjusted HR = 2.624, 95% CI, 1.280 to 5.380, $P = 0.008$), but not associated with major bleeding ($P = 1.000$) and thrombocytopenia (adjusted HR = 2.167, 95% CI, 0.750 to 6.263, $P = 0.153$) (**Table 2**). Considering death as a competing event, a competing risk model analysis using the Fine-Gray test was conducted to explore the association between AC and bleeding events or thrombocytopenia. Finally, the AC group had no significantly higher risk of bleeding events (Fine-Gray test, $P = 0.500$) or thrombocytopenia (Fine-Gray test, $P = 0.911$) than the non-AC group when using death as a competing event in the model.

## Clinical Subgroup Stratification

In-hospital mortality between the AC and the non-AC groups was compared in individuals stratified according to ARDS

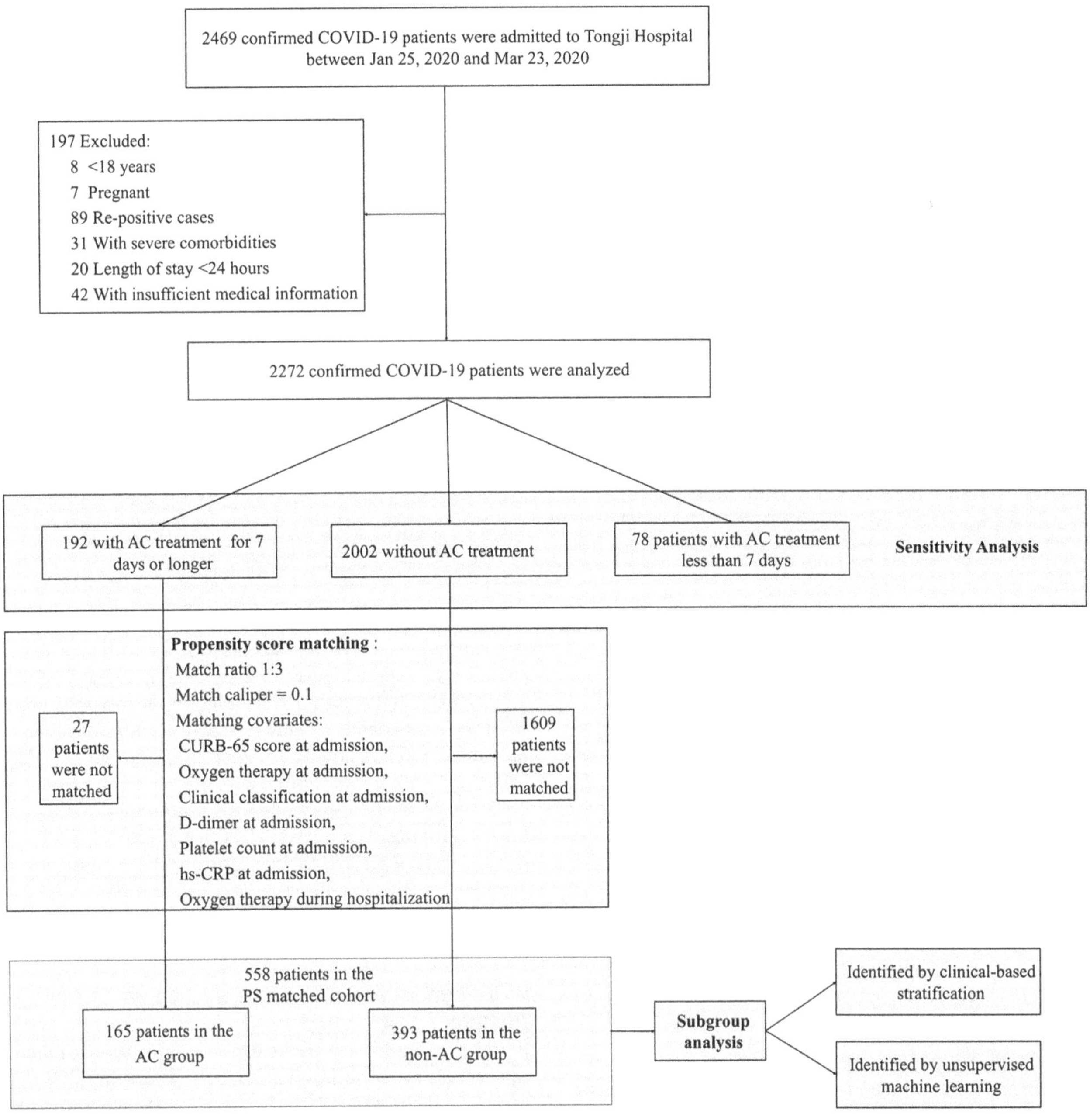


**FIGURE 1** | Flow diagram of the study. COVID-19, Coronavirus Disease 2019; AC, anticoagulation; hs-CRP, high sensitivity C-reactive protein; PS, propensity score.

classification, COVID-19 clinical classification, and D-dimer levels at both hospital admission and during hospitalization. At hospital admission, AC treatment was associated with lower in-hospital mortality in subgroups of mild ARDS (adjusted odds ratio [OR] = 0.005, 95% CI, 0.000–0.174, $P = 0.004$), severe COVID-19 cases (adjusted OR = 0.076, 95% CI, 0.024–0.236, $P < 0.001$) and patients with a D-dimer level $\geq 0.5\,\mu g/mL$ (adjusted OR = 0.042, 95% CI, 0.003–0.603, $P = 0.020$). During the hospital stay, AC treatment was associated with lower in-hospital mortality among patients who developed to severe ARDS (adjusted OR = 0.046, 95% CI, 0.013–0.157, $P < 0.001$) or critical COVID-19 (adjusted OR = 0.095, 95% CI, 0.034–0.266, $P < 0.001$) (**Figure 3**).

The interaction effect between AC treatment and the subgroups was also analyzed by logistic regression (**Supplementary Table 2**). An interaction effect was observed between the subgroups identified by ARDS at admission ($P < 0.001$) or clinical classification at admission ($P < 0.001$) and AC treatment.

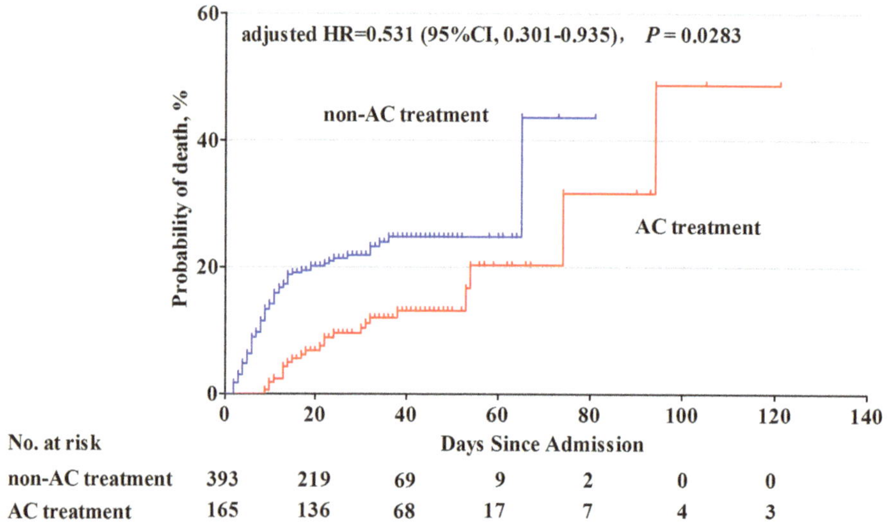


**FIGURE 2 |** Cumulative probability of death in COVID-19 patients with and without AC treatment. Patients with AC treatment had a lower probability of in-hospital mortality than those without AC treatment (adjusted* HR = 0.531, 95% CI: 0.301–0.935, $P = 0.0283$). *Adjusted for time-dependent AC exposure and baseline covariates including age, smoking, comorbidities, white blood cells, D-dimer, lactate dehydrogenase, urea, antiviral therapy, intravenous immunoglobulin, convalescent plasma therapy, and oxygen therapy in hospitalization. HR, hazard ratio; CI, confidence interval; AC, anticoagulation.

## PAM Clustering Analysis

### The Optimal Number of Clustering Determination

BIC and AIC scores were used to automatically select the best number of clusters K for our model. As shown in **Figure 4**, we tried to find the optimal K by conducting an exhaustive search of the possible K values. By and large, the results from AIC and BIC are proportional. BIC score suggests that four clusters are optimal. For the AIC score, a shape "elbow point" is also indicated at four, after four the decrease is becoming notably smaller. Even though a better fitness of the data might be achieved by increasing the number of clusters, an additional cost will be needed including the over-fitting issue and the complexity of interpreting clinically plausible subgroups. Therefore, four clusters were selected to be optimal in this work.

### Clinical Features of Patients' Subgroups

The clinical features of the four clusters are shown in **Tables 4, 5** and **Figure 5**. Patients in clusters 1 and 2 were non-critical cases. Patients in clusters 1 and 2 had no ARDS at admission then developed mild ARDS during the hospital stay. They mainly needed nasal cannula oxygenation at admission as well as during hospitalization. Within these non-critical clusters, cluster 1 was characterized by the youngest age (51 years, IQR 39–63) and had the least number of comorbidities (0, IQR 0–1). Compared to clusters 1 and 2, clusters 3 and 4 were critical cases. In laboratory testing results at admission, both clusters 3 and 4 had significantly higher neutrophils count, lower lymphocytes and platelets count, higher lactate dehydrogenase and hs-CRP, higher urea and creatinine, elevated prothrombin time and D-dimer. In vital signs, clusters 3 and 4 had significantly lower peripheral blood oxygen saturation and respiratory rate at admission. Either at admission or during the hospital stay, both clusters 3 and 4 had significantly more severe levels of ARDS and need a higher level of oxygen therapy. Notably, cluster 4 exhibited as the most critical sub-phenotype. Compared to cluster 3, patients in cluster 4 had significantly excessive inflammation (elevated white blood cells, neutrophils and lactate dehydrogenase), organ dysfunction (higher total bilirubin and urea), severe coagulopathy (elevated prothrombin time and D-dimer), unstable hemodynamics (higher rate of vasopressor use) and neurologic dysfunction (disturbance of consciousness). Compared to the other three clusters, cluster 4 had severe ARDS either at admission or during the hospital stay. As a result, cluster 4 also needed the highest level of oxygen therapy accordingly.

### AC Treatment and Outcomes in Different Patients Clusters

In the non-critical cluster (clusters 1 and 2), we found no significantly lower in-hospital death risk associated with AC treatment (**Figure 6**). In cluster 3, patients who received AC treatment had a significantly lower in-hospital mortality than those who did not receive this treatment (adjusted OR = 0.027, 95% CI, 0.005 to 0.134, $P < 0.001$). However, patients in cluster 4, who had elevated inflammation biomarkers and even severe multi-organ dysfunction, did not benefit from AC treatment. For safety endpoint, AC treatment was not associated with increasing bleeding events (**Figure 6**). In addition, the interaction effect was found between the AC treatment and sub-phenotypes identified by PAM clustering ($P < 0.001$, **Supplementary Table 2**).

## DISCUSSION

COVID-19 infections have affected patients globally. The ISTH pointed out that COVID-19 patients develop a clinically

**TABLE 1** | Patients Baseline Characteristics and Treatments in propensity score matched cohort.

| | No. (%) | | | |
|---|---|---|---|---|
| | Total (*n* = 558) | AC treatment (*n* = 165) | Non-AC treatment (*n* = 393) | *P*-value |
| Age, median (IQR), years | 66 (56, 73) | 69 (60, 78) | 65 (53, 71) | <0.001 |
| **Gender** | | | | |
| Male | 307 (55.0) | 91 (55.2) | 216 (55.0) | 0.967 |
| Female | 251 (45.0) | 74 (44.8) | 177 (450) | |
| Current smoking | 40 (7.2) | 18 (10.9) | 22 (5.6) | 0.026 |
| Comorbidities | 354 (63.4) | 124 (75.2) | 230 (58.5) | <0.001 |
| Diabetes | 118 (21.1) | 41 (24.8) | 77 (19.6) | 0.165 |
| Hypertension | 247 (44.3) | 90 (54.5) | 157 (39.9) | 0.002 |
| Cardiovascular disease | 71 (12.7) | 31 (18.8) | 40 (10.2) | 0.005 |
| CODP | 45 (8.1) | 20 (12.1) | 25 (6.4) | 0.023 |
| Chronic kidney disease | 19 (3.4) | 6 (3.6) | 13 (3.3) | 0.845 |
| Chronic liver disease | 18 (3.2) | 4 (2.4) | 14 (3.6) | 0.487 |
| Autoimmune disease | 8 (1.4) | 2 (1.2) | 6 (1.5) | 1.000 |
| Immunosuppression | 2 (0.4) | 0 (0) | 2 (0.5) | 1.000 |
| Malignancy | 21 (3.8) | 3 (1.8) | 18 (4.6) | 0.118 |
| **Oxygen therapy at admission** | | | | |
| Without oxygen inhalation | 100 (17.9) | 25 (15.2) | 75 (19.1) | 0.206 |
| Nasal cannula | 375 (67.2) | 110 (66.7) | 265 (67.4) | |
| Face mask with reservivor bag | 46 (8.2) | 20 (12.1) | 26 (6.6) | |
| High-flow nasal cannula | 4 (0.7) | 2 (1.2) | 2 (0.5) | |
| Non-invasive ventilation(bi-level) | 20 (3.6) | 4 (2.4) | 16 (4.1) | |
| Invasive mechanical ventilation | 13 (2.3) | 4 (2.4) | 9 (2.3) | |
| **ARDS at admission** | | | | |
| No ARDS | 331 (59.3) | 85 (51.5) | 246 (62.6) | 0.067 |
| Mild | 120 (21.5) | 45 (27.3) | 75 (19.1) | |
| Moderate | 71 (12.7) | 25 (15.2) | 46 (11.7) | |
| Severe | 36 (6.5) | 10 (6.1) | 26 (6.6) | |
| **Clinical classification at admission** | | | | |
| Moderate | 62 (11.1) | 18 (10.9) | 44 (11.2) | 0.537 |
| Severe | 459 (82.3) | 139 (84.2) | 320 (81.4) | |
| Critical | 37 (6.6) | 8 (4.8) | 29 (7.4) | |
| CURB-65 score at admission | 1 (0, 2) | 1 (0, 2) | 1 (0, 1) | 0.099 |
| qSOFA score at admission | 0 (0, 1) | 0 (0, 1) | 0 (0, 1) | 0.608 |
| **Initial laboratory parameters, median (IQR)** | | | | |
| White blood cells, $\times 10^9$/L | 6.29 (4.89, 8.58) | 7.15 (5.40, 9.57) | 5.97 (4.60, 8.02) | <0.001 |
| Neutrophils, $\times 10^9$/L | 4.71 (3.12, 7.04) | 5.65 (4.06, 7.78) | 4.24 (2.90,6.37) | <0.001 |
| Lymphocytes, $\times 10^9$/L | 0.90 (0.60, 1.31) | 0.84 (0.60, 1.15) | 0.94 (0.61, 1.34) | 0.060 |
| Platelets, $\times 10^9$/L | 217.0 (153.0, 291.3) | 209.0 (143.5, 278.0) | 219.0 (159.0, 293.0) | 0.129 |
| Total bilirubin, mmol/L | 9.6 (7.2, 13.7) | 10.7 (7.0, 14.8) | 9.4 (7.2, 13.1) | 0.072 |
| Lactate dehydrogenase, U/L | 321.0 (237.0, 450.3) | 357.0 (262.5, 468.0) | 313.0 (228.0, 434.5) | 0.002 |
| Urea, mmol/L | 5.0 (3.6, 7.0) | 5.2 (4.1, 7.4) | 4.8 (3.4, 6.8) | 0.019 |
| hs-CRP, mg/L | 43.6 (13.0, 102.0) | 50.9 (1.0, 112.7) | 36.9 (10.6, 99.0) | 0.009 |
| Prothrombin time, s | 14.0 (13.4, 15.0) | 14.1 (13.5, 15.2) | 14.0 (13.4, 14.9) | 0.142 |
| D-dimer, mg/mL | 1.36 (0.58, 2.98) | 2.22 (1.11, 6.21) | 1.11 (0.56, 2.58) | <0.001 |
| Creatine | 72 (58, 89) | 74 (59, 90) | 71 (58, 89) | 0.707 |
| Antiviral therapy | 522 (93.5) | 162 (98.2) | 360 (91.6) | 0.004 |
| **Other treatments** | | | | |
| Intravenous immunoglobulin | 186 (33.3) | 82 (49.7) | 104 (26.5) | <0.001 |
| Corticosteroid | 276 (49.5) | 107 (64.8) | 169 (43.0) | <0.001 |
| Convalescent plasma | 22 (3.9) | 15 (9.1) | 7 (1.8) | <0.001 |

*(Continued)*

**TABLE 1** | Continued

| | No. (%) | | | |
|---|---|---|---|---|
| | **Total (*n* = 558)** | **AC treatment (*n* = 165)** | **Non-AC treatment (*n* = 393)** | ***P*-value** |
| **Oxygen therapy in hospitalization** | | | | |
| Without oxygen inhalation | 6 (1.1) | 1 (0.6) | 5 (1.3) | <0.001 |
| Nasal cannula | 328 (58.8) | 85 (51.5) | 243 (61.8) | |
| Face mask with reservivor bag | 43 (7.7) | 15 (9.1) | 28 (7.1) | |
| High-flow nasal cannula | 25 (4.5) | 8 (4.8) | 17 (4.3) | |
| Non-invasive ventilation(bi-level) | 79 (14.2) | 15 (9.1) | 64 (16.3) | |
| Invasive mechanical ventilation | 72 (12.9) | 36 (21.8) | 36 (9.2) | |
| ECMO | 5 (0.9) | 5 (3.0) | 0 (0) | |

*Variables represented the poorest value of the first day at admission. AC, anticoagulation; IQR, interquartile range; COPD, Chronic obstructive pulmonary disease; ARDS, acute respiratory distress syndrome; qSOFA, quick sequential organ failure assessment; hs-CRP, high sensitive C reacting protein; ECMO, extracorporeal membrane oxygenation.*

**TABLE 2** | Primary and secondary outcomes of PS matched cohort.

| | No. (%) | | | | | |
|---|---|---|---|---|---|---|
| | **Total (*n* = 558)** | **AC group (*n* = 165)** | **Non-AC group (*n* = 393)** | **Crude HR (95% CI)** | **Adjusted* HR (95% CI)** | **Adjusted* HR for time-dependent AC exposure (95% CI)** |
| **Primary outcomes** | | | | | | |
| In-hospital mortality | 107 (19.2) | 23 (13.9) | 84 (21.4) | 0.450 (0.278–0.727) | 0.249 (0.143–0.436) | 0.531 (0.301–0.935) |
| **Secondary outcomes** | | | | | | |
| Bleeding events | 121 (21.7) | 42 (25.5) | 79 (20.1) | 0.673 (0.460–0.984) | 0.675 (0.413–1.104) | 3.187 (1.846–5.504) |
| Major bleeding | 4 (0.7) | 0 (0) | 4 (1.0) | 0.017 (0–58.149) | – | – |
| CRNMB | 32 (5.7) | 17 (10.3) | 15 (3.8) | 1.339 (0.663–2.705) | 1.149 (0.465–2.839) | 3.713 (1.446–9.532) |
| Bloody sputum | 9 (1.6) | 3 (1.8) | 6 (1.5) | 0.628 (0.155–2.544) | 0.201 (0.008–4.896) | 0.958 (0.051–18.063) |
| Positive FOBT/GOBT | 5 (0.9) | 4 (2.4) | 1 (0.3) | 4.011 (0.447–35.976) | – | – |
| Microscopic hematuria | 80 (14.3) | 25 (15.2) | 55 (14.0) | 0.597 (0.370–0.965) | 0.443 (0.232–0.846) | 2.624 (1.280–5.380) |
| Thrombocytopenia | 79 (14.2) | 25 (15.2) | 54 (13.8) | 0.608 (0.372–0.993) | 0.665 (0.334–1.327) | 2.167 (0.750–6.263) |

**Adjusted for baseline covariates including age, smoking, comorbidities, white blood cells, D-dimer, lactate dehydrogenase, urea, antiviral therapy, intravenous immunoglobulin, convalescent plasma therapy, and oxygen therapy in hospitalization. PS, propensity score; AC, anticoagulation; HR, hazard ratio; CI, confidence interval; CRNMB, clinically relevant non-major bleeding; FOBT, fecal occult blood test; GOBT, gastric occult blood test.*

**TABLE 3** | Hazard ratio for in-hospital mortality in the full cohort by AC treatment duration, dosage and type in sensitivity analyses.

| | **No. of in-hospital death/total no. (%)** | **Crude HR (95% CI)** | **Adjusted* HR (95% CI)** | **Adjusted* HR for IPTW model# (95% CI)** |
|---|---|---|---|---|
| Non-AC treatment | 91/2002 (4.5) | Reference | Reference | Reference |
| **Duration** | | | | |
| AC treatment <7 days | 44/78 (56.4) | 13.600 (9.482–19.507) | 3.424 (2.242–5.230) | 1.018 (0.742–1.399) |
| AC treatment for 7 days or longer | 38/192 (19.8) | 2.881 (1.943–4.272) | 0.864 (0.560–1.335) | 0.164 (0.104–0.260) |
| **Dosage** | | | | |
| Low dose thromboprophylaxis | 43/176 (24.4) | 4.354 (3.020–6.277) | 1.387 (0.923–2.085) | 0.498 (0.329–0.754) |
| Intermediate dose thromboprophylaxis | 21/55 (38.2) | 6.702 (4.153–10.816) | 1.492 (0.870–2.560) | 0.349 (0.224–0.545) |
| Therapeutic dose anticoagulation | 18/39 (46.2) | 6.959 (4.131–11.723) | 1.575 (0.905–2.742) | 0.225 (0.132–0.384) |
| **Type** | | | | |
| LMWH | 80/262 (30.5) | 5.120 (3.878–7.162) | 1.432 (1.004–2.043) | 0.382 (0.271–0.537) |
| Non-LMWH | 2/8 (25.0) | 3.590 (0.866–14.884) | 2.029 (0.482–8.538) | 0.094 (0.019–0.466) |

**Adjusted for baseline covariates including age, gender, levels of platelets count, prothrombin time, D-dimer, total bilirubin, lactate dehydrogenase, urea, and high-sensitivity C reactive protein.*

*#Covariates in IPTW model: level of oxygen therapy, clinical classification, high-sensitivity C reactive protein and D-dimer levels, Platelet count at admission, CURB-65 score at hospital admission, and the highest level of oxygen therapy during hospitalization.*

*AC, anticoagulation; HR, hazard ratio; CI, confidence interval; IPTW, inverse probability of treatment weighting analysis; LMWH, low molecular weight heparin.*

| Subgroup | AC no. of events/total no. (%) | Non-AC no. of events/total no. (%) | Crude Odds Ratio(95%CI) |
|---|---|---|---|
| ARDS at admission | | | |
| No ARDS | 8/85 (9.4) | 17/246 (6.9) | 1.400 (0.581-3.371) |
| Mild | 9/45 (20.0) | 20/75 (26.7) | 0.688 (0.282-1.677) |
| Moderate | 2/25 (8.0) | 25/46 (54.3) | 0.073 (0.015-0.347) |
| Severe | 4/10 (40.0) | 22/26 (84.6) | 0.121 (0.023-0.634) |
| ARDS in hospitalization | | | |
| No ARDS | 0/21 (0) | 0/126 (0) | - |
| Mild | 0/53 (0) | 0/114 (0) | - |
| Moderate | 0/27 (0) | 2/43 (4.7) | - |
| Severe | 23/64 (35.9) | 82/110 (74.5) | 0.192 (0.098-0.373) |
| Clinical classification at admission | | | |
| Moderate | 3/18 (16.7) | 1/44 (2.3) | 8.600 (0.830-89.122) |
| Severe | 18/139 (12.9) | 58/320 (18.1) | 0.672 (0.380-1.189) |
| Critical | 2/8 (25.0) | 25/29 (86.2) | 0.053 (0.008-0.363) |
| Clinical classification in hospitalization | | | |
| Moderate | 0/1 (0) | 0/4 (0) | - |
| Severe | 0/103 (0) | 1/283 (0.4) | - |
| Critical | 23/61 (37.7) | 83/106 (78.3) | 0.168 (0.084-0.336) |
| D-dimer at admission, mg/mL | | | |
| D-dimer<0.5 | 0/8 (0) | 5/86 (5.8) | - |
| D-dimer≥0.5 | 23/157 (14.6) | 79/307 (25.7) | 0.495 (0.297-0.826) |
| 0.5≤D-dimer<2.5 | 9/80 (11.3) | 40/204 (19.6) | 0.520 (0.239-1.128) |
| 2.5≤D-dimer<5.0 | 4/33 (12.1) | 15/46 (32.6) | 0.285 (0.085-0.959) |
| D-dimer≥5.0 | 10/44 (22.7) | 24/57 (42.1) | 0.404 (0.168-0.975) |
| Over all | 23/165 (13.9) | 84/393 (21.4) | 0.596 (0.361-0.985) |

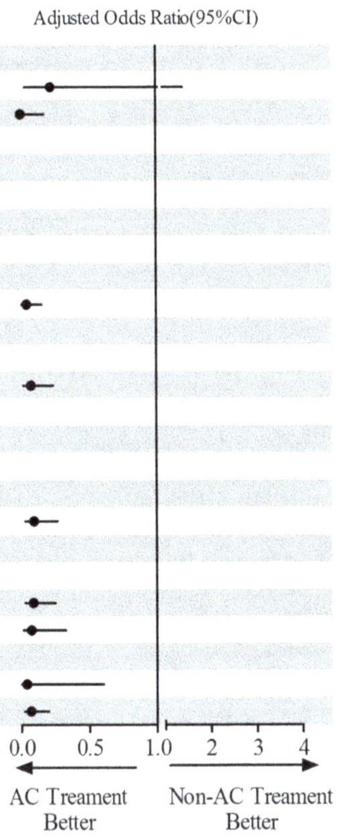


**FIGURE 3 |** Subgroup analysis based on clinical stratification of in-hospital mortality between AC treatment and non-AC treatment patients. The multivariate logistic regression analysis adjusted for baseline covariates including age, smoking, comorbidities, white blood cells, D-dimer, lactate dehydrogenase, urea, antiviral therapy, intravenous immunoglobulin, convalescent plasma therapy, and oxygen therapy in hospitalization. ARDS, acute respiratory distress syndrome; AC, anticoagulation.

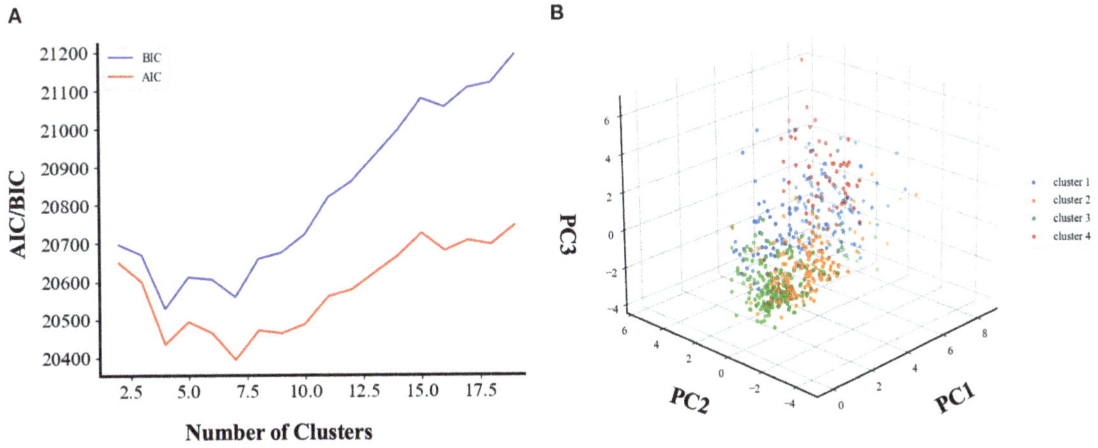


**FIGURE 4 |** Model selection and cluster visualization. The selection of the best number of clusters K is based on BIC and AIC score. K = 4 was chosen after comparing the BIC score of models with different number of clusters by unsupervised clustering analysis. For AIC score, K = 4 is also a good choice for the trade-off between model complexity and the fitting of the data. **(A)** Unsupervised clustering analysis for choosing the best number of clusters. BIC, Bayesian information criteria; AIC, Akaike information criterion. **(B)** Three-dimensional visualization of clustering results. We visualize our clustering results in three-dimensional space. The high dimensional training data was projected into three-dimensional space by using principal component analysis. PC, Principal component.

**TABLE 4** | Variables included in the PAM-based clustering model.

| | Cluster 1 ($n$ = 144) | Cluster 2 ($n$ = 203) | Cluster 3 ($n$ = 158) | Cluster 4 ($n$ = 53) | $P$-value |
|---|---|---|---|---|---|
| Age | 51 (39, 63) abc | 69 (62, 76) | 67 (59, 74) | 68 (63, 72) | <0.001 |
| Gender | a | de | | | |
| Female | 42 (29.2, −4.4) | 156 (76.8, 11.4) | 38 (24.1, −6.2) | 15 (23.8, −2.6) | <0.001 |
| Male | 102 (70.8, 4.4) | 47 (23.2, −11.4) | 120 (75.9, 6.2) | 38 (71.7, 2.6) | |
| No. of comorbidities | 0 (0,1) abc | 1 (0, 2) | 1 (0, 2) | 1 (1, 2) | <0.001 |
| **Initial laboratory parameters** | | | | | |
| White blood cells, ×109/L | 5.62 (4.47, 7.81) c | 5.97 (4.89, 7.60) e | 6.61 (4.72, 8.84) f | 11.38 (8.96, 15.77) | <0.001 |
| Neutrophils, ×109/L | 3.79 (2.62, 5.44) bc | 4.22 (3.03, 5.71) de | 5.46 (3.47, 7.74) f | 10.55 (7.64, 14.68) | <0.001 |
| Lymphocytes, ×109/L | 1.27 (0.90, 1.58) bc | 1.06 (0.77, 1.42) de | 0.61 (0.46, 0.82) | 0.51 (0.36, 0.76) | <0.001 |
| Platelets, ×109/L | 283 (223, 342) abc | 226 (177, 296) de | 161 (127, 222) | 157 (102, 216) | <0.001 |
| Total bilirubin, mmol/L | 8.9 (6.4, 12.1) bc | 8.3 (6.4, 12.1) de | 11.6 (8.3, 14.4) f | 14.6 (10.6, 23.4) | <0.001 |
| Lactate dehydrogenase, U/L | 258 (205, 320) bc | 284 (224, 344) de | 444 (333, 524) f | 601 (458, 795) | <0.001 |
| Urea, mmol/L | 3.95 (3.10, 5.28) bc | 4.60 (3.30, 5.70) de | 6.35 (4.70, 9.20) f | 9.80 (6.60, 13.85) | <0.001 |
| Creatinine, μmol/L | 70 (58, 82) bc | 63 (54, 78) de | 83 (66, 101) | 91 (75, 121) | <0.001 |
| hs-CRP, mg/L | 17.0 (6.7, 55.6) bc | 17.0 (5.9, 43.3) de | 109.8 (69.9, 162.3) | 112.3 (71.4, 186.3) | <0.001 |
| Prothrombin time, s | 13.7 (13.2, 14.2) bc | 13.8 (13.2, 14.3) de | 14.5 (13.8, 15.4) f | 16.2 (15.1, 17.6) | <0.001 |
| D-dimer, mg/mL | 0.91 (0.39, 2.10) bc | 1.17 (0.58, 2.59) de | 1.58 (0.86, 3.01) f | 21.00 (2.72, 21.00) | <0.001 |
| Hemoglobin, g/L | 131 (120, 141) a | 119 (109, 128) de | 131 (120, 141) | 132 (117, 142) | <0.001 |
| **At admission** | | | | | |
| Oxygen therapy | bc | de | f | | |
| Without oxygen inhalation | 32 (22.2, 1.6) | 47 (23.2, 2.4) | 20 (12.7, −2.0) | 1 (1.9, −3.2) | <0.001 |
| Nasal cannula | 105 (72.9, 1.7) | 147 (72.4, 2.0) | 103 (65.2, −0.6) | 20 (37.7, −4.8) | |
| Face mask with reservoir bag | 3 (2.1, −3.1) | 8 (3.9, −2.8) | 23 (14.6, 3.4) | 12 (22.6, 4.0) | |
| High-flow nasal cannula | 1 (0.7, 0) | 0 (0, −1.5) | 1 (0.6, −0.1) | 2 (3.8, 2.8) | |
| NIV | 2 (1.4, −1.6) | 0 (0, −3.4) | 6 (3.8, 0.2) | 12 (22.6, 7.8) | |
| IMV | 1 (0.7, −1.5) | 1 (0.5, −2.2) | 5 (3.2, 0.8) | 6 (11.3, 4.6) | |
| Vasopressor | 0 (0, −1.9) c | 0 (0, −2.4) e | 2 (1.3, −0.6) f | 8 (15.1, 7.7) | <0.001 |
| Disturbance of consciousness | 0 (0, −3.0) c | 2 (1.0, −2.9) e | 6 (3.8, −0.4) f | 16 (30.2, 9.8) | <0.001 |
| $SpO_2$ | 97 (95, 98) bc | 97 (95, 99) de | 93 (86, 96) | 90 (79, 96) | <0.001 |
| Respiratory rate, /min | 20 (20, 22) bc | 20 (20, 22) de | 20 (20, 25) | 25 (20, 32) | <0.001 |
| Heart rate, /min | 92 (84, 105) a | 86 (77, 99) d | 96 (86, 109) | 88 (78, 113) | <0.001 |
| MAP, mmHg | 97 (90, 104) | 97 (89, 106) | 96 (89, 107) | 99 (91, 107) | 0.771 |
| **During hospitalization** | | | | | |
| Oxygen therapy | bc | de | f | | |
| Without oxygen inhalation | 4 (2.8, 2.3) | 2 (1.0, −0.2) | 0 (0, −1.5) | 0 (0, −0.8) | <0.001 |
| Nasal cannula | 121 (84.0, 7.1) | 173 (85.2, 9.6) | 34 (21.5, −11.2) | 0 (0, −9.1) | |
| Face mask with reservoir bag | 8 (5.6, −1.1) | 13 (6.4, −0.9) | 22 (13.9, −0.9) | 0 (0, −2.2) | |
| High-flow nasal cannula | 4 (2.8, −1.1) | 6 (3.0, −1.3) | 14 (8.9, 3.1) | 1 (1.9, −1.0) | |
| NIV | 3 (2.1, −4.8) | 1 (0.5, −7.0) | 57 (36.1, 9.3) | 18 (34.0, 4.3) | |
| IMV | 3 (2.1, −4.5) | 8 (3.9, −4.8) | 27 (17.1, 1.9) | 34 (64.2, 11.7) | |
| ECMO | 1 (0., −0.3) | 0 (0, −1.7) | 4 (2.5, 2.6) | 0 (0, −0.7) | |
| Vasopressor | 3 (2.1, −5.7) bc | 7 (3.4, −6.6) de | 43 (27.2, 3.8) f | 45 (84.9, 13.5) | <0.001 |
| Lowest $SpO_2$ | 95 (93, 96) bc | 95 (92, 96) de | 89 (77, 94) f | 67 (56, 80) | <0.001 |

*Quantitative variables are expressed as medians (interquartile ranges). Categorical variables are expressed as No. (%, adjusted standardized residuals). It is considered that the difference between the actual frequency and the expected frequency of this value is statistically significant if the absolute value of the adjusted standardized residual is >2. Bonferroni correction for multiple comparison was used in the comparison of cluster analysis results. The letters "a" to "f" indicate a significant difference between two group, respectively (a = cluster 1 vs. cluster 2, b = cluster 1 vs. cluster 3, c = cluster 1 vs. cluster 4, d = cluster 2 vs. cluster 3, e = cluster 2 vs. cluster 4, f = cluster 3 vs. cluster 4. PAM, partitioning around medoids; hs-CRP, high sensitivity C-reactive protein; NIV, noninvasive ventilation (bi-level); IMV, invasive mechanical ventilation; $SpO_2$, peripheral blood oxygen saturation; MAP, mean arterial pressure; ECMO, extracorporeal membrane oxygenation.*

**TABLE 5 |** Outcome and variables not included in the PAM-based clustering model.

| | **Cluster 1** (*n* = 144) | **Cluster 2** (*n* = 203) | **Cluster 3** (*n* = 158) | **Cluster 4** (*n* = 53) | ***P*-value** |
|---|---|---|---|---|---|
| **Symptoms** | | | | | |
| Fever | 120 (83.3, 0.4) | 159 (78.3, −1.8) | 135 (85.4, 1.2) | 45 (84.9, 0.5) | 0.306 |
| Cough | 109 (75.7, 0.1) | 145 (71.4, −1.6) | 123 (77.8, 0.9) | 43 (81.1, 1.0) | 0.367 |
| Expectoration | 66 (45.8, 0.3) | 86 (42.4, −0.8) | 75 (47.5, 0.8) | 22 (41.5, −0.5) | 0.746 |
| Shortness of breath | 74 (51.4, −1.7) | 117 (57.6, 0.1) | 100 (63.3, 1.8) | 29 (54.7, −0.4) | 0.210 |
| Myalgia | 27 (18.8, −0.8) | 38 (18.7, −1.0) | 41 (25.9, 1.8) | 11 (20.8, 0) | 0.332 |
| Fatigue | 48 (33.3, −0.3) | 68 (33.5, −0.3) | 57 (36.1, 0.5) | 19 (35.8, 0.2) | 0.942 |
| Diarrhea | 23 (16.0, −2.2) | 50 (24.6, 0.9) | 39 (24.7, 0.7) | 14 (26.4, 0.7) | 0.177 |
| Nausea/vomiting | 17 (11.8, −0.7) | 29 (14.3, 0.4) | 23 (14.6, 0.5) | 6 (11.3, −0.5) | 0.842 |
| **At admission** | | | | | |
| $FiO_2$ | 0.30 (0.27, 0.30) bc | 0.30 (0.27, 0.30) de | 0.36 (0.30, 0.42) f | 0.51 (0.38, 0.63) | <0.001 |
| SBP, mmHg | 124 (117, 136) ac | 131 (121, 143) | 131 (120, 146) | 135 (122, 151) | 0.004 |
| DBP, mmHg | 81 (76, 90) | 79 (72, 87) | 78 (73, 88) | 80 (72, 88) | 0.258 |
| CURB-65 score | 0 (0, 1) abc | 1 (1, 1) de | 1 (1, 2) f | 2 (2, 3) | <0.001 |
| ARDS at admission | bc | de | f | | |
| No ARDS | 108 (75.0, 4.4) | 170 (83.7, 8.9) | 49 (31.0, −8.6) | 4 (7.5, −8.1) | <0.001 |
| Mild | 29 (20.1, −0.5) | 26 (12.8, −3.8) | 55 (34.8, 4.8) | 10 (18.9, −0.5) | |
| Moderate | 5 (3.5, −3.9) | 6 (3.0, −5.2) | 41 (25.9, 5.9) | 19 (35.8, 5.3) | |
| Severe | 2 (1.4, −2.9) | 1 (0.5, −4.3) | 13 (8.2, 1.1) | 20 (37.7, 9.7) | |
| **Initial laboratory parameters** | | | | | |
| Hematocrit, % | 38 (34, 40) a | 35 (32, 38) de | 37 (34, 40) | 38 (34, 41) | <0.001 |
| ALT, U/L | 28 (19, 48) a | 20 (13, 36) d | 29 (17, 47) | 24 (19, 41) | <0.001 |
| AST, U/L | 27 (20, 38) bc | 23 (18, 34) de | 40 (28, 62) | 41 (26, 56) | <0.001 |
| Total protein, g/L | 69.6 (66.2, 73.5) bc | 68.0 (64.6, 72.7) de | 65.9 (62.5, 70.5) | 63.3 (60.8, 69.9) | <0.001 |
| Albumin, g/L | 35.7 (31.5, 39.5) bc | 34.4 (31.4, 38.3) de | 31.4 (28.4, 34.2) | 29.3 (26.7, 31.8) | <0.001 |
| Globulins, g/L | 33.3 (29.9, 37.8) b | 33.5 (30.1, 37.1) d | 34.9 (31.4, 39.1) | 34.8 (31.5, 39.1) | 0.003 |
| **During hospitalization** | | | | | |
| Highest $FiO_2$ | 0.30 (0.30, 0.36) bc | 0.33 (0.30, 0.36) de | 0.66 (0.45, 1.00) f | 1.00 (0.70, 1.00) | <0.001 |
| ARDS during hospitalization | bc | de | f | | |
| No ARDS | 62 (43.1, 5.3) | 83 (40.9, 5.9) | 2 (1.3, −8.5) | 0 (0, −4.6) | <0.001 |
| Mild | 60 (41.7, 3.6) | 80 (39.4, 3.7) | 27 (17.1, −4.2) | 0 (0, −5.0) | |
| Moderate | 11 (7.6, −2.1) | 22 (10.8, −0.9) | 35 (22.2, 4.3) | 2 (3.8, −2.0) | |
| Severe | 11 (7.6, −7.1) | 18 (8.9, −8.6) | 94 (59.5, 9.1) | 51 (96.2, 10.7) | |
| In-hospital mortality | 2 (1.4, −6.3) bc | 6 (3.0, −7.4) de | 52 (32.9, 5.2) f | 47 (88.7, 13.5) | <0.001 |
| Survival time, days | 23 (17, 34) abc | 31 (18, 40) e | 31 (14, 44) f | 10 (6, 17) | <0.001 |
| Bleeding events | 21 (14.6, −2.4) bc | 31 (15.3, −2.8) de | 51 (32.3, 3.8) | 18 (34.0, 2.3) | <0.001 |
| Major bleeding | 0 (0, −1.2) | 0 (0, −1.5) | 4 (2.5, 3.2) | 0 (0, −0.7) | 0.021 |
| CRNMB | 6 (4.2, −0.9) | 7 (3.4, −1.8) | 14 (8.9, 2.0) | 5 (9.4, 1.2) | 0.070 |
| Bloody sputum | 2 (1.4, −0.2) | 2 (1.0, −0.9) | 5 (3.2, 1.8) | 0 (0, −1.0) | 0.378 |
| Microscopic hematuria | 12 (8.3, −2.4) bc | 21 (10.3, −2.0) de | 34 (21.5, 3.0) | 13 (24.5, 2.2) | <0.001 |
| Positive FOBT/GOBT | 1 (0.7, −0.3) | 2 (1.0, 0.2) | 1 (0.6, −0.4) | 1 (1.9, 0.8) | 0.713 |
| Thrombocytopenia | 5 (3.5, −4.3) bc | 7 (3.4, −5.5) de | 37 (23.4, 3.9) f | 30 (56.6, 9.3) | <0.001 |

*Quantitative variables are expressed as medians (interquartile ranges). Categorical variables are expressed as No. (%, adjusted standardized residuals). It is considered that the difference between the actual frequency and the expected frequency of this value is statistically significant if the absolute value of the adjusted standardized residual is >2. Bonferroni correction for multiple comparison was used in the comparison of cluster analysis results. The letters "a" to "f" indicate a significant difference between two group respectively (a = cluster 1 vs. cluster 2, b = cluster 1 vs. cluster 3, c = cluster 1 vs. cluster 4, d = cluster 2 vs. cluster 3, e = cluster 2 vs. cluster 4, f = cluster 3 vs. cluster 4. PAM, partitioning around medoids; $FIO_2$, fraction of inspired oxygen; SBP, Systolic blood pressure; DBP, Diastolic blood pressure; ARDS, acute respiratory distress syndrome; ALT, Alanine aminotransferase; AST, Aspartate aminotransferase; CRNMB, clinically relevant non-major bleeding; FOBT, fecal occult blood test; GOBT, gastric occult blood test.*

significant coagulopathy, characterized by thrombocytopenia, mildly prolonged prothrombin time, and elevated serum D-dimer levels (27). Recent research indicates that coagulopathy is not only common in COVID-19 patients but is also associated with increased mortality (9). The potential mechanism for the development of coagulopathy in COVID-19 patients may

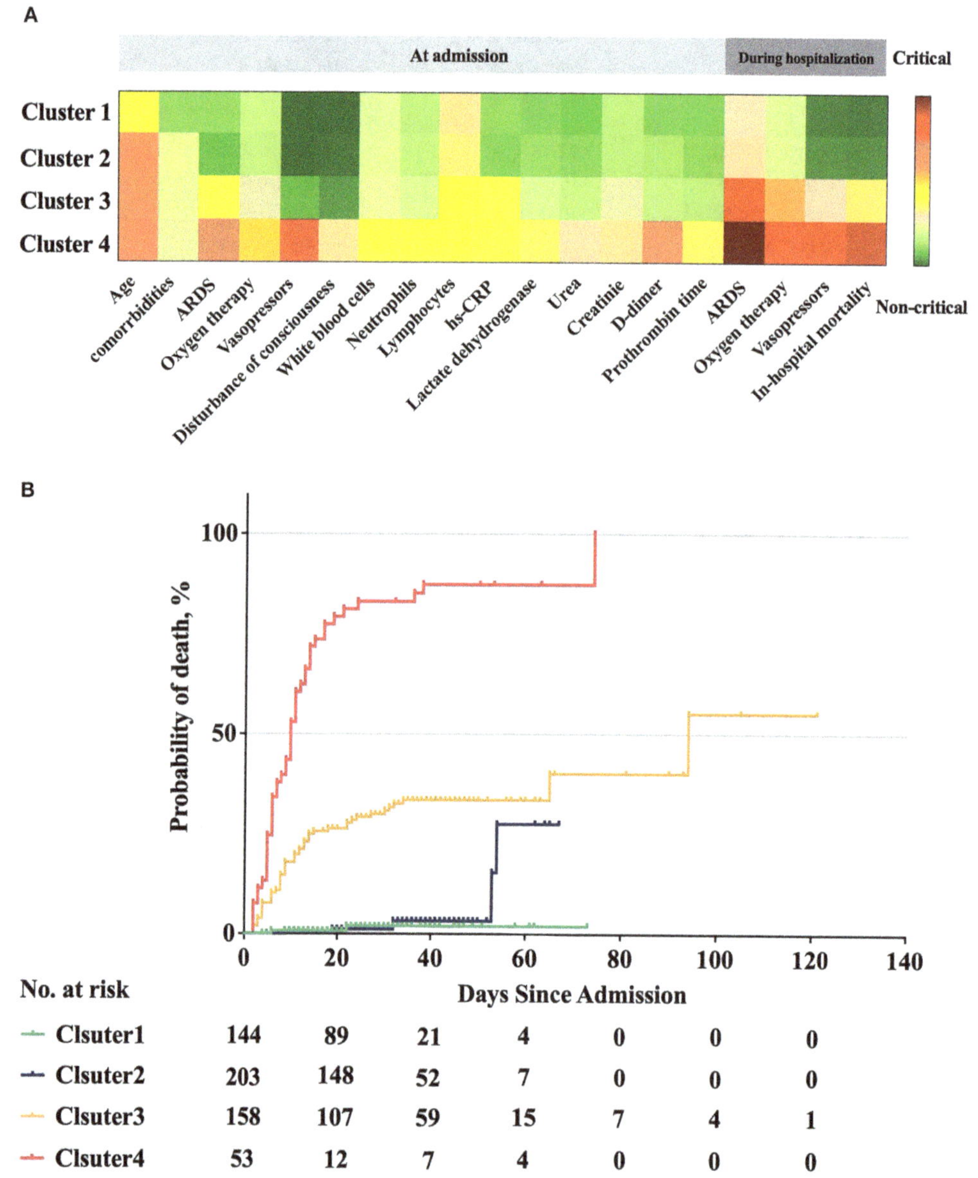


**FIGURE 5 |** Clinical characteristics and probability of death of the four clusters. Clusters 1 and 2 were non-critical cases from admission to discharge and they showed lower probability of death. Cluster 3 had significant higher in hospital mortality and probability of death than clusters 1 and 2, but lower than that in cluster 4. Cluster 4 had the highest in hospital mortality and probability of death, and there were significant differences with the other three clusters. **(A)** Clinical characteristics of four clusters. Some of the significant clinical features are plotted for each cluster. The features are displayed by color-coded heatmap with normalized values. **(B)** Comparison of probability of death between four clusters. There was statistically significant difference in the survival distribution between any two groups ($P < 0.001$), except that there was no statistically significant difference in the survival distribution of cluster 1 and cluster 2 (Log-Rank test, $P = 0.512 > 0.008$).

be related to endothelial cell dysfunction (37) and hypoxia-induced thrombosis (38) following a SARS-CoV-2 infection. Because the endothelium plays an important role in regulating hemostasis, fibrinolysis, and vessel wall permeability, endothelial dysfunction in pulmonary microvessels may act as a trigger for immunothrombosis, resulting in coagulopathy. Histological analysis of pulmonary vessels in COVID-19 patients shows more widespread thrombosis with microangiopathy compared to that observed in patients with influenza. Based on this preliminary evidence, AC treatment may be beneficial for COVID-19 patients by inhibiting thrombin generation and thereby reducing mortality. The ISTH suggests that a prophylactic dose of LMWH should be considered in all patients without contraindications. Moreover, the Chinese Diagnosis and Treatment Protocol for COVID-19 Patients (Version 8.0) also suggested using AC treatment in selected patients. However, these recommendations require additional clinical evidence to determine the association between AC treatment and the outcome of COVID-19 patients,

| Clusters | AC *no. of events/total no. (%)* | Non-AC *no. of events/total no. (%)* | Crude Odds Ratio(95%CI) |
|---|---|---|---|
| **In-hospital mortality** | | | |
| Cluster 1 | 1/27 (3.7) | 1/117 (0.9) | 4.462 (0.270, 73.680) |
| Cluster 2 | 4/64 (6.3) | 2/139 (1.4) | 4.567 (0.814, 25.612) |
| Cluster 3 | 8/61 (13.1) | 44/97 (45.4) | 0.182 (0.078, 0.423) |
| Cluster 4 | 10/13 (76.9) | 37/40 (92.5) | 0.270 (0.047, 1.549) |
| **Bleeding events** | | | |
| Cluster 1 | 4/27 (14.8) | 17/117 (14.5) | 1.023 (0.314, 3.328) |
| Cluster 2 | 8/64 (12.5) | 23/139 (16.5) | 0.720 (0.303, 1.712) |
| Cluster 3 | 24/61 (39.3) | 27/97 (27.8) | 1.682 (0.853, 3.316) |
| Cluster 4 | 6/13 (46.2) | 12/40 (30.0) | 2.000 (0.554, 7.216) |

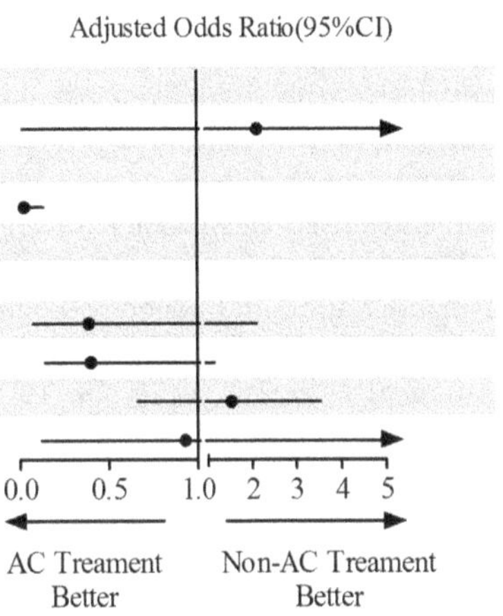


**FIGURE 6** | Comparing of in-hospital mortality and bleeding events between AC treatment and non-AC treatment patients based on unsupervised machine learning. AC, anticoagulation.

and also to clarify the indications, contradictions and optimal duration, dose, and time to use AC. We conducted this matched cohort study using a comprehensive source of COVID-19 patients. In general, results showed that receiving AC treatment was associated with a decreased in-hospital mortality in these patients. Although patients who received AC treatment exhibited a significant increase in CRNMB and microscopic hematuria, they had no increase in the incidence of major bleeding. A clinical subgroup analysis was also carried out to identify patient subgroups who receive greater benefit from AC treatment. At hospital admission, patients of severe COVID-19 clinical cases, patients with mild ARDS or patients who had a D-dimer level $\geq 0.5$ µg/mL were more likely to benefit from AC therapy. During hospitalization, patients who developed severe ARDS or critical COVID-19 cases were more likely to benefit from AC therapy (**Figure 3**). Results of clusters identified by unsupervised machine learning revealed similar results as of clinical subgroups. Critical patients of cluster 3 could benefit from AC treatment whereas non-critical patients in clusters 1 and 2 did not. Nevertheless, a sub-phenotype (cluster 4) exhibited even severe multiple organ dysfunction and excessive inflammation might not benefit from AC therapy.

To date, several research works have investigated systemic AC therapy in COVID-19 patients (9–13, 39). Although the results generally suggested that AC treatment was associated with lower mortality of COVID-19 patients, a constant instruction for clinic application was not easy to conclude. Several possible reasons are worth to be noted. As a retrospective cohort study, imbalance of baseline covariates, covariates related to outcome and covariates related to exposure assignment might lead to biased results. Among the existing studies, some studies used propensity score methods for reducing the effects of confounding (12, 39), some did not (9, 10). In our study, we applied PSM which yield a relatively balanced cohort. We also did IPTW analysis, another propensity score method, to detect the selective bias potentially caused by PSM in the full cohort. The results from PS matched cohort and IPTW analysis in the full cohort both revealed that AC treatment was associated with lower death risk. We also noted that, without the PS method, either the crude results or baseline-adjusted results will lead to an adverse conclusion. Immortal time is a gap period between exposure (usually the span after cohort follow-up) and initiation of follow-up (20). This might cause potential immortal time bias and exaggerate the association between the exposure and outcome. As a result, we carried out a Cox proportional hazards model with a time-dependent manner for the drug exposure in this study.

Another key question concerns the confounders involving various durations, dosages and types of AC treatment. In a retrospective cohort study from the Mount Sinai Health System (11), the duration of hospitalization (median 5 days, IQR 3–8 days) and the course of AC treatment (median 3 days, IQR 2–7 days) were relatively short. Within the current consensus on anticoagulant therapy for venous thromboembolism, it is generally considered that patients with confirmed deep vein thrombosis or pulmonary embolism need LMWH treatment for at least 5 days followed by Dabigatran or Edoxaban (40). As a new disease without comprehensive study until now, to determine the optimal duration, type and dosage of AC treatment need more evidence. In our study, we conducted a series of sensitivity analyses to investigate the relationship between outcome and AC treatment duration, dosage and type. We found that AC treatment for 7 days or longer was associated with a lower death risk while AC treatment for <7 days was not. Low dose thromboprophylaxis, intermediate dose thromboprophylaxis and therapeutic dose anticoagulation were all associated with lower death risk. Although we recorded detailed AC treatment type, the majority was LMWH (**Supplementary Figure 1**), we only investigated LMWH and non-LMWH for sensitivity analyses here. It is revealed that both LMWH and non-LMWH treatment were associated with a lower death rate.

The heterogeneity of the research population is another vital confounder that influences the results. In our study, we analyzed a full cohort of unselected patients from two designated hospitals including mild to critical cases. In general, we found that AC treatment was associated with low mortality, which had a constant result with the previous studies. Furtherly, we investigated who might benefit from AC treatment in subgroup analyses. The stratification criteria used in our study included the most frequently used classification of clinical severity of the COVID-19 patients. It is well-known that hypoxia is a core clinical manifestation and major pathophysiology change that contributes to the death of COVID-19 patients (41–43). The classification of both ARDS (18, 29, 44) and COVID-19 clinical severity classification (17, 45) indicates the severity of hypoxia and accordingly, they are used frequently by clinicians to evaluate and triage patients and to decide major treatments (e.g., levels of oxygen therapy). As a result, we stratified patients according to ARDS classification, COVID-19 clinical classification, and D-dimer levels at both hospital admission and during hospitalization. By this strategy, we found that, at admission, severe cases of COVID-19 clinical classification, mild ARDS cases and patients with a D-dimer level $\geq$0.5 μg/mL may benefit from AC. While during the hospital stay, critical cases and severe ARDS cases may benefit from AC. These results were in constant with Sun et al.' study (9) with severe cases and subgroup analysis from Shen et al. (39) and CORIST Studies (12).

Clustering the study population may help minimize the influence of heterogeneity on the results. The traditional way to categorize patients is based on pre-defined standards. The standards are usually defined by a group of experienced experts with a strong background and prior knowledge in the medical area. Therefore, the procedure for generating the standards alone takes considerable effort and time. In addition, these standards cannot easily be quickly established or updated for a new situation in a short period, which was apparent when we faced this new pandemic, COVID-19. Unsupervised clustering algorithms in machine learning offer another perspective to perform the identification of data subclasses. Unsupervised clustering approaches can achieve more stable and robust clustering results without any prior knowledge of the meaning of each variable in the data. In addition, it may also identify some intrinsic correlations between the variables which sometimes cannot be easily noticed by human experts. Considering the heterogeneity of COVID-19 patients, an innovative strategy was carried out to identify subphenotype of patients who exhibited distinct clinical characteristics and respond to certain treatment using unsupervised learning approach (46). To this end, a four-class PAM-based clustering model was established, representing four distinct COVID-19 patient subphenotypes with different clinical characteristics. In particular, clusters 1 and 2 were non-critical cases with significantly lower mortality. Patients in these two clusters did not benefit from AC treatment. Clusters 3 and 4 were critical cases both exhibited significant abnormal laboratory testing results at admission and unstable vital sign. Cluster 3 had mild to moderate ARDS at admission and progressed to severe ARDS during the hospital stay. Patients in cluster 3 can benefit from AC treatment and had no significant increase in bleeding events. Compared to cluster 3, cluster 4 was the most critical cases and has the highest mortality. A novel result by the clustering approach was that, among these most critical patients (clusters 4), who had moderate or severe ARDS at admission and developed severe ARDS during the hospital stay, AC treatment was not associated with a lower death risk. Further characteristic analysis of these clusters revealed cluster 4 was characterized by multiple organ dysfunction and excessive inflammation. This led us to conclude that critical COVID-19 patients with these features cannot benefit from AC treatment. Recently, an open-label, adaptive, multiplatform, randomized control trial was published (14), with the researchers noting that the initial strategy of therapeutic-dose anticoagulation did not result in a greater probability of survival in critically ill COVID-19 patients (defined as COVID-19 that led to the receipt of ICU-level respiratory or cardiovascular organ support in an ICU) compared to usual-care thromboprophylaxis. This result was different from our clinical subgroup analysis but similar to the phenotypes of clusters 4 in our unsupervised clustering analysis.

Analysis of safety endpoints showed that although the risk of bleeding events, including CRNMB and microscopic hematuria, were higher in the AC group compared to the non-AC group, there was no significant difference in the risk of major bleeding events or thrombocytopenia between the two groups. In brief, the above findings suggested that the use of AC treatment for 7 days or longer in hospitalized COVID-19 patients was associated with increased CRNMB and microscopic hematuria but not with other bleeding events, especially major bleeding. These key observations are consistent with those reported in recent studies (11, 39). Although the competing risk model analysis in this study revealed that there was no significant difference in bleeding risk between the AC and non-AC groups when considering death as a competitive event, the increase of CRNMB still reminds clinicians should be more cautious when using anticoagulation treatment.

This study had several limitations. Firstly, as a retrospective cohort study, imbalanced confounders and selective bias may exist. Large-scale, multicenter, randomized, controlled trials are urgently needed to fully assess the efficacy of AC in patients with COVID-19. Besides, our unsupervised clustering model did not take the importance of each variable into consideration, as it treated all the variables equally as numerical values and measured the similarity between patients based on geometric distance. However, the variables could have completely different semantic meanings. Therefore, it is still necessary for human experts to inspect the clustering results to make sure that the results are explainable. Future work could be to intrinsically integrate the importance of clinic variables into the similarity measurements of unsupervised cluster models.

## CONCLUSION

COVID-19 patients who received AC treatment for 7 days or longer had a significantly lower in-hospital death risk but not higher risk of major bleeding. Through the clinical subgroup analysis, critically ill patients were more likely to benefit from AC treatment. Specifically, the unsupervised machine learning model revealed that, within critically ill COVID-19 patients, patients characterized by multiple organ dysfunction (neurologic, circulation, coagulation, kidney and liver dysfunction) and excessive inflammation may not benefit from AC treatment.

## ETHICS STATEMENT

This retrospective cohort study was approved by the ethics committee of Tongji Medical College, Huazhong University of Science and Technology (No. 2020-S220). The clinical trial was registered and verified by the Chinese Clinical Trial Registry (ChiCTR2000039855).

## AUTHOR CONTRIBUTIONS

YB, YL, SW, and SL conceptualized the paper. YB, ZH, and SL had full access to all of the data in the study and take responsibility for the integrity of the data and the accuracy of the data analysis. HD and JC performed the unsupervised clustering analysis by machine learning and established the clustering model. YB, YL, ZH, YFa, GY, SY, YW, JL, YFe, LX, YZ, and ZY contributed to the acquisition, analysis, and interpretation of data. YB and YL drafted the manuscript. HD and JC drafted the clustering model part of the manuscript. PZ and SL helped revise the manuscript. YB, SW, and JH did the statistical analysis. SL and YB obtained the fundings. SL attests that all listed authors meet authorship criteria and that no others meeting the criteria have been omitted. YB and SL supervised the study and are the guarantors. All authors contributed to the critical revision of the manuscript for important intellectual content and gave final approval of the version to be published.

## ACKNOWLEDGMENTS

The authors thank all the included patients and their families, physicians, nurses, dieticians, and all staff.

## REFERENCES

1. Asselah T, Durantel D, Pasmant E, Lau G, Schinazi RF. COVID-19 discovery, diagnostics and drug development. *J Hepatol.* (2021) 74:168–84. doi: 10.1016/j.jhep.2020.09.031
2. Huang C, Wang Y, Li X, Ren L, Zhao J, Hu Y, et al. Clinical features of patients infected with 2019 novel coronavirus in Wuhan, China. *Lancet.* (2020) 395:497–506. doi: 10.1016/S0140-6736(20)30183-5
3. Ackermann M, Verleden SE, Kuehnel M, Haverich A, Welte T, Laenger F, et al. Pulmonary vascular endothelialitis, thrombosis, and angiogenesis in Covid-19. *N Engl J Med.* (2020) 383:120–8. doi: 10.1056/NEJMoa2015432
4. Fox SE, Akmatbekov A, Harbert JL Li G, Quincy Brown J, Vander Heide RS. Pulmonary and cardiac pathology in African American patients with COVID-19: an autopsy series from New Orleans. *Lancet Respir Med.* (2020) 8:681–6. doi: 10.1016/S2213-2600(20)30243-5
5. Magro C, Mulvey JJ, Berlin D, Nuovo G, Salvatore S, Harp J, et al. Complement associated microvascular injury and thrombosis in the pathogenesis of severe COVID-19 infection: a report of five cases. *Transl Res.* (2020) 220:1–13. doi: 10.1016/j.trsl.2020.04.007
6. Ding Y, Wang H, Shen H, Li Z, Geng J, Han H, et al. The clinical pathology of severe acute respiratory syndrome (SARS): a report from China. *J Pathol.* (2003) 200:282–9. doi: 10.1002/path.1440
7. Nicholls JM, Poon LLM, Lee KC, Ng WF, Lai ST, Leung CY, et al. Lun pathology of fatal severe acute respiratory syndrome. *Lancet.* (2003) 361:1773–8. doi: 10.1016/S0140-6736(03)13413-7
8. Ng DL, Al Hosani F, Keating MK, Gerber SI, Jones TL, Metcalfe MG, et al. Clinicopathologic, immunohistochemical, and ultrastructural findings of a fatal case of middle east respiratory syndrome coronavirus infection in the United Arab Emirates, April 2014. *Am J Pathol.* (2016) 186:652–8. doi: 10.1016/j.ajpath.2015.10.024
9. Tang N, Bai H, Chen X, Gong J, Li D, Sun Z. Anticoagulant treatment is associated with decreased mortality in severe coronavirus disease 2019 patients with coagulopathy. *J Thromb Haemost.* (2020) 18:1094–9. doi: 10.1111/jth.14817
10. Ayerbe L, Risco C, Ayis S. The association between treatment with heparin and survival in patients with Covid-19. *J Thromb Thrombolysis.* (2020) 50:298–301. doi: 10.1007/s11239-020-02162-z
11. Paranjpe I, Fuster V, Lala A, Russak AJ, Glicksberg BS, Levin MA, et al. Association of treatment dose anticoagulation with in-hospital survival among hospitalized patients with COVID-19. *J Am Coll Cardiol.* (2020) 76:122–4. doi: 10.1016/j.jacc.2020.05.001
12. Di Castelnuovo AF, Costanzo S, Iacoviello L. Heparin in COVID-19 patients is associated with reduced in-hospital mortality: the multicentre Italian CORIST Study. *Thromb Haemost.* (2021) 121:1054–65. doi: 10.1055/a-1347-6070
13. Evans EL, Povstyan OV, De Vecchis D, Macrae F, Lichtenstein L, Futers TS, et al. Impact of anticoagulation prior to COVID-19 infection: a propensity score–matched cohort study. *Blood.* (2020) 136:140–4. doi: 10.1182/blood.2019004174
14. Investigators R-C. Investigators ACA, Investigators A, Goligher EC, Bradbury CA, McVerry BJ, et al. Therapeutic Anticoagulation with Heparin in Critically Ill Patients with Covid-19. *N Engl J Med.* (2021) 385:777–89. doi: 10.1056/NEJMoa2103417
15. American Society of Hematology. *COVID-19 and VTE/Anticoagulation: Frequently Asked Questions.* (2021). Available online at: https://www.hematology.org/%20covid-19/covid-19-and-vte-anticoagulation (accessed April 12, 2021).
16. National Institutes of Health. *COVID-19 Treatment Guidelines.* (2021). Available online at: https://www.covid19treatmentguidelines.nih.gov./antithrombotic-therapy/ (accessed April 12, 2021).
17. National Health Commission of the People's Republic of China. *Diagnosis and Treatment Protocol for COVID-19 Patients (Trial Version 8).* (2020). Available online at: http://www.nhc.gov.cn/yzygj/s7653p/202008/0a7bdf12bd4b46e5bd28ca7f9a7f5e5a.shtml (accessed August 19, 2020).
18. Force ADT, Ranieri VM, Rubenfeld GD, Thompson BT, Ferguson ND, Caldwell E, et al. Acute respiratory distress syndrome: the Berlin Definition. *JAMA.* (2012) 307:2526–33. doi: 10.1001/jama.2012.5669
19. World Health Organization. *Clinical Management of Severe Acute Respiratory Infection When Novel Coronavirus (2019-nCoV) Infection Is Suspected: Interim Guidance.* (2020). Available online at: https://www.who.int/publications/i/item/10665-332299 (accessed April 12, 2021).
20. Suissa S. Immortal time bias in pharmaco-epidemiology. *Am J Epidemiol.* (2008) 167:492–9. doi: 10.1093/aje/kwm324
21. Schulman S, Kearon C; Subcommittee on Control of Anticoagulation of the Scientific and Standardization Committee of the International Society on Thrombosis and Haemostasis. Definition of major bleeding in clinical investigations of antihemostatic medicinal products in non-surgical patients. *J Thromb Haemost.* (2004) 3:692–4. doi: 10.1111/j.1538-7836.2005.01204.x
22. Kaatz S, Ahmad D, Spyropoulos AC, Schulman S. Subcommittee on Control of Anticoagulation. Definition of clinically relevant non-major bleeding in studies of anticoagulants in atrial fibrillation and venous thromboembolic disease in non-surgical patients: communication from the SSC of the ISTH. *J Thromb Haemost.* (2015) 13:2119–26. doi: 10.1111/jth.13140

23. Thachil J, Tang N, Gando S, Falanga A, Cattaneo M, Levi M, et al. ISTH interim guidance on recognition and management of coagulopathy in COVID-19. *J Thromb Haemost.* (2020) 18:1023–6. doi: 10.1111/jth.14810
24. Neill AM, Martin IR, Weir R, Anderson R, Chereshsky A, Epton MJ, et al. Community acquired pneumonia: aetiologyand usefulness ofseveritycriteriaon admission. *Thorax.* (1996) 51:1010–6. doi: 10.1136/thx.51.10.1010
25. Ware LB, Matthay MA. The acute respiratory distress syndrome. *New Engl J Med.* (2000) 342:1334–49. doi: 10.1056/NEJM200005043421806
26. Riviello ED, Kiviri W, Twagirumugabe T, Mueller A, Banner-Goodspeed VM, Officer L, et al. Hospital incidence and outcomes of ARDS using the Kigali modification of the Berlin definition. *Am J Respir Crit Care Med.* (2016) 193:52–9. doi: 10.1164/rccm.201503-0584OC
27. Singer M, Deutschman CS, Seymour CW, Shankar-Hari M, Annane D, Bauer M, et al. The Third international consensus definitions for sepsis and septic shock (Sepsis-3). *JAMA.* (2016) 315:801–10. doi: 10.1001/jama.2016.0287
28. Aggarwal CC, Hinneburg A, Keim DA. On the surprising behavior of distance metrics in high dimensional space. In: *International Conference on Database Theory.* Berlin: Springer (2001). p. 420–34.
29. Weakliem, David L. A critique of the Bayesian information criterion for model selection. *Sociol Methods Res.* (1999) 27:359–97. doi: 10.1177/0049124199027003002
30. Austin PC. An introduction to propensity score methods for reducing the effects of confounding in observational studies. *Multivariate Behav Res.* (2011) 46:399–424. doi: 10.1080/00273171.2011.568786
31. Lim WS, van der Eerden MM, Laing R, Boersma WG, Karalus N, Town GI, et al. Defining community acquired pneumonia severity on presentation to hospital: an international derivation and validation study. *Thorax.* (2003) 58:377–82. doi: 10.1136/thorax.58.5.377
32. Kuss O, Blettner M, Borgermann J. Propensity score: an alternative method of analyzing treatment effects. *Dtsch Arztebl Int.* (2016) 113:597–603. doi: 10.3238/arztebl.2016.0597
33. Geleris J, Sun Y, Platt J, Zucker J, Baldwin M, Hripcsak G, et al. Observational study of hydroxychloroquine in hospitalized patients with Covid-19. *N Engl J Med.* (2020) 382:2411–8. doi: 10.1056/NEJMoa2012410
34. Chen C, Chen C, Yan JT, Zhou N, Zhao JP, Wang DW. Analysis of myocardial injury in patients with COVID-19 and association between concomitant cardiovascular diseases and severity of COVID-19. *Zhonghua Xin Xue Guan Bing Za Zhi.* (2020) 48:567–71. doi: 10.3760/cma.j.cn112148-20200225-00123
35. Liang W, Liang H, Ou L, Chen B, Chen A, Li C, et al. Development and validation of a clinical risk score to predict the occurrence of critical illness in hospitalized patients with COVID-19. *JAMA Intern Med.* (2020) 180:1081–9. doi: 10.1001/jamainternmed.2020.2033
36. Wu C, Chen X, Cai Y, Xia J, Zhou X, Xu S, et al. Risk factors associated with acute respiratory distress syndrome and death in patients with coronavirus disease 2019 pneumonia in Wuhan, China. *JAMA Intern Med.* (2020) 180:934–43. doi: 10.1001/jamainternmed.2020.0994
37. Gando S, Levi M, Toh CH. Disseminated intravascular coagulation. *Nat Rev Dis Primers.* (2016) 2:16037. doi: 10.1038/nrdp.2016.37
38. Gupta N, Zhao YY, Evans CE. The stimulation of thrombosis by hypoxia. *Thromb Res.* (2019) 181:77–83. doi: 10.1016/j.thromres.2019.07.013
39. Shen L, Qiu L, Liu D, Wang L, Huang H, Ge H, et al. The association of low molecular weight heparin use and in-hospital mortality among patients hospitalized with COVID-19. *Cardiovasc Drugs Ther.* (2021) 4:1–8. doi: 10.1007/s10557-020-07133-3
40. Schulman S, Konstantinides S, Hu Y, Tang LV. Venous thromboembolic diseases: diagnosis, management and thrombophilia testing: observations on NICE guideline [NG158]. *Thromb Haemost.* (2020) 120:1143–6. doi: 10.1055/s-0040-1712913
41. Somers VK, Kara T, Xie J. Progressive hypoxia: a pivotal pathophysiologic mechanism of COVID-19 pneumonia. *Mayo Clin Proc.* (2020) 95:2339–42. doi: 10.1016/j.mayocp.2020.09.015
42. Grasselli G, Zangrillo A, Zanella A, Antonelli M, Cabrini L, Castelli A, et al. Baseline characteristics and outcomes of 1591 patients infected with SARS-CoV-2 admitted to ICUs of the Lombardy Region, Italy. *JAMA.* (2020) 323:1574–81. doi: 10.1001/jama.2020.5394
43. Xie J, Covassin N, Fan Z, Singh P, Gao W, Li G, et al. Association between hypoxemia and mortality in patients with COVID-19. *Mayo Clin Proc.* (2020) 95:1138–47. doi: 10.1016/j.mayocp.2020.04.006
44. Ferrando C, Suarez-Sipmann F, Mellado-Artigas R, Hernandez M, Gea A, Arruti E, et al. Clinical features, ventilatory management, and outcome of ARDS caused by COVID-19 are similar to other causes of ARDS. *Intensive Care Med.* (2020) 46:2200–11. doi: 10.1007/s00134-020-06251-8
45. Nicastri E, Petrosillo N, Ascoli Bartoli T, Lepore L, Mondi A, Palmieri F, et al. National Institute for the Infectious Diseases "L. Spallanzani", IRCCS Recommendations for COVID-19 clinical management. *Infect Dis Rep.* (2020) 12:8543. doi: 10.4081/idr.2020.8543
46. Calfee CS, Delucchi K, Parsons PE, Thompson BT, Ware LB, Matthay MA, et al. Subphenotypes in acute respiratory distress syndrome: latent class analysis of data from two randomised controlled trials. *Lancet Respir Med.* (2014) 2:611–20. doi: 10.1016/S2213-2600(14)70097-9

# Permissions

All chapters in this book were first published by Frontiers; hereby published with permission under the Creative Commons Attribution License or equivalent. Every chapter published in this book has been scrutinized by our experts. Their significance has been extensively debated. The topics covered herein carry significant findings which will fuel the growth of the discipline. They may even be implemented as practical applications or may be referred to as a beginning point for another development.

The contributors of this book come from diverse backgrounds, making this book a truly international effort. This book will bring forth new frontiers with its revolutionizing research information and detailed analysis of the nascent developments around the world.

We would like to thank all the contributing authors for lending their expertise to make the book truly unique. They have played a crucial role in the development of this book. Without their invaluable contributions this book wouldn't have been possible. They have made vital efforts to compile up to date information on the varied aspects of this subject to make this book a valuable addition to the collection of many professionals and students.

This book was conceptualized with the vision of imparting up-to-date information and advanced data in this field. To ensure the same, a matchless editorial board was set up. Every individual on the board went through rigorous rounds of assessment to prove their worth. After which they invested a large part of their time researching and compiling the most relevant data for our readers.

The editorial board has been involved in producing this book since its inception. They have spent rigorous hours researching and exploring the diverse topics which have resulted in the successful publishing of this book. They have passed on their knowledge of decades through this book. To expedite this challenging task, the publisher supported the team at every step. A small team of assistant editors was also appointed to further simplify the editing procedure and attain best results for the readers.

Apart from the editorial board, the designing team has also invested a significant amount of their time in understanding the subject and creating the most relevant covers. They scrutinized every image to scout for the most suitable representation of the subject and create an appropriate cover for the book.

The publishing team has been an ardent support to the editorial, designing and production team. Their endless efforts to recruit the best for this project, has resulted in the accomplishment of this book. They are a veteran in the field of academics and their pool of knowledge is as vast as their experience in printing. Their expertise and guidance has proved useful at every step. Their uncompromising quality standards have made this book an exceptional effort. Their encouragement from time to time has been an inspiration for everyone.

The publisher and the editorial board hope that this book will prove to be a valuable piece of knowledge for researchers, students, practitioners and scholars across the globe.

# List of Contributors

**Hui Chen and Jun Wang**
Department of Critical Care Medicine, The First Affiliated Hospital of Soochow University, Soochow University, Suzhou, China

**Zhu Zhu**
Department of General Surgery, the Affiliated Suzhou Science & Technology Town Hospital of Nanjing Medical University, Suzhou, China

**Nan Su**
Department of Respiratory and Critical Care Medicine, the First Affiliated Hospital of Soochow University, Soochow University, Suzhou, China

**Jun Gu**
Department of Respiratory Medicine, Affiliated Hospital of Nantong University, Nantong, China

**Shu Lu**
Department of Intensive Care Unit, Affiliated Hospital of Nantong University, Nantong, China

**Li Zhang**
Department of Respiratory Medicine, Zhongda Hospital Southeast University, Nanjing, China

**Xuesong Chen**
Department of Respiratory and Critical Care Medicine, the First Affiliated Hospital of Nanjing Medical University, Nanjing, China

**Lei Xu**
Department of Emergency Medicine, the Affiliated Hospital of Xuzhou Medical University, Xuzhou, China

**Xiangrong Shao**
Department of Respiratory Medicine, the Affliliation Hospital of Yangzhou University, Yangzhou, China

**Jiangtao Yin**
Department of Intensive Care Unit, the Affiliated Hospital of Jiangsu University, Zhenjiang, China

**Jinghui Yang**
Department of Critical Care Medicine, Sir Run Run Hospital, Nanjing Medical University, Nanjing, China

**Baodi Sun**
Department of Emergency, Sir Run Run Hospital, Nanjing Medical University, Nanjing, China

**Yongsheng Li**
Department of Intensive Care Medicine, Tongji Medical College, Tongji Hospital, Huazhong University of Science and Technology, Wuhan, China

**Yohei Hirano**
Department of Emergency and Critical Care Medicine, Juntendo University Urayasu Hospital, Chiba, Japan

**Keito Shinmoto**
Department of Internal Medicine, Tokyo bay Ichikawa Urayasu Medical Center, Chiba, Japan

**Yohei Okada**
Department of Primary Care and Emergency Medicine, Graduate School of Medicine, Kyoto University, Kyoto, Japan

**Kazuhiro Suga**
Department of Mechanical Engineering, Faculty of Engineering, Kogakuin University, Tokyo, Japan

**Jeffrey Bombard and Shogo Murahata**
Dowell Co., Ltd., Hokkaido, Japan

**Manoj Shrestha**
DeerWalk Japan, Tokyo, Japan

**Patrick Ocheja**
Graduate School of Informatics, Kyoto University, Kyoto, Japan

**Aiko Tanaka**
Department of Anesthesiology and Intensive Care Medicine, Osaka University Graduate School of Medicine, Osaka, Japan

**Kyongsik Yun**
Computation and Neural Systems, California Institute of Technology, Pasadena, CA, United States

**Jihoon Oh**
Department of Psychiatry, College of Medicine, Seoul St. Mary's Hospital, The Catholic University of Korea, Seoul, South Korea

**Tae Ho Hong**
Division of Hepato-Biliary and Pancreas Surgery, Department of Surgery, College of Medicine, Seoul St. Mary's Hospital, The Catholic University of Korea, Seoul, South Korea

**Eun Young Kim**
Division of Trauma and Surgical Critical Care, Department of Surgery, College of Medicine, Seoul St. Mary's Hospital, The Catholic University of Korea, Seoul, South Korea

**Xuan Song**
Division of Pulmonary and Critical Care Medicine, Department of Medicine, Mayo Clinic, Rochester, MN, United States
Intensive Care Unit, Liaocheng Cardiac Hospital Affiliated to Shandong First Medical University Shandong, China
Intensive Care Unit, DongE Hospital Affiliated to Shandong First Medical University, Shandong, China

**Timothy J. Weister**
Anesthesia Clinical Research Unit, Mayo Clinic, Rochester, MN, United States

**Yue Dong and Rahul Kashyap**
Department of Anesthesiology and Perioperative Medicine, Mayo Clinic, Rochester, MN, United States

**Kianoush B. Kashani**
Division of Nephrology and Hypertension, Department of Medicine, Mayo Clinic, Rochester, MN, United States

**Xueyuan Huang**
Department of Blood Transfusion, The Third Xiangya Hospital, Central South University, Changsha, China

**Yongjun Wang**
Department of Blood Transfusion, The Second Xiangya Hospital, Central South University, Changsha, China

**Bingyu Chen**
Department of Transfusion, Zhejiang Provincial People's Hospital, Hangzhou, China

**Yuanshuai Huang**
Department of Transfusion, The Affiliated Hospital of Southwest Medical University, Luzhou, China

**Xinhua Wang**
Department of Transfusion, Beijing Aerospace Center Hospital, Beijing, China

**Linfeng Chen**
Department of Transfusion, Beijing Shijitan Hospital, Capital Medical University, Beijing, China

**Xianjun Ma**
Department of Blood Transfusion, Qilu Hospital of Shandong University, Jinan, China

**Le-Ping Liu, Yan-Wei Luo, Hang Dong and Rong Gui**
Department of Blood Transfusion, The Third Xiangya Hospital of Central South University, Changsha, China

**Miao Wu and Jie Wei**
Department of Emergency, Renmin Hospital of Wuhan University, Wuhan, China

**Xianjin Du**
Department of Critical Care Medicine, Renmin Hospital of Wuhan University, Wuhan, China

**Raymond Gu**
Department of Surgery, State University of New York Upstate Medical University, Syracuse, NY, United States

**Qin-Yu Zhao**
Department of Blood Transfusion, The Third Xiangya Hospital of Central South University, Changsha, China
College of Engineering and Computer Science, Australian National University, Canberra, ACT, Australia

**Jing-Chao Luo, Huan Wang, Shen-Ji Yu, Kai Liu, Yi-Jie Zhang and Guo-Wei Tu**
Department of Critical Care Medicine, Zhongshan Hospital, Fudan University, Shanghai, China

**Zhe Luo**
Department of Critical Care Medicine, Zhongshan Hospital, Fudan University, Shanghai, China
Department of Critical Care Medicine, Xiamen Branch, Zhongshan Hospital, Fudan University, Xiamen, China

**Longxiang Su, Shengjun Liu, Hao Wang, Dongkai Li, Huan Chen, Xiang Zhou and Yun Long**
Department of Critical Care Medicine, State Key Laboratory of Complex Severe and Rare Diseases, Peking Union Medical College, Peking Union Medical College Hospital, Chinese Academy of Medical Sciences, Beijing, China

**Zheng Xu, Fengxiang Chang, Yingying Ma and Na Hong**
Digital Health China Technologies Co., Ltd., Beijing, China

**Huizhen Jiang**
Department of Information Center, State Key Laboratory of Complex Severe and Rare Diseases Peking Union Medical College, Peking Union Medical College Hospital, Chinese Academy of Medical Sciences, Beijing, China

**Weiguo Zhu**
Department of Information Center, State Key Laboratory of Complex Severe and Rare Diseases Peking Union Medical College, Peking Union Medical College Hospital, Chinese Academy of Medical Sciences, Beijing, China
Department of Primary Care and Family Medicine, State Key Laboratory of Complex Severe and Rare Diseases, Peking Union Medical College, Peking Union Medical College Hospital, Chinese Academy of Medical Sciences, Beijing, China

**Philipp K. Buehler, Anique Herling, Stephanie Klinzing, Pedro David Wendel Garcia, Michael Karbach, Elisabeth Schaubmayr, Reto A. Schuepbach and Daniel A. Hofmaenner**
Institute of Intensive Care Medicine, University Hospital Zurich, Zurich, Switzerland

**Nadine Bienefeld**
Department of Management, Technology and Economics, Work & Organizational Psychology, ETH Zurich, Zurich, Switzerland

**Stephan Wegner and Quentin Lohmeyer**
Department of Mechanical and Process Engineering, ETH Zurich, Zurich, Switzerland

**Shi Zhang, Zhonghua Lu, Zongsheng Wu, Wei Chang, Feng Liu, Jianfeng Xie and Haibo Qiu**
Jiangsu Provincial Key Laboratory of Critical Care Medicine, Department of Critical Care Medicine, Zhongda Hospital, School of Medicine, Southeast University, Nanjing, China

**Yi Yang**
Department of Clinical Medicine, Gansu University of Traditional Chinese Medicine, Lanzhou, China
Jiangsu Provincial Key Laboratory of Critical Care Medicine, Department of Critical Care Medicine, Zhongda Hospital, School of Medicine, Southeast University, Nanjing, China

**Jiang Wu**
Department of Blood Transfusion, Renji Hospital Affiliated to Shanghai Jiao Tong University, Shanghai, China

**Zi-Wei Chen**
Department of Laboratory Medicine, The Third Xiangya Hospital of Central South University, Changsha, China

**Yong-Jun Wang**
Department of Blood Transfusion, The Second Xiangya Hospital of Central South University, Changsha, China

**Yibing Zhu**
Medical Research and Biometrics Center, National Center for Cardiovascular Diseases, Fuwai Hospital, Chinese Academy of Medical Sciences and Peking Union Medical College, Beijing, China
Department of Emergency, Guang'anmen Hospital, China Academy of Chinese Medical Sciences, Beijing, China

**Guowei Wang**
School of Computer Science and Technology, Wuhan University of Technology, Wuhan, China

**Renqi Yao**
Department of Burn Surgery, The First Affiliated Hospital of Naval Medical University, Shanghai, China
Translational Medicine Research Center, Fourth Medical Center and Medical Innovation Research Division of the Chinese People's Liberation Army (PLA) General Hospital, Beijing, China

**Chao Ren**
Translational Medicine Research Center, Fourth Medical Center and Medical Innovation Research Division of the Chinese People's Liberation Army (PLA) General Hospital, Beijing, China

**Ge Chen and Wei Li**
Medical Research and Biometrics Center, National Center for Cardiovascular Diseases, Fuwai Hospital, Chinese Academy of Medical Sciences and Peking Union Medical College, Beijing, China

**Xin Jin**
Yidu Cloud Technology Inc., Beijing, China

**Junyang Guo**
Beijing Big Eye Xing Tu Culture Media Co., Ltd., Beijing, China

**Shi Liu**
School of Information Science and Engineering, Hebei North University, Shijiazhuang, China

**Hua Zheng, Yan Chen and Bin Du**
Medical ICU, Peking Union Medical College Hospital, Peking Union Medical College and Chinese Academy of Medical Sciences, Beijing, China

**Qianqian Guo**
Department of Anesthesiology, Peking University Shougang Hospital, Beijing, China

**Lin Li**
School of Computer Science and Technology, Wuhan University of Technology, Wuhan, China

**Xiuming Xi**
Department of Critical Care Medicine, Fuxing Hospital, Capital Medical University, Beijing, China

**Huibin Huang**
Department of Critical Care Medicine, Beijing Tsinghua Changgung Hospital, School of Clinical Medicine, Tsinghua University, Beijing, China

**Yang Li and Qian Yu**
Academy for Advanced Interdisciplinary Studies, Peking University, Beijing, China

**Zongqing Lu, Jin Zhang, Jianchao Hong, Jiatian Wu, Wenyan Xiao, Tianfeng Hua and Min Yang**
The 2nd Department of Intensive Care Unit, The Second Affiliated Hospital of Anhui Medical University, Hefei, China
The Laboratory of Cardiopulmonary Resuscitation and Critical Care Medicine, The Second Affiliated Hospital of Anhui Medical University, Hefei, China

**Ming-Cheng Chan**
Division of Critical Care and Respiratory Therapy, Department of Internal Medicine, Taichung Veterans General Hospital, Taichung, Taiwan
Central Taiwan University of Science and Technology, Taichung, Taiwan
The College of Science, Tunghai University, Taichung, Taiwan

**Wen-Cheng Chao**
Department of Critical Care Medicine, Taichung Veterans General Hospital, Taichung, Taiwan
Department of Computer Science, Tunghai University, Taichung, Taiwan
Department of Automatic Control Engineering, Feng Chia University, Taichung, Taiwan

**Ming-Yen Lin, Chi-Chun Li and Pin-Hsiu Lin**
Department of Information Engineering and Computer Science, Feng Chia University, Taichung, Taiwan

**Jiun-Long Wang**
Division of Chest Medicine, Department of Internal Medicine, Taichung Veterans General Hospital, Taichung, Taiwan
Department of Life Sciences, National Chung-Hsing University, Taichung, Taiwan

**Chieh-Liang Wu**
Department of Critical Care Medicine, Taichung Veterans General Hospital, Taichung, Taiwan
Department of Industrial Engineering and Enterprise Information, Tunghai University, Taichung, Taiwan
Artificial Intelligence Studio, Taichung Veterans General Hospital, Taichung, Taiwan
Colledge of Medicine, National Chung Hsing University, Taichung, Taiwan

**Kai Zhang, Wei Cui and Gensheng Zhang**
Department of Critical Care Medicine, Second Affiliated Hospital, Zhejiang University School of Medicine, Hangzhou, China

**Shufang Zhang**
Department of Cardiology, Second Affiliated Hospital, Zhejiang University School of Medicine, Hangzhou, China

**Yucai Hong and Zhongheng Zhang**
Department of Emergency Medicine, Sir Run-Run Shaw Hospital, Zhejiang University School of Medicine, Hangzhou, China

**Yu Liu**
Key Laboratory of Intelligent Computing & Signal Processing, Ministry of Education, Anhui University, Hefei, China

**Guina Liu**
Department of Periodical Press and National Clinical Research Center for Geriatrics, West China Hospital, Sichuan University, Chengdu, China
West China School of Medicine, Sichuan University, Chengdu, China

**Nian Li**
Department of Medical Administration, West China Hospital, Sichuan University, Chengdu, China

**Lingmin Chen**
Department of Anesthesiology and National Clinical Research Center for Geriatrics, West China Hospital, Sichuan University and The Research Units of West China (2018RU012), Chinese Academy of Medical Sciences, Chengdu, China

**Yi Yang**
Department of Clinical Medicine, Gansu University of Traditional Chinese Medicine, Lanzhou, China

**Yonggang Zhang**
Department of Periodical Press and National Clinical Research Center for Geriatrics, West China Hospital, Sichuan University, Chengdu, China
Chinese Evidence-based Medicine Center, West China Hospital, Sichuan University, Chengdu, China
Nursing Key Laboratory of Sichuan Province, Chengdu, China

**Ming-Hao Luo**
Shanghai Medical College, Fudan University, Shanghai, China

**Peng Sun**
Artificial Intelligence Institute, Shanghai Jiao Tong University, Shanghai, China

**Huiqing Ge**
Department of Respiratory Care, Sir Run Run Shaw Hospital, Zhejiang University School of Medicine, Hangzhou, China
Regional Medical Center for National Institute of Respiratory Diseases, Bethesda, MD, United States

**Kailiang Duan, Jimei Wang and Liuqing Jiang**
Department of Respiratory Care, Sir Run Run Shaw Hospital, Zhejiang University School of Medicine, Hangzhou, China

**Lingwei Zhang, Yuhan Zhou, Luping Fang and Qing Pan**
College of Information Engineering, Zhejiang University of Technology, Hangzhou, China

**Leo M. A. Heunks**
Department of Intensive Care Medicine, Amsterdam UMC, Amsterdam, Netherlands

**Shu-Fang Liu and Sou-Jen Shih**
Department of Nursing, Taichung Veterans General Hospital, Taichung, Taiwan

**Tian-Li Yu and Chih-Hung Chang**
Department of Electrical Engineering, National Taiwan University, Taipei, Taiwan

**Shih-Fang Yang Mao, Yueh-Se Li and Chia-Chen Chen**
Electronic and Optoelectronic System Research Laboratories, Industrial Technology Research Institute, Hsinchu, Taiwan

**Hui-Jiun Chen**
Department of Critical Care Medicine, Taichung Veterans General Hospital, Taichung, Taiwan
Colledge of Medicine, National Chung Hsing University, Taichung, Taiwan
Department of Automatic Control Engineering, Feng Chia University, Taichung, Taiwan
Big Data Center, National Chung Hsing University, Taichung, Taiwan

**Jinzhang Li and Hongjia Zhang**
Department of Physiology and Pathophysiology, School of Basic Medical Sciences, Capital Medical University, Beijing, China
Department of Cardiac Surgery, Beijing Anzhen Hospital, Capital Medical University, Beijing, China
Beijing Lab for Cardiovascular Precision Medicine, Beijing, China

**Ming Gong**
Department of Cardiac Surgery, Beijing Anzhen Hospital, Capital Medical University, Beijing, China
Beijing Lab for Cardiovascular Precision Medicine, Beijing, China

**Yashutosh Joshi**
Department of Cardiothoracic Surgery, St Vincent's Hospital, Sydney, NSW, Australia

**Lizhong Sun**
Department of Cardiac Surgery, Beijing Anzhen Hospital, Capital Medical University, Beijing, China

**Lianjun Huang**
Department of Interference Diagnosis and Treatment, Beijing Anzhen Hospital, Capital Medical University, Beijing, China

**Ruixin Fan**
Department of Cardiovascular Surgery, Guangdong Provincial People's Hospital, Guangzhou, China

**Tianxiang Gu**
Department of Cardiac Surgery, First Affiliated Hospital, China Medical University, Shenyang, China

**Zonggang Zhang**
Department of Cardiac Surgery, People's Hospital of Xinjiang Uygur Autonomous Region, Urumqi, China

**Chengwei Zou**
Department of Cardiovascular Surgery, Shandong Provincial Hospital Affiliated With Shandong First Medical University, Jinan, China

**Guowei Zhang**
Department of Cardiovascular Surgery, The First Affiliated Hospital of Harbin Medical University, Harbin, China

**Ximing Qian**
Department of Cardiac Surgery, School of Medicine, Sir Run Run Shaw Hospital, Zhejiang University, Hangzhou, China

**Chenhui Qiao**
Department of Cardiovascular Surgery, The First Affiliated Hospital of Zhengzhou University Zhengzhou, China

**Yu Chen**
Department of Cardiac Surgery, Peking University People's Hospital, Beijing, China

**Wenjian Jiang**
Department of Cardiac Surgery, Beijing Anzhen Hospital, Capital Medical University, Beijing, China
Beijing Lab for Cardiovascular Precision Medicine, Beijing, China
Department of Cardiothoracic Surgery, St Vincent's Hospital, Sydney, NSW, Australia

**Xuandong Jiang, Yun Wang, Yuting Pan and Weimin Zhang**
Intensive Care Unit, Dongyang Hospital of Wenzhou Medical University, Jinhua, China

**Yi Bian, Yue Le, Zhigang He, Ye Wang, Shanshan Yu, Yu Fang, Gang Yu, Jianmin Ling, Yikuan Feng, Liuniu Xiao, Yingfang Zheng and Shusheng Li**
Department of Emergency Medicine, Tongji Medical College, Tongji Hospital, Huazhong University of Science and Technology, Wuhan, China
Department of Critical Care Medicine, Tongji Medical College, Tongji Hospital, Huazhong University of Science and Technology, Wuhan, China

**Han Du**
Germany Research Center for Artificial Intelligence, Saarland Informatics Campus, Saarbrücken, Germany

**Junfang Chen**
Intelligent Medicine Research Center, Greater Bay Area Institute of Precision Medicine (Guangzhou), Fudan University, Guangzhou, China

**Ping Zhang**
Department of Neurology, Tongji Medical College, Tongji Hospital, Huazhong University of Science and Technology, Wuhan, China

**Sheng Wei**
Ministry of Education Key Laboratory of Environment and Health, Department of Epidemiology and Biostatistics, School of Public Health, Tongji Medical College, Huazhong University of Science and Technology, Wuhan, China

**Jiao Huang and Zhen Yu**
Center for Evidence-Based and Translational Medicine, Zhongnan Hospital of Wuhan, Wuhan, China
Department of Critical Care Medicine, Renmin Hospital of Wuhan University, Wuhan, China

# Index

www.ingramcontent.com/pod-product-compliance
Lightning Source LLC
LaVergne TN
LVHW082203200926
848484LV00008B/2204
* 9 7 9 8 8 8 7 4 0 0 8 7 7 *